① WML2

CEFN C
M

✔ KT-178-785

Cefn Coed Library

Z000687

Withdrawn from stock 16/4/24

Acclaim for previous editions

'... clearly written, well edited ....readable, stimulating and highly recommended to all those whose work involves treatment of psychological distress.' *Medical Education*

'This nicely presented book is an excellent vehicle to encourage proper ongoing debate on these crucial issues. One looks forward to further revisions. I am sure it will continue to find a place on the shelves of mental health workers, whether they be in clinical or academic posts.' *International Clinical Psychopharmacology*

'In 1981, the first edition of this book was well received—rightly so, because it contained a rich mixture of well-argued papers. This new edition is very good value.' *Bulletin of Medical Ethics*

'... a splendid book. Every psychiatrist would be the better for reading it, both for the information contained and the thoughts provoked.' *Australian and New Zealand Journal of Psychiatry*

'I commend Drs Bloch and Chodoff for a well-edited, well-organized, readable and useful addition to the psychiatric literature.' *American Journal of Psychiatry*

'... a welcome contribution to the literature of psychiatric ethics ... the papers are excellently written and include comprehensive bibliographies.' *Journal of Medical Ethics*

'... The editors are to be congratulated on a most successful conclusion to a formidable project.' *Psychosocial Medicine*

OXFORD MEDICAL PUBLICATIONS

Psychiatric Ethics

Oxford University Press makes no representation, express or implied, that the drug dosages in this book are correct. Readers must therefore always check the product information and clinical procedures with the most up-to-date published product information and data sheets provided by the manufacturers and the most recent codes of conduct and safety regulations. The authors and the publishers do not accept responsibility or legal liability for any errors in the text or for the misuse or misapplication of material in this work.

Psychiatric Ethics

THIRD EDITION

Edited by

SIDNEY BLOCH
Associate Professor and Reader in Psychiatry,
University of Melbourne

PAUL CHODOFF
Clinical Professor of Psychiatry,
George Washington University,
Washington DC

and

STEPHEN A. GREEN
Clinical Professor of Psychiatry,
Georgetown University,
Washington DC

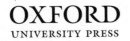

OXFORD
UNIVERSITY PRESS

OXFORD

UNIVERSITY PRESS

Great Clarendon Street, Oxford OX2 6DP

Oxford University Press is a department of the University of Oxford
and furthers the University's aim of excellence in research, scholarship,
and education by publishing worldwide in

Oxford New York

Athens Auckland Bangkok Bogota Buenos Aires Calcutta
Cape Town Chennai Dar es Salaam Delhi Florence Hong Kong Istanbul
Karachi Kuala Lumpur Madras Madrid Melbourne Mexico City Mumbai
Nairobi Paris São Paulo Singapore Taipei Tokyo Toronto Warsaw
and associated companies in
Berlin Ibadan

Oxford is a registered trade mark of Oxford University Press

Published in the United States
by Oxford University Press Inc., New York

© S. Bloch, P. Chodoff, and S. Green, 1999

The moral rights of the authors have been asserted

First edition published 1981
Second edition published 1991
Reprinted 1991, (with corrections) 1993, 1994
Third edition published 1999

All rights reserved. No part of this publication may be reproduced,
stored in a retrieval system, or transmitted, in any form or by any means,
without the prior permission in writing of Oxford University Press.
Within the UK, exceptions are allowed in respect of any fair dealing for the
purpose of research or private study, or criticism or review, as permitted
under the Copyright, Designs and Patents Act, 1988, or in the case of
reprographic reproduction in accordance with the terms of licences
issued by the Copyright Licensing Agency. Enquiries concerning
reproduction outside those terms and in other countries should be sent to
the Rights Department, Oxford University Press,
at the address above.

This book is sold subject to the condition that it shall not, by way
of trade or otherwise, be lent, re-sold, hired out, or otherwise circulated
without the publisher's prior consent in any form of binding or cover
other than that in which it is published and without a similar condition
including this condition being imposed on the subsequent purchaser.

British Library Cataloguing in Publication Data
Data available

Library of Congress Cataloging in Publication Data
Psychiatric ethics / edited by Sidney Bloch, Paul Chodoff, and Stephen
Green. – 3rd ed.
(Oxford medical publications)
Includes bibliographical references and index.
1. Psychiatric ethics.   I. Bloch, Sidney.   II. Chodoff, Paul.
III. Green, Stephen A., 1945–   .   IV. Series.
RC455.2.E8P75 1999   174'.2–dc21   98-24779
ISBN 0 19 262900 X (Hbk)   ISBN 0 19 262899 2 (Pbk)

Typeset by Downdell, Oxford
Printed in Great Britain on acid free paper by
Bookcraft (Bath) Ltd,
Midsomer Norton, Avon

Contents

Abbreviations

AAPL	American Academy of Psychiatry and Law
ACT	Assertive Community Treatment
ADHD	attention-deficit hyperactivity disorder
AIDS	autoimmune deficiency syndrome
AMA	American Medical Association
APA	American Psychiatric Association
APP	amyloid precursor protein
APS	Australian Psychological Society
CMHC	community mental health clinic
CPA	Canadian Psychiatric Association
CPA	Care Programme Approach
DSM	Diagnostic and Statistical Manual (APA)
ECT	electroconvulsive therapy
ELSI	ethical, legal, and social implications
EP	extrapyramidal
epr	electronic patient record
FMS	false-memory syndrome
FTC	Federal Trade Commission
GP	general practitioner
HIV	human immunodeficiency virus
HMO	health maintenance organization
HoNOS	Health of the Nation Outcome Scales
ICD	International Classification of Diseases (WHO)
IPSS	International Pilot Study of Schizophrenia
IRB	institutional review board
JCAHO	Joint Commission of Healthcare Organizations
MCO	managed-care organization
MODY	maturity onset diabetes of the young
NAMI	National Alliance for the Mentally Ill
NH&MRC	National Health and Medical Research Council (Australia)
NHS	National Health Service
PACT	Prescribing analysis and costs
PAS	physician-assisted suicide
PCC	Professional Conduct Committee
PTSD	post-traumatic stress disorder
QOL	quality of life

QALY	quality-adjusted-life years
RANZCP	Royal Australian and New Zealand College of Psychiatrists
SSDI	Social Security Disability Insurance
SSI	Supplemental Security Income
SSRI	selective serotonin reuptake inhibitor
US	United States (of America)
WHO	World Health Organization
WMA	World Medical Association
WPA	World Psychiatric Association

Contributors

Tom L. Beauchamp, PROFESSOR OF PHILOSOPHY and SENIOR RESEARCH SCHOLAR
Georgetown University, Washington DC, USA

Sidney Bloch, ASSOCIATE PROFESSOR and READER IN PSYCHIATRY
University of Melbourne, Australia

Paul Brown, CONSULTANT PSYCHIATRIST
Pierre Janet Centre, Melbourne, Australia

Paul Chodoff, CLINICAL PROFESSOR OF PSYCHIATRY
George Washington University, Washington DC, USA

Norman Daniels, GOLDTHWAITE PROFESSOR OF RHETORIC
Tufts University, Medford, USA

Allen R. Dyer, PROFESSOR OF PSYCHIATRY AND BEHAVIORAL SCIENCES
East Tennessee State University, Johnson City, TN, USA

Anne Farmer, PROFESSOR OF PSYCHIATRY
University of Wales College of Medicine, Cardiff, UK

K. W. M. Fulford, PROFESSOR OF PHILOSOPHY AND MENTAL HEALTH
University of Warwick, Coventry; and
HONORARY CONSULTANT PSYCHIATRIST
University of Oxford, Warneford Hospital, Oxford, UK

Glen O. Gabbard, CALLOWAY DISTINGUISHED PROFESSOR OF PSYCHO-ANALYSIS AND EDUCATION
The Menninger Clinic, Topeka, USA

Philip Graham, formerly PROFESSOR OF CHILD PSYCHIATRY
Institute for Child Health, University of London, London, UK

Stephen A. Green, CLINICAL PROFESSOR OF PSYCHIATRY
Georgetown University, Washington DC, USA

Thomas G. Gutheil, PROFESSOR OF PSYCHIATRY
Harvard Medical School, Boston, MA, USA

David Heyd, CHAIM PERELMAN PROFESSOR OF PHILOSOPHY
The Hebrew University of Jerusalem, Israel

Jeremy Holmes, CONSULTANT PSYCHOTHERAPIST
Department of Psychiatry, North Devon District Hospital, Barnstaple, and
Southmead Hospital, Bristol, UK

David I. Joseph, CLINICAL PROFESSOR OF PSYCHIATRY
George Washington University, Washington DC, USA

Kevin V. Kelly, CLINICAL PROFESSOR OF PSYCHIATRY
Cornell University Medical College, New York, USA

Peter McGuffin, PROFESSOR OF PSYCHOLOGICAL MEDICINE
University of Wales College of Medicine, Cardiff, UK

Harold Merskey, EMERITUS PROFESSOR OF PSYCHIATRY
University of Western Ontario, London, Ontario, Canada

Robert Michels, WELSH McDERMOTT UNIVERSITY PROFESSOR OF PSYCHIATRY
Cornell University Medical College, New York, USA

David F. Musto, PROFESSOR OF CHILD PSYCHIATRY and HISTORY OF MEDICINE
Yale School of Medicine, New Haven, USA

Joseph Onek, ATTORNEY
Washington DC, USA

Catherine Oppenheimer, CONSULTANT PSYCHIATRIST
Department of Psychiatry of Old Age, Warneford Hospital, Oxford, UK

Christos Pantelis, ASSOCIATE PROFESSOR OF PSYCHIATRY
University of Melbourne; and Mental Health Research Institute, Melbourne,
Australia

Russell Pargiter, CONSULTANT PSYCHIATRIST
University of Tasmania, Hobart, Australia

Roger Peele, CLINICAL PROFESSOR OF PSYCHIATRY
George Washington University, Washington DC, USA

Walter Reich, YITZHAK RABIN MEMORIAL PROFESSOR OF INTERNATIONAL
AFFAIRS, ETHICS AND HUMAN BEHAVIOUR
George Washington University, Washington DC, USA

James E. Sabin, ASSOCIATE CLINICAL PROFESSOR OF PSYCHIATRY
Harvard Medical School; and
CO-DIRECTOR
Center for Ethics in Managed Care, Harvard, USA

George Szmukler, CONSULTANT PSYCHIATRIST AND MEDICAL DIRECTOR
Bethlem and Maudsley Hospitals, London, UK

John Wing, EMERITUS PROFESSOR OF SOCIAL PSYCHIATRY
Institute of Psychiatry, University of London, London, UK

1

Introduction

Sidney Bloch, Paul Chodoff, and Stephen Green

In the last edition of *Psychiatric Ethics* (1991), we launched the introductory chapter with this question: Why a book on psychiatric ethics? We then countered the arguments commonly raised in debating this issue and which rest on the premise that serving the best interests of patients or respecting the dignity of people generally pre-empt ethical complications. We suggested that psychiatrists could all too easily and usually unwittingly disregard ethical aspects of their professional task, despite the need to make vital moral decisions in every facet of their work.

At the end of the 1990s we are confident that most, if not all, of our colleagues would agree that raising the question of the need for this type of volume is unnecessary. The concrete reality of a third edition over a period spanning the 1980s and 1990s, and with the prospect of its continuing role in the next century, points to a coming of age of the discourse of ethics in psychiatry.

We can identify ample evidence of this welcome development in international psychiatry: regular conferences and symposia on the subject; the incorporation of ethical themes into the conference programmes of general psychiatry and the subspecialties; frequent publication of journal articles and book chapters on diverse facets of the field; the advent of the new journal *Philosophy, Psychiatry and Psychology*; and the creation of special interest groups in national associations like the Royal College of Psychiatrists and the Royal Australian and New Zealand College of Psychiatrists.

Psychiatric ethics has attained a firm place in the affairs of psychiatrists universally; its future is secure, and this prospect a source of immense encouragement to those who see the subject as paramount for the ongoing welfare of the profession. In the last edition, we devoted several pages to the reasons for these progressive developments. The interested reader is referred to that edition for a detailed account. Suffice to comment, an increased professional commitment to accountability, in parallel with a growing 'consumer' movement (and, we hope, a mutual sense of partnership), has paved the way for a creative engagement with the ethical dimension.

Ethics: its boundaries in this book

Ethics, derived from the Greek *ethikos*, meaning 'disposition', has a philosophical home in the discourse of moral philosophy, the study of conduct with respect to whether an action is right or wrong, and to the goodness and badness of the motives and ends of the action (Chapter 3). Moral philosophers set out to show how value judgements are arrived at and tackle the question of whether ethical propositions can be proven. They examine concepts like good, bad, right, wrong, should, ought, justice, duty, obligation, responsibility, and many other evaluative terms. A basic premise is that where people have a choice of one or another course of action and their activities are not entirely proscribed, the question follows as to whether the decision made and the action chosen are right or wrong.

In wrestling with these questions, the philosopher may offer a theory—this is the most general level of ethics. Several classic models have been proposed and some won support. The *utilitarian* position, for example, has exerted a profound influence with its emphasis on the consequences of acts, on the balance between good and bad consequences, between benefits and harms. A person should choose to act in a way that leads to the best outcome, by recognizing the interests of all the people who will be affected by that action. The final consequence would be the greatest possible welfare of all concerned.

A competing theory is the *deontological*, with its central notion that certain acts are inherently wrong, and can never be made right, and that moral judgements are universally applicable. Murder of an innocent person, for example, is judged to be always wrong. Religious morality is typically of this type—for instance, the Bible is regarded as the sole guide to moral conduct. Rawls' theory of justice has proved appealing to many people in the latter part of this century. His core thesis is that morality is made up of those principles chosen by the rational person (that is the person who acts in his own interests) with the crucial proviso that he makes judgements behind a 'veil of ignorance'—that is, he is unaware of the position he would have in a society in which his principles would operate. Any self-interest is in this way avoided by choosing moral principles while situated behind the 'veil'.

While these theories may be entirely coherent and thoroughly well-argued, the question still arises as to how they apply to concrete day-to-day situations. We could argue that for psychiatrists who face challenging and complex circumstances, every situation is unique and precludes the application of general principles or guidelines of conduct. Adherence to this 'situational' or case-by-case approach has the virtue of appreciating the special features involved but its considerable disadvantage is its exhausting quality, calling as it does on the psychiatrist to reach an ethical position vis-à-vis every one of his patients, their families, and his colleagues. Such an onslaught of incessant moral decision-making would soon lead to a paralysis of clinical action.

Despite the uniqueness argument, we surmise that most ethically demanding situations recur regularly in the psychiatrist's pursuits and are amenable to systematic consideration and action. But an immediate caveat follows: ethical dilemmas are not resolved by easy, ready-made remedies—as the chapters in this book demonstrate (although some contributors do express personal judgements about some of the ethical problems they discuss). Instead, the approach entails describing problems as clearly as possible so that their nature and complexity can be fully appreciated, a process that paves the way for reasoned ethical judgements.

It is always tempting, but equally hazardous to assist the psychiatrist by offering guidelines for ethical conduct. Immutable ethical rules are simply not available. Rather ethical decision-making depends on the individual in association with professional peers and their well-considered reflections to act in morally appropriate ways. Guidelines may be set but are, unlike laws, unenforceable. Moreover, a code of ethics or conduct can only be expressed in general terms. Psychiatrists remain responsible for making ethical decisions in specific cases.

When we spoke earlier about the use of the term ethics in the context of moral philosophy we also alluded to the practical dimension. A perusal of the 23 chapters that follow clearly reveals that psychiatrists grapple with problems which they encounter every day. Although these problems differ according to the type of psychiatry practised, certain themes are pervasive. These include: how to assess the moral costs and benefits of their actions; how to maintain confidentiality in the face of competing loyalties; how to seek patients' consent for a procedure or treatment; how to define the boundaries of their professional task without recourse to hubris or undue timidity; how to strike a balance between the ethos of contractual equality and a benevolent paternalism; how to satisfy the interests of patients, their families, and the broader community especially when they clash; how to avoid discriminating against or exploiting patients; and how to advocate for patients, many of whom are disenfranchised and powerless. As editors, we hope that this new edition will help to shed light on these themes which so impinge on the practising psychiatrist, and in which elements of the human, the contingent, and the ambiguous take precedence over purely scientific and clinical aspects.

Finally, we wish to point out how the third edition differs from its predecessors. We believe our selection of topics cover the central ethical issues facing the contemporary psychiatrist. Since the second edition we have had the opportunity to observe the field and to witness further developments and, as a result, we have added six new chapters.

One new noteworthy subject is the ethical dimension of community psychiatry. With the universal trend to speed up the closure of the old-style mental hospitals (dealt with in Chapter 20 by Peele and Chodoff), has come a flurry of challenges to the clinician practising in the framework of the community. These are examined by Szmukler in Chapter 17. The two chapters should be read in conjunction with each other. Linked to this radical transformation in the way psychiatric care is provided in the late 1990s are the implications for how best to organize relevant services, especially for a highly vulnerable group of patients and their principal caregivers, their families. Sabin and Daniels highlight the pertinent justice issues, in particular how limited resources should be allocated from an ethical standpoint. Green tackles a specific attempt to deal with resource allocation, managed health care. Dominating the medical environment generally in the United States, managed care in its various guises is beginning to infiltrate the medical care systems in other countries, raising a plethora of ethical issues which call for assiduous scrutiny.

As Farmer and McGuffin point out, psychiatric genetics has been riding on the crest of a wave since the 1980s and will undoubtedly transform psychiatric research and clinical practice. In terms of both the research problems thrown up hitherto and the clinical implications of the emerging findings, the psychiatric profession will have to ponder long and hard on how to traverse uncharted moral territory.

The territorial metaphor leads us conveniently to mention another new chapter, on boundary violations. Although these have been carefully teased out, especially the perils of sexual exploitation of patients, the subject has continued to attract much attention, probably paralleling the prominent publicity paid to actual cases. Glen Gabbard, who has been at the forefront of the research into the offending psychiatrist, presents his views in a chapter that combines scholarship and empathy. The sixth new chapter relates to boundary violations from the perspective of attempts by psychiatric associations to identify measures to contain sexual and other forms of exploitation. On a more positive note, codes of ethics and codes of conduct have earned growing recognition as a suitable means for psychiatry to achieve self-regulation. Bloch and Pargiter consider the history, purpose, and forms of ethical codes and their potential role in psychiatry.

In this outline of new material, we should briefly comment on chapters which appeared in the second edition but which we have now either amalgamated or omitted. The 1991 volume ended with three chapters devoted to various forms of abuse of psychiatry—in Nazi Germany, the former Soviet Union, and Japan. These are now fortunately part of history; nevertheless, we need to remind ourselves constantly of psychiatry's vulnerability to misuse. Readers interested in detailed accounts of any of the three cases can turn to the pertinent chapters in the second edition, although all these instances of abuse are dealt with in summary fashion by Chodoff in Chapter 4 and aspects of the political abuse of psychiatry in the former USSR by Reich in Chapter 10.

The social dimension of psychiatric ethics, previously a separate chapter, finds its way into several chapters of this edition, particularly those by Dyer, Szmukler, Peele and Chodoff, and Bloch and Pargiter. Ethical aspects of sexuality and sex therapy have been brought under the rubric of psychotherapy ethics while deinstitutionalization and involuntary treatment are now dealt with in the same chapter.

We had envisaged a chapter on repressed memory and the so-called false-memory syndrome but were foiled by our inability to identify a contributor who was both a scholar of the subject and sufficiently detached from the controversies that have been raging throughout the 1990s. We suspect that the ethical issues are simply too new and too 'hot' to be handled dispassionately at the moment (we anticipate a chapter in the fourth edition!). In the interim Chodoff, Reich and Holmes have outlined some preliminary thoughts on various aspects of the topic in their respective chapters.

It is a pleasure to thank our contributors, both veteran (some authors have stayed with the project since initially approached in 1979!) and new, for their commitment to our objective of producing a comprehensive, scholarly but yet practical volume. Practising psychiatrists for the most part, they bring a sharp eye to ethical facets of professional research or practice with which they are intimately familiar. We have sought contributors from many parts of the world in order to recruit a 'star cast' but also to reflect the fact that the ethical dimension of psychiatry crosses all national boundaries. On the other hand some contributors have opted to weave a universal fabric with clinical, legal and Governmental illustrations drawn from their own countries. In this regard, we invite readers to draw on their own experience in journeying through the book and to compare this with the particulars selected by our authors.

Our gratitude goes to the staff at Oxford University Press—Diana Waha, Sheila Sellars, Richard Marley, and Martin Baum who have been unswervingly supportive of *Psychiatric ethics*. This third edition is testimony to their dedication to our objectives.

The three editors (Paul Chodoff and Sidney Bloch warmly welcome Stephen Green to the editorial team) are grateful to their respective families—Selma, Felicity, Leah, David, Aaron, Madeleine, Jessica and Julia for 'being there', especially when deadlines loomed. Sidney Bloch expresses his warm appreciation to the Hebrew University for providing a perfect intellectual environment while he was a Visiting Professor during the academic year 1997–98.

Finally, we pay tribute to the many thousands of our colleagues who have adopted *Psychiatric ethics* in diverse ways since its first appearance in 1981. It is most heartening for us to note that the book has contributed to the ethical dimension of psychiatric practice and research, whether as a personal text, as a textbook in training or as a reference. We hope the new edition will meet the expectations of readers both old and new and that it will continue to play a helpful role in the ethical reflections and actions of psychiatrists and other mental health professionals.

Melbourne and Washington
October 1998

S.B.
P.C.
S.G.

2

A historical perspective

David F. Musto

Three factors underlie the ethical questions which at all times have preoccupied those delegated to help the mentally ill: the role of the therapist, the nature of mental disease, and the cultural, religious, and even political environment in which patient and therapist coexist. Since the 1970s these factors and the formal study of psychiatric ethics have been explicitly analyzed and have become almost a new subspecialty. Before the mid-twentieth century, however, few such formal studies existed. This lack of attention is understandable, since the profession of psychiatry developed as a medical specialty only recently, and since for much of the last century the codes discussed and adopted for general medicine appeared to have served psychiatry well. The dramatic changes in the scope of psychiatry since the Second World War, however, have brought ethical issues peculiar to it into sharp focus.

The governing factors listed above have varied widely in Western medical tradition since Hippocrates. What we call issues in psychiatric ethics during that time must represent the imposition of categories familiar to us, such as informed consent and 'right to be treated', onto a historical record for which these terms are not entirely appropriate. In reviewing the past we will be looking for ethical concepts deemed pertinent by medical or other cultural authorities when the behavior of a person was judged to be grossly abnormal and to require treatment or limitation of freedom. Social control in a broad sense could be justified as the theme for a study of psychiatric ethics; but in this brief survey the subjects will be studied in the traditional medical context. The realization that ethical issues transcend medicine—and therefore psychiatry—constitutes a fundamental change in outlook that has marked the recent rise of interest. Restriction of the subject to the context of the history of medicine is a concession to space, not a judgment on its proper boundaries. A convenient starting-point is the Greco–Roman period.

Greco–Roman period

It would be an error to consider the Hippocratic Oath as representing Greek or Roman medical practice. The tradition of Hippocratic thinking was akin to Pythagoreanism, a school of thought with strict moral precepts whose tenets more resembled later Christian principles than the flexible mores of Hellenistic practices which, for example, condoned abortion and suicide.[1] The Oath does include, however, some of the earliest affirmations of confidentiality and the primacy of the patient's health:

Whatever houses I may visit, I will come for the benefit of the sick, remaining free of all intentional injustice, of all mischief and in particular of sexual relations with both female and male persons, be they free or slaves.

What I may see or hear in the course of the treatment or even outside of the treatment in regard to the life of the men, which on no account one must spread abroad, I will keep to myself holding such things shameful to be spoken about.[2]

Insanity is not mentioned in the Oath. In the Greek world there appears to have been little legal provision for the insane, although Roman law did provide for trusteeship of an incompetent person's property and other restrictions of his rights. Mental illness as well as drunkenness were conditions that could decrease a defendant's criminal responsibility, although such decisions appear to have been made by judges without the advice of a physician or other expert on mental illness.[3]

Treatment of the insane in the ancient Western world ranged from such harsh methods, described by Celsus (first century of the Christian era), as purgation, bleeding, beatings, and cold baths to milder policies advocated by Soranus (first and second centuries), which are similar to the moral therapy espoused, although rarely practised, in the early nineteenth century: esteem for the patient, relative freedom of movement, and kind treatment.

Just as a range of restraints on freedom can be identified in these early approaches to mental illness, so the causes advanced for insanity extended from divine intervention to organic or natural factors. When ethical issues are drawn from this period, the vague edges of the definition of insanity and various responses to it make firm statements about these issues difficult. Clearly, for those who were treated medically, evidence suggests that harshness of treatment or limitations of freedom were the prerogative of the physician, and that the patient and his family had little to say about either. Furthermore, the major determinant in the form of therapy depended on the custodian's faith in a particular school of medicine, or perhaps in a lack of faith in any medical treatment and, instead, a dependence on religious intervention.

The marks of insanity were simple: strange, violent, suicidal, or homicidal behavior that did not have a likely explanation from the observer's point of view. Bizarre explanations from the patient would only confirm the judgment of the family or other authorities. Treatment might be painful or harmful, but the physician administered it with a clear conscience because his theory of medicine required certain courses of action. In these instances ethical problems may exist for us, but did not for the confident physician or the patient's faithful custodian or, perhaps, even for patients themselves. The random manner in which those considered insane received care continued for centuries until more formal and elaborate systems evolved, first with hospitals and, much later and only since the twentieth century, with the varieties of care possible when a large mental health profession exists.

The Middle Ages and the Renaissance

The Middle Ages brought no medical advance to the insane; rather, the major influence on attitudes toward the mentally ill emanated from religion. For example, the Prophet Mohammed revealed that the insane are the beloved of God and especially chosen by him to declare the truth. This attitude, taken with the founding of hospitals in the Moslem world and the establishment of an enlightened medical profession, suggests that Islam was disposed towards humane care of the ill. Because of the Prophet's statement, the status of the patient was elevated to at least the same level as that of the therapist, a rare event in the history of psychiatry.[4]

Jewish tradition, as stated in the Talmud, portrayed the insane as victims of a disease, not of possession.[5] Christian religious orders provided humane, though limited, treatment for the deranged, but outside the monasteries Europeans had diminishing resources for care as the Roman Empire was gradually eroded. The ensuing anarchy apparently was responsible for an increase in gaolings, beatings, and torture among the insane. Compounding their misfortune, schisms among Christians led to an increase in the mal-treatment of patients by equating deviant opinions with demonic possession and heresy.[6] Among competing religious factions little concern was shown for the rights of heretics whom we would now consider sane, and certainly no more concern was shown for those whose disordered fantasies and opinions were thought the product of heresy. Yet it would be unfair and misleading to suggest that European Christian attitudes toward the insane were characterized by a belief in demonic possession which had to be rooted out by the most severe methods. Toward the end of the Middle Ages, hospitals for the mentally ill were founded; humane physicians and caregivers did exist, and their numbers were to multiply in the sixteenth and seventeenth centuries.[7]

At the same time, legal care for the insane seems to have been in some specific instances balanced and thoughtful. This is the conclusion of Richard Neugebauer,[8] who studied judicial records regarding 'natural fools' and those judged *non compos mentis* in England from the thirteenth to the seventeenth centuries. These records do not support the accepted belief that the era was cruel and dominated by demonological explanations of mental retardation and disorder. There was a growing pattern of reasonable distinctions between congenital and temporary conditions, protection of the property and interests of those judged incompetent, and a disinclination to be punitive or cruel.

In monastic hospitals the insane received good care, in keeping with the dictum of St Benedict that 'care of the sick is to be placed above and before every other duty'.[9] With suppression of the monastic orders in Protestant countries and confiscation of their property, care of patients suffered. Still,

even taking into account the existence of a few hospitals and of legal protection, the Middle Ages offered only a random and unpredictable response to
insanity. The ethical context in which decisions were taken was the religious
tradition of the locality. This could mean emphasis on charity and understanding, or it could justify severe measures if demonic possession were
suspected. It is probably reasonable to generalize that during this time a person
with bizarre behavior and beliefs was seldom classified as a 'patient', and,
moreover, that no broad consensus existed for what we think of as humane
treatment. The low level of institutional and public health care for all health or
social problems meant that the overall quality of treatment for the mentally ill
would be as low as that for other illnesses, such as leprosy and communicable
diseases.

The seventeenth century to the French Revolution

The two centuries preceding the French Revolution were a period of increased
hospital building but no significant improvement in caring for the mentally ill.
The traditional religious view of mental illness was progressively balanced by
advances in anatomy and physiology which suggested that it was the product
of organic change. Humane treatment, however, seems to have been related
more to culturally inspired responses than to organic explanations of disordered behavior or beliefs. An assumption that a lesion in the brain or other
part of the body caused mental illness brought contrasting treatment. Powerful
and destructive therapies were justified on the grounds that they were required
for the correction of specific lesions, while milder treatments were advocated
because of the belief that strenuous applications would impair the natural
capacity of the body or mind to heal the lesion and restore health.

Mild treatment, though, appears to have been rare in the great hospitals that
were built before the French Revolution, with the exception of those administered by religious orders. The rise of the sciences stimulated new explanations for the body's functions: mechanical, physical, and chemical theories
challenged the Galenic tradition of four humors whose balance brought health.
New theories fostered new regimens: strong medicines, bleeding, purgation,
and blistering competed with methods such as isolation, beatings, and instilling fear. Faith in theory continued to outweigh empirical considerations
based on the actual effects of the patient's treatment. In general, eighteenth-
century therapists considered their task difficult and in need of rough
procedures.

The American and French Revolutions gave a new importance to the
individual in terms of his rights in the secular order. This importance rivaled
the religious tradition of immortality and equality before God. In the late
eighteenth century, particularly in France, mental illness was considered the
result of a wrongly ordered society: the patient was the victim of an exploitative social environment. The attitude that placed blame on society exonerated

the ill person; it also suggested that care could take on a social form and promoted optimism as to the outcome—at least in the heyday of revolutionary fervor.

Philippe Pinel, so often honored for removing the chains from patients, was not totally original in his efforts, but he did adopt and promote more humane attitudes than his predecessors. The basis for his action in the 1790s was faith in the Revolution and one of its corollaries—the expectation that an improved society would result in fewer patients and great improvement in those already interned. He did not abolish authority over his patients—in fact, he was quite firm—but he believed that communication with them in as egalitarian a manner as possible was in keeping with the spirit of the French Republic and also beneficial to their health. Pinel was confident that few restraints were necessary if patients were treated with fundamental regard to their individuality and self-respect.[10]

In contrast, George III of Great Britain, who suffered a relapse of his mental condition in 1788, received traditional rugged care and close restraint because his physicians were determined he should receive the best care that their theories commanded: wild behavior required a strong antidote. Even the King could not escape what we would today consider cruel treatment. Whatever anxiety the physicians felt about the King's response to their care, their consciences were untroubled. Pinel was equally at ease when he moved in the direction of more benign treatments. In both instances the physician had virtually absolute control over his patient.

Benjamin Rush, the father of American psychiatry, introduced improvements for patients under his care at the Pennsylvania Hospital in Philadelphia. As usual in the movement toward less confining treatments, reformers faced the problem of the hyperactive and threatening patient. Rush, whose own son was long a patient at the hospital, devised restraints like the 'tranquilizer chair', which prevented movement that could cause further damage to the patient, while reducing blood-flow to the brain—required by his theory of insanity. His goal was to ensure that necessary restraint and treatment created no unintended or undesirable effects.[11]

The nineteenth century

In the nineteenth century, ethical formulations for the medical profession were promulgated in many countries. In 1803, for example, Dr Thomas Percival published a formal statement on medical ethics (see Chapters 3 and 6). Percival's immediate goal was the establishment of a code of ethics and etiquette for the Manchester Infirmary, in order to reduce controversy among the attending physicians. His comments, however, on mental patients in asylums such as existed on the Infirmary grounds, reveal the conflict between humane care and the need to preserve order. His attitude is not far different from that of Pinel or Rush when he writes:

The law justifies *the beating of a lunatic, in such a manner as the circumstances may require*. But it has been before remarked that a physician, who attends an asylum for insanity, is under an obligation of honor as well as of humanity to secure to the unhappy sufferers, committed to his charge, all the tenderness and indulgence compatible with steady and effectual government. And the strait waistcoat, with other improvements in modern practice, now preclude the necessity of coercion by corporal punishment. [Percival's italics][12]

Although he wished to be kind, he believed the physician with special knowledge of the insane could take actions that might appear harsh to young and uninformed physicians. 'Certain cases of *mania*', he wrote, 'seem to require a *boldness of practice* which a young physician of sensibility may feel a reluctance to adopt.' When this occurs, the novice 'must not yield to timidity, but fortify his mind by the councils of his more experienced brethren of the faculty'. Yet Percival could not let his advice admit of too severe an interpretation, for he warned that 'it is more consonant to probity to err on the side of caution than of temerity'.[13] Repeatedly, these advocates of humane care faced the problem of keeping order in hospitals and regulating the admission of patients. Percival strongly favored strict inspection of asylums for proper care and for assurance that no one was admitted without a certificate signed by a physician, surgeon, or apothecary. He emphasized the provision for writs of *habeas corpus* and other legal protection of hospital inmates. Here then are two aspects of care of the insane in which ethical problems arise: whether detention is justified, and whether care given during detention is as humane as possible.

Often the adoption of ethical codes in the nineteenth century was related to the advent of professionalism, whereby standards were set for members of a professional organization who were distinguished from physicians or laymen outside the organization. Medical etiquette was a prominent feature of these codes, which regulated procedures for consultation, details about fees and relations with fellow physicians. Through statutory laws and third-party payment procedures, society later would begin to control aspects of practice that physicians had first governed through internal professional standards. But in the 1800s, especially in the United States, professionalism was not a concern of the state, and jurisdictions had few or no licensing powers. So many schools of medical practice existed that the need to distinguish among them became a matter of pride for their adherents as well as a source of economic advantage. Thus physicians established a variety of medical associations, each of which set codes of conduct and standards.

When the American Medical Association was founded in 1847 its members adopted a code of ethics based on Percival's work.[14] The Association did not become a powerful medical organization until the twentieth century, but its code of ethics is representative of mid-nineteenth-century concerns about proper clinical practice. The first section stresses the physician's high moral obligation, the need for secrecy, the requirement that a physician see a patient through to the end of his illness—whether to cure or to death—balancing hope with realistic warnings to the family. There followed a long section, entirely missing from Percival, entitled 'Obligations of patients to their physicians'. The patient should choose a properly trained physician, provide all relevant information, follow the regimen prescribed, and after recovery 'entertain a just and enduring sense of the value of the services rendered him by his physician'.[15]

Later sections of the code detail courtesies of physicians to one another and the qualifications of a regular physician. The title of the last chapter is 'Of the duties of the profession to the public, and the obligations of the public to the profession'. The relationship of physicians to coroners, guidelines for dispensing free service, and the need to educate the public regarding quackery are stated; yet, in distinction to the detailed treatment in Percival's work, there is no discussion of medical practice within hospitals, and the only reference to insane asylums is in a list of various institutions in which medical authorities must have an interest, such as hospitals, schools, and prisons.

Hooker's contribution

In 1849, two years after adoption of the American Medical Association code, Worthington Hooker, a Connecticut physician, published what is increasingly recognized as a pioneer study of medical ethics in the United States, *Physician and patient; or, a practical view of the mutual duties, relations and interests of the medical profession and the community.*[16] The titles of the chapters, 'Skill in medicine', 'Popular errors', 'Quackery', 'Good and bad practice', 'Influence of hope in the treatment of disease', 'Truth in our intercourse with the sick', and 'Moral influence of physicians' reflect his ethical concerns. Two chapters, 'Mutual influence on mind and body in disease' and 'Insanity', particularly merit our attention. Hooker, like Percival, advocated removal of the mentally ill to a retreat, and reliance upon a 'regimen, or the regulation of their occupations and amusements, bodily and mental, and very little indeed upon medicine'. Hooker deplored the practice, which he admitted was widespread, of intentionally deceiving the insane, or any other patient. He recommended early treatment, and that its costs should be shared by the town and state of the patient's residence. On the subject of how best to determine whether a person is insane, Hooker approved of the French system, in which a committee of experts made the decision after an examination conducted over several days. He regretted that, in his experience, police and prison authorities too often had the final decision, and, in some instances, regarded the advice of physicians as interference. 'Such having been the opinion and practices of our courts of justice', Hooker reflected, 'it is not strange that the rights of the insane have often been trampled on'.[17] In the matter of who might commit an insane person to institutional care, he noted that in Connecticut and Massachusetts it was the civil authorities, not physicians, who made the decision. Even worse, these authorities often committed someone only after he had performed some dangerous act. 'With such defects in the provision of the law', Hooker concluded, 'it is no wonder that the community is occasionally shocked with outrageous, even fatal acts by insane persons, who through neglect have been permitted to go at large.'[19] In keeping with his desire for early treatment in cases of insanity, he suggested that those suspected of being insane be examined by a 'standing commission of lunacy ... composed of physicians who are properly qualified'.[20]

Dr Hooker had sought to introduce expertise into decisions regarding insanity, and this is by and large what occurred in the century after his advocacy. He saw application of knowledge by professionals as increasing the rights of the committed and reducing the error during commitment procedures. It is worth noting that he did not favor waiting until an overt, dangerous act had been committed before acting on behalf of the community and the patient. He was unaware of the present-day argument that cultural bias might distort professional judgment, or that reserving the decision about confinement entirely to medical practitioners might abridge legal protection for the patient.

Hospital as a human warehouse

For several generations thereafter few issues other than the justification for commitment and the humaneness of care were raised regarding psychiatric patients. Such currently significant concerns as the ethics of behavior-control can be dissected away from the practices and concerns of 1800, but only with difficulty. The rights of the committed patient were few, and the primitive state of what we might call the psychiatric profession of the time meant that treatment consisted chiefly in admission to a hospital and residence there until reversion to a normal state, improvement, withdrawal by relatives, or death. The chief question for those who worried about the quality of care was how to conduct a paternalistic relationship kindly, effectively, and efficiently. Personal attention to a patient was expensive, and required great devotion on the part of individual caregivers and hospital authorities. Attempts to make contact with patients through close, kind supervision, mutual respect, and a wholesome environment—'moral therapy'—could not survive waves of pessimism about the curability of mental illness, the overloading of caregivers with patients, and the degradation of hospitals to the status of human warehouses. These conditions obtained in the mid-nineteenth century in many countries. Attention to ethical questions suffered as the possibility of substantial reform declined.[21]

Superintendents of American institutions for the insane, who formed an organization in 1844 (later to become the American Psychiatric Association), argued especially for the right to make most decisions about their patients, from commitment to the way the hospital was organized. This body, antedating the American Medical Association, testifies to the special role these physicians had assumed within the profession. Increasingly isolated from medical practice in general, the superintendents saw themselves as experts in a field too often neglected financially, misunderstood by the community, and requiring extraordinary powers of insight and judgment. Harassed by patients' complaints of maltreatment and wrongful commitment, the superintendents were more concerned to protect themselves from legal encroachment than they were about the veracity of these accounts. To the extent that an asylum attempted moral management (to use a term of Pinel's), which was also a goal of the English reformers William and Samuel Tuke at the York Retreat, an uplifting and healthy environment was created for the patient.[22] One could hardly find fault with trying to improve the conditions of patients, the authorities believed; and if better conditions did not exist, the cause lay in inadequate financial support from governments, not with the managers of the asylums. Worry over behavior modification did not exist, nor did the experts wonder whether they were guided by cultural bias in designing a healthy mental environment. In fact, American psychiatrists of the time commonly found the origin of illness in disobedience or ignorance of what now could be called New England Protestant principles of conduct.[23]

The Packard case

An occasional dramatic error in commitment became a popular cause, stimulating the creation of new laws and procedures. Particularly noteworthy was the case of Mrs E. P. W. Packard who was committed in 1860 by her husband, a clergyman, to an Illinois institution on the grounds that she held dangerous religious beliefs. Her husband was a strict fundamentalist, and feared that his wife would poison the minds of their children with liberal ideas. After some years the trustees freed Mrs. Packard; but her troubles were not over. Her husband imprisoned her in her own home, and sought to have her recommitted. Finally, in 1864, a trial was held at which she was declared sane. She then embarked on a campaign to make commitment for the expression of opinions an impossibility, 'no matter how absurd these opinions may appear to others'.[24] Events like Mrs. Packard's wrongful detention seemed to give credibility to claims against the hospital superintendents, although the latter vowed that such miscarriages were extremely rare. As one anonymous writer in the *American Journal of Insanity* explained:

There can be no clashing or division of interest between the public and the institutions. They are one and the same, and no officer of any public institution can have any possible object in receiving or retaining any sane person in an asylum.[25]

Experimenting with new procedures

While the psychiatric profession and the mental hospitals in the United States were becoming established and stimulating a body of law and precedent regarding the care of the ill, increased experimentation with new procedures and operations raised other ethical questions within the profession and among the laity. Prominent among the questioners were those severe critics of nineteenth-century medicine, the antivivisectionists.[26] Three instances of what we today might consider abuses of research in Ohio, Maryland, and Ontario led to harsh criticism from physicians in North America and Great Britain. It is noteworthy that the condemnation came first and strongest from peers, illustrating the alertness of professional self-regulation. These experiments were not representative of contemporary treatment. On the other hand, one should be aware that the high-minded aspirations of asylum superintendents in fact probably did not reflect the reality of day-to-day existence in mental hospitals. Published reports and admonitions are not good guides to the routine practice of psychiatry.

The Ohio experiment was published in the eminent *American Journal of Medical Science* in 1874. Dr Roberts Bartholow studied the effect of stimulating the exposed surface of a patient's brain electrically through her ulcerated skull. A few days later the patient died, but Dr Bartholow denied that the experiment was related to her death.[27] However, the *British Medical Journal* criticized his procedure and conclusions.[28] The editor was reaffirming Claude Bernard's comment in his *Introduction to the study of experimental medicine*:

It is our duty and our right to perform an experiment on man whenever it can save his life, cure him or gain him some personal benefit. The principle of medical and surgical morality, therefore, consists in never performing on man an experiment that might be harmful to him to any extent, even though the result might be highly advantageous to science, that is, to the health of others.[29]

In a reply,[30] Dr Bartholow tried to justify his actions, but acknowledged that the procedure was injurious to the brain; and he stated that he would not repeat such an experiment.

Reports such as that of Bartholow became a refrain in the antivivisectionist literature as examples of experimenters meddling with the bodies of poor patients while observing great caution toward fee-paying patients. The antivivisectionists saw a similarity between charity patients and laboratory animals: they opposed experiments on both, and sought to arouse the public through dramatic reports.[31]

In 1897, Dr George Rohé, superintendent of a Maryland hospital for the insane, reported on his research of operating on female pelvic organs in order to relieve insanity. He based this treatment on such diagnoses as hysteroepilepsy melancholia, puerperal insanity, and mania, and claimed a recovery rate of about one-third.[32] Similar operations were reported by Dr A. T. Hobbs of the Asylum for the Insane at London, Ontario.[33]

Reproaches against Drs Rohé and Hobbs appeared in the same issue of the *British Medical Journal* that had published their papers. Dr James Russell argued that there was no scientific basis for the widespread belief that gynecological problems lay at the root of insanity in many women.[34] 'The relation of gynaecology to psychiatry has been pretty thoroughly discussed in late

years, and the general consensus of opinion gathered from alienists and neurologists alike is that ... to extol it as a great curative method in the treatment of
insanity is nothing short of absurdity.'[35] The procedures closely approached
criminality, since the women could not understand their possible consequences.
Dr Russell even queried 120 physicians in Great Britain and in America and
found, as presumably he had suspected, that few believed female organs were
associated with insanity or that any operation on them would be beneficial.
The operations did not meet the test of conformity with current standards of
medical practice.

Dr Rohé's reply to Dr Russell's severe and sarcastic criticism was very weak;
he had been misunderstood, and reasserted his claim for a cure of insanity. Dr
Hobbs, 'in reply, repudiated the idea that he ever approved of operative
interference unless there was actual disease'.[36]

In looking back over the nineteenth century—keeping in mind that we are
considering, rather narrowly, antecedents to the modern psychiatric profession—we see that the growth of mental hospitals and the increase in their
inmates, the decline in most instances of 'moral therapy', and a deterioration in
the relations between physicians and patients were all evidence of an atmosphere of pessimism about the ultimate cure of mental illness. This pessimism, in
spite of advances in understanding syphilis, alcoholism, and other specific
causes of mental illness, overshadowed ethical concerns, and caused them to
appear unimportant. A further consequence was that patients who displayed
bizarre behavior were relegated by some caregivers to a less than fully human
status. Even reformers like Benjamin Rush described such patients as animal-
like and fit for being 'broken' like wild animals.[37] In the twentieth century, and
especially since the Second World War, there have been powerful changes in
most of these perceptions, as new concepts and sensitivities about the activities
of psychiatrists have arisen.

The twentieth century

If an atmosphere of pessimism prevailed through most of the nineteenth
century about the possibility of finding a cure for mental illness, by the
twentieth century psychiatry and other mental health professions were evolving
and manifesting new optimism about the future of their disciplines. This
optimism, in the face of the hundreds of thousands of patients with poor
prognoses and without adequate care, was based on developments in both
biological research and psychodynamic and social psychiatry. In the application of these new treatments paternalism was still evident. Physicians decided
whether to pursue an innovation and to whom to apply it; they would meet
few institutional or professional obstacles. Psychiatry and its related disciplines sharply changed their focus from long-term care for the mentally ill to
therapy and the search for cures. They also became increasingly skeptical about
the beneficial aspects of mental hospitals despite a massive increase in the

number of institutionalized patients between 1880 and 1960.[38] They moved from passively accepting those brought to them to actively seeking ways in which they might help the entire community. The public health model applied to psychiatry appeared to some to be the fulfilment of a great goal of providing treatment for everyone, not just those who could afford a private psychiatrist or who were forced to enter a great warehouse for mental incompetents. In the United States, this new role lay behind efforts to increase the number of psychiatrists and the establishment of a nation-wide network of community mental health centers in the 1960s.

The crisis of confidence in psychiatry's authority

Since mid-century several developments have conspired to dampen this optimism about psychiatry's potential and have also raised important ethical issues. Some of these trends are either no longer at work today or have receded into the background. The misuse of psychiatry in the service of totalitarian states (see Chapters 4 and 10 which cover, in part, the cases of Nazi Germany and the former Soviet Union) undoubtedly shook public confidence in psychiatry. The collapse of communism in Eastern Europe has led to a revival of professional standards for psychiatry in that part of the world. The extensive use of psychosurgery for certain diagnoses between 1935 and the mid-1950s throughout the developed world also served to weaken confidence in psychiatry. In England, Wales, and the United States alone, as a conservative estimate, approximately 30 000 patients received lobotomies and related procedures during this period.[39] Enthusiasm for these new therapies was created by a number of factors, including the difficulty in finding a cure for schizophrenia, overcrowded asylums, competition between psychiatrists and neurologists, confidence in the success of biological research in other fields of medicine and, last but not least, the media.[40] Growing opposition to these procedures and the development of new psychotropic drugs brought an end to psychosurgery's heyday.

Yet another trend was the anti-psychiatry movement. Anti-psychiatrists have existed as long as there has been psychiatry, but they gathered considerable strength for the first time in the anti-authoritarian atmosphere of the 1960s.[41,42] Sociologist Erving Goffman and philosopher Michel Foucault published influential works questioning the nature of psychiatric institutions.[43,44] Moreover, psychiatrists themselves led the most radical attacks against the pathological nature of schizophrenia (R. D. Laing)[45] and, in the case of Thomas Szasz, even the existence of mental illness itself. Szasz argued that it was unethical to restrict the actions of patients without their consent. He saw psychiatrists who so impose their 'help' as policemen and gaolers, mental hospitals that confine such persons as prisons, and the insanity defense as a mechanism whereby offenders try to avoid responsibility for their acts and the courts evade their duty to punish.[46,47] Research in the last decades of the twentieth century indicating that many serious mental illnesses have biological or genetic determinants has helped refute the argument that such illnesses are merely social constructs.

However, the impact of these trends, and especially the anti-psychiatry movement, on public opinion has been long lasting. Since mid-century the public has become increasingly suspicious of the authority of a professional élite and the standards for behavior and deviancy which they have promulgated. The accuracy of expert opinion is less an issue now than the prior issue of whether experts have any right to prescribe norms of behavior or to modify behavior without the full consent and understanding of the patient.

On the other hand, three other developments since mid-century retain contemporary relevance for psychiatric ethics: doubts about the efficacy of psychotherapy, the 'new economics' of medicine, and finally the potential for good and ill of new types of organic treatments, especially drug therapy.

New ethical issues in psychiatric practice

There has been a veritable 'assault on Freud' since the 1950s which charges that psychotherapy is unscientific, its claims unverifiable, and its success based at best on a 'placebo' effect. Studies suggest that psychotherapy is effective in dealing with many types of neurotic states, but much about how and why this is so remains to be proven clinically.[48] However, this uncertainty, along with the continued development of alternative, low-cost treatment possibilities in the form of new psychoactive drugs, has raised ethical questions for doctors about both the legitimacy of psychotherapy on the one hand and the possible overuse of drug treatment on the other. There is also increasing recognition within the profession that both psychotherapy and the psychotherapist are anything but value-neutral.[49] Ethical and effective care must take into account the 'unscientific' value systems of both doctor and patient, including religious beliefs and cultural differences. Therapists themselves have fallen from their previous privileged position in the sense that their own conduct is under more intense scrutiny than ever, especially in regard to sexual contact with patients.[50]

There have also been significant economic pressures on the mental health disciplines in the twentieth century that have created ethical dilemmas. In 1980 the philosopher William J. Winslade identified a long-standing conflict between utilitarian thinking, characterized by cost-effective treatment often relying on behavioral control by drugs, and values advocating individually tailored, possibly long-term, and expensive care.[51]

The desire to cut public expenses, along with the notion shared by both pro- and anti-psychiatrists alike around mid-century that most patients could be cared for more humanely outside of mental hospitals, led to the creation of community mental health centers and large-scale deinstitutionalization in the United States after 1960. This triumph of autonomy over paternalism has forced many of the mentally ill into daily living situations that they are ill-suited to cope with. The 'new economics' has also inserted insurance companies between doctors and patients on an unparalleled level. These companies normally demand detailed information about patients, which often puts therapists in the uncomfortable position of having to decide between protecting the patient's confidentiality or complying with insurance requirements. 'Managed care' has created a similar dilemma by insisting on treatment options that are the most cost-effective and 'medically necessary' at a time when psychiatrists find themselves competing with therapists from other mental health fields and having to justify to the public the uses of their own discipline, especially psychotherapy.[52] The desire to cut mental health costs in order to provide care to as many as possible is both noble and, given current financial constraints felt by the public sector in most industrialized nations, probably inevitable, but it raises serious ethical challenges for psychiatry.

In recent decades biological psychiatry has continued to make tremendous strides and has revolutionized our understanding of brain function and chemistry. Organic treatments based on newly developed drugs seem to hold great promise but raise very serious ethical issues. Many of the same forces that led to the overapplication and misuse of psychosurgery earlier in the century— the physician's desire to provide quick, effective, economical care that does not require institutionalization, rivalry between medical disciplines, overconfidence about the potential of new technologies to treat intractable diseases, and public enthusiasm—are at work in regard to the new psychotropic drugs and may lead to their overuse. The ethical implications of possible future 'designer drugs' that produce significant changes in personality on demand are of course enormous, as is the question of who should prescribe them.

Codes of ethics

As a result of these developments, psychiatrists have devoted more attention to ethical issues and professional standards than ever before. The tragic abuse of medicine during the Second World War led to the *Nuremberg Statement*— rules for medical research—which was subsequently incorporated into the *Declaration of Helsinki* (see Appendix). In 1948 the World Medical Association promulgated the *Declaration of Geneva* (see Appendix) and, a year later, the *International code of medical ethics*, which was designed to be a model for national medical codes. These two texts are modern restatements of the Hippocratic Oath. Within psychiatry itself, the World Psychiatric Association adopted the *Declaration of Hawaii* in 1977 (see Appendix). This was the first ethical code designed specifically for psychiatrists.[53] It responded both to the misuse of psychiatry by the state in the USSR[54] and to the aggressive public health and paternalistic stances in Western psychiatry. To cite a few of the *Declaration*'s statements: it calls for disclosure of diagnosis and discussion of alternative therapies with the patient, requires that detained patients should have an avenue of appeal, and calls for the seeking of patients' consent to any treatment, with third-party consent in cases of patients' incapacity. Some national psychiatric associations have formulated their own ethical codes. The American Psychiatric Association, for example, adopted the *Principles of medical ethics* of the American Medical Association, and in 1973 produced a text, the *Principles of medical ethics with annotations especially applicable to psychiatry*.[55,56] (See Appendix) This text (last revised in 1995), unlike the *Declaration of Hawaii*, does not advocate an essentially egalitarian relationship between therapist and patient. Rather, its emphasis—demonstrating its direct descent from Hippocratic tenets—is on the need for the psychiatrist to merit and maintain the trust of patients and other professionals alike.

Psychiatry is in an era of unprecedented professional development yet finds itself in a crisis in its relations with patients and the public. In this quandary the welfare of the profession depends on sound analysis of ethical questions. These questions seem to lose some of their urgency when the scientific underpinning of the profession appears solid. In fact, concern about ethical issues from both within the profession and from the public seem to have stood in inverse relation to overall confidence about the state of the mental health disciplines. Should psychiatry continue to move towards a greater reliance on organic treatment for its authority and further towards faith in a genetic basis for behavior, powerful and broad professional control over the destinies of others may reappear.

References

1. Edelstein, L.: The Hippocratic Oath, text, translation and interpretation, in *Ancient medicine*, ed. O. Temkin and C. L. Temkin. Baltimore, Johns Hopkins University Press, 1967, pp. 17–18.
2. Ibid., p. 6.
3. Rosen, G.: *Madness in society: chapters in the historical sociology of mental illness.* Chicago, University of Chicago Press, 1968, pp. 125–8.
4. Mora, G.: History of psychiatry, in *Comprehensive textbook of psychiatry*, ed. A. M. Freedman and H. I. Kaplan. Baltimore, Williams and Wilkins, 1967, p. 12. For a dissenting view, see: Mobaraky, G. H.: Islamic view of mental disorders (Letter to the editor). *American Journal of Psychiatry* **146**:561, 1989.
5. Mora, ibid. p. 5.
6. Ackerknecht, E. H.: *A short history of psychiatry*, trans. S. Wolff. New York, Hafner, 1968, p. 17.
7. Mora, G.: History of psychiatry, in *Comprehensive textbook of psychiatry*, ed. A. M. Freedman and H. I. Kaplan. Baltimore, Williams and Wilkins, 1967, pp. 16–17.
8. Neugebauer, R.: Treatment of the mentally ill in medieval and early modern England: a reappraisal. *Journal for the History of Behavioural Science* **14**:158–69, 1978.
9. Ellenberger, H. F.: Psychiatry from ancient to modern times, in *American handbook of psychiatry*, 2nd edn, vol. 1, ed. S. Arieti. New York, Basic Books, 1974, p. 14.

10. Hunter, R. and Macalpine, I.: *Three hundred years of psychiatry 1535–1860: a history presented in selected English texts.* London, Oxford University Press, 1963, pp. 602–10.
11. Dain, N.: *Concepts of insanity in the United States, 1789–1865.* New Brunswick, NJ, Rutgers University Press, 1964, pp. 18–19, 23.
12. Percival T.: *Medical ethics* (1803), ed. C. D. Leake. Huntington, NY, Robert E. Krieger, 1975, p. 126.
13. Ibid., p. 89.
14. Code of medical ethics adopted by the National Medical Convention in Philadelphia, June, 1847, in Hooker, W. L.: *Physician and patient; or, a practical view of the mutual duties, relations and interests of the medical profession and the community (1849).* New York, Arno Press. 1972, pp. 440–53.
15. Ibid., p. 444.
16. Hooker. W. L.: *Physician and patient; or, a practical view of the mutual duties, relations and interests of the medical profession and the community (1849).* New York, Arno Press, 1972. See also Musto, D. F.: Worthington Hooker (1806–1867): physician and educator. *Connecticut Medicine* **48**:569–74, 1984.
17. Ibid., p. 334.
18. Ibid., p. 340.
19. Ibid., p. 342.
20. Ibid., p. 342.
21. Musto, D. F.: Therapeutic intervention and social forces: historical perspectives, in *American handbook of psychiatry*, vol. 5, ed. S. Arieti. New York, Basic Books, 1975, pp. 34–42.
22. Hunter, R. and Macalpine, I.: *Three hundred years of psychiatry 1535–1860. A history presented in selected English texts.* London, Oxford University Press, 1963, pp. 602–10, 684–90.
23. Grob, G. N.: *Mental institutions in America: social policy to 1875.* New York, Free Press, 1973, pp. 160–1.
24. Packard, Mrs E. P. W.: *Marital power exemplified in Mrs. Packard's trial, and self-defense from the charge of insanity; or three years' imprisonment for religious belief, by the arbitrary will of a husband with an appeal to the Government to so change the laws as to protect the rights of married women.* Hartford, Connecticut, Case, Lockwood, 1866, p. 55.
25. *American Journal of Insanity* **29**:302, 1872.
26. Harvey, J.: Human experimentation in the nineteenth century. Unpublished manuscript. Harvard University, 1977. (I am indebted to Ms Harvey for calling my attention to this reference in psychosurgery)
27. Bartholow, R.: Experimental investigations into the functions of the human brain. *American Journal of Medical Science* **67**:305–13, 1874.
28. *British Medical Journal* **i**:687, 1874.
29. Bernard, C.: *An introduction to the study of experimental medicine* (1865), trans. H. C. Greene. New York, Henry Schuman, 1949, p. 101.
30. Bartholow, R.: Experiments on the functions of the human brain. *British Medical Journal* **i**:727, 1874.
31. French, R. D.: *Antivivisection and medical science in Victorian society.* Princeton, Princeton University Press, 1975.
32. Rohe, G. E.: The etiological relation of pelvic disease in women to insanity. *British Medical Journal* **ii**:766–9, 1897.
33. Hobbs, A. T.: Surgical gynaecology in insanity. *British Medical Journal* **ii**:769–70, 1897.

34. Russell, J.: The after-effects of surgical procedure on the generative organs of females for the relief of insanity. *British Medical Journal* **ii**:770–7, 1897.
35. Ibid., p. 770.
36. Ibid., p. 774.
37. Deutsch, A.: *The mentally ill in America (1938)*. New York, Columbia University Press, 1949.
38. In the United States, the 1880 census listed 91 997 insane persons out of a total population of 50 million. By 1940, the population in the continental United States increased to around 133 million, but the number of patients in American public mental hospitals alone expanded fivefold to 450 000. Grob, G. N.: *Mental illness and American society, 1875–1940*. Princeton, New Jersey, Princeton University Press, 1983.
39. Swayze, V. W.: Frontal leukotomy and related psychosurgical procedures in the era before antipsychotics (1935–1954): a historical overview. *American Journal of Psychiatry* **152**:505–15, 1995.
40. Valenstein, E. S.: *Great and desperate cures. The rise and decline of psychosurgery and other radical treatments for mental illness*. New York, Basic Books, 1986.
41. Postel, J. and Allen, D. F.: History and anti-psychiatry in France, in *Discovering the history of psychiatry*, ed. M. S. Micale and R. Porter. New York, Oxford University Press, 1994, pp. 384–414.
42. Dain, N.: Psychiatry and anti-psychiatry in the United States, in *Discovering the history of psychiatry*, ed. M. S. Micale and R. Porter. New York, Oxford University Press, 1994, pp. 415–44.
43. Goffman, E.: *Asylums*. Harmondsworth, Penguin, 1968.
44. Foucault, M.: *Madness and civilization: a history of insanity in the age of reason (1961)*. New York, Random, 1965.
45. Laing, R. D.: *The divided self (1960)*. Baltimore, Penguin, 1971.
46. Szasz, T. S.: *The myth of mental illness: foundations of a theory of personal conduct (1961)*. New York, Harper and Row, 1974.
47. Szasz, T. S.: *The manufacture of madness: a comparative study of the Inquisition and the mental health movement*. New York, Harper and Row, 1970.
48. Holmes, J.: Editorial review. The assault on Freud. *Current Opinion in Psychiatry* **9**:175–6, 1996.
49. Holmes, J.: Values in psychotherapy. *American Journal of Psychotherapy* **50**: 259–73, 1996.
50. Gabbard, G. O.: Lessons to be learned from the study of sexual boundary violations. *American Journal of Psychotherapy* **50**:311–22, 1996.
51. Winslade, W. J.: Ethics and ethos in psychiatry: historical patterns and conceptual changes. Unpublished paper presented at the American College of Psychiatrists, Annual Meeting, San Antonio, Texas, 6 Feb. 1980.
52. Chodoff, P.: Ethical dimensions of psychotherapy: a personal perspective. *American Journal of Psychotherapy* **50**:298–310, 1996.
53. Blomquist, C. D. D.: From the Oath of Hippocrates to the Declaration of Hawaii. *Ethics in Science and Medicine* **4**:139–49, 1977.
54. See, for example, Bloch, S. and Reddaway, P. *Russia's political hospitals*. London, Gollancz, 1977 and *Soviet psychiatric abuse*. London, Gollancz, 1984.
55. Moore, R. A.: Ethics in the practice of psychiatry—origins, functions, models, and enforcement. *American Journal of Psychiatry* **135**:157–63, 1978.
56. The principles of medical ethics with annotations especially applicable to psychiatry. *American Journal of Psychiatry* **130**:1057–64, 1973.

3

The philosophical basis of psychiatric ethics

Tom L. Beauchamp

The moral problems discussed in this book have emerged from professional practice in psychiatry. The objective of this chapter is to provide an understanding of philosophical ethics that will be sufficient for reading other chapters and sufficient to appreciate the relevance of philosophical investigations for psychiatric ethics.

Morality

The terms 'ethical' and 'moral' are here treated as identical in meaning, but 'morality' and 'moral philosophy' (as well as 'ethical theory') are given different meanings. The term 'morality' refers to widely shared social conventions about right and wrong that form a stable communal consensus in all moral communities. Morality comprehends many standards of conduct that we refer to as 'moral rules', 'human rights', and virtues. The core parts of morality exist before their acceptance by individuals, who learn about moral responsibilities and moral ideals as they grow up. They also eventually learn to distinguish the general morality that holds for all persons—what I will call the common morality—from rules binding only members of special groups, such as physicians.

The common morality

The morality shared by all morally serious persons in all societies is not *a morality*; it is simply morality. It is universal because it contains ethical precepts found wherever morality is found. In recent years, the favored category has been human rights,[1] but parts of morality are also found in standards of obligation and virtue. These norms constituting our shared morality might well be called 'morality in the narrow sense', because the morality we share in common is only a small slice of the entire moral life. Morality in the broad sense includes divergent moral norms and positions that spring from particular cultural, philosophical, and religious roots.

Many people are curious about and even skeptical of the idea of a common morality. They think that virtually nothing is shared across cultures and different moral traditions. This is a confusion of the broad and narrow senses of 'morality'. While the broad sense allows for ample diversity and disagreement, the narrow sense simply captures what we all already know and appreciate about morality. The following are examples of universal precepts that all morally serious persons share in common: Tell the truth; Respect the privacy of others; Protect confidential information; Obtain consent before invading another person's body; Do not kill; Do not cause pain; Do not steal or otherwise deprive of goods; Prevent harm from occurring to others.

It is no objection to these rules to note that in some circumstances they can be validly overridden by other norms with which they conflict. All norms can be validly overridden in some circumstances in which they compete with other moral claims. For example, we might not tell the truth in order to prevent someone from killing another person; and in order to protect the rights of one person, a person might have to disclose confidential information about another person. Principles, duties, and rights are not unbending standards. They are general norms that must be balanced with other norms and made specific for circumstances.

Moral justification

Because we have a good grasp of features of the common morality, we generally have no difficulty in deciding whether to act morally. We make moral judgments through appeals to rules, cases, moral exemplars, and the like. These moral beacons work well as long as we are not asked to justify our judgments. However, when we experience moral problems, we begin moral deliberation. In reaching a moral judgment, any agent should be prepared to defend the judgment by a process of giving moral reasons—often referred to as moral justification. The reasons we finally accept, therefore, express the conditions under which we believe some course of action is warranted.

The objective of justification is to establish one's case by presenting sufficient grounds for action or belief. One might attempt a justification by appealing to pre-existing rules, such as those listed above or those in codes of ethics. One might also appeal to authoritative institutional agreements and practices or to the moral convictions in which we have the highest confidence in the common morality. In each case, appeals are made to the best moral reasons for the proposed course of action. Justification also requires that all relevant and obtainable information be acquired and that one be impartial in the process of moral deliberation. One's reasons must be impartially selected and impartially applied, while remaining sensitive to moral conflicts as well as conflicts with legal obligations, religious traditions, and the like.

A reason can be a good reason without being sufficient for justification, and an attempted justification is not always a successful justification. For example, a good reason for involuntarily committing certain mentally ill persons to institutions is that they present a clear and present danger to other persons. By contrast, a reason for commitment that is sometimes offered as a good reason, but which many people consider a bad reason (because it involves a deprivation of liberty), is that some mentally ill persons present a clear and present danger to themselves, or because they require treatment for a serious mental disorder.

If someone holds that involuntary commitment on grounds of danger to self is a good reason and is solely sufficient to justify commitment, that person should be able to give some account of why this reason is good and sufficient. That is, the person should be able to give further justifying reasons for the belief that the reason offered is good and sufficient. The person might refer, for example, to the dire consequences for the mentally ill that will occur if no one intervenes. The person might also invoke certain principles about the moral importance of caring for the needs of the mentally ill. In short, the person is expected to give a set of reasons that amounts to an argued defense of his or her perspective.

Thus far, we have been concerned primarily with the justification of moral judgments, but philosophers are no less concerned with the justification of ethical theories. These theories can be helpful when reflecting on psychiatric ethics, and they are often invoked in the literature of the field.

Classical ethical theories

My objective in this section and the next is not to defend ethical theory or to argue that it has the capacity to resolve problems in psychiatry, but to explicate several types of theory. I will concentrate on utilitarianism, Kantianism, virtue ethics, the ethics of care, and casuistry.

Utilitarian theories

To utilitarians, the object of morality is to promote human welfare by minimizing harms and maximizing benefits. They regard an action or practice as right if it leads to the greatest possible balance of good consequences or to the least possible balance of bad consequences. Utilitarians defend *the principle of utility*, which asserts that we ought always to produce the maximal balance of positive value over disvalue. There are four essential features of utilitarianism that may be extracted from the reasoning of utilitarians:[2]

1. *The principle of utility.* First, actors are obliged to maximize the good: we ought always to produce the greatest possible balance of value. This leads to questions of how we should understand the good or the valuable.

2. *The standard of goodness.* The goodness or valuable nature of consequences is to be measured by items that count as primary goods or basic utilities.

Many utilitarians agree that we ought to produce values that do not vary from person to person. But other utilitarians interpret the good as that which is subjectively desired or wanted, and in this account the satisfaction of desires or wants is the goal of moral actions.

3. *Consequentialism*. All utilitarian theories decide which actions are recommended entirely by reference to the consequences of the actions, rather than by virtue of any intrinsic moral features they may have, such as truthfulness or fidelity.

4. *Impartiality (Universalism)*. Finally, in a utilitarian theory all parties affected must receive equal and impartial consideration.

A significant dispute has arisen among utilitarians over whether the principle of utility is to be applied to *particular acts* in particular circumstances or to *rules of conduct* that determine which acts are right and wrong. For the rule utilitarian, actions are justified by appeal to rules such as, 'Don't deceive' and 'Don't break promises'. These rules are themselves justified by appeal to the principle of utility. An act utilitarian simply justifies actions directly by appeal to the principle of utility.

Many philosophers object to act utilitarianism, charging its exponents with basing morality on mere expediency. On act-utilitarian grounds, they say, it is desirable for a psychiatrist to disclose confidential information to a family or the police if it would relieve a family or society of a burden thereby leading to the greatest good for the greatest number. Many opponents of act utilitarianism have argued that strict rules must be maintained—e.g. the rules of confidentiality that psychiatrists have traditionally supported. These apparently desirable rules can be justified by the principle of utility, so utilitarianism need not be abandoned if act utilitarianism is judged unworthy.

Rule utilitarians hold that rules have a central position in morality and cannot be compromised by the demands of particular situations. Compromise would threaten rules, whose effectiveness is judged by determining whether the observance of a given rule would, in theory, maximize social utility better than any substitute rule (or having no rule). Utilitarian rules are, in theory, firm and protective of all classes of individuals, just as human rights firmly protect all individuals. Still, we should ask whether rule-utilitarian theories differ substantially from act utilitarianism. Dilemmas often arise that involve conflicts among moral rules, for example, rules of confidentiality conflict with rules protecting individual or social welfare. If there are no rules to resolve these conflicts, perhaps the rule-utilitarian theory simply collapses into the act-utilitarian theory.

Kantian theories

A second type of theory has been called *deontological*, but is now increasingly called *Kantian* because of its origins in the theory of Immanuel Kant. He held that acts are morally praiseworthy only if the person's motive for acting is to perform a true duty. It is not good enough that one happens to perform the morally correct action, because one could perform it from self-interested motives having nothing to do with morality. For example, if a psychiatrist spends long hours to rescue a desperately troubled patient only because he or she fears a spouse will otherwise not pay the fees, and not because of a belief in the importance of performing the act itself, then the psychiatrist acts rightly but deserves no moral credit for doing so.

Morality, in this conception, provides a rational framework of universal principles and rules that constrain and guide everyone. Kant's supreme principle, called 'the moral law' and 'the categorical imperative', is expressed in several ways in his writings. In his first formulation, the principle is, 'I ought never to act except in such a way that I can also will that my maxim should become a universal law'.[3] Kant's view is that wrongful practices, including invasion of privacy, theft, and manipulative suppression of information are 'contradictory'; that is, they are not consistent with what the very duties they presuppose. Consider cases of lying. The universalization of rules that allow lying would entitle everyone to lie to you, just as you could lie to them. Such rules are inconsistent with the practice of truth-telling that they presuppose.

Kant states his categorical imperative in another and distinctly different formulation. This form may be more widely quoted and endorsed in contemporary ethics than the first form, and certainly it is more frequently invoked in biomedical ethics. This formulation stipulates that, 'One must act to treat every person as an end and never as a means only'.[4] Thus, one must treat persons as having their own autonomously established goals. It has been widely said that Kant is arguing categorically that we can never treat another as a means to our ends. This interpretation, however, misrepresents his views. He argues only that we must not treat another exclusively as a means to our own ends. When adult human research subjects are asked to volunteer, for example, they are treated as a means to a researcher's ends. However, they are not exclusively used for others' purposes, because they do not become mere servants or objects. Their consent justifies using them as means to the end of research. Kant's imperative demands only that persons in such situations be treated with the respect and moral dignity to which all persons are always entitled, including the times when they are used as means to the ends of others.

Alternatives to classical theories

Utilitarianism and Kantianism have been dominant models in ethical theory throughout much of the twentieth century. None the less, recent philosophical writing has often focused on the need to supplement or replace these theories. Proposed replacement theories are: (1) virtue theories; (2) the ethics of care; and (3) casuistry. The first two are of substantive importance for psychiatric ethics, and the third contains practical ideas about method in ethics.

Virtue ethics

Virtue ethics descends from the classical Greek tradition of ethics represented by Plato and Aristotle,[5] who regarded the cultivation of virtuous traits of character as the central feature of the moral life. This approach investigates the role of a person's characteristic motivational structure. A conscientious person, for example, not only has a disposition to act conscientiously, but a morally appropriate desire to be conscientious. The person characteristically has a moral concern and reservation about acting in a way that would not be conscientious. Having only the motive to act in accordance with a rule of obligation is not morally sufficient for virtue. In addition, one needs virtues such as conscientiousness.

Consider persons who always perform obligations because they are obligations, but who intensely dislike having to allow the interests of others to be taken into account. These individuals do not cherish, feel congenial toward, or think fondly of others, and treat them as they should only because obligation requires it. Imagine a psychiatrist who always meets his or her moral responsibilities while acting from motives and desires such as fear of professional disrespect. This psychiatrist has come to detest working and hates having to spend time with every patient who comes through the door. He cares not at all about being of service to people, but wishes only to make money. Although this individual meets moral responsibilities, something in his or her character is morally lacking. The admirable compassion, commitment, and conscientiousness guiding the lives of many dedicated health professionals is absent in this person.

Virtue ethics may seem only of intellectual interest, but it has practical value in that a morally good person with right desires or motives is more likely to understand what should be done, to perform required acts, and to form moral ideals than would a morally bad or indifferent person. A trusted person has an ingrained motivation and desire to do what is right and to care about whether it is done. Whenever the feelings, concerns, and attitudes of others are the morally relevant matters, rules and principles are not as likely as human warmth and sensitivity to lead a person to notice what should be done. From this perspective, virtue ethics is at least as fundamental in the moral life as principles of basic obligation.

The ethics of care

The 'ethics of care' extends some themes in virtue ethics about the centrality of character, but it focuses on features of close personal relationships such as sympathy, fidelity, love, and friendship. Noticeably absent in this theory are universal moral rules and impartial calculations. The care perspective views universality and impartiality in the traditional theories as cutting away too much of morality. Lost in the distance of impartiality is the warmth involved in caring about what is closest to us and mixed with our own personal and professional lives. In seeking the blindness of justice that we expect in courts, we may be made morally blind and indifferent to special needs. So, although impartiality is a moral virtue in some contexts, it may be a moral vice in others.

Defenders of the ethics of care find principles of obligation often to be irrelevant or ineffectual. A defender of principles could say that principles of care, compassion, and kindness structure our understanding of when it is appropriate to respond in caring, compassionate, and kind ways, but there is something *ad hoc* about this claim. It seems to capture our moral experience best to say that we rely on our emotions, our capacity for sympathy, our sense of friendship, and our knowledge of how caring people behave.

Additional reasons exist for thinking that a morality centered on care can be a robust presence in professional ethics such as psychiatric ethics. It is difficult to express the precise responsibilities of a health-care professional adequately through principles and rules. We can state how caring physicians and nurses should respond in encounters with patients, but such generalizations will often not be subtle enough to give sound guidance for the next patient. Behavior that in one context is caring seems to intrude on privacy or be offensive in another context. The ethics of care fits this context of relationships, whereas many other theories seem poorly equipped for it. The care perspective is especially important for roles such as parent, friend, physician, and nurse, where contextual response, attentiveness to subtle clues, and discernment are more likely to be relied upon than is conformity to rules.

Casuistry

A third alternative to classical theories has been labeled 'casuistry'. It focuses on decision-making using particular cases, where the judgments arrived at rely on judgments reached in prior cases. Casuists are skeptical of the power of principles and theory to resolve problems in specific cases. They think that many forms of moral thinking and judgment do not involve appeals to general guidelines, but rather to narratives, paradigm cases, and precedents established by previous cases.[6]

Consider the way a physician thinks in making a judgment and then a recommendation to a patient. Many individual factors, including the patient's medical history, the physician's successes with other similar patients, paradigms of expected outcomes, and the like will play a role in formulating a judgment and recommendation to this patient, which may be very different from the recommendation made to the next patient with the same malady. The casuist views moral judgments and recommendations similarly. One can make successful moral judgments of agents, actions, and policies, casuists say, only when one has an intimate understanding of particular situations and an appreciation of treating similar cases similarly.

An analogy to case law is helpful in understanding the casuist's point. In case law, the normative judgments of courts of law become authoritative, and it is reasonable to hold that these judgments are primary for later judges who assess other cases—even though the particular features of each new case will be different. Matters are similar in ethics. Normative judgments about certain cases emerge through case comparisons: a case under current consideration is placed in the context of a set of cases that shows a family resemblance, and the similarities and differences are assessed. The relative weight of competing values is presumably determined by the comparisons to analogous cases. Moral guidance is provided by an accumulated mass of influential cases, which represent a consensus in society and in institutions reached by reflection on cases. That consensus then becomes authoritative and is extended to new cases.[7]

Cases such as *Tarasoff* have been enormously influential in psychiatry. Writers have used it to reach decisions about the case that can serve as a form of authority for decisions in new cases. Features of their analyses have then been discussed throughout the literature of biomedical ethics, and they become integral to the way we think and draw conclusions in the field.[8] However, *Tarasoff* is a dubious choice to illustrate the casuistic method.[9] For *Tarasoff* or any other case to work well, it must be believed that decisions can be reached in new cases by a process of comparing similar cases. Many unique features in *Tarasoff* make it difficult to use the case for purposes of generalization to other cases. Casuistry is a potentially useful method for psychiatric ethics, but it is important to choose cases carefully and to test them systematically by closely comparing similarities and differences.

At first sight, casuistry seems strongly opposed to the frameworks of principles and theory in traditional moral theory. However, closer inspection of casuistry shows that its primary concern is with an excessive reliance in recent philosophy on impartial, universal action-guides. Two casuists, Albert Jonsen and Stephen Toulmin, write that '*good* casuistry ... applies general principles to particular cases with discernment'. As a history of similar cases and similar judgments mounts, we become more confident in our general judgments. A 'locus of moral certitude' arises in the judgments, and the stable elements crystallize into tentative principles. As confidence in these generalizations increases, they are accepted less tentatively and moral knowledge develops.[10]

From this perspective, ethical theory is desirable: case-based judgment is, as Baruch Brody puts it, only the first stop on the road to moral knowledge. The next stop is theory formation. The goal is to find a theory that coherently systematizes these judgments, explains them, and provides help in dealing with other cases.[11] So understood, casuistry is not inconsistent with classical ethical theory; it simply places an emphasis on practical decision-making, rather than featuring a general theory.

A framework of moral principles

The common morality, we saw earlier, contains numerous moral precepts. These precepts are supported by principles that are basic in biomedical ethics. These principles are generally accepted in classical ethical theories[12] and seem to be presupposed in traditional medical codes, which have relied heavily upon the implications of the general principle 'Do no harm'. But there are other general principles of no less importance.

Ideally, a set of general principles will serve as an analytical framework of basic principles that expresses the general values underlying rules in the common morality and guidelines in professional ethics. Elsewhere James Childress and I have defended four clusters of moral principles that can serve this function:[13]

(1) respect for autonomy (respecting the decision-making capacities of autonomous persons);

(2) nonmaleficence (avoiding the causation of harm);

(3) beneficence (providing benefits and balancing benefits against risks);

(4) justice (fairness in the distribution of benefits and risks).

These principles do not form a moral system or theory, but they do provide a framework through which we can identify and reflect on moral problems. The framework is abstract and spare, and moral thinking and judgment must take account of other considerations. Abstract principles simply do not contain sufficient content to address the nuances of moral circumstances, as professional guidelines, such as those governing psychiatry, clearly show.[14] Often the most prudent course is to search for more information about cases and policies, rather than to try to decide prematurely on the basis of either principles or some general theoretical analysis. More information sometimes will resolve problems and in other cases will help fix which principles are most important in the circumstances. Many solutions will conform to principles in so far as possible, while recognizing that compromises in situations of conflict often are justified.

Principles provide a starting point for moral judgment and policy evaluation, but they do not treat the subtleties of moral problems. Below I will discuss the need for specification of principles and how they can be overridden by other moral principles. For now, however, I will concentrate on the principles themselves, especially their meaning and moral implications.

Respect for autonomy

Respect for autonomy is a frequently mentioned moral principle in psychiatric ethics. It is rooted in the liberal moral and political tradition of the importance of individual freedom and choice. In moral philosophy personal autonomy refers to personal self-governance: personal rule of the self by adequate under-standing while remaining free from controlling interferences by others and from personal limitations that prevent choice. 'Autonomy' thus means freedom from external constraint and the presence of critical mental capacities such as understanding, intending, and voluntary decision-making capacity.[15]

To respect an autonomous agent is to recognize with due appreciation that person's capacities and perspective, including his or her right to hold certain views, to make certain choices, and to take certain actions based on personal values and beliefs. The moral demand that we respect the autonomy of persons can be expressed as a principle of respect for autonomy: autonomy of action should not be subjected to control by others. The principle provides the basis for the right to make decisions, which in turn takes the form of specific autonomy-related rights.

Many issues in psychiatric ethics concern failures to respect a person's autonomy, ranging from manipulative underdisclosure of pertinent informa-tion to non-recognition of a refusal of medical interventions. For example, in the debate over whether autonomous, informed patients have the right to refuse medical interventions, the principle of respect for autonomy suggests that an autonomous decision to refuse interventions must be respected. Although it was not until the late 1970s that psychiatry and law gave serious attention to rights to refuse for patients such as those involuntarily committed, this is no reason for thinking that respect for autonomy as now understood is only a recent addition to our moral perspective. It simply means that the implications of this principle were not widely appreciated until recently (and may still not be well understood).

During and after the 1970s, requirements of informed consent gained a foothold in medicine, and they seem to be justified by obligations of respect for autonomy.[16] These requirements have generated a number of moral problems in psychiatric ethics. For example, it would seem that a psychiatrist cannot rightfully impose treatment on a non-dangerous but mentally disturbed person, but also cannot accept a consent to treatment by such a person as autonomous. If autonomy is required to authorize treatment, then the treatment would not be authorized even if it would be beneficial. What, if anything, warrants the treatment? Should guardian consent be sought? Are the medical benefits themselves an adequate moral basis for proceeding?[17]

The principle of respect for autonomy also applies in quite simple exchanges in the psychiatric world, such as listening carefully to patients' questions, answering the questions in the detail that respectfulness would demand, and not treating patients in a patronizing fashion. To respect the autonomy of each self-determining agent is to recognize him or her as entitled to such treatment, with a due regard to their considered evaluations and view of the world. Psychiatric patients are, of course, often in a particularly vulnerable position when mental problems, such as depression, impair their understanding, judg-ment, or ability to think clearly—raising questions about their competence to make choices. Psychiatrists caring for such patients can also be in the difficult position of overruling what the patient wants in ways that seem to directly challenge their right to make choices. This leads to the subtle problem of how to care for patients respectfully and without rendering them fearful or threatened.

Controversial problems with the principle of respect for autonomy, as with all moral principles, arise when we must interpret its significance for particular contexts and determine precise limits on its application and how to handle situations when it conflicts with other moral principles. Many controversies involve questions about the conditions under which a person's right to autonomous expression demands actions by others. They also involve questions about the restrictions society may rightfully place on choices by patients or subjects when these choices conflict with other values. If restriction of the patient's autonomy is in order, the justification will always rest on some competing moral principle such as beneficence or justice. Many interesting cases in psychiatry are problems of medical paternalism, which are addressed below.

Nonmaleficence

Since the days of Hippocrates, physicians have avowed that they would do their patients no harm. Among the most quoted principles in the history of codes of medical ethics is the maxim *primum non nocere*: 'Above all, do no harm'.[18] British physician Thomas Percival furnished the first developed modern account of health-care ethics, in which he maintained that a principle of non-maleficence fixes the physician's primary obligations and triumphs even over respect for the patient's autonomy in a circumstance of potential harm to patients:

To a patient ... who makes inquiries which, if faithfully answered, might prove fatal to him, it would be a gross and unfeeling wrong to reveal the truth. His right to it is suspended, and even annihilated; because ... it would be deeply injurious to himself, to his family, and to the public. And he has the strongest claim, from the trust reposed in his physician, as well as from the common principles of humanity, to be guarded against whatever would be detrimental to him.[19]

Similar ideas have been many times repeated in classical medical writings and codes, and there can be little doubt that many basic rules in the common morality are requirements to avoid causing a harm. They include rules such as, 'Do not kill'; 'Do not cause pain'; 'Do not disable'; 'Do not deprive of pleasure'; 'Do not cheat'; and 'Do not break promises'.[20] Similar, but more specific prohibitions are found across the literature of biomedical ethics, each grounded in the principle that intentionally or negligently caused harm is a fundamental moral wrong.[21]

There are many issues of nonmaleficence in psychiatry—some involving blatant abuses of persons and others involving subtle and unresolved questions. Blatant examples of failures to act nonmaleficently are found in the use of psychiatry to classify political dissidents as mentally ill, thereafter treating them with harmful drugs and incarcerating them with insane and violent persons.[22] More subtle examples are found in the use of psychotropic medications for the treatments of aggressive and destructive patients. These common treatment modalities are helpful to many patients, but they can be harmful to others. Careless psychiatrists can also cause harm when they fail to take an adequate history, prescribe an improper dosage of medicine, fail to monitor and treat side-effects, and the like.[23]

A sensitive and consequential question about nonmaleficence in psychiatry has been raised by Paul S. Appelbaum in his investigation of 'the problem of doing harm' through psychiatric testimony in criminal contexts and civil litigation—for example by omitting information in the context of a trial, after which a more severe punishment is delivered to the person than likely would have been delivered. Appelbaum presents the generic problem for psychiatric ethics as a straightforward one of nonmaleficence:

If psychiatrists are committed to doing good and avoiding harm, how can they participate in legal proceedings from which harm may result? If, on the other hand, psychiatrists in court abandon medicine's traditional ethical principles, how do they justify that deviation? And if the obligations to do good and avoid harm no longer govern psychiatrists in the legal setting, what alternative principles come into play? ... Are psychiatrists in general bound by the principles of beneficence and nonmaleficence?[24]

This general problem extends beyond forensic ethics to subtle regions of therapeutic ethics—for example, when assessments of competence are made and involuntary commitment is advocated.[25] In each case, harms are balanced against benefits, which takes us to the subject of beneficence and its massive role in psychiatry.

Beneficence

A no less core value in medicine is that the welfare of patients is the goal of health care. Medicine's context and justification are found in clinical diagnoses and therapies aimed at the promotion of health by cure or prevention of disease. General obligations in the moral life as well as specific duties in professional ethics requiring positive assistance may be clustered under the single heading of 'beneficence'. The principle of beneficence requires us to help others further their important and legitimate interests, often by preventing or removing possible harms.[26]

The basic roles and concepts that give substance to the principle of beneficence in medicine are as follows: The positive benefits the physician is obligated to seek all involve the alleviation of disease and injury. The harms to be prevented, removed, or minimized are the pain, suffering, and disability of injury and disease. The range of benefits a psychiatrist may help provide include helping patients find appropriate forms of financial assistance and helping them gain access to health care or research protocols. Sometimes the benefit is for the patient, at other times for society. Presumably such acts are required when the benefits are substantial and can be provided with minimal risk to the psychiatrist; one is not under an obligation of beneficence in all circumstances of risk.

An analysis of beneficence, broadly conceived, could lead to utilitarian demands of sacrifice and extreme generosity in the moral life, for example, giving a kidney for transplantation or donating bone marrow. The precise scope or range of acts required by the obligation of beneficence therefore needs to be limited, but drawing a precise line has proved to be difficult. Fortunately, we do not need a resolution in the present context. That we are morally obligated on some occasions to benefit others—at least in professional roles such as medicine and research—is not controversial.

Ordinary moral intuitions, as well as those of physicians, often suggest that certain duties not to cause harm to others are more compelling than duties to benefit them. However, this hierarchical ordering rule is not sanctioned by either morality or ethical theory. A harm inflicted may be negligible or trivial, whereas the harm to be prevented may be substantial: saving a person's life by a therapeutic intervention often outweighs the harms (as well as the disrespect for autonomy) caused by involuntary institutionalization. One of the motivations for separating non-maleficence from beneficence is that they themselves conflict when one must either avoid harm or bring aid—and cannot do both. If the weights of the two principles can vary, as they can, there can be no mechanical rule asserting that one obligation must always outweigh the other.

Those engaged in both medical practice and research know that risks of harm presented by interventions must be weighed against possible benefits for patients, subjects, and the public. The physician who professes to 'do no harm' is not pledging never to cause harm, but rather to strive to create a positive balance of goods over inflicted harms. This is recognized in the Nuremberg Code, which enjoins: 'The degree of risk to be taken should never exceed that determined by the humanitarian importance of the problem to be solved by the experiment'.

Justice

Every civilized society is a cooperative venture structured by moral, legal, and cultural principles that define the terms of social cooperation. Justice has been the most widely discussed subject. A person has been treated justly if treated according to what is fair, due, or owed. For example, if equal political rights are due all citizens, then justice is done when those rights are accorded. The term *distributive justice* refers to fair, equitable, and appropriate distribution in society, determined by justified norms of distribution that structure part of the terms of social cooperation. Usually this term refers to the distribution of primary social goods, such as economic goods and fundamental political rights. But burdens are also within its scope. Paying for forms of national health insurance is a distributed burden; Medicare checks and grants to do research are distributed benefits.[27]

There is no single principle of justice. Somewhat like principles under the heading of beneficence, there are several principles, each requiring specification in particular contexts. Philosophers have also developed diverse theories of justice that provide material principles and that defend the choice of principles. These theories attempt to be more specific than the formal principle by elaborating how people are to be compared and what it means to give people their due. Egalitarian theories of justice emphasize equal access to primary goods; libertarian theories emphasize rights to social and economic liberty; and utilitarian theories emphasize a mixed use of such criteria so that public and private utility are maximized. These three theories of justice all capture some of our intuitive convictions about justice, each with a different use of principles.

The role of managed care in psychiatric practice has raised many issues of distributive justice in recent years (see Chapter 18). For example, which forms of mental suffering create legitimate claims for coverage by health insurance, and what is the role of the notion of 'medical necessity' in making such determinations?[28] These are essentially questions of fairness, and the obligations of justice created by our answers to them often intersect with moral principles.

An example is found in the question, 'When is it legitimate to circumvent a system of insurance restrictions that a psychiatrist believes to be unfair?' A study by Dennis H. Novack and colleagues indicates that 68 per cent of polled physicians who perceived an insurance scheme to be unfair were willing to make false statements to third-party payers in order to secure payments for their patients. However, among this 68 per cent of responding physicians, 85 per cent insisted that their act would not involve 'deception'.[29] The study suggests that physicians feel strongly enough about injustices of current payment systems that they will make false statements to counterbalance an imbalance, and then will view what they have done as not a matter of deception or lying because the act is morally justified. The economics-driven context in which psychiatry is currently practiced poses many similar problems of justice.[30]

Problems of justice in conflict with other commitments and loyalties is not infrequent in psychiatry. Another example has been reported in adolescent consultation psychiatry when a consulting psychiatrist discovered a serious surgical failure that caused the death of a troubled 16-year-old youth. The consulting psychiatrist had information that the family did not have and would not be given, although the information was in the chart. Here denial of information seemed more than a failure to acknowledge the parents' right to the information; it seemed an injustice because they would be denied the opportunity to pursue reparation. The psychiatrist therefore disclosed the surgical complication to the youth's mother.[31]

The nature and function of moral principles

The prima facie character of principles, rules, and rights

W. D. Ross developed a theory intended to assist us in resolving problems of conflict between principles. His views are based on an account of what he calls prima facie duties, which he contrasts with actual duties. A prima facie duty is a duty that is always to be acted upon unless it conflicts on a particular occasion with an equal or stronger duty. A prima facie duty is always right and binding, all other things being equal; it is conditional on not being overridden or outweighed by competing moral demands. One's *actual* duty, by contrast, is determined by an examination of the respective weights of competing prima facie duties in particular situations.

Imagine that a psychiatrist has confidential information about a patient who is also an employee in the hospital where the psychiatrist practices. The employee is seeking advancement in a stress-filled position, but the psychiatrist has good reason to believe this advancement would be devastating for both the employee and the hospital. The psychiatrist has duties of confidentiality, non-maleficence, and beneficence in these circumstances: should the psychiatrist break confidence? Could the matter be handled by making this disclosure only to the hospital administrator and not to the personnel office? Can such disclosures be made consistent with one's general commitments to confidentiality? Addressing these questions through a process of moral justification is required to establish one's actual duty in the face of these conflicts of prima facie duties.

One Professor of Psychiatry, Howard D. Kibsi, has asserted that there is only one exception to the duty of confidentiality: 'when the clinician is directed by a court of law to disclose information'.[32] Because confidentiality is a prima facie duty, this thesis is both too broad and too narrow.[33] It is too broad, because being directed by a court of law may not be a justification for psychiatrists to disclose confidential information, just as it is not for journalists or members of the clergy. The thesis is too narrow, because there are many circumstances under which the duty of confidentiality may be overridden by compelling circumstances, such as coercion of the psychiatrist by the patient or awareness of a massive public danger presented by the patient. The idea that we can list the exceptions to moral rules—one or more, general or professional —is almost always an unrealistic hope.

Although no philosopher or professional code has successfully presented a system of moral rules that is free of conflicts and exceptions, this fact is not cause for either skepticism or alarm. Prima facie duties reflect the complexity of the moral life, in which a hierarchy of rules and principles is impossible. The problem of how to weight different moral principles remains unresolved, as does the best set of moral principles to form the framework of biomedical ethics. None the less, the four general categories of prima facie principles discussed in the previous section have proven serviceable as a basic starting point and source for reflection on cases and problems. The main difficulty with these principles and with prima facie duties, as we will now see, is that in many contexts they must be specified.

Specification and moral reform

Practical moral problems often cannot, as we noticed earlier, be resolved by appeal to such general principles. These practical problems typically require that we make our general norms suitably specific.[34] To be practical, moral principles must be made specific for a context and must make room for considerations of feasibility and institutional policies. Even specific norms are often too indeterminate and need further specification.[35] A simple example of specification of commitments to obtain consent is found in the following provision in the *Ethical guidelines for the practice of forensic psychiatry* of the American Academy of Psychiatry and the Law: 'The informed consent of the subject of a forensic evaluation is obtained when possible. Where consent is not required, notice is given to the evaluee of the nature of the evaluation. If the evaluee is not competent to give consent, substituted consent is obtained in accordance with the laws of the jurisdiction.'[36]

Another problem in biomedical ethics has been handled by the following specification, which is often found in the literature of medical ethics: 'Research investigators must put the welfare of subjects ahead of scientific knowledge gained from studies'. This has the ring of a good specification (of commitments to subject welfare and to the obligation to perform good research), and also appears to be a good hierarchical rule. However, we should be prepared to find that some forms of research—for example, some forms of non-therapeutic research with volunteers—do not and cannot put the welfare of subjects ahead of the goal of scientific knowledge, because there is significant risk involved and no immediate prospect of benefit for the subjects. One must then specify further that obtaining good study results from research can be justified by an adequate informed consent from competent volunteers, even though there is risk and no immediate prospect of benefit.[37]

Such progressive specification is central to biomedical ethics, especially in the formulation of institutional and public policy. A typical example of a problem most psychiatrists have or will face arises from our earlier discussion of autonomy. It would be morally wrong to override refusals of treatment in the case of many psychiatric patients, but it seems legitimate to override refusals by those who are marginally competent, temporarily confused, and the like when a significant medical benefit is at stake. It would be too wooden a doctrine to say that a refusal must always be accepted, but it would be arbitrary to accept some refusals and not accept others without reasonable criteria that allow one to differentiate the circumstances in which refusals may be overridden. To determine the conditions under which a patient's autonomy can and should be enhanced by providing further information and the conditions under which information should be withheld from other patients is to engage in specification, because the precise nature and limits of commitments to principles of respect for autonomy and beneficence are made more specific. Proposed specifications can, of course, be tested in practice and can and should be discussed with other professionals who face a similar range of patients and circumstances.

We cannot reasonably expect that strategies of specification will function as a cure-all for our deepest problems of moral conflict. Specification will not always eliminate competing proposals for the resolution of contingent conflicts. In problematic cases, several specifications will emerge that are well-defended proposals for resolution. None the less, specification, together with a moral justification that defends one's chosen specification, is essential for professional ethics; and when a specification is developed from a solid base of information and clinical experience, it stands a good chance of handling a range of cases in a justifiable manner.

Professional morality

Medical paternalism

The principles of respect for autonomy and beneficence sometimes conflict, giving rise to the problem of paternalism. The word 'paternalism' refers to treating individuals in the way that a parent treats his or her child. In biomedical ethics the word is more narrowly used to apply to treatment that restricts individual autonomy: paternalism is the intentional limitation of the autonomy of one person by another, where the person who limits autonomy appeals exclusively to grounds of benefit for the person whose autonomy is limited. The essence of paternalism is an overriding of a person's autonomy on grounds of providing them with a benefit—in medicine, a medical benefit. In psychiatry, the obligations of beneficence that would warrant paternalism are typically professional obligations of care.

Examples of paternalism in medicine include involuntary commitment to institutions for treatment, intervention to stop 'rational' suicides, resuscitating patients who have asked not to be resuscitated, withholding medical information that patients have requested, compulsory psychiatric care, and denial of an innovative therapy to patients who wish to try it.[38] Such paternalism has been under attack in recent years, especially by defenders of the autonomy rights of patients. The latter hold that physicians intervene too often and assume too much paternalistic control over patients' choices.

Philosophers and lawyers have generally supported the view that the autonomy of patients is the decisive factor in the patient–physician relationship and that interventions can be valid only when patients are in some measure unable to make voluntary choices or to perform autonomous actions. The point is that patients can be so ill that their judgments or voluntary abilities are significantly affected, or because they are incapable of grasping important information about their case, thus being in no position to reach carefully reasoned decisions about their medical treatment or their purchase of drugs. Beyond this form of intervention, many have argued, paternalism is not warranted.

However, paternalism also has defenders, even under some conditions in which autonomous choice is overridden. Any careful proponent of a principle of paternalism will specify precisely which goods and needs deserve paternalistic protection and the conditions under which intervention is warranted. Some have argued that one is justified in interfering with a person's autonomy only if the interference protects the person against his or her own actions where those actions are extremely and unreasonably risky (for example, refusing a life-saving therapy in non-terminal situations) or are potentially dangerous and irreversible in effect (as some drugs are). According to this position, paternalism is justified if, and only if, the harms prevented from occurring to the person are greater than the harms or indignities (if any) caused by interference with his or her liberty and if it can be universally justified, under relevantly similar circumstances, always to treat persons in this way.

Psychiatrists frequently exhibit paternalistic beliefs or advance arguments that appear to accept the appropriateness of various forms of paternalism. An example is the widespread tendency of psychiatrists to commit persons dangerous to themselves even in the complete absence of psychotic symptoms.[39] Another example is found in the conflict between social activists who defend the liberty rights of homeless persons and psychiatrists who believe that many of the homeless should be protected against harms that they might do to themselves or should be provided benefits they would not attempt to secure for themselves, even if involuntary civil commitment is required.

One major source of the difference between supporters and opponents of paternalism rests on the emphasis each places on capabilities for autonomous action by patients making 'choices'. Supporters of paternalism tend to cite examples of persons of diminished or compromised capacity, for example chronic alcoholic and clinically depressed, suicidal patients. Opponents of paternalism focus on persons who are capable of autonomous choice but have been socially restricted in exercising their capacities. Examples include those involuntarily committed to institutions largely because of eccentric behavior and those who might rationally elect to refuse treatment in life-threatening circumstances. One critical element of this controversy thus concerns the quality of understanding, of voluntariness, and also of consent or refusal by the persons whose autonomy might be restricted by such policies.

There can be little serious doubt that some forms of paternalism are unjustifiable interventions, but it is an open question whether minor forms of withholding information and manipulation to treatment are justified in light of massively important goals, such as life-saving therapies and prevention of suicide. The nuances of each case will involve a balancing of different factors, and it will serve moral reflection not to assume from the outset that paternalism in general is either justified or unjustified. Such polar thinking can do more harm to patients and professionals alike than more deliberate approaches in which we reason through the case.

Ethics in professional life

Just as there is a general common morality that is accepted by all morally serious persons, so most professions contain, at least implicitly, a professional morality with standards of behavior that are widely accepted by those in the profession. The recent interest in sexual activity between psychotherapists and patients, for example, arose in a context in which moral views were already widely present in the profession. In professional contexts many moral guidelines are transmitted informally, but formal instruction and attempts at the codification of professional morality have increased in recent years. Psychiatrists now widely acknowledge, for example, the need to conform to the American Psychiatric Association's *Principles of medical ethics*,[40] as well as more specialized guides such as the American Academy of Psychiatry and the Law's *Ethical guidelines*.[41]

Such codes are sometimes defended by appeal to general principles or other norms in the common morality. Usually, however, professional codes are attempts to explicate the inchoate morality already widely accepted in the profession. This morality includes responsibilities to patients and research subjects (such as informed consent, privacy, and confidentiality), and responsibilities to society (such as avoiding conflicts of interest and meeting legal obligations), responsibilities to colleagues, employers, and funding sources (such as reporting unacceptable behavior and conditions in the profession).

The internal morality accepted by psychiatrists and various attempts to improve it will be discussed elsewhere in this volume. Here only one precaution deserves special notice: legal obligations and the guidelines of professional associations are often accepted as the primary moral authorities, and many members of professions believe that these laws and guidelines establish what ethically should be done. A problem with this way of framing standards of professional conduct comes in its bottom line: conduct acceptable under laws and codes is judged acceptable in general. Ignored is that the conduct may be inappropriate by standards of morality that are independent of the law, such as the standards of the common morality and ethical theory that have been discussed throughout this chapter.

Although case law, statutory law, and professional associations have established influential guidelines for reflection on both legal and moral obligations, moral standards must be distinguished from legal and peer standards. The law and often professional associations primarily specify permissible conduct (what one has a right to do), whereas morality specifies obligatory and ideal conduct (what it is right to do and what it is best to do). Moreover, issues of legal liability and practicability within the litigation process demand that legal and professional requirements be very different from moral requirements and often less rigorous in their moral demands.

Despite an important intersection between morals and law, the law is not the repository of our moral standards and values, even when the law is concerned with areas of moral conduct such as medical ethics. The law also rarely specifies forms of conduct directly applicable to professions such as psychiatry. The law rightly backs away from attempting to legislate against everything that is morally wrong and rarely addresses questions such as appropriate peer censure.

Medicine and law also have starkly different orientations. The law is concerned about the occurrence of harm and negligence, deprivation of liberty, liability, deterrence, and the like. Medicine is concerned with avoiding harms and providing benefits to individuals and society. These different orientations create situations in which many conflicts emerge between law and medical practice. Physician-assisted suicide is one current and controversial example. Such assistance is generally prohibited in law and in medical codes. But even if this form of assistance is prohibited by these guidelines, it does not follow from a moral point of view that one should necessarily obey the law or one's professional peers. If there is moral justification for helping some patients, then their physicians do nothing morally wrong in acting to help them.

This perspective leaves room for justified moral non-conformity to state laws and evasive non-compliance with prohibitions recommended by professional associations.[42] Carefully considered acts of non-compliance and moral non-conformity in helping patients can be morally defensible, despite the prima facie obligation to obey the law and professional codes. Physicians often feel bound by the law and by the ethical code of their profession. True, they are bound, but only by prima facie duties.[43] To accept this position is not to accept a radical account of moral obligation. It is simply to acknowledge that morality has its own standards, and that in a conflict with law or professional guidelines, morality may rightly prevail.

References and Notes

1. See, for example, Ronald Dworkin: *Taking rights seriously*. Cambridge, MA, Harvard University Press, 1977; Judith Jarvis Thomson: *The realm of rights*, Cambridge, MA, Harvard University Press, 1990; Ruth Macklin: *Universality of the Nuremberg Code*, in *The Nazi Doctors and the Nuremberg Code*,

ed. George J. Annas and Michael Grodin, New York, Oxford University Press, 1992, pp. 240–57.

2. For utility-centered theory, see John Stuart Mill: *Utilitarianism*, in *Collected works of John Stuart Mill*, vol. 10, ed. John M. Robson. Toronto, University of Toronto Press, 1969; Peter Singer: *Practical ethics*, 2nd edn, Cambridge University Press, 1993; Richard B. Brandt: *Morality, utilitarianism, and rights*. Cambridge University Press, 1992; Shelly Kagan: *The limits of morality*. Oxford, Clarendon Press, 1989; R. G. Frey, ed.: *Utility and rights*, Minneapolis, University of Minnesota Press, 1984; James Griffin: *Well-being: its meaning, measurement, and importance*. Oxford, Clarendon Press, 1986; Samuel Scheffler, ed.: *Consequentialism and its critics*. Oxford University Press, 1988.

3. Immanuel Kant: *Foundations of the metaphysics of morals*, trans. Lewis White Beck. Indianapolis, IN, Bobbs-Merrill, 1959, pp. 37–42.

4. Ibid., p. 47.

5. See esp. Aristotle: *Nicomachean ethics*, trans. T. Irwin. Indianapolis, Hackett, 1985.

6. Albert R. Jonsen: Casuistry as methodology in clinical ethics. *Theoretical Medicine* **12** (December 1991); Jonsen and S. Toulmin: *Abuse of casuistry*. Berkeley, University of California Press, 1988.

7. John D. Arras: Principles and particularity: the role of cases in bioethics. *Indiana Law Journal* **69**:983–1014 (Fall 1994) (with two replies); and Getting down to cases: the revival of casuistry in bioethics. *Journal of Medicine and Philosophy* **16**:29–51, 1991.

8. See, for example, James C. Beck, ed: *Confidentiality versus the duty to protect: foreseeable harm in the practice of psychiatry*. Washington, American Psychiatric Press, 1990, esp. Chapters 7 and 9; A. A. Stone: The *Tarasoff* decision: suing psychiatrists to safeguard society. *Harvard Law Review* **90**:358–78, 1976; Loren H. Roth and Alan Meisel: Dangerousness, confidentiality, and the duty to warn. *American Journal of Psychiatry* **134**:508–11, 1977; Jaime Paredes, Dale Beyerstein, Barry Ledwidge, and Claudio Kogan: Psychiatric ethics and ethical psychiatry. *Canadian Journal of Psychiatry* **35**:600–3; Loretta Kopelman: Moral problems in psychiatry, in *Medical Ethics*, 2nd edn, ed. Robert M. Veatch. Boston, Jones and Bartlett, 1997, pp. 290–3; Martin L. Smith and Kevin P. Martin: Confidentiality in the age of AIDS: a case study in clinical ethics. *Journal of Clinical Ethics* **4**:236–41, 1993, esp. 238f; James C. Beck: Violent patients and the *Tarasoff* duty in private psychiatric practice. *Journal of Psychiatry and Law* **13**:361–76, 1985; David L. Goldman and Therese Jacob: Anatomy of a second generation Tarasoff case. *Canadian Journal of Psychiatry* **36**:35–8, 1991.

9. See the arguments to this effect in Athena Beldecos and Robert M. Arnold: Gathering information and casuistic analysis. *Journal of Clinical Ethics* **4**:241–45, 1993; Roderick W. Pettis and Thomas G. Gutheil: Misapplication of the Tarasoff duty to driving cases: a call for a reframing of theory, *Bulletin of the American Academy of Psychiatry and the Law* **21**:263–75, 1993.

10. Jonsen and Toulmin: *Abuse of casuistry*. Berkeley, University of California Press, 1998, pp. 16–19, 66–7; Jonsen: Casuistry and clinical ethics. *Theoretical medicine*, pp. 67, 71.

11. See Baruch Brody: *Life and death decision making*. New York, Oxford University Press, 1988, p. 13.

12. Some reservations about them have been expressed in the alternative accounts discussed in the previous section, as well as in some literature in biomedical ethics. For reservations: see *Principles of health care ethics*, ed. Raanan Gillon and Ann

Lloyd. London, John Wiley, 1994; Stephen Toulmin: The tyranny of principles. *Hastings Center Report* **11**, 1981; K. Danner Clouser and Bernard Gert: A critique of principlism, *Journal of Medicine and Philosophy* **15**:219–36, April 1990; K. Danner Clouser: Common morality as an alternative to principlism, *Kennedy Institute of Ethics Journal* **5**, 1995.

13. *Principles of biomedical ethics*, 4th edn, Chapters 3–6. New York, Oxford University Press, 1994.

14. For a good example of a code with abstract principles that make only minimal commitments, see: Ethical guidelines for the practice of forensic psychiatry. *American Academy of Psychiatry and the Law* as revised October, 1991, pp. 1–5.

15. For autonomy-based theory, see Robert Nozick: *Anarchy, state, and utopia*. New York, Basic Books, 1974; H. Tristram Engelhardt, Jr.: *The foundations of bioethics*, 2nd edn. New York, Oxford University Press, 1996; Joel Feinberg: *The moral limits of the criminal law*. New York, Oxford University Press, 1984–87; Jay Katz: *The silent world of doctor and patient*. New York, Free Press, 1984; James F. Childress: The place of autonomy in bioethics. *Hastings Center Report* **20**:12–16, January/February 1990.

16. See Ruth R. Faden and Tom L. Beauchamp: *A history and theory of informed consent*. New York, Oxford, 1986.

17. See the interesting example of this problem in Mircea Sigal: Involuntary hospitalization—medical or judicial authority. *Israel Journal of Psychiatry and Related Sciences* **31**:254–60, 1994.

18. See Albert R. Jonsen: Do no harm: axiom of medical ethics, in *Philosophical and medical ethics: its nature and significance*, ed. Stuart F. Spicker and H. Tristram Engelhardt, Jr. Dordrecht, D. Reidel, 1977, pp. 27–41.

19. Thomas Percival: *Medical ethics; or a code of institutes and precepts, adapted to the professional conduct of physicians and surgeons*. Manchester, S. Russell, 1803, pp. 165–6. Percival's work was the pattern for the American Medical Association's (AMA) first code of ethics in 1847.

20. See Bernard Gert: *Morality*. New York, Oxford, 1988, esp. p. 6; and Charles Culver and Bernard Gert: *Philosophy in medicine: conceptual and ethical issues in medicine and psychiatry*. New York, Oxford, 1982.

21. See, for example, Nancy Davis: The priority of avoiding harm, in *Killing and letting die*, ed. Bonnie Steinbock. Englewood Cliffs, NJ, Prentice-Hall, 1980, pp. 172–214; Paul Ramsey and Richard A. McCormick, S. J., ed.: *Doing evil to achieve good: moral choice in conflict situations*. Chicago, Loyola University Press, 1978; Willard Gaylin, Leon Kass, Edmund Pellegrino, and Mark Siegler: Doctors must not kill. *Journal of the American Medical Association* **259**:2139–40, 1988.

22. See, for example, Sidney Bloch and Peter Reddaway: *Soviet psychiatric abuse: the shadow over world psychiatry*. Boulder, Colo., Westview Press, 1984, esp. Ch. 1.

23. For the legal implications of these failures see Robert M. Wettstein: Legal and ethical issues, in *Handbook of aggressive and destructive behavior in psychiatric patients*, ed. Michel Hersen, Robert T. Ammerman, and Lori A. Sisson. New York, Plenum Press, 1994, pp. 113–28.

24. Paul S. Appelbaum: The parable of the forensic psychiatrist: ethics and the problem of doing harm. *International Journal of Law and Psychiatry* **13**:249–59, 1990, esp. 250–1.

25. See the similar and broad range of questions discussed in Ruth Macklin: A perspective on ethics in forensic psychiatry, in *Critical issues in American psychiatry and the law*, vol. 2, ed. Richard Rosner, New York, Plenum Press, 1985, 19–39.

26. For a strong statement of the importance of beneficence for biomedical ethics, see Edmund Pellegrino and David Thomasma: *For the patient's good: The restoration of beneficence in health care.* New York, Oxford University Press, 1988.

27. For accounts of justice that have deeply influenced contemporary biomedical ethics, see John Rawls: *A theory of justice.* Cambridge, Harvard University Press; Norman Daniels: *Just health care.* New York, Cambridge University Press, 1985; Allen Buchanan: Health-care delivery and resource allocation, in *Medical ethics*, 2nd edn, ed. Robert Veatch. Boston, Jones and Bartlett, 1997; Daniel Callahan: *Setting limits: medical goals in an aging society.* New York, Simon & Schuster, 1987.

28. See James E. Sabin and Norman Daniels: Determining 'medical necessity' in mental health practice. *Hastings Center Report* **24**, 5–13, 1994.

29. Dennis H. Novack, *et al.*: Physicians' attitudes toward using deception to resolve difficult ethical problems. *Journal of the American Medical Association* **261**:2980–5, 1989. See also Norman Daniels: Why saying no to patients in the United States is so hard: cost containment, justice, and provider autonomy. *New England Journal of Medicine* **314**:1380–3, 1986.

30. See E. Haavi Morreim: The new economics of medicine: special challenges for psychiatry. *Journal of Medicine and Philosophy* **15**:97–119, 1990.

31. Jonathan Bloomber, Janet Wozniak, Norman Fost, Donald N. Medearis, and David B. Herzog: Ethical dilemmas in child and adolescent consultation psychiatry. *Journal of the American Academy of Child and Adolescent Psychiatry* **31**:557–61, 1992.

32. Howard D. Kibsi [Letter]: Sexton's psychiatrist violated ethics. *New York Times* August 9, 1991, p. A26.

33. On the complicated balancing involved in judgments of confidentiality, see Loretta M. Kopelman: Moral problems in psychiatry, op. cit.; James C. Beck: When the patient threatens violence: an empirical study of clinical practice after Tarasoff. *Bulletin of the American Academy of Psychiatry and the Law* **10**:189–201, 1982; Martin L. Smith and Kevin P. Martin: Confidentiality in the age of AIDS: a case study in clinical ethics. *Journal of Clinical Ethics* **4**:236–41, 1993; Edgar L. Lipton: The analyst's use of clinical data, and other issues of confidentiality. *Journal of the American Psychoanalytic Association* **39**:967–85, 1991; James C. Beck, ed., *Confidentiality versus the duty to protect: foreseeable harm in the practice of psychiatry*, op. cit.; Robert L. Goldstein: When doctors divulge: is there a 'threat from within' to psychiatric confidentiality? *Journal of Forensic Sciences* **34**:433–8, 1989; Martha A. Carpenter: The process of ethical decision making in psychiatric nursing practice. *Issues in Mental Health Nursing* **12**:179–91, 1991.

34. Henry S. Richardson: Specifying norms as a way to resolve concrete ethical problems. *Philosophy and Public Affairs* **19**:279–310, 1990.

35. Some useful reflections on the limits in psychiatry of the four principles mentioned previously, and the need for their specification, is found in K. W. M. Fulford and Tony Hope: Psychiatric ethics: a bioethical ugly duckling, in *Principles of health care ethics*, ed. Raanan Gillon and Ann Lloyd, op. cit.: 681–95.

36. As revised October, 1991, p. 2.

37. Many of the problems of psychiatric research that would have to be explored in any well-specified research ethics are explored in Timothy Howell and Robert L. Sack: The ethics of human experimentation in psychiatry: toward a more informed consensus. *Psychiatry* **44**:113–32, 1981.

38. For analyses of various problems of paternalism in psychiatry, see L. Kjellin and T. Nilstun: Medical and social paternalism: regulation of and attitudes towards

compulsory psychiatric care. *Acta Psychiatrica Scandinavica* **88**:415–19, 1993; Ernle W. D. Young, James C. Corby, and Rodney Johnson: Does depression invalidate competence?: consultants' ethical, psychiatric, and legal considerations. *Cambridge Quarterly of Healthcare Ethics* **2**:505–15, 1993; Maurice Lipsedge: Choices in psychiatry, in *Doctors' decisions: ethical conflicts in medical practice*, ed. G. R. Dunstan and Elliot A. Shinebourne, New York, Oxford University Press, 1989, 145–53; Harold I. Schwartz, and Loren H. Roth: Informed consent and competency in psychiatric practice, in *Review of Psychiatry*, vol. 8, Washington DC, American Psychiatric Press, 1989, 409–31; H. Tristram Engelhardt, Jr. and Laurence B. McCullough: Ethics in psychiatry, in *American handbook of psychiatry*, 2nd edn, vol. 7, ed. S. Arieti and H. K. H. Brodie, New York, Basic Books, 1981, 795–818.

39. See the documentation in the study by R. Michael Bagby, Judith S. Thompson, Susan E. Dickens, and Michiko Nohara: Decision making in psychiatric civil commitment: an experimental analysis. *American Journal of Psychiatry* **148**:28–33, 1991.

40. *Principles of medical ethics with annotations especially applicable to psychiatry*, Washington DC, American Psychiatric Association, 1995.

41. Ethical guidelines for the practice of forensic psychiatry, op. cit., pp. 1–5.

42. See James F. Childress: Civil disobedience, conscientious objection, and evasive noncompliance: a framework for the analysis and assessment of illegal actions in health care. *Journal of Medicine and Philosophy* **10**:63–83, 1985.

43. See the discussion of this problem in psychiatry in Robert G. Weinstock, Gregory G. Leongt, and J. Arturo Silva: Opinions by AAPL forensic psychiatrists on controversial ethical guidelines: a survey. *Bulletin of the American Academy of Psychiaty and the Law* **19**:237–48, 1991.

4

Misuse and abuse of psychiatry: an overview

Paul Chodoff

This chapter will be devoted to an account of how the misuse and abuse of psychiatry give rise to ethical problems. In it I shall allude to and adumbrate a number of the issues to be treated more fully in later chapters. I shall also take advantage of my half century as a psychiatric practitioner to venture some observations on how things have changed during that period.[1]

Psychiatrists today are increasingly aware that they practice within a fairly well-defined ethical framework, and that derelictions will lead to unpleasant consequences, sometimes severe. But this degree of interest in and concern about ethical matters was not evident when I began my career in the post-World War II era. At that time there was very little discussion about ethical standards and transgressions among colleagues, and, in contrast to the plethora we see today, few articles and no books on psychiatric ethics. Indeed, this lack was a motivating force behind the production of the 1st edition of *Psychiatric ethics* in 1981.

What are the reasons for such a marked shift in what might be called the moral climate within which psychiatrists now work? I do not believe that my current colleagues are finer persons or more virtuous than those of the past. Rather they have become more conscious of what they should or should not do, and what will happen to them if they err. One factor in the change has been the pronounced shift away from the previously prevailing paternalistic model ('father knows best—you should do what he tells you and not complain') of the doctor–patient relationship.[2] A different model now prevails (at least theoretically), one in which the patient has moved away from being a subject of paternalism, towards what might be called a contractual relationship with the doctor, who will be held accountable for incompetent or unacceptable behavior. This means that, like anyone else engaging in activities sanctioned by society and which involve a certain degree of power, psychiatrists must be able to provide responsible answers to questions about the scope, legitimacy, and effectiveness of what they do, and provide machinery to redress errors or wrongs.

As I have increasingly become aware of the need to be accountable to society and to the patient, so have I, along with my colleagues, had to keep in mind that the patient I am dealing with is an autonomous agent who must be informed about what is going on between us and give assent or refusal. This state of affairs marks a considerable change from the somewhat apocalyptic view of Jonas Robitscher in 1980[3]—that the psychiatrist operates in relative immunity from the necessity to account for himself. It should be pointed out, however, that there seems to be something of a backlash against what might be called the tyranny of autonomy, which has itself led to some questionable consequences.[4]

Another factor accounting for current greater ethical vigilance is the dethronement of science from its former position of unquestioned authority, especially at a time when the whole concept of authority is under scrutiny. Add the extreme litigiousness currently so characteristic of at least American society, and there is little wonder that psychiatry is now practiced in an atmosphere in which dissatisfied patients are likely to take legal action or refer to ethics committees psychiatrists' behavior which previously might have been passed over.

Also playing a role is the vast change in the economic underpinning of psychiatric practice as signaled by third-party payment and managed care.[5] Only someone who has been in practice for as long as I have, starting at a time when the financial transaction between the patient and myself consisted of a simple two-party process of billing and direct payment, can appreciate the magnitude of the changes. These have contributed to the current perception of the doctor, including the psychiatrist, as more of a business person than a caring professional worthy of respect and forebearance.

Finally, at least for American psychiatrists and whether as cause or effect, the *Principles of medical ethics with annotations especially applicable to psychiatry*, which first appeared in 1973,[6] and have been frequently revised since, now play a significant role in focusing attention on the ethical dimensions of professional behavior.

Misuse (improper use that may have a bad effect) and abuse (perverse use with implications of maltreatment) are inevitable perils for all institutions involving fallible humans. Given the rainbow of motivations that influence human behavior, given the unpredictable influence of chance and circumstance on events, it could not be otherwise. This generalization certainly applies to psychiatry, a complicated enterprise only partially monitored by the canons of science and operated by men and women of vastly differing backgrounds. It is also pertinent that, to a greater extent than the rest of medicine, psychiatry operates in an interface between responsibilities to the patient and/or obligations to the society or to the government, and this further complicates the position of the psychiatrist when faced with ethical decisions.

Psychiatrist power

It will be the thesis of this chapter that the principal engine behind the misuse and abuse of psychiatry is the significant amount of power the psychiatrist wields. This is manifest in two overlapping ways: directly in the doctor–patient treatment relationship, and as a possible hazard of the psychiatrist's role as intermediary between persons who are putatively mentally disordered and governmental and non-governmental institutions with an interest in their dispositions. Psychiatric power is itself ethically neutral: it may be employed for the benefit of patients and the public but it can also be harmful. This potentially ambiguous role of psychiatric power transcends national and ideological boundaries. Thus, the widely quoted statement of Jonas Robitscher in 1980 that the psychiatrist is 'one of the most important non-governmental decision makers in modern life'[3] can be balanced by the assertion of Professor M. Kabanov, Director of the Bechterev Institute in Leningrad, in 1988, that 'in no sphere of health care do medics possess such rights as in psychiatry'.[7]

What are the sources of this power? First, psychiatrists are physicians, and, as such, are the custodians of the keys of life and death for their patients, a heritage to which is attached the ancient identification of physician as priest. As acceptance of religion has attenuated, its place has been taken to some extent by science: the priest's position has become combined with that of the scientist, but in both roles doctors are the objects of the dependent yearnings of frightened people who willingly attribute to their physicians an omnipotence that will spare them pain, even save their lives. But when psychiatrists operate primarily in the psychotherapeutic rather than the psychopharmacological domain, they dispose of additional power in a relationship which is very likely to involve intimate matters, often secret and painful. The asymmetrical nature of this intimacy augments, sometimes to an intense degree, the transference elements regularly present between physicians and patients. These transference misreadings tend to increase the patient's dependence on the powerful psychiatrist. This power is present whether or not the psychiatrist wishes to avoid exercising it. It will have its effects, either beneficial or harmful.

The cardinal ethical principle here is that abuse of psychiatry occurs whenever psychiatrists exploit the clinical relationship for their own purposes. These may be for sexual gratification, for the satisfaction of certain pathological needs, or for financial gain.

Direct doctor–patient relationship

Sexual exploitation

Sexual acting out usually, but not always, between a male psychiatrist and female patient has been catapulted into distressing and unwelcome prominence in recent years both within the profession and in the eyes of the public. The subject will be dealt with fully in Chapter 8 by Glen Gabbard. In my recollection, ethical derelictions of this kind were not taken so seriously in the heady post-World War II days when psychoanalysis was in a position of almost regal ascendency. Although not condoned, such behavior was not likely to result in serious difficulties for the therapist—more an occasion for scandalized gossip than for sanctions. A case in point is Freud's tolerant attitude about the sexual relations between Jung and his former patient, Sabrina Spielrein. Another example is the Anne Sexton case[8] in which the sexual involvement of one of her therapists with the poet resulted in no official action or condemnation. Ironically illustrative of how things have changed, an earlier therapist, who had been therapeutically helpful to Ms Sexton, had to combat charges after her death that he had violated the principles of confidentiality in his relationship with her.

It is worth noting that a more stringent attitude about sexual offenses of this kind has been contributed to greatly by the rise of the women's movement with its demands for equality and autonomy. However, the pendulum seldom swings in one direction without going too far, and I believe that a possible overreacton can be seen in the 1995 position of the American Psychiatric Association Ethics Committee that any post-treatment sexual encounter between a therapist and former patient is always unethical.[9] The case can be made that this ruling counters the principle of respect for autonomy, by implying that the patient, usually a woman, is always in the thrall of a dominant male therapist and incapable of making an independent decision. The whole subject of boundary violations[10] in the form of non-sexual physical contact between therapist and patient presumably for the purpose of comfort or solace, partakes of the same ambivalence (see Chapter 8). On the one hand is the need to avoid the slippery slope and, on the other, the possibility that therapeutically beneficial spontaneity may be inhibited.

Psychopathological exploitation

The use of therapist power to procure gratification of psychopathological needs can be responsible for more subtle ethical derelictions than those in the sexual sphere.[11] These may not rise to the level necessary to be brought to the attention of an ethics committee, but they violate the dictum of the American psychiatrist, Jeremy Lazarus: 'The doctor is obligated to do what is in the patient's best interest and not what is in the doctor's best interest.'[12] Exploitation can take various forms. Is the choice between drug treatment and psychotherapy always motivated by considerations of the patient's best interest or may it be influenced by the psychiatrist's interests and skills? The same question may arise when one mode of psychotherapy is chosen over another. An attempt to extract every last detail of a sexual encounter may have as its primary purpose voyeuristic, sadistic satisfaction for the therapist. Although, undoubtedly, patient identification with the values and behavior of therapists can be beneficial, exploitation rather than benefit will be the outcome if therapists fool themselves and misuse their power to impose their own possibly inappropriate set of values. Separating such value impositions from useful therapeutic strategy can be difficult, particularly in what has been called 'the ethical minefield of marital and family therapy.'[13]

'False memory' controversy

The above question, whether therapists are imposing false values and beliefs on patients is at the center of what has become a firestorm of conflict, involving not only the world, of psychotherapy (see Chapter 11) and psychiatry, but also the legal profession and the public. Here I refer to the false memory vs recovered memory dispute. On the one side are those who hold that a variety of adult psychopathological states including, but not restricted to, multiple personality disorder, have their ultimate origin in episodes of childhood sexual abuse which have been repressed, and, on the other, those who question these claims and believe that they are largely iatrogenic artifacts. The conflict has been fierce and unrelenting, leaving little room for compromise. As a consequence of these allegations, fathers of purported victims and workers in child-care institutions, have been accused, prosecuted, and sometimes jailed. Many of the charges have been based on information emerging from therapeutic encounters in which suggestion and hypnosis may have played a considerable role. Some of these sentences have been overturned by Appeals' courts, and there have even been instances in which damages have been awarded against therapists accused of responsibility for the charges. There is a real possibility that certain therapists have been so overcome by their zeal as to behave un-ethically in these instances. An interesting side-effect is the opportunity that this episode has afforded certain critics[14] to raise questions about such basic psychoanalytic doctrines as repression.

Although all the evidence is not yet in on this tangled matter, it can be stated that while therapists may be acting benevolently and in the best interests of patients and society when their efforts lead to the exposure of real instances of child abuse, the probability seems to be increasing that a significant number of these allegations are untrue or exaggerated. We may be dealing with what Richard Gardner has labeled 'sexual abuse hysteria'.[15]

Financial exploitation

Harm can be done when the doctor–patient relationship is compromised not only for sexual or psychopathological gratification but also through the lure of Mammon. The question of when the desire for financial security becomes a dominating rather than a reasonable component of therapeutic decisions is not easily determined. Choice of treatments is influenced not only by skills and interests, as mentioned previously, but also, certainly, by financial considerations. An ethical hazard arises when this is the main reason for a decision but is falsified or fudged. Here we have a troubling contrast between the therapist as healer and as business person, a danger pointed out by Edmund Pellegrino, speaking of the medical profession generally:

Today our profession faces the unenviable choice between two opposing moral orders, one based on the primacy of our ethical obligations to the sick, the other on a primacy of self interest in the market place. These two orders are not fundamentally reconcilable. Like it or not the profession will be forced to choose between them. (personal communication, 1995)

Effect of third-party payment

At this point, speaking from the perspective of someone who began practice when payment for services (as it was in Freud's day) was an entirely out-of-pocket, two-party fee for service transaction, one of the most momentous changes has been the gradual replacement of the two-party by a three-party system of payment.[16] The changes have been, of course, primarily economic, but certainly not without ethical implications. One incidental effect of the introduction of a third-party into many treatment decisions has been the significant curtailment and complication of the power that psychiatrists wielded when all transactions were between patients and themselves. Nowhere is this seen more clearly than in the direct and immediate danger posed to confidentiality by third-party involvement.[5] No longer can psychiatrists unquestionably promise confidentiality to patients, because, in order to secure reimbursement, certain diagnostic and sometimes other extensive information must be released to the insurance carrier. The resultant ethical dilemma entails discomfort and resentment among practitioners, and is a significant component of their negative attitude towards third-party payers. It needs to be said that although protecting the patient is paramount, this value may come into conflict with the value of accountability to the public. Also, considerations of self interest may not be entirely lacking if it is necessary to fudge diagnoses in order to establish medical necessity. Ethical issues with respect to confidentiality will be discussed in Chapter 7.

Managed care

The other sea change I have witnessed has been the various forms of limiting and monitoring treatment that have received the label of managed care, and which has so changed practice conditions as to render them almost unrecognizable from what they were in the 1950s. Like third-party payment, of which it is in a sense an extension, although the impact of managed care is primarily economic, it carries with it important and disturbing ethical implications. These will be fully dealt with in Chapter 19, but here I venture a few observations.

The restrictive effects of managed care are felt with particular severity by psychiatrists who are predominantly psychotherapists. They are outraged when arbitrary limitations and meddlesome interferences are imposed, and insist that ethically they must defend their patients' needs for adequate treatment. However, the intrusions of managed care, although unwelcome, do raise troublesome questions about some aspects of psychotherapy: the extent to which some patients fit within the medical model and thus can qualify for reimbursement by meeting the criterion of medical necessity, the scope and efficacy of psychotherapy, and the professional qualifications necessary to qualify as a competent practitioner. To buttress their claims that they oppose the restrictions of managed care in the interests of their patients and not of themselves, psychotherapists need to attend to these issues. Ethical aspects of psychotherapy is the subject of Chapter 11.

Divided loyalties

I turn now to ways other than the direct doctor–patient relationship through which psychiatric power can be corrupted into misuse and abuse. These occur when psychiatrists operate in a situation of divided loyalty, when their allegiance is split, on the one hand, between the patients under their care, as avowed in the Hippocratic Oath, and, on the other, certain institutions, either governmental or non-governmental, which employ psychiatrists or exert control over them.

Most modern societies have gradually, over the years, bestowed upon psychiatrists a significant role in important decisions based on the presence or absence of disordered mental functioning. These include decisions about whether: to hospitalize certain individuals against their will; to declare people accused of crimes to be competent to be tried and punished or to be freed of responsibility; to guide and monitor the punishment of criminals; to compel soldiers in time of war to continue combat or to exempt them; to require conformance to certain duties of citizenship, like being drafted for military service; and to allow or to refuse payment in connection with disability claims by presumably disabled workers.

All of these situations, many of which will be discussed in later chapters, attenuate the psychiatrist's primary responsibility to his patient and may put him in the uncomfortable position of being a double agent.[17] Parenthetically, this is even true in the therapeutic relationship where, under constraints like the *Tarasoff* decision, psychiatrists must acknowledge they can not promise absolute confidentiality.

In certain situations, psychiatrists may attempt to avoid the double-agent conflict by denying that services are rendered in the context of a doctor–patient relationship, and by claiming that they are acting only on behalf of their employers. The considerable debate about the ethical legitimacy of this position applies to psychiatrists who, in the United States, perform reviews for managed-care companies. It has generated so much acrimony that review psychiatrists have been the subject of complaints to an American Psychiatric Association (APA) District Branch ethics committee.

Another instance of the divided loyalties dilemma for psychiatrists in the United States derives from the statement in the APA *Principles of medical ethics* that: 'A psychiatrist should not be a participant in a legally authorized execution'. The interpretation of this principle has been the subject of a serious and even passionate disagreement about the responsibility of the psychiatrist in capital cases with regard to such issues as declaring the accused not fit to stand trial, or deciding to treat or not to treat a condemned criminal suffering a mental illness which disqualifies him for execution. These issues will be discussed in Chapter 16.

As indicated above, it is clear that the problem of divided loyalty occurs in many areas of practice, but the most serious instances occur when the psychiatrist is under an obligation to the state or government to make a decision about the disposition of a putative sufferer from mental disorder. Although the interests of patient and state may coincide, such an outcome is by no means inevitable. Every psychiatrist in this position must understand that a point can be reached when he must decide whether the patient's needs and rights can ethically be subordinated to the state's requirements. Beyond this point there is a danger that psychiatrists may be instrumental in allowing their profession to degenerate into a system of social control, even of oppression. The twentieth century has seen two horrendous instances of how psychiatric power can be perverted and corrupted by totalitarian states to inflict great damage and even death on innocent people. Although fortunately now of historical interest only, this volume would not be complete without at least brief accounts of these psychiatric nightmares (see the second edition of *Psychiatric ethics* for fuller accounts).

Soviet abuse of psychiatry

The misuse of psychiatry by converting various forms of dissent and unacceptable social behavior into spurious diagnoses of mental illness and then transfering them into the criminal justice or civil commitment systems began in the Soviet Union under the Stalin regime (although there were foreshadowings as far back as Tsarist times).[18] But it was not until Khrushchev came to power that this practice, scornfully described by one of the dissidents as 'the government using the fig leaf of psychiatry as a reliable coverup for the imprisonment of people with minds of their own'[19] reached a crescendo and continued at a high level for two decades thereafter. The victims were primarily political dissenters, but also included nationalists, religious believers, would-be emigrants, and people who might be called 'nuisances'. Various forms of political activity, such as taking part in a proscribed public demonstration or even possessing a forbidden book, could lead to arrest or civil commitment. In the case of the former, instead of a trial on a criminal charge the accused would be subjected to a psychiatric examination, often conducted by a psychiatric team from the Serbsky Forensic Psychiatric Institute in Moscow. With the report that the accused suffered from mental illness and thus was not accountable for his actions, a trial to determine the validity of this finding was held. But this trial was a charade. Relatives and friends could not attend, the nominal defense attorney had almost no power, and invariably the opinion of the psychiatric panel was accepted. The accused then became a 'patient', and was incarcerated within a system of special hospitals that were in fact psychiatric prisons, often for long periods of time, sometimes for years. Release depended often on recantation of their beliefs and a pledge not to repeat former behavior. Sometimes they were 'treated' with powerful neuroleptic drugs for purposes clearly punitive rather than therapeutic, and they were in the unpleasant proximity of genuinely criminally insane patients confined in the same institutions. Even after discharge the 'ex-patient' was kept under constant surveillance and their activities were severely limited.

The extent to which psychiatry could be perverted and manipulated for state purposes is illustrated by the case of General Piotr Grigorenko.[19] Grigorenko, a dedicated Communist from youth, undertook a military career and distinguished himself during World War II. He rose to the rank of Major General, received advanced degrees and numerous decorations. However, recognizing the violations of human rights in the then USSR, he became an activist and advocate. Arrested in 1964, he underwent the procedures previously described and was forcibly interned in a psychiatric hospital for 15 months. On discharge, he was expelled from the Communist Party, deprived of his pension, and forced to work as a porter. Rearrested in 1969, he was cleared by a psychiatric panel in Tashkent, but was then re-examined by the 'hired guns' from the Serbsky Institute, who, after cursory examination, found that Grigorenko suffered from a condition characterized by 'reformist ideas, overestimation of his own personality, affective intensity, and a conviction of the rightness of his actions'. Diagnosed as suffering from a paranoid personality with signs of cerebral arteriosclerosis, he was again involuntarily hospitalized under brutal conditions. It is of interest that years later, after he had been discharged and allowed to leave the former USSR and emigrate to the United States, he was re-examined by a team of distinguished American psychiatrists who found him to be entirely free of mental disorder.[20]

The purpose of the Soviet state in sponsoring and orchestrating this misuse of psychiatry was to discredit legitimate dissent by labeling it as insanity. What can be said about the motivations and behavior of the Soviet psychiatrists involved in the process? First, it is necessary to consider the ideological underpinnings that influenced Soviet psychiatrists just as it did all other Soviet citizens. In the USSR, at least in principle, unlike the Western democracies, obligations to the state took precedence over the rights of the individual. The Marxist–Leninist creed maintained that with the elimination of the class struggle, serious conflict between the individual and the state would no longer exist; the state now entirely represented and embodied the interests of all citizens. Upon graduation from medical school, the Soviet psychiatrist, like all Soviet physicians, took, not the Hippocratic Oath but rather the Physicians' Oath of the Soviet Union pledging the new doctor to work in the interests of the society, to be 'guided by Communist morality', and to be responsible to the Soviet state as well as to serve the welfare of patients. With this kind of indoctrination, a core of belief could exist that dissent was destructive and could occur only under the influence of pathological thinking.

Action on the basis of this belief was facilitated for Soviet psychiatrists by their adherence to the idiosyncratic but compelling diagnostic system formulated by the influential Soviet psychiatrist, Professor Andrei Snezhnevsky. This is discussed by Reich in Chapter 10, but it needs to be said here that the Snezhnevsky system made it easy to classify dissenters as suffering such illnesses as 'sluggish schizophrenia', a diagnosis not disqualified by 'seeming normality' and 'absence of symptoms', or, as is illustrated by the case of General Grigorenko, by a panoply of human characteristics mislabeled as symptoms.

A capsular summary of the justification for Soviet psychiatry during these years is contained in a statement by Nikita Khrushchev in 1959 as follows:

A crime is a deviation from generally recognized standards of behavior, frequently caused by mental disorder. Can there be nervous disorders among certain people in Communist society? Evidently yes. If that is so, then there may also be offences which are characteristic of people with abnormal minds. To those who might start calling for opposition to Communism on this basis, we can say that clearly the mental state of such people is not normal.[21]

Can we take this declaration seriously, or may we be forgiven if, more cynically, we label it as an exercise in 'hypodenial' (a combination of hypocrisy and refusal to acknowledge facts)? For it is also pertinent to note that Soviet psychiatrists had few alternatives to doing what they were told, or at least being quiet about what they saw, since they earned their livings as employees of the state through the Ministry of Health. Income and professional advancement could come only through governmental approval, and there were no independent Soviet psychiatric societies to support dissenters.

In fact, the vast majority of Soviet psychiatrists acquiesced but did not participate in this perverse system of abuse; a few at the top were actively involved, and a minuscule number bravely defied (and received) punishment to reveal what was happening.

Notwithstanding the increasingly vehement protest by psychiatrists throughout the world, particularly under the aegis of the World Psychiatric Association, the Soviet perversion continued, involving thousands of victims, until slowly and finally sputtering to a halt as Communism collapsed in the former Soviet Union.

The Soviet experience offers an appalling example to psychiatrists. Although no longer occurring anywhere on anything like the massive scale that took place in the Soviet Union, it is still a temptation for totalitarian or corrupt regimes to rid themselves of troublesome objectors through the mental illness gambit. Instances have been reported in Cuba and Turkmenistan.[22] The continued vigilance of individual psychiatrists and organizations like Amnesty International and the International Geneva Initiative will be required to keep this blight on psychiatry under control.

'Double agents' in the West

Can psychiatrists in the United States and the West, generally, be held free of the charge that they too have abrogated the rights of patients in the interests of social control? Thomas Szasz[23] maintains that the very existence of their profession as an instrument for treating non-existent mental illnesses, and for imposing conformity by using psychiatric diagnoses to stigmatize unconventional behavior, is proof that such a charge is justified. Without accepting this sweeping indictment, it can be acknowledged that including too many varieties of the vast range of human behavior under psychiatric rubrics may lead to a constriction of spontaneity and freedom, even to absurdity. Note the case of a few years ago in which the malevolent effect of a kind of cake called 'Twinkies' in inhibiting free will was argued as a defense against a charge of murder. We can be warned by the use of 'sluggish schizophrenia' in the former Soviet Union as a diagnosis under which 'seemingly normal' individuals were confined to hospitals. Furthermore, examples can be cited (outstandingly the Ezra Pound case) in which psychiatrists may also have acceded to professional and state pressure by subjecting patients under criminal charges to prolonged hospitalization on the basis of dubious clinical criteria.

Manipulation of diagnostic labels for other than scientific purposes or to facilitate treatment-planning often occurs in connection with the double-agent problem when the loyalty of psychiatrists to their patients is in conflict with their allegiance to the institutions they represent. This is likely to occur in military or prison settings, and also when legal issues are at stake, as in criminal trials, especially with the insanity defense. This problem assumes a certain poignancy because psychiatrists asked to make such decisions may be performing functions approved by state and society, but at the same time are placed at moral risk that they may be damaging their patients' interests.

There are exceptions, however, to the rule that the pressure to manipulate diagnoses usually originates from the state or the institution which employs the psychiatrists. Thus, as I can attest from personal observation and participation, during the Vietnam War potential draftees were sometimes given very questionable psychiatric diagnoses that kept them from being drafted, and before *Roe* v *Wade* (1973), the US Supreme Court decison that permitted abortion under certain conditions, pregnant women were afforded psychiatric warrant for abortions on the grounds of doubtful suicidal potential. In these examples, the psychiatrists were presumably acting not for the state but rather for their patients, thus raising the morally interesting question whether exclusive concentration on patients' wishes to the neglect of legitimate societal or state requirements can be considered an improper use of psychiatric power, and thus fall into the misuse or abuse category, in a way that can be seen as the opposite of what occurred in the former USSR. An urgent and increasingly intense example of this conflict can be seen in the behavior of psychiatrists who feel themselves to be between a rock and a hard place as they endeavor to defend their patients' interests (and sometimes their own) under the market-oriented economics of third parties and managed care (see Chapter 19).

Nazi abuse of psychiatry

The consequences for the victims of psychiatric misuse in the former Soviet Union were dire, but in Nazi Germany, German psychiatrists were even more culpable, since they were significantly involved in the early stages of the fatal chain of events starting with sterilization and 'euthanasia' of mentally ill patients, that climaxed in the gassings in the Nazi death camps. The question immediately arises, as put by Sidney Bloch,[21] 'as to how a psychiatric fraternity with a tradition for scholarship stretching back to the mid-nineteenth century could collaborate with the Nazi leadership in such heinous practices as the compulsory sterilization and the murder (erroneously called euthanasia) of tens of thousands of chronically mentally ill and mentally handicapped people'. The process, ineluctably leading to the worst disaster of the disastrous twentieth century, began long before the Nazis came to power when German scientists and psychiatrists, along with their confreres in some Western countries, (including Switzerland and Sweden as 1997 newspaper stories have revealed), became intoxicated with the idea of improving racial stock through selective breeding in accordance with the then esteemed 'science' of eugenics. It is discomforting to recall that in the early part of this century, German scientists and physicians were looking admiringly on the sterilization laws passed by a number of states in the United States under which thousands of mentally ill patients were involuntarily sterilized.[24]

According to the post-war testimony of Hitler's personal physician, Karl Brandt, Hitler decided even before 1933 that he would one day try to eliminate the mentally ill.[24] Thus, the enthusiasm to foster racial hygiene by 'eliminating life unworthy of life' was supported and blessed by the Nazis shortly after Hitler came to power when laws were passed implementing the sterilization of the mentally ill, particularly those with a supposed genetic defect. After some hundreds of thousands of such operations, sterilization was succeeded by 'euthanasia' of defective children, and the mentally ill and intellectually re-tarded in October 1939. Some 70 000 were killed in psychiatric hospitals until the program was officially called off after clerical protest in August 1941. However, even after this exposure, patients in psychiatric hospitals, although no longer killed directly, were hastened to death through neglect and starvation. A further step on the road to Auschwitz occurred with what has been called the 'medicalization of anti-Semitism', including the precepts of another pseudoscience—criminal biology—as Jews became defined as genetically diseased, a cancer that had to be eliminated to restore the health of the German people. It is chilling to reflect on, and difficult to understand, the assent and participation of the German psychiatric profession, including such eminences as Carl Schneider in this complete perversion of their profession and their Hippocratic Oath. Psychiatric protest was almost non-existent.

Possibly complementing the pseudoscientific rationalizations and the deadly pressure from the Nazi leaders, another explanation for this behavior of Nazi psychiatrists has been suggested by Robert Lifton[25] in the form of a psychological formulation which he terms 'doubling'—defined as 'the division of the self into two functioning wholes, so that a part self acts as an entire self'. Thus, the Auschwitz doctor supervising the gas chambers during the day, in the evenings could luxuriate in his role of affectionate father and pet lover. Whether this formulation has validity or is something of an excuse for inexcusable behavior, as critics have alleged, it is quite clear that a straight line exists from psychiatric activities directed against the mentally ill to the killing of Jews and Gypsies in the camps, and that German psychiatrists unswervingly traversed this path. In fact, the killing in the psychiatric hospitals was carried out with equipment that, along with responsible doctors and technicians, was transferred in late 1941 to the death camps to begin their work of eliminating Jews and other mongrel specimens of 'life unworthy of life'.

Although it may be hoped that the Nazi Holocaust will never be repeated, there is cause for concern in the phenomenon of 'ethnic cleansing', based on stereotyping of enemy groups such as occurred in the Bosnian conflict during the mid-1990s. Also, the pseudoscientific reasoning and rationalizations employed to justify the Holocaust have troubling implications for such current concerns as physician-assisted suicide and resource allocation. Both of these subjects will be discussed in Chapters 21 and 18, respectively.

Japanese psychiatric abuse

The following material is largely derived from the chapter by Timothy Harding[26] in the 2nd edition of *Psychiatric ethics*. A third form of national abuse, very different from the Nazi and Soviet varieties, occurred in Japan during the period following World War II until reform in the late 1980s. As post-war economic and social changes rendered the previous tradition of home care for the mentally ill in Japan more difficult, there was an increasing need for institutional treatment. Because of governmental prejudice against developing public medicine, the passage of a series of laws led to a state of affairs in which the care of the mentally ill came largely to be relegated to the private sector through governmental subsidies and low interest loans which encouraged private investment. The result was a sustained growth in the psychiatric population in Japan at a time when there was a steady decrease in every other industrialized country. Most hospitals were located in remote rural areas, a situation reminiscent of that in the US during the early part of this century. Almost all admissions were involuntary. There was little legal protection for patients, hospitals were understaffed and rehabilitation services insufficient. Abuses were widespread, patients were maltreated or beaten, and many were kept for long periods in horrendous conditions. Sometimes (reminiscent of the Soviet practice) they were given large doses of neuroleptics with little or no therapeutic intent. The hospitals were predominantly profit-making enterprises that provided, at best, little more than custodial care. As one embittered Japanese psychiatrist stated, 'If psychiatry is run as business, profits come before patients', a conclusion, incidentally, that ominously echoes the previously quoted statement of Dr Pellegrino and may also apply to some managed care organizations in the US. As Professor Harding observed,[26] 'This form of abuse can be termed psychiatric abuse by economic motives'. As the Soviet misuse was an evil deriving from communism, Japanese abuse cannot be separated from capitalism.

The reform movement culminating in a new law of 1988 seems to have been effective in materially improving conditions for the mentally ill in Japan, although discharged mental patients apparently still bear a stigma so that, for instance, they may not be allowed to enter a public bath.

The Japanese abuse, here described, may serve as a warning beacon for developments in the United States in the 1990s where some for-profit mental hospital decisions seem to be weighed toward the comfort of the investor rather than the comfort of the patient. If this trend continues, we may be heading towards a time when the patient will be dealt with as an economic entity rather than treated as a suffering human being.[27] Conversely, it is also relevant to conditions in the US to note that Japanese reformers were concerned to avoid what they saw as the deplorable consequences of deinstitutionalization by so limiting the criteria for involuntary hospital admissions that it would be difficult to provide adequate inpatient treatment for those mentally ill patients who required it.

Deinstitutionalization

We are all familiar with the corrupting potential of power; it has been my thesis throughout this chapter that this truism applies to the power allotted to psychiatrists. I have illustrated how this may happen—both in the doctor–patient relationship and in situations where a psychiatrist plays an inter-mediary role between patients and institutions, governmental or otherwise. I now reverse my field and want to make the case that absence of power, or power inefficiently applied, can also have maleficient consequences.

In the early part of my 50 years in practice, psychiatrists could too easily hospitalize people diagnosed as mentally ill against their will, sometimes with loose diagnoses, and without sufficient regard for autonomy and individual civil rights. Such patients were often confined in large institutions that were bitterly and rightfully characterized as human warehouses. An ethically motivated protest against this state of affairs by psychiatrists and, especially, civil liberties lawyers, was increasingly effective so that the procedures of involuntary hospitalization underwent profound changes. These changes were one important factor in a precipitous drop in the population of state and government hospitals. Thus, in 1946, St Elizabeths Hospital in Washington DC had 7468 patients, and still almost 7000 in 1955, whereas in 1997 its patient population had plummeted to 800. But as the vicissitudes of involuntary hospitalization illustrate,[28] it is a sad but ironically accurate commentary on human behavior that good intentions often lead to bad results. In this case we can point to revolving door admissions, hospital stays too brief to stabilize patients, and, especially, to the massive deinstitutionalization of mental patients since the 1980s. The effects can readily be seen in many large cities in several countries as discharged mentally ill persons now comprise a substantial segment of the homeless, tramping our streets like 'Tom O'Bedlams, living, no one cared how, and dying, no one cared where'. As pungently put by Dr E. Fuller Torrey,[29] 'deinstitutionalization has been a psychiatric Titanic!'

Although certainly a complicated phenomenon with many roots, one of the puissant reasons for this fiasco is the shift away from *parens patriae* criteria for commitment, to criteria making dangerousness to self or others the principal determinant of eligibility for involuntary hospitalization. Having failed to resist this trend towards reliance on dangerousness as the main criterion for involuntary hospitalization, with its corollary that the concept of a humane and protective asylum (literally meaning refuge) has become stigmatized, psychiatrists must share the responsibility for its consequences. As one who has lived through and witnessed the profound change in rules governing involuntary hospitalization, I aver that psychiatrists can be charged with being ethically delinquent in their responsibility to their patients. Involuntary hospitalization and deinstitutionalization are the subjects of Chapter 20.

Speculation about the future

I turn now from a retrospectively charged survey of important issues in psychiatric ethics in the late 1990s to venture a few remarks about what we might expect in the future, and what we can do to maintain decent and proper behavior among psychiatrists. As I remarked at the beginning, I have witnessed an increasing interest in ethical issues among my colleagues. I have little doubt that this will continue, will become an even more prominent feature of our professional identities, and be reflected in psychiatric training programs, as discussed in Chapter 24.

Since human nature is unlikely to change dramatically, we will continue to see the kinds of perversions of power that stain doctor–patient relationships, although these may occur less frequently as concern for autonomy and informed consent continue to exert their influence. I would venture that we will see fewer derelictions in the sexual sphere as such boundary violations become increasingly subject to appropriate sanctions and publicity.

I believe that the major ethical dilemma looming before us, one which I have alluded to in several contexts and which is bound to become more urgent, is the conflict between our Hippocratic duty to our patients as the virtually exclusive determinant of our clinical actions, and our obligations to various aspects of the larger community in which we live and work. Fierce and undivided loyalty to the patient is still the rallying cry of most psychiatrists on the grounds, as put most forcefully by Alan Stone,[30] that the doctor–patient relationship 'is the basic building block of trust in medicine. All of our ethical obligations derive from that relationship to our patients.' There is no doubt that the constraints, sometimes arbitrary and unreasonable, imposed by managed care, impair the ability of psychiatrists to treat patients according to their best judgment and justify the profession's protests, as do, assuredly, legitimate concerns about basing health care on market forces impelled primarily by the profit motive rather than patient welfare. However, for ethical balance, we must take into account whether considerations of self-interest are also playing a role in the Hippocratic fervor of psychiatrists.

Although a minority, there are those who voice concern that the individualism that dominates our culture, with its almost insatiable demand for health care, must have limits imposed on it for the overall good of society. Contrasting what she terms an individual-oriented ethic with a societal ethic, Austad[31] points out that under the former, the psychiatrist's primary loyalty is to the patient whereas under the societal ethic, the needs of the patient are tempered by the needs of society as a whole. Dr Christine Cassel[32] has even suggested that the Hippocratic Oath may need to be revised to reflect a commitment to population-based health.

A spectre lurking behind the managed-care debate is the largely unacknowledged role of managed care in providing a crude form of health care rationing. Rationing may be necessary[33] because of the escalation of health-care costs as a consequence of the almost limitless expansion of the concept of health, and, if I may venture a personal judgment, the refusal of the US to embark upon a centralized national medical program. If rationing is inevitable, psychiatrists will be confronted with a host of knotty ethical issues such as what forms of treatment should be limited, who should be subject to rationing, and who should make the decisions.

Promoting moral behavior among psychiatrists

The increased concern for the ethical dimensions of psychiatric practice carries with it the obligation of our profession to teach and promote moral behavior. One way to accomplish this is through courses in ethics in medical school, psychiatric training programs, and postgraduate courses as discussed by Michels and Kelly in Chapter 24. Although ethics is the study of morality rather than morality itself, courses in ethics promote self-scrutiny about pertinent issues and increase awareness about gray areas that otherwise might remain unexplored. Formal codes of ethics play an important role in guiding moral behavior among practitioners; they are discussed in Chapter 6 by Bloch and Pargiter. Such codes, of course, vary from time to time and place to place, but always serve the purposes of raising moral consciousness and providing a means of education and a tool in self-regulation. They also provide a basis to investigate possible violations of ethical standards and to impose sanctions. Current examples of such codes are the *Principles of medical ethics with special annotations for psychiatry* in the US,[6] and the code of the Royal Australian and New Zealand College of Psychiatrists.[34]

Having been active in the operations of an American Psychiatric Association District Branch Ethics Committee for a number of years, I can attest to the difficulties of attempting to formalize and, in a sense, 'legalize' acceptable standards. As a result of this experience, however, I believe that the care and seriousness with which possible ethical derelictions are being catalogued, investigated, and, if necessary, punished, is of value both to the psychiatric profession and to the public that its practitioners serve.

Finally, perhaps whimsically, we may refer back to the Aristotelean tradition of virtue ethics[35]. May we hope that our profession, with its compelling intellectual stimulation, and its attraction to people motivated to help others, to benefit society, and not to shrink from self-scrutiny, will meet the requirements put forth by Thomas Percival[36] in the nineteenth century about 'the ineradicability of the physician's character as guarantor of the patient's good and welfare', and by Sigmund Freud, that our relationships with patients should be grounded on 'a love of truth, precluding sham and deceit'.[37]

References

1. Chodoff, P.: Ethical dimensions of psychotherapy: a personal perspective. *American Journal of Psychotherapy* **50**:298–309, 1996.
2. Chodoff, P.: Paternalism vs autonomy in medicine and psychiatry. *Psychiatric Annals* **8**:320, 1983.
3. Robitscher, J: *The powers of psychiatry*. New York, Houghton-Mifflin, 1980.
4. Veatch, R M, Gaylin, W. and Steinboch, B.: Can the moral commons survive autonomy? *Hastings Center Report* **26**:41–7, 1996.
5. Chodoff, P.: Effects of the new economic climate on psychotherapeutic practice. *American Journal of Psychiatry* **144**:1293–7, 1987.
6. *The principles of medical ethics with annotations especially applicable to psychiatry.* Washington DC, American Psychiatric Association, 1973.
7. Kabanov, M.: Psychiatry defended: reforms suggested, *Federal Broadcast Information Service–Soviet* **88**:107, 1988.
8. Chodoff, P.: The Anne Sexton biography: the limits of confidentiality. *Journal of the American Academy of Psychoanalysis* **20**:639–44, 1992.

9. *The principles of medical ethics with annotations especially applicable to psychiatry,* Washington DC, American Psychiatric Association, Section 2:1, 1995.
10. Epstein, R.: *Keeping boundaries: maintaining safety and integrity in the psychotherapeutic process.* Washington, DC, American Psychiatric Press, 1994.
11. Gruenberg, P. B.: Nonsexual exploitation of patients: an ethical perspective. *Journal of the American Academy of Psychoanalysis* **23**:425–34, 1995.
12. Lazarus, J.: quoted in *Psychiatric News* Nov. 5, 1993.
13. Lakin, M.: *Ethical issues in the psychotherapies.* Oxford, Oxford University Press, 1988.
14. Crews, F.: The memory wars: Freud's legacy in dispute. New York Review of Books, 1995.
15. Gardner, R.: Sex abuse hysteria. *Creative Therapeutics.* Creskill, NJ, 1991.
16. Chodoff, P.: Psychiatry and the fiscal third-party. *American Journal of Psychiatry* **135**:1141–7, 1978.
17. Hastings Center Report: In the service of the state: the psychiatrist as double agent 8(Supp):1–23, 1978.
18. Bloch, S. and Reddaway, P.: *Psychiatric terror.* New York, Basic Books, 1977.
19. Chodoff, P.: Involuntary hospitalization of political dissenters in the Soviet Union. *Psychiatric Opinion* **11**:5–19, 1974.
20. Reich, W.: Grigorenko gets a second opinion. *New York Times*, May 13, 1979.
21. Quoted in Bloch, S.: Psychiatry: An impossible profession? *Australian and New Zealand Journal of Psychiatry* **31**:172–83, 1997.
22. Kaplan, A.: Geneva initiative offers political abuse of psychiatry, fosters professional development. *Psychiatric Times*, April 1997.
23. Szasz, T.: *Psychiatric Slavery.* New York, Free Press, 1977
24. Proctor, R. N.: *Racial hygiene.* Cambridge, MA, Harvard University Press, 1988.
25. Lifton, R. J.: *The Nazi doctors.* New York, Basic Books, 1986.
26. Harding, T.: Ethical issues in the delivery of mental health services, in *Psychiatric ethics*, 2nd edn, ed. S. Bloch and P. Chodoff. Oxford University Press, 1991, pp. 473–92.
27. Bittker, T. E.: The industrialization of American psychiatry. *American Journal of Psychiatry* **142**:149–54, 1985.
28. Chodoff, P.: The case for involuntary hospitalization of the mentally ill. *American Journal of Psychiatry* **133**:496–500, 1976.
29. Torrey, E. F.: *Out of the shadows: confonting America's mental illness crisis.* New York, Wiley, 1997.
30. Stone, A.: quoted in *Psychiatric News* p. 27, 4.
31. Austed, C.S.: *Is long term psychotherapy unethical?* San Francisco, Jossey-Bass, 1996.
32. Cassel, C. K.: quoted in *Psychiatric News* p. 50, May 2, 1997.
33. Gaylin, W.: Health unlimited. *Wilson Quarterly* pp. 38–42, 1996.
34. Bloch, S. and Pargiter, R.: Developing a code of ethics for psychiatry, in *Codes of ethics and the professions*, ed. M. Coady and S. Bloch. Melbourne, Melbourne University Press, 1996, pp. 193–225.
35. Beauchamp, T. and Childress, J.: *Principles of biomedical ethics*, 4th edn. Oxford, Oxford University Press, 1994.
36. quoted in ref. 35, p. 198.
37. Freud, S.: *Analysis terminable and interminable*, Standard Edition, vol 23. London, Hogarth, 1978, pp. 211–53.

5

Psychiatry as a profession

Allen R. Dyer

Psychiatry as a profession is inevitably caught up in our culture's attempt to determine what is meant by a profession and how professions should be defined and regulated. Psychiatrists need to be clear about their own self-understanding, especially as they apply to professional goals. Should psychiatry seek to advance the standing of its guild by emphasizing its new technological prowess, or should it seek to rehabilitate its image as a profession by emphasizing the traditional ethical values of humanistic service? Are these goals compatible or exclusive? Before we can answer these basic questions, we need to reflect on the defining features of professions in general.

Ever since university professors (the first were the masters at the University of Paris) were allowed to incorporate in the thirteenth century, there has been much ambiguity in the understanding of a profession.[1] Originally the word 'profession' meant to profess religious vows. One was called to the 'discipline' in the same way as disciples were called to their master for a vocation of service. From the Middle Ages, however, professions became increasingly organized into guild-like fraternities and correspondingly criticized for placing their own economic interests on an equal plane with their ideals of public service.

A profession may be defined by:

(1) its knowledge, technology, and expertise; or
(2) its ethics and values.[2]

Habits of modern thought might lead us to conclude that this is an either/or choice. Clearly for psychiatry as for medicine generally, technology has become increasingly important, even central in some people's minds. Medicine is usually understood to mean *allopathic* treatment with drugs and procedures the favored treatment modalities. The recent primary care thrust has reopened consideration of medicine as a more holistic approach to healing. Talking again becomes an important part of healing. It is important to recognize that ethics is fundamental to professional definition. Technology is useful as long as it serves ethical ends, but not as an end in itself. Indeed, knowledge, technology, and expertise are not commodities to be bartered in the marketplace, but skills which all may be used to ethical ends. Medical technology falls under the purview of professional values.

Ethical issues pervade professional life. All aspects of professional development involve ethics. Entry into a profession (usually through admission to a professional school) involves ethics at least implicitly in the choice of candidates who have demonstrated a work ethic in achieving academically, and perhaps explicitly as well in attempts to select candidates of character, reflecting the values of the profession. Ethics may be part of the education formally in the curriculum, but more implicitly in the socialization to the norms of the profession. Finally, ethics is involved in professional discipline, even resulting in expulsion of those members who violate the code of ethics.

Medicine as a profession grounded in particular values goes back to the fourth century BCE (before the Christian (or Common) Era) and specifically to the Hippocratic Oath. The Oath is a remarkable document, not so much in answering ethical questions posed by modern medicine, but in framing those questions. It is often noted dismissively that the Oath is anachronistic and offers little useful guidance to the modern physician. The Oath does indeed provide limited help for those expecting a catalogue of rules. On the other hand, it is valuable in defining goals of medicine by articulating key principles, most notably those of beneficence and its corollary, the principle of non-maleficence (*primum non nocere*, first do no harm). At a time when many other factors (especially economic) demand the physician's attention, the greatest liability of the Oath may ironically be its greatest asset, namely its antiquity. The Oath provides an ethical perspective that questions many assumptions of modern culture; it offers a vantage point transcending the pressures of social and political expediency.

The second paragraph of the Oath articulates the classical understanding of a profession organized around its ethics:

To hold him who has taught me this art as equal to my parents and to live my life in partnership with him, and if he is in need of money to give him a share of mine, and to regard his offspring as equal to my brothers in male lineage and to teach them this art—if they desire to learn it—without fee and covenant; to give a share of precepts and oral instruction and all the other learning to my sons and to the sons of him who has instructed me and to pupils who have signed the covenant and have taken an oath according to the medical law, but to no one else.[3]

We note here the origins of what we now understand as the professional organization of physician-healers. The profession is organized around its teachers, and the relationship between them and their students; teacher and student are like family, including the bonds of dependency. The Oath has been criticized as exclusionary (by those who view medicine as a commodity) for not making instruction available to all. Again this may be more a virtue than a shortcoming since it makes 'signing the covenant and taking an oath according to medical law' a requirement of receiving instruction. Entry into the profession thus calls for a commitment to shared values.

The anti-trust challenge to the profession

I have referred above to the professions in terms of core ethical principles which define them. Most basic of these (elaborated in the next section) is the principle of trustworthiness, the ability to win a people's trust by showing them personal integrity. Trust has the religious connotations of belief and faith. It has the psychological connotation of confidence and dependency. It also has a legal meaning with an entirely different connotation. Trust also means monopoly, a combination of firms or corporations for the purpose of reducing competition and controlling prices throughout a business or industry.

The medieval ambiguity in the notion of a profession comes to focus in the modern anti-trust laws. Codes of ethics which highlight the trust-promoting feature of professional life, from the Hippocratic Oath to most of the codes of the world's professional associations, stress that their members should elicit and maintain the trust of those seeking their help. The profession of these vows is quite different from business or corporate interests, which are governed by anti-trust or anti-monopoly laws.

In the United States, for instance, the Sherman anti-trust law, passed in 1890, states succinctly that, 'Any contract, combination, or conspiracy in restraint of trade is illegal'. Left to the courts to interpret, they held for 85 years that the 'learned professions' were exempt from the anti-trust laws, which applied only to business and industry. By 1975, however, it was not uncommon to refer to health care as an industry. Although patients still consulted doctors, they often obtained their care from institutions, which were increasingly concerned with the financial aspects of delivering high-cost, 'high-tech' medical services. In 1975 the US Supreme Court ended the learned professions' exemption through the *Goldfarb* decision.

Goldfarb, a Washington attorney, wanted to buy a house and as an attorney himself, knew that one did not need the brightest or most expensive legal mind to search the title. He thus went shopping for the cheapest attorney but found the fees they were charging were all the same. 'Restraint of trade', he claimed, and took his fellow attorneys to court. The Supreme Court concurred. Soon after its decision ending the learned professions' exemption, the Federal Trade Commission (FTC), which had been waiting in the wings and expecting this result, entered suit against the American Medical Association (AMA), holding that they were in restraint of trade because their code of ethics prohibited advertising. Medical prices were high, the FTC contended, because doctors were prohibited from advertising, thus keeping patients from shopping for the 'best deals'.

The Supreme Court decided in favour of the FTC in 1982, inaugurating the era of advertising by physicians and other professionals. Medicine, in effect, was transformed from a profession into a trade. The AMA could no longer adopt a code of ethics without approval from the FTC. More crucial than the issue of advertising, the FTC won regulatory jurisdiction over the medical profession.[4-6]

We might lament a significant loss in this decision, on ethical grounds. Professional advertising, however, was not the cardinal issue in this case. The defense of the AMA did not address the reasons underlying the prohibition of professional advertising (actually 'solicitation of patients', which is what had been proscribed). It was assumed that medicine would try to maintain a monopoly on health care, but do so in a way which was not in restraint of trade. We are left with the question: What distinguishes a profession from a trade? If medicine is to be considered a profession, what does that mean?

The ethical definition of a profession

The nineteenth and twentieth centuries have witnessed numerous occupational groups seeking to attain the professional status occupied by the paradigm professions of medicine, law, and the clergy. Sociologists observing this phenomenon have identified the formula by which professionalization occurs. The process first entails specialization, namely acquisition of technical skill and expertise; but these attributes do not suffice to establish a group as a profession. An occupation wishing to exercise professional authority must then find a basis to assert exclusive jurisdiction, link skill and this jurisdiction to identifiable standards of training, and then convince the public that its services are uniquely trustworthy.[7]

The evolution of professions usually involves a number of steps, including first becoming a full-time occupation; the establishing of the first training school, the first university school, the first local professional association, and then a national professional association; state licensing laws; and ultimately, the development of a formal code of ethics.

Established professions by these criteria include accounting, architecture, engineering, dentistry, law, and medicine. Developing professions would include librarianship, nursing, optometry, pharmacy, school teaching (often organized as a trade with trade unions), and social work. New professional groups are city management, town planning, and hospital administration.

The theme of trustworthiness is a pivotal consideration in the definition of a profession, in that it bridges the epistemological gulf between the idea of a profession as defined by its expertise and a profession as defined by its ethics. In order to be worthy of trust a professional must be both knowledgeable and ethical.

Codes of ethics, of course, do not assure ethical behavior of the members of a professional group, but they attempt in various ways to promote ethical standards through entry, education, and exit.

1. *Entry*: admission standards look to the character of the person seeking to enter the profession. In England, prospective barristers have been required to dine with their would-be colleagues at the Inns of Court. On these occasions their fellows could determine their suitability to join the profession. Even emphasis on grades and board scores involves an ethical dimension, the work ethic; though hopefully admissions committees look beyond such tangible manifestations of ability and willingness to work.

2. *Education* does not mean merely the teaching of ethics in the form of a curriculum. The curriculum itself reflects the values of the profession. Medicine's bifurcated curriculum, basic science, and clinical clerkships, reveals professional divisions in psychiatry, and also conceals deeper divisions in medicine overall. Ethics education occurs not only as a didactic enterprise but is an integral part of the socialization process in professional life. One learns the values of the professional culture by living them with ethically committed members of that profession. Formal ethics is a way of reflecting on those experiences.

3. *Exit* refers to professional discipline. Professions reserve the right and the responsibility to discipline members who fail to adhere to certain standards of ethics specified in their codes. Professions are ambivalent about policing their own members; and control of licensure is held by external statutory bodies. However, it is also important that professions themselves take discipline seriously in order to maintain both their own integrity and the public trust.

Codes of ethics are far more than administrative documents. They are certainly more than a list of rules by which a member of a professional group can identify and exclude those exhibiting deviant behavior. A code also serves to symbolize the principles by which a professional group defines itself. As such the code reflects values, although these cannot always be explicitly stipulated. Any list of rules would be found wanting by such expectations. If it were possible to make clinical judgments this way, we could take a good law book and a good enough computer algorithm and dispense with a professional altogether. The role of the professional is to personalize care.

The Hippocratic Oath in eight succinct statements outlines the values of the medical profession over the past 24 centuries. It defines for the first time the physician as healer, specializing in caring for the sick, uninterested in and forswearing any other possibilities in relation to those who seek help. For the first time in history, according to the anthropologist, Margaret Mead, the authority to heal was vested in a practitioner who was not also a shaman with the power to harm.[8] The sole purpose of the Hippocratic physician was to promote health, foreshadowing the modern conception of a profession.

A recurring theme in the rhetoric of the Oath is the imperative to benefit the patient. Although such language sounds paternalistic to the modern ear, we do not expect patients to be so self-sufficient as to take complete care of themselves. The autonomy of the patient, however, is respected and she is actively involved in decision-making wherever possible.

Psychiatry as a profession has attended to these nuances of the doctor–patient relationship in a manner which may serve as a model for other professions. There is probably no better statement of the doctor–patient relationship than Freud's classic papers on transference. We are cautioned to appreciate and fully understand that the patient inevitably develops strong feelings toward the doctor, that these feelings are more a function of the role of the physician, and that they are 'not to be attributed to the charms of his own person'.[9] Tempting as it may be to believe the flatterer or frustrating as it may be to bear the brunt of a patient's anger, it is important to recognize the possibility that these feelings may have been brought into the relationship rather than stem from it. Furthermore, Freud's psychoanalytic work requires physicians to scrutinize their own conduct for clues to understand the patient's responses. This applies not only to psychoanalytic treatment since such dynamics occur in all intimate relationships. No aspect of psychiatry nor any aspect of medicine can rely solely on the application of technique without an appreciation of the dynamics of the relationship between doctor and patient.

Threats to the professional relationship

The current revolution in health-care organization and financing, at least in the US, is calling into question not only many of the traditional assumptions of medical ethics, but assumptions about the doctor–patient relationship, the nature of health and disease, and even the role of persons in a society. It is not just about economic values; it is also about human values. The most sobering change is the erosion of a dyadic person-to-person, doctor–patient relationship. Doctors in the new environment are being transformed into 'providers'; patients into 'consumers'; and any number of 'third parties' claim an interest in what transpires between them.

In the economic model of marketplace transactions, much more is at stake than how the funding is managed. The metaphor of 'health care as an industry' jeopardizes the healing process. Health care is reduced to physical interventions that take place in a constrained period. Physicians become merely providers and technicians, and patients consumers and recipients of technology. The two groups are likely to be strangers to one another. Medicine is transformed from a human service into a commodity.

In the interest of efficiency and reducing cost, these transformations might seem warranted but the evolving practices must be subjected to ethical scrutiny. Certainly much of what we witness is not ethically justifiable, nor does it serve the ends it was purported to serve. Changing medicine from profession to trade by the Federal Trade Commission was justified as a cost-saving measure on the grounds that extending consumer choice (through advertising) would reduce costs. The value placed on this autonomy, however, set the stage for a transformation in which consumers enjoy little choice about the health care they receive. Health care has become an investment opportunity where vast sums have been siphoned away from service delivery into the pockets of executives and shareholders of mega-corporations. The 'market' solution has been a non-solution to this point in that it has only succeeded in lowering costs without adequately addressing quality of service or the distribution and allocation of resources. The resultant unregulated (or underregulated) market resembles the lawlessness of the post-Civil War, American frontier, or early stages of industrialization, the era of the 'robber barons', where efficiencies and wealth were achieved at the cost of environmental pollution and human suffering. In such markets the goal of business is to make profits for the owners or shareholders with no direct accountability in terms of the services provided.

An interesting irony arises for physicians in the context of these changes. Many of those who operated in the former 'cottage industry' often favored free-market approaches, forgetting that limiting medical practice to licensed physicians was itself a form of regulation. A truly free market would allow patients to contract with any practitioner they might choose and also to purchase drugs freely. The constraints on such freedoms were the scientific and ethical standards of the profession. These standards, inevitably imperfect, were so thoroughly a dimension of medical consciousness as to be taken for granted (when all discussion of value began to focus on economic considerations).

Ethically minded physicians are inevitably in conflict with a system designed to limit or deny the care necessary for their patients. While recognizing that resources are finite, they must struggle to do the best possible job for the individual patient without compromising their integrity. Managed care could provide a useful framework for ethical practice by reviewing medical necessity, but without any inherent accountability it becomes a pretext to cut services in order to make money for investors. Many aspects of managed care, such as gag rules prohibiting physicians from discussing treatment options with their patients, are fraudulently unethical. Such policies do not enhance consumers' choice (even the choice of paying out of pocket), but diminish their autonomy. They directly undermine the goal of informed consent, a key feature of the respect for autonomy. Gag rules place the physician in the position of double agent, without the possibility of disclosure. It is difficult for the physician to say, 'Trust me', or even 'Consumer, beware'. Many of the practices of managed care, like misleading advertising or incomplete disclosure, are more subtly unethical. And some features such as limiting who may serve on panels may be in restraint of trade. They are certainly not pro-competitive. Managed care, an ethically unstable response to the health-care financing dilemma, must be subjected to thoroughgoing ethical evaluation.

The modern impasse

The traditional understanding of a profession, as we have discussed, places great emphasis on ethics. Here ethics is symbolized by codes of ethics, but these codes also serve to remind professionals of virtues which may guide their actions. Virtue comprises both good intent and good faith, ideals which are elusive in day-to-day practice. References to virtue almost sound suspect to the modern ear. 'Accountability' has virtually supplanted 'virtue' as a way of assuring proper conduct. Virtue aspires to ideals which cannot be perfectly met, while accountability holds someone to a standard which has been explicitly specified. Where virtue is lofty, even precarious, accountability tends to function at the lowest common denominator. A patient would hope that professions would aspire to the highest ideals of virtue. By contrast, a health-care organization seeking a 'technician' for management of a capitated population would hold that technician accountable through bureaucratic control.

A profession, as defined by its ethics, must attend carefully to the people allowed to assume the responsibilities and accompanying privileges of professional activity. Deciding who shall be accepted and monitoring the performance of members are pivotal tasks of all professional organizations. Control of entry and exit has been traditionally viewed as paramount for professional self-regulation. I would argue that such activities are impossible to pursue satisfactorily without a concept of virtue. If medicine extends beyond mere technical expertise, then some understanding of 'virtue' or 'character' are essential attributes of a physician whether acknowledged explicitly or not.

I would further venture that the juxtaposition of virtue and accountability is a feature of what we might call a 'modern' outlook, which has certain recognizable features, particularly the desire for explicitness and an intolerance of ambiguity. As the possibility of a post-modern culture begins to emerge at the end of the twentieth century, we can gain a perspective on 'modernity' as it applies to professional life. Modernity is a set of identifiable cultural assumptions, which can no longer be taken for granted but which must be scrutinized in order to respond to and define that which will follow.

The post-modern alternatives

By no means do I want to imply that post-modernism is a recognizable culture entity or even that what is often discussed as post-modernism will be the cultural norm of the twenty-first century. In speculating about post-modernism and its likely effects on professions, we have the difficult, dual task of understanding historical change as it occurs and at the same time being unflinchingly honest with ourselves about our most cherished assumptions. It would not be an exaggeration to suggest that we are witnessing a revolution in health care. We should also realize that the revolution in health care is part of a larger revolution in social thinking tantamount to a paradigm change of the sort Thomas Kuhn described in *The structure of scientific revolutions.*[10] Moreover, we may conjecture that the cultural shift we are experiencing is a transition from modern culture to post-modern culture (see Jameson,[11] Kolb,[12] Gergen,[13] and Eberle[14] for contributions to the subject). Little consensus prevails as to what post-modernism will entail. It is simply too soon to tell. None the less, the medical profession, including psychiatry, would be distinctly advantaged if it were to respond to the challenges involved by reconceptualizing core issues.

In Table 5.1 I summarize features commonly associated with modernity: secularism, free-market forces, constitutional democracy, civil rights, nationalism, bureaucracy, industrialization (efficiency), capitalism, science and technology, rational thought and progress. Many of the tensions experienced in professional ethics stem from the tension in how to think about and experience the process of valuing in the modern paradigm. While many of the features of the old modern age are comfortably familiar and some perhaps worth defending, they cannot be taken for granted.

There are at least two distinct strains of post-modernism. The intellectual movement most often identified with post-modernism, *deconstructionism*, seeks to undermine the unities and certainties of the modern age on the grounds that they are artificial constructions of a false, impersonal scientism in which human experience is made the object of detached analysis. Often using linguistic innovations, such as talking about 'psychiatries' instead of 'psychiatry' to emphasize the plurality of opinion within a discipline, deconstructionism attacks traditional values. Deconstructionism is typically post-individual, post-patriarchal, and post-humanist. Depending on where you stand, deconstructionism is either unnerving or exciting.

An alternative form of post-modernism I would like to identify may be called 'post-critical', after the philosophy of Michael Polanyi. Polanyi also pointed out that modern science, as usually understood, purports to be objective, the observer detached and value-neutral. But, in fact, genuine science never

Table 5.1 Features commonly associated with modernity

Secular society	Freemarket
	Constitutional democracy
	Civil rights
	Nationalism
	Bureaucratic administration
	Industrialization—efficiency
	Capitalism
	Science and technology
	Rational thought
	Progress

proceeds in this manner, but depends on the judgments of a committed knower. Science for Polanyi is neither objective nor subjective, but rather personal. Hence he has entitled his major work, *Personal knowledge: toward a post-critical philosophy.*[15] Moreover, scientific tradition plays a salient role in the understanding of the scientific community.

I raise these epistemological notions since they have a bearing on how ethics is to be understood. Ethics explicitly articulated is always in tension with more tacitly understood principles. The tensions permeating this chapter may be appreciated in the context of the larger, cultural tensions of which they are manifestations. Striving for explicitness is very much a feature of the modern outlook, but useful as it is, explicitness does not take us far enough. Ethics must also deal with the nuances of human experience. Table 5.2 highlights the tension between the modern and post-modern positions.

We may anticipate the post-modern by identifying the distinguishing features of modernity and even better appreciate the paradigm shift we are experiencing by examining what preceded modernity. Table 5.3 suggests a perspective on this development. Notable in pre-modern thinking is the focus on human experience and the human dimension. In the more deconstructive approaches to post-modernism, this dimension drops out, but in approaches which stress the role of tradition (such as Polanyi's post-critical philosophy), the recovery of the human dimension lost in modernity becomes an inherent part of the post-modern enterprise. For example, in post-modern approaches to art and architecture, we see the reintroduction of the human form and of human scale. Pre-modern art was representational; pictures told stories. Modern art abandoned these representations in favor of abstract and expressionistic ideas. Modern architecture, grand and impersonal, forced us to adapt to monolithic skyscrapers, huge black boxes, in which humans were but cogs in a machine; post-modern architecture reintroduces the human element. Whimsical touches such as oversize arches, pediments, columns, and windows serve, even in large buildings, as reminders of places of human meeting.

Table 5.2   Functions of ethics

Modern account	Post-modern or (post-critical) account
Universal	Contextual
Impersonal	Personal
Atemporal	Historical
Acultural	Cultural
Based on obligation	Based on integrity
Enforced by control, suasion, or sanction	Enforced by willing assent, trust in a convivial order or community

Table 5.3 A perspective on paradigmatic development

Pre-modern	Pre-scientific Ecclesiastical authority Magical thinking Focus on human experience
Modern	Emphasizes the individual and the search for a sytematic, scientific *certitude*
Post-modern	(a) *Deconstructive* Undermines the unities and closures found in mdodern thought (b) *Post-critical* Makes use of modern achievement and offers new freedoms

These humanistic, communitarian and historical elements in continuity with tradition offer hopeful and exciting possibilities for the future of medicine. Medicine in the modern paradigm has been a technological marvel, but focusing on the body as a machine has left an impersonal coldness that has created the host of ethical dilemmas we have come to identify within the domain of bioethics (not to mention an economic nightmare). It is the possibility of recovering the human dimension in medicine that suggests a useful direction for post-modernism in medicine. In addition, looking back to the contribution of the pre-modern age, we are better placed to appreciate the role of the Hippocratic tradition in contemporary medicine. Though it is sometimes criticized for being anachronistic, its true value becomes apparent in the way that it provides a perspective of enduring values by which the shortcomings of modern expediency may be judged.

While health care in the modern era focused on fixing the broken machine, we may anticipate and hope that in the post-modern era healing in the broadest sense will again come to the fore. We see classical roots of this expectation in the Greek tradition of the therapy of the word, which formed the basis,

Table 5.4 Evolution of medical practice

Old paradigm (Modern)	New paradigm (Post-modern)
Acute illness—hospital based	Chronic illness—community based
Curative—physician centered	Preventative—doctor–patient partnership
Prototype—young, white male	Cultural diversity

explicitly and implicitly, in the talking cure especially as developed by Freud. We also witnessed in the bifurcation of modern psychiatry, the split of mind and body and the cleavage between psychological and biological approaches. I use the past tense emphatically because I want to underscore the importance of a more integrative approach for the psychiatry of the future.

George Engel in 1977 issued a call for a 'new' medical model, the bio–psycho–social.[16] Two decades later this newness has come to be taken for granted and the radical nature of the original proposal forgotten. As we have progressed in appreciating the impact of stress on human beings and the complex interaction of mind and body, the integration of the biological, psychological, and social does not seem as revolutionary as it did in the 1970s when biological reductionism held sway. We may hope for a realization of a genuine bio–psycho–social approach in psychiatry, even more appropriately conceptualized as a bio–psycho–social–*spiritual* model. I include the spiritual realm not only in a narrowly religious sense, but also to cover the transcendent. We can appreciate spirituality in medicine, for example, in some treatment approaches to substance abuse, which affirm a recognition of a 'force greater than myself' not necessarily defined in a specific manner. We recognize something beyond self in friendships, families, fellowships, communities. In this sense spirituality is post-narcissistic.

Otto Guttentag may be highlighting this approach in another way in his reference to an 'anthropological medical model'.[17] This broader scope reminds us of the core purpose of medicine: to provide a service to benefit the patient.

When placed in the context of defining a profession, such considerations as the spiritual and the anthropological, might seem obvious, but the bifurcations run so deeply in psychiatry, medicine, and the Cartesian world, that we may all too easily slip into accepting dualities (like mind versus body or psychological versus biological) that really make no sense. It is epistemological nonsense to accept such dichotomous positions. Polanyi suggests that strict objectivity in science (leading to these divisions which plague psychiatry) is ultimately misleading. In an important paper entitled 'Life transcending physics and chemistry',[18] he argues that one cannot understand a machine by reducing it to its parts. The workings of a grandfather clock, for example, cannot be explained by giving an account of its components. Similarly, the meaning of life cannot be explained by dissecting out its elements.

Psychiatry, of all the professions, should be prepared to understand this message. The knowledge patients share of themselves is received by fellow human beings who ideally are trained to grasp not only the recital of symptoms but also the meaning of symbolic communication. Nothing frustrates patients more than feeling they are not being listened to, their stories not being heard, and their inner world not being understood.

Finally, we might approach the question of what defines psychiatry by asking the question upside-down. If psychiatry is not a profession, what is it? The alternatives suggest only partial answers. Psychiatry is a science, an applied science. Psychiatry is a medical specialty. Psychiatry is a trade. Each of these partial answers begs, however, for a more comprehensive view. Psychiatry can best be understood as a profession, seeking to apply science but best defined by values located in a human context.

References

1. Post, Seymour G.: Parisian masters as a corporation, 1200-1246. *Spectrum* **9**: 421–45, 1934.
2. Dyer, Allen R.: *Ethics and psychiatry: toward professional definition.* Washington DC, American Psychiatric Press, 1988.
3. Edelstein, Ludwig: The Hippocratic Oath. Text, translation, and interpretation. *Bulletin of the History of Medicine* (Suppl. 1), 1943, p. 3. Also in Edelstein, L.: *Ancient medicine.* Baltimore, Johns Hopkins University Press, 1967. (also see Appendix)
4. Greenhouse, J.: Justices uphold right of doctors to solicit trade. *New York Times*, p. 10, 24 March, 1982.
5. Lee, R. E.: Application of antitrust laws to the profession. *Journal of Legal Medicine* **1**:143–53, 1979.
6. Havighurst, Clark: Antitrust enforcement in the medical services industry: what does it all mean? *Milbank Memorial Fund Quarterly/Health and Society* **58**:89-124, 1980.
7. Wilensky, H.: The professionalization of everyone? *American Journal of Sociology* **70**:13ff, 1964.
8. Margaret Mead, quoted in M. Levine: *Psychiatry and ethics.* New York, George Braziller, 1972, pp. 324–5.
9. Freud, S.: Observations on transference love, in *Standard Edition*, vol. XII, London, Hogarth Press, 1958, p. 161.
10. Kuhn, Thomas S.: *The structure of scientific revolutions*, 3rd edn. Chicago, University of Chicago Press, 1996.
11. Jameson, Frederick: *Postmodernism, or the cultural logic of late capitalism.* Durham, NC, Duke University Press, 1991.
12. Kolb, David: *Postmodern sophistications: philosophy, architecture, and tradition.* Chicago, University of Chicago Press, 1992.
13. Gergen, Kenneth J.: *The saturated self: dilemmas of identity in contemporary life.* New York, Basic Books, 1991.
14. Eberle, G.: *The geography of nowhere: finding one's self in the postmodern world.* Kansas City, MO, Sheed and Ward, 1994.
15. Polanyi, Michael: *Personal knowledge: toward a post-critical philosophy.* London, Routledge & Kegan Paul, 1952. Also New York, Harper and Row, 1964.
16. Engel, George L.: The need for a new medical model: a challenge for biomedicine. *Science* **196**:129–36, 1977.
17. Guttentag, Otto: On defining medicine. *The Christian Scholar*, **XLVI**:200–11, 1963.
18. Polanyi, M.: Life transcending physics and chemistry. *Chemical and Engineering News* **45**:54ff, 1967.

6

Codes of ethics in psychiatry

Sidney Bloch and Russell Pargiter

Psychiatry as a branch of the well-established profession of medicine has throughout its history been influenced by codes of ethics; none the less it remains unclear what role such codes should play in determining clinical practice. In this chapter we explore this question by tracing the evolution of ethical codes in medicine from Hippocrates to the present; comparing the different forms codes assume; discussing the diverse purposes to which they can be put including the raising of moral consciousness, protecting the 'guild', as a means of education and as a tool in self-regulation. We use the code of ethics of the Royal Australian and New Zealand College of Psychiatrists to illustrate some of these themes.

An historical context

One means to understand contemporary developments in codes of ethics in psychiatry is to examine their historical context. A range of salient questions arise. Why did it take centuries following the Hippocratic Oath (generally acknowledged as the first code of medical ethics) for the creation of a code specifically for psychiatrists? Were previous codes (Hippocratic and others), typically generic in character, deemed adequate? Were the specific features inherent in psychiatric practice not sufficiently clear to the ethicist? More cynically, were the mentally ill seen as so deviant, tantamount to being depicted as non-human, that in an approach to their care, essentially custodial until the nineteenth century, an ethical dimension was regarded as superfluous? (See Foucault[1] for an intriguing account of the ostracism of the mentally ill from the sixteenth century onwards.) Was it only in the wake of the professionalization of psychiatry that particular ethical concerns of the 'new' corporate group could be identified (e.g. the forerunner of the American Psychiatric Association was only established in 1844 and that of the British College of Psychiatrists in 1853).

An obvious launching point in tracing out the evolution of ethical codes in medicine is the Oath of Hippocrates.[2] Probably written around 400 BC by his students, the Oath comprises a series of vows of a religious nature, influenced by a Pythagorean cult which was associated with the Pythagorean School of Medicine. According to the Oath, the physician is enjoined to view himself as a member of a noble fraternity which entails the twin obligations of honouring his teachers, virtually as parental figures, and teaching and nurturing succeeding generations of physicians. So profound is the Oath that the gods and goddesses are recruited to witness this commitment. The language in this section reflects the code's solemnity, even its sacredness. The contemporary doctor would no doubt perceive both the form and content as arcane and precious. Similar criticism however cannot be made of the latter half which deals with the specific ethical questions and includes firm rules. Thus, for instance, the doctor should preserve patients' confidences, resist exploiting them sexually, and not perform procedures which exceed this expertise.[†]

Perhaps the most outstanding characteristic of the oath is its paternalism, embodied unambiguously in the phrase: 'I will keep them [patients] from harm and injustice'. The doctor is obliged to assume complete responsibility for the patient, secure in the sense that he is a member of a noble profession supported in his actions by his fellows.

Despite its pagan context and archaic form the Oath provides both an ethos for professional activities and, innovatively, a series of specific rules of medical conduct. Perhaps, for these reasons, it has stood the test of time.[3] The Oath's use in some medical schools upon graduation testifies to this, but more confirmatory of its influence is its common citation in clinico-ethical discourse. The development of Christianity and Islam saw modification of the Greek form of the Oath into versions more suited to those religions with, for example, substitution of the Greek gods by Christian and Muslim theology.

By contrast with the enduring impact of the Hippocratic Oath, other ancient medical codes are today little more than curiosities. Yet, their existence suggests that efforts to codify ethical principles in medicine took place in a variety of cultures, each linked to a prevailing ethos. Three representative codes are illustrative—Indian, Hebrew, and Persian oaths. The *Caraka Samhita*,[4] a medical text written by an Indian physician in the first century AD, contains an oath for medical students. Like the Oath of Hippocrates, it comprises a series of vows. The student swears to treat his patients considerately and not to take advantage of them. More specific injunctions cover sexual exploitation, keeping abreast of medical knowledge, and confidentiality.

The *Book of Asaph Harofe*[5] is the oldest known Hebrew medical text and like the *Caraka Samhita* contains an oath for medical students to be sworn upon graduation. Asaph ben Berachyahu, a Jewish physician, practised in Syria or Mesopotamia, probably in the sixth century AD. Again, we note reference to a ban on sexual exploitation and the need to maintain confidences. Much of the oath however is religious in character, the student urged to place his trust in God, the ultimate source of mercy and knowledge.

[†] Based on our chapter, Developing a code of ethics for psychiatry, in *Codes of ethics and the professions*, ed. M. Coady and S. Bloch. Melbourne, Melbourne University Press, pp. 193–225, 1996.

A similar emphasis on the Divine typifies the text on medical ethics by Haly Abbas,[6] a tenth century Persian physician. While revealing his respect for Hippocrates, Abbas urges the doctor to regard God as omniscient and thus as the fountainhead of wisdom. As with Hippocrates, the teacher must be revered and the needs of the following medical generation safeguarded. A benevolent, compassionate attitude is called for in treatment. More specific references are made, *inter alia*, to confidentiality, sexual exploitation, and continuing education.

Several centuries passed before the development of additional codes of medical ethics. In 1617, for example, Chen Shih-Kung,[7] a Chinese physician, incorporated a statement on medical ethics in his manual on surgery. He includes five 'commandments' united by the theme of respect for the dignity of patients. A more precise list of duties constitutes the ethical statement conceived in 1770 by the Persian, Mohamed Hosin Aghili.[8] Among the 23 duties are forerunners of contemporary ethical obligations in medicine. For instance, the doctor should consult a colleague if his expertise proves insufficient; he should not persist with an obviously ineffective remedy but consider applying an alternative; he should not impugn the reputation of fellow practitioners; and he should share his knowledge with the public at large (other obligations covered in previous codes are also included).

The most notable contribution to the codification of medical ethics since the Renaissance was undoubtedly made by the English physician, Thomas Percival. Because of his pivotal role as a source of contemporary medical ethical thinking, we need to examine carefully his *Code of institutes and precepts adapted to the professional conduct of physicians and surgeons*, published in 1803 and, in essence, a manual of medical ethics and etiquette.[9]

The provenance of the Code is of considerable interest. Percival, a noted physician, moralist, and devout Christian, was requested in 1791 to prepare a code of conduct to facilitate the resolution of a divisive conflict then raging in the Manchester Infirmary over who should ultimately be responsible for patient care. Within a few months, he had submitted a document which later comprised the first four chapters of his manual. Dealing with professional conduct in the hospital setting, this chapter is more akin to a code of practice than to a code of ethics (a distinction we explore later) but yet suffused with Judeo-Christian principles. In the dedication to his son, then a medical student, Percival refers to the wise man acting on 'determinate principles' and of the good man ensuring that these principles are 'conformable to rectitude and virtue'; several of the precepts themselves incorporate a religious dimension. The sixth, for example, states an important role for moral and religious influences in healing the sick and for their promotion in the hospital's milieu. Elsewhere, in a reference to the treatment of women with syphilis, Percival is forthright, even judgemental, in condemning 'immoderate passions and vicious indulgences'. However, he hastily complements this homily with an appeal to his colleagues to adopt benevolent principles, including forgiveness, 'favourable to reformation and to virtue'. (Interestingly, no mention is made in the document of male patients with syphilis.) In a more secular but still virtue-based vein, Percival urges his colleagues to assume a tender stance by responding as sensitively to patients' feelings as to their symptoms.

A substantial portion relates to issues of proper practice, even pointing out matters like the requirement for audit and quality assurance, e.g. the standard of drugs should be optimal (equally the quality of the wine used as medication!); wards should not be overcrowded; a hospital register should be maintained to record all variety of data in order to enhance 'medical science'; and the effectiveness of new treatments should be diligently monitored.

Given the Code's origin in a vehement disputation among the medical staff, it is not surprising that several precepts relate to intercollegiate matters. Thus, surgeons and physicians should acknowledge their respective areas of expertise, consult with one another about complicated cases, desist from impugning the reputation of colleagues, and respect the opinions of all medical staff including the most junior.

Relatively little attention is paid to duty-based principles which tend to be at the forefront of contemporary codes of ethics and which even had a place in ancient codes. For instance, confidentiality receives the briefest mention. This is perhaps attributable to pressure on Percival to ameliorate strained professional relationships; obligations to the patient were evidently subsidiary. Such imbalance is also reflected in the Code's unduly paternalistic character which even includes a reference to 'condescension with authority as to inspire the minds of the patients with gratitude, respect and confidence'. Furthermore, the patient is not entitled to select a physician of his own choice; devious practices to achieve such preference entails 'falsehood' on their part and 'produces unnecessary trouble' (presumably for the medical establishment and the hospital bureaucracy). In a thoughtful essay, Edmund Pellegrino[10] concedes that grounds do exist for levelling criticism against Percival's protective posture of his profession and the corresponding scant regard for patient autonomy; the arguments of notable commentators like Jay Katz[11] and Veatch[12] are introduced as a part of the appraisal of Percival's contribution. In his summation, Pellegrino generously suggests that Percival's chief accomplishment was in devising a novel approach to the prevention and management of professional conflict. He reminds us that Percival neither set out to produce a treatise on medical ethics nor claimed expertise in formal ethical reasoning. Rather, as a devout Christian, he regarded Judeo-Christian tenets as central to proper practice. Thus, in his *Medical ethics*, necessarily virtue-based, the thrust is the 'ineradicability of the physician's character as guarantor of the patient's good and welfare'. The corollary is clear: one is a good physician because one is a good person.

We commented earlier upon the dialectic of virtue versus duty as a primary integrating concept in the codification of ethical practice in medicine and will return to this theme. In the interim we may conveniently quote Pellegrino[10] in his assessment of Percival's work and its context:

Percival teaches us how a virtuous man of the 18th century ought to interpret his obligations to his patients, his hospital and his society. We know how different is our cultural and social milieu from his. To suggest a resuscitation of all of Percival's axioms would be a sentimental anachronism at best, and a dangerous reinforcement of some of medicine's less admirable tendencies.

Yet beneath the emphasis on intra-professional relationships, and the emphasis on how a Christian gentleman should behave, there is a viable ethic, many of whose elements are neither time nor culture-bound. It is the lesson of this ethic and its call to personal virtue and character that a 18th century physician can teach us.

Percival—a bridge to the twentieth century

Reference to time and culture is a convenient springboard to chart developments in codes of medical ethics during the rest of the nineteenth and in the twentieth centuries. One key event was the establishment of the American Medical Association (AMA) in 1847 and its adoption that year of a code derived from Percival.[13] It focused on the disarray in which American medicine found itself. With legislation on registration and regulation muddled, the patient encountered a variety of practitioners all of whom claimed expertise but among whom were quacks and charlatans. The formidable task facing the AMA was to ferret out pseudo-practitioners and so enable properly trained doctors to represent the profession.

A principle purpose of the Code therefore was to reflect a decent standard of American medicine and inspire the public's confidence in it. Subsequently, when statutory measures displaced this purpose, the code served as a duty-based document with a sharper focus on the patient and a more pronounced ethical foundation. The current version has been condensed to seven principles, with annotations, concerned with the respect for the patient's dignity, confidentiality, continuing medical education, the education of the public, and medicine's contribution to an improved community.

A century elapsed before a further key development, the Nuremberg medical trials (*US* v. *Karl Brandt et al.*, 1946).[14,15] The Tribunal's decision included a pioneering statement of principles relevant to research on human beings which centred on the process of informed consent and a notion that the anticipated results of research should justify its execution. Although confined to medical research the statement's mere existence coupled with awareness of the horrific medical crimes paved the way for the creation of the World Medical Association (WMA), designed to enhance ethical standards of clinical and research practice.

As in the case of the AMA's production of a code as a first task, so the WMA produced, in 1948, the *Declaration of Geneva* (see Appendix). The document is a contemporary version of the Oath of Hippocrates, emphasizing such aspects as respect for teachers and colleagues and treatment of patients without consideration of religion, race, nationality, or sociopolitical status. A year later, the WMA produced a more typically duty-oriented code which called on doctors to maintain the highest standard of professional conduct, and to avoid a series of practices deemed unethical. Rather revealingly, the authors seemed as preoccupied with pragmatic issues like fees and self-advertisement as they did with ethical aspects such as confidentiality and interprofessional respect.

In the wake of the WMA's efforts, many national medical associations devised codes for their own membership. For example the Australian Medical Association produced a code in 1964, the Soviet Union in 1971.

Specific codes for psychiatrists

As part of these national developments, a small number of psychiatric organizations became aware of the particular ethical dilemmas encountered by their members, but it was not until 1973 that the first code specific to psychiatry was produced, by the American Psychiatric Association (APA).[16] Three years earlier, the APA had requested its Ethics Committee to devise a code suited to psychiatrists. The AMA however insisted that psychiatrists, as medical practitioners, were bound by its ethical principles. Thus the APA could supplement but not subtract from those principles. The AMA had set a precedent by incorporating into its Code a series of annotations, including vignettes of ethical violation, derived from case studies. The APA followed suit, devising a set of new annotations 'especially applicable to psychiatry'.

The Canadian Psychiatric Association (CPA),[17] in a comparable procedure, applied the Canadian Medical Association's Code of Ethics as a source of ethical principles for its Code, adding annotations along the lines of the APA.

These initiatives were atypical of the psychiatric profession as a whole, other national psychiatric organizations ostensibly not yet prepared, for reasons about which we can only speculate, to imitate their North American counterparts. Developments within the World Psychiatric Association (WPA), the main international body, in the mid-1970s may account for the minimal level of activity at a national level. A WPA conference on ethical aspects of psychiatry was convened in 1976 in London, the first of its kind. There, Clarence Blomquist,[18] Professor of Medical Ethics at the Karolinska Institute in Stockholm, provided an historical context for the question of whether and how the WPA should adopt an international code expressly for psychiatrists. This erudite contribution paved the way for a code launched a year later at the WPA's World Congress in Honolulu.

The *Declaration of Hawaii* (see Appendix) consists of guidelines deemed to be the minimal requirements for ethical standards in psychiatry. The declaration is mostly duty-based with the psychiatrist urged to: serve the best interests of the patient; offer the best available treatment; obtain informed consent before performing a procedure or treatment; apply professional skills and knowledge only for legitimate diagnostic and therapeutic purposes (the Soviet misuse of psychiatry for political purpose whereby mentally-well, political and religious dissenters in the former USSR were confined to mental hospitals as a state-inspired means to suppress dissent was much to the forefront at the time);[19] preserve the patient's confidences; and obtain informed consent when requesting a patient's participation in teaching.

A number of clinical circumstances were highlighted to which the psychiatrist had to pay heed: the patient's incompetence by virtue of mental illness to provide informed consent; the vulnerability of psychiatry to political or other forms of misuse; and the possibility of a non-therapeutic relationship such as an assessor in forensic psychiatry.

Although a laudable initiative, the *Declaration of Hawaii* was, and remains, relatively inaccessible for the vast majority of psychiatrists. The reason is straightforward. Since the WPA comprises member societies rather than individual members, and the Code has not been incorporated into the statutes of national psychiatric bodies, it would not have been readily obtainable even by the interested psychiatrist.

Notwithstanding, the APA and CPA have been joined by only a minuscule number of other national groups since Honolulu, including the Royal Australian and New Zealand College of Psychiatrists[20] and the Russian Society of Psychiatrists.[21]

With this historical sketch in mind, we move to a conceptual level by considering the chief potential purposes of codes in psychiatry (many points however apply to medicine in general).

Potential purpose of codes of ethics in psychiatry

We can differentiate from our historical overview four principal purposes, namely:

(1) to protect and promote the professional status of psychiatrists;

(2) as an intrinsic part of a process of self-regulation;

(3) to sensitize psychiatrists to the ethical dimension of their work; and

(4) to serve as a tool in professional education.

Although not mutually incompatible, it is apparent through an examination of codes of ethics in medicine that an emphasis on any one purpose tends to be associated with a de-emphasis of the other three; this applies particularly to the first and second categories. Let us consider each in turn.

In a code principally designed *to protect and promote the welfare of the profession* for which it has been devised, the tendency is for a guild-based instrument whereby the members determine paternalistically and independently of patients' interests, the nature and scope of their obligations. An element of condescension is inherent here, a sense that the doctor knows best. This is well epitomized, for instance, in Percival's[9] code when he actually deploys the term 'condescension' coupling it with authority. These qualities purportedly inspire patients to feel confident and respectful of their doctors. As noted earlier, a similar sense of paternalism pervades the Oath of Hippocrates.

A code of this kind is usually regarded in one of two diametrically opposed ways—either as self-serving or as a means of binding a group of professionals into a cohesive force. The two positions can be summarized in the following way. The critic would claim, along with George Bernard Shaw, that: 'All professions are conspiracies against the laity'. Thus, with the professional's foremost priority the preservation of status and power, a code of ethics is only relevant in so far as it assists in fulfilling this requirement. Any reference to patients is incidental to the doctor's self-interest. Patients are infantilized in this model, permitted a slender role in assuming responsibility for their welfare. They are deprived in particular of a voice in medical decision-making which is regarded by the guild-oriented codifier as a professionally driven obligation. Jay Katz[11] in his influential treatise on the doctor–patient relationship has highlighted what he avers are the asymmetrical features of this association and their deleterious effect on the medical profession.

A contrary view, enshrined in almost all codes prior to the Nuremberg period, reflects the profession's view of itself as the embodiment of a noble tradition of commitment and dedication. Medicine is not simply an occupation but a life-long participation in a process of professing skills and ensuring corresponding expertise is maintained. As Everett Hughes[22] points out:

Professionals profess. They profess to know better than others the nature of certain matters, and to know better than their clients what ails them or their affairs. This is the essence of the professional idea and the professional claim. Since the professional does profess he asks that he be trusted. ... The client is to trust the professional; he must tell him all such secrets which bear upon the affairs at hand. He must trust his judgement and skill. In return, the professional asks protection from any unfortunate consequences of his professional actions; he and his fellows make it very difficult for anyone outside—even civil courts—to pass judgement upon one of their number. Only the professional can say when his colleague makes a mistake.

In these latter comments, Hughes introduces an essential dimension of the profession as self-protective. In his essay from which the above quote is taken, he elaborates on this theme when referring the professional's crucial need for 'close solidarity' and a sharing of an 'ethos of its own'. In this context, we can reiterate a point made earlier about life-long commitment and dedication.

In terms of codes which parallel this position, the pre-eminent features is a vow to establish a covenant with the profession itself and thus with fellow members. As we saw in the historical section, this is precisely what the ancient codes stressed; the pertinent passage of the Oath of Hippocrates[2] is clearly illustrative:

To hold him who has taught me this art as an equal to my parents and to live my life in partnership with him, and if he is in need of money to give him a share of mine, and to regard his offspring as equal to my brothers in male lineage and to teach them this art— if they desire to learn it—without fee and covenant; to give a share of precepts and oral instruction and all the other learning to my sons and to the sons of him who has instructed and to pupils who have signed the covenant and have taken an oath according to the medical law, but to no one else.

The aforementioned comments concerning professional solidarity, a particular ethos and an advantageous positions to detect the peer who has erred also relate to the second potential purpose of a code of ethics, as part of the processes of self-regulation. Typically the professional prizes autonomy in all facets of his endeavours. In psychiatry, this includes clinical freedom, namely the capacity to exercise professional judgement independently albeit in tandem with accepted conventions of clinical practice.[23] Clinical initiatives are valued provided they are not so idiosyncratic as to jeopardise proper standards of care.[24] A related freedom enables the practitioner to entertain novel possibilities whether in the realm of theory or clinical application. In similar vein, research is esteemed as a pivotal means to develop and enhance skill and expertise.

These freedoms are, however, subject to constraints from within the profession. Solidarity calls for allegiance to specified norms and commitment to mutual respect. Members who behave deviantly disrupt the cohesiveness of the group. Their actions need to be curtailed lest they harm peers.

In making these comments in this way, we are aware of an implicit value judgement which echoes the earlier criticism levelled against the medical profession as predominantly self-interested. And indeed, it can be said that a code aids a self-regulating process to prevent the profession's exposure to sanctions by external authorities like statutory bodies, government bureaucracies, and the civil courts.[25]

Contrastingly a positively connoted view holds that self-regulation linked to a code contributes to the protection of the patient rather than the corporate group. The code encapsulates duties regarded as central to proper clinical practice. Such a duty-driven document, in contrast to a virtue-based one, purportedly provides guidelines to the profession but stops short of being unduly prescriptive or restrictive. Standards of practice can even be enhanced through the application of a code coupled with self-regulation by demanding more of the doctor than mere compliance with a set of legal rules or regulations.

As Pellegrino suggests,[26] standards for judging professional behaviour range along a continuum from least to most stringent. A code has the potential to elevate standards from a minimalist ethics in which the sole constraint is a set of legal rules to a more rigorous level. Ethical principles and associated moral rules, both code-derived, call for a higher level of moral commitment— to an intermediate standard in Pellegrino's classification. The most demanding standards exceed this intermediate level by requiring the fulfilment of a virtue-based ethical code; thus beneficence supplements duty, even to the point of personal cost, and altruism supplants self-interest.

The corollary of this range of possibilities, in the context of self-regulation, is the balance between duty and virtue encompassed in a code. At first sight, it would appear as if a combination is most preferable. Further reflection however reveals a potential disharmony in that duty-based code enjoins the professional to comply with what amounts to a set of guidelines, whereas a virtue-based code signals the desiderata of certain qualities like compassion, honesty and benevolence, each of which however resists ready definition and characterization. Virtue is a complex matter which has long exercised and challenged the greatest of minds. Even Plato[27] was obliged to resort to a rhetorical question when tackling it in the Meno:

Can you tell me, Socrates, whether virtue is acquired by teaching or by practice; or if neither by teaching nor practice, then whether it comes to man by nature or in what other way?

This brief discussion of virtue serves to introduce the third possible purpose of a code, its capacity to *promote moral sensitivity*. A sensitizing role combined with a structuring one (the clarification of moral issues arising in practice) are defined by Clouser[28] as basic to all codes. Use of the phrase 'moral sensitivity' is intentional in that it obviates the snag of how to handle the concept of virtue. By moral sensitivity we refer to a state of receptiveness in which professionals are open to impressions of an ethical kind through an alertness to moral quandaries inherent in their task. These quandaries necessarily exercise 'clinico-ethical consciousness' although their impact may range from negligible to profound, depending on various personal and situational factors.

A code may raise the level of moral sensitivity through at least two mechanisms: (a) its actual existence influences the professional in a non-specific fashion by acting as a regular prod in the event of a discomforting or baffling clinical encounter which encompasses a moral dimension; and (b) aspects of a code's content, certainly for psychiatrists, are bound to resonate with their experience of such critical issues as involuntary hospitalization, preventing suicide, occupying ambiguous roles as in forensic psychiatry, and obtaining informed consent in the case of the incompetent patient.[29]

Thus, Michels and Kelly (see Chapter 24) in their chapter on teaching psychiatric ethics refer to an attitude-related goal whereby trainees become sensitized to the ethical aspects of their task that might otherwise be construed as scientific or technical. In the same vein, Thompson[30] specifies the need to promote sensitivity and awareness of moral complexity in clinical practice. These authors highlight the centrality of professionals' (trainee and trained) active experiencing of, and involvement with the ethical dimension of their practice, and regard this as a necessary though not sufficient aspect of the ethically minded person. Lacking in the moral sensitizing function are other components equally important in a moral framework, namely moral reasoning, moral decision-making and corresponding action.[31] The final purpose of a code as an *educational* tool in psychiatric ethics is to contribute to an understanding of these three components. Although codes generally steer clear of didacticism, study of their principles may enable an appreciation that even complex moral problems are subject to systematic, critical analysis.[32] Thus, students can learn to arrive at moral decisions by rational argument, justifying their premises and views.[33] Through a code, students also may become acquainted with salient concepts in moral philosophy which constitute a basis for ethical reasoning.

Codes containing detailed annotations such as those of the APA and the RANZCP can further serve the educational process by demonstrating the vulnerability of even the most lofty principles, leading to their necessarily varied application and, in some circumstances, to their inappropriate use, e.g. when two principles collide.

Pari passu, the psychiatrist may learn how to recognize the utility of a code by considering how a specific ethical quandary encountered in practice is handled by the principles and annotations comprising the code. Although a code may influence psychiatrists in their day-to-day moral decision-making, the fulfilment of the sensitizing and educational functions as outlined is only likely to take place when the corporate group stresses the pivotal place of a code in its ethos. This may occur either implicitly or through an emphasis on ethics in training and subsequent continuing education.

Forms of codes

Codes can take various forms but these can be reduced to covenants (oaths are essentially similar), codes of practice, codes of conduct, and codes of ethics.

The best known example of a covenant is the Hippocratic Oath, restated in modern form in the *Declaration of Geneva*. Codes may also be declaratory as exemplified by the WMA's series of declarations—*Geneva* on medical practice (1948) (see Appendix), *Helsinki* on clinical research (1964) (see Appendix), *Oslo* on therapeutic abortion (1970), *Sydney* on determination of death (1968), and *Tokyo* on torture (1975).

The form may be determined by its implicit purpose; this may be virtue-driven (usually in covenants and oaths), reactive and deterrent (e.g. the Nuremberg trial statement), or duty-driven as in procedural and regulatory codes. Most codes infer or state principles of which those relating to patient care and professional integrity constitute the core. Additionally, codes variously cover duties to society, disciplinary procedures, and, increasingly and more specifically, the protection of 'consumers' (patients). The spectrum on which they may be primarily constructed range from giving space to the virtuous to the deterrence of potential offenders.

From this account we are able to differentiate two approaches to the codi-fication of valued professional behaviour—what we may refer to as genuine

ethical codes and codes of conduct or practice (these latter terms are synonymous for our purposes). Having previously touched on the former we can
summarize their essential features as follows: codes of ethics, which include
inter alia covenants, oaths, declarations, and sets of principles, are rooted in
tenets of moral philosophy. Whatever the balance between virtue and duty,
moral precepts are at the heart of such codes. In the case of duty, obligations
and responsibilities are ethically grounded.

Consider the duty to preserve a patient's confidences. This derives from the
principle of respect for privacy; the doctor keeps the patient's secrets out of
an obligation to safeguard his right not to have his world intruded upon.
In deontological terms, respect for privacy is linked closely to respect for
autonomy and both are regarded as fundamental moral requirements. For the
consequentialist, as Gillon[34] aptly summarizes, confidentiality is predicated on
the notion that:

> ... people's better health, welfare, the general good, and overall happiness are more
> likely to be attained if doctors are fully informed by their patients, and this is more likely
> if doctors undertake not to disclose their patients' secrets. Conversely, if patients did
> not believe that doctors would keep their secrets then either they would not divulge
> embarrassing but potentially medical important information, thus reducing their
> chances of getting the best medical care, or they would disclose such information and
> feel anxious and unhappy at the prospect of their secrets being made known.

Even when pragmatic implications are woven into code with an associated prescriptive quality, their source remains the original moral requirement.
Thus, in the case of confidentiality, the code may incorporate complex
qualifications including the need to breach confidentiality; but the annotations do not detract from the moral framework within which they arise (we
return to confidentiality in order to demonstrate the form of code selected by
the RANZCP).

A code of practice (or conduct) contrasts sharply with a code of ethics in
respect to points made in preceding paragraphs. Although the objectives of the
two forms of code may be similar—to promote good professional conduct—
their premises differ. In the case of a code of practice, moral principles *per se*
are not fundamental to its construction or compliance although they may
feature implicity. Instead, a code of practice assumes a prominent pragmatic
function, comprising a set of rules or regulations or standards 'designed to
control behaviour, products and procedures within a particular ... area of
activity'.[35]

In the area of mental health, for instance, the professional may be offered
specific guidelines as to how he should pursue his task. The boundaries
between clinical guidelines (as might be embodied in a quality assurance
programme), rules, regulations, and standards to be achieved tend to be
blurred. A compounding factor is the legal status of the code. On the one hand,
a professional group might determine in an entirely voluntary way that a code

of practice suits its requirements for setting and maintaining standards; on the other hand, the code may be imposed by an external body through legal or quasi-legal means.

Two examples will illuminate these various possibilities. A code of practice was laid before the British Parliament in 1989 pursuant to the 1983 Mental Health Act.[36] The code was indeed foreshadowed in the 1983 legislation inasmuch as a health commission was required to ensure the psychiatric profession's proper implementation of the Mental Health Act. Accordingly, the code is devised particularly with the object of addressing elements of the Act. Take personal searches as illustrative. The code contains four statements on conducting a search of a patient; these are of rules and guidelines but are wedded to provisions in the Act. Thus, authorities should ensure the development of a legally validated operational policy; a search, if on lawful grounds, should occur with a patient's consent and have 'due regard for [his] dignity'; if consent is not given, a search should be legally justified and 'should be carried out with the minimum force necessary . . .'; and the patient should be informed about the location of belongings removed from him. As can be noted, the requirements for certain practices are stipulated precisely and have a legal flavour, but the legal dimension of the code overall is left ambiguous. The psychiatrist has only the following crucial introductory statement as a signpost: 'This Act [the 1983 Mental Health Act] does not impose a legal duty to comply with the Code but failure to follow the Code could be referred to in evidence in legal proceedings.'

Unlike the preceding example, a code of practice may be adopted voluntarily by a professional body as a means of setting certain standards for its members. The body may then extend this function by linking the code to an internal disciplinary procedure. The Australian Psychological Society (APS)[37] exemplifies this model in its 'Code of professional conduct' (adopted in 1968 with subsequent revisions in 1986, 1990 1994, and 1997). The APS's Committee on Ethical and Professional Standards bears the responsibility for dealing with complaints against a member whether initiated by a consumer, a colleague or a member of another professional body. In this context, the Code is 'involved', i.e. the complainant specifies that one (or more) of its provisions 'has been or is being violated'. No doubt because of this quasi-judicial quality the Code's principles are elaborated upon in considerable detail and are prescriptive. For instance, the psychologist is provided with nine firm guidelines concerning assessments procedures with clients, 15 referable to the consulting relationship, 11 for conducting research, and so on.

This foray into the different forms that codes can take reveals the multiple purposes to which they can be put, ranging from a set of 'motherhood is good' statements to a quasi-legal document. With this aspect of codes and preceding sections on an historical context and a conceptual framework dealt with, we are now in a position to illustrate these facets by examining the RANZCP's Code of Ethics.

The RANZCP's code as illustrative

As we have seen an historical and a philosophical approach applied to codes of ethics are valuable for their illumination and comprehension. The opportunity follows to appraise critically the principles formulated and their con-temporaneous application. The shaping of abstract principles by pragmatic considerations is no better revealed than in ethics as applied to psychiatry. In the following section we illustrate, using the RANZCP's code, the process whereby skeletal principles are fleshed out with the substance that typifies clinical practice with all its doubts dilemmas, and human frailties.

The concept underlying the code of ethics created specifically for Australasian psychiatrists not only derives from the need to re-emphasize the bond between psychiatry as a branch of medicine and the medical profession as a whole but also to explicate ethical aspects of particular significance to psychiatrists. Alongside these considerations there is a need to provide a clear guide to psychiatrists in an increasingly complex and rapidly changing society. Codes in the distant past were relatively simple: an exhortatory statement of principles whose implementation were clear-cut. The Renaissance, and the agricultural, industrial, political, and technological revolutions have all contributed to a society in which application of ethics in all fields, and certainly including psychiatry, has become so complicated that codes have had to be extended to cover the many situations that arise—and even then often serve only to clarify the dilemmas rather than to resolve them.[38]

The opportunity to understand the rationale and purpose of a code was provided fortuitously by the governing council of the RANZCP when it requested its Ethics Committee in 1990 to formulate a code of ethics. Until then the College had relied upon the non-specific code of the Australian Medical Association and was also guided, albeit at a distance, by the more specific 'Principles of medical ethics with annotations especially applicable to psychiatry' of the APA (see Appendix).[16]

Underlying reasons for the decision are difficult to pinpoint but several factors probably influenced the College. The interface between profession and society had come under critical scrutiny reflecting on the values and integrity of psychiatrists individually and inevitably on the profession as a whole. It had become clear that the codes on which the College had relied no longer fulfiled the function of giving psychiatrists unambiguous guidelines in areas relevant to their speciality. This unease at the College's lack of a specific code may well have been related to the notorious Chelmsford Hospital 'deep sleep' therapy cases which first surfaced officially in 1980. Several patients died either as a result of this outmoded treatment or through suicide in the immediate after-math of being a patient at Chelmsford. During the subsequent painfully slow and intermittent progress of the numerous complaints, allegations, and trials culminating in a Royal commission,[39] an enduring thread of accusation un-ravelled against the profession as represented by the College; its members felt disadvantaged in not having a specific document with which it could defend itself. Other concerns sprouted on this seed-bed of discomforture, in particular accusations of sexual impropriety of psychiatrists towards their patients. In the State of New South Wales a statutory Health Complaints Unit pursued these matters vigorously, eventually passing them on to the State's Medical Board. Here a number of cases were proven and the offending psychiatrists deregistered.

In addition the College was concerned by the number of members brought to its attention who seemed confused about or unaware of a psychiatrist's ethical obligations. It was noted that sister professions such as psychology already had codes. The formation of a body to monitor clinical activities of the College fellows, including continuing medical education and quality assurance, resulted in the creation of a Board of Practice Standards; this group required a clearly articulated ethical base on which to function. In the face of the community's apparent loss of confidence in the profession and pressures for internal re-organization, a code was as necessary a foundation as the RANZCP's revision of its basic objectives. The task fell naturally to the Ethics Committee which over many years had prepared a series of ethical guidelines but whose moral source derived from various documents of comparable institutions and organisations such as the Australian Medical Association, the APA, and the WPA.

Paradoxically, in determining the nature of a code, the Ethics Committee had to consider what it was not. As we discussed earlier, there are several contenders in the field comprising codes of practice (e.g. Department of Health, Mental Health Act 1983)[36] and codes of conduct (e.g. Australian Pharmaceutical Manufacturers Association).[40] In examining these documents the committee appreciated their links to ethical principles but concluded that these were not explicitly articulated and the codes tended to be regulatory with a marked disciplinary overtone. The committee also noted that some professions are more readily regulated than others. Psychiatry, dealing as it does with the vagaries of human behaviour, requires that professional judgement be given greater latitude whilst ensuring at the same time that ethical principles are rigorously adhered to.

Although an Objective of the College's Memorandum and Articles of Association[41]

To cultivate and maintain high principles and standards of practice and ethics in respect of psychiatry, to promote fair, honourable and proper practice and discourage and suppress malpractice or misconduct therein, to settle doubtful points of practice and questions of professional usage, to protect the honour, good reputation, interests and work of the College, to consider complaints against members or associates, to define the grounds upon which a member or associate may be expelled, suspended or subjected to other disciplinary measures and to establish procedures for expelling, suspending or otherwise disciplining members and associates whether consequent upon a complaint or otherwise refers broadly to ethical and disciplinary aspects, the governing council had clearly distinguished between these by establishing a new body, the Professional Conduct Committee (PCC) (quite separate from the Ethics Committee). Until the advent of the PCC the Ethics Committee had functioned at times as a *de facto* complaints body in its advisory role. It was this experience that deterred the Committee from selecting a regulatory type of code, clearly separating ethical guidelines from the procedure of their implementation including where necessary by disciplinary action.

In trying to achieve the practice of high-quality psychiatry the College had to ensure a balance between the competing elements of compassion, competence, efficiency, and effectiveness. It would be an error to assume that any one of these represents ethics. In this respect other arms of the College deal with clinical standards, competence and effectiveness. These considerations and structure influenced the Ethics Committee only to include in the Code general indications of those ethical obligations which would ensure that various aspects of practice referred to were addressed while, at the same time, retaining clinical relevance. This illustrates an ever-present tension in the committee's deliberations—to formulate a code which was not minimalist in its expectations yet was not so aspirational as to have little application to day-to-day practice. Although pragmatic these principles initially drove the committee's reasoning rather than a systematic study of moral philosophy.

The Ethics Committee's procedure

Having established this provisional rationale the committee created a framework in 1992 on which the code was to be devised. The model of the APA (*The principles of medical ethics with annotations especially applicable to psychiatry*)[16] was adopted, comprising a preamble, a statement of principle, and annotations to each of the principles which enlarge upon their relevance to diverse aspects of clinical practice. A total of 14 principles under three headings, relating to patient, psychiatrist, and society, were formulated; as the annotations were critically developed the headings were deleted and the principles reduced from 14 to 9, without loss of point or purpose.

To illustrate the way the committee pursued these tasks, we focus on the principle and annotations of confidentiality (see Table 6.1) as they reflect well the changing interface between a principle and its application in a world where technology and societal demands create uncertainty. The principle was formulated without difficulty having been a feature of all codes since Hippocrates.[2] In keeping with our determination to distil principles into succinct yet clear statements, that on confidentiality was reduced to the bare essentials. This principle is considerably shorter than the Hippocratic injunction and the language less arcane than in the *Declaration of Geneva* (see Appendix). The principle lost its prominence in the *Declaration of Hawaii* (see Appendix) by becoming entangled in several related issues. Instead, these are reflected in nine annotations with references to problems raised by technology, the changing

Table 6.1   Principle three

Psychiatrists shall hold information about the patient in confidence.

1   In the face of the complex and extensive organisational structure of contemporary psychiatric practice, the widespread use of photocopied material and facsimile, computerised clinical records and data banks, the increased demand for accountability from various sources, and the highly personal and sensitive nature of the information obtained from patients, psychiatrists are obliged to respect their patient's right to confidentiality and to safeguard all information associated with the psychiatrist–patient relationship.

2   Confidentiality cannot always be absolute. A careful balance must be maintained between preserving confidentiality as a fundamental aspect of clinical practice and the need to breach it on rare occasions in order to promote the patient's optimal interests and care, and/or the safety or other significant interests of third parties.

3   It is reasonable that clinical information, including case notes, may need to be shared with colleagues and other health professionals in order to provide optimal care and treatment (for example between clinical members of a multidisciplinary team or when a second opinion is sought). Wherever possible, the patient should be informed carefully regarding the limits of confidentiality, as part of the process of obtaining consent. In special circumstances, where the patient is incapable of understanding the concept of confidentiality and its limits (for example the severely mentally ill, the elderly, mentally infirm, and young children), consent should be obtained, if possible, from the patient's relatives or guardian. Psychiatrists may need to impress on other professionals with whom they share information about a patient that the ethical requirement for confidentiality is fundamental to proper medical practice.

4   Information about the patient obtained from other sources (for example relatives, friends, employer, teacher) is subject to the same principles of confidentiality as information obtained from the patient.

5   Whilst upholding the principle of confidentiality, psychiatrists must do so within the constraints of the law and with regard to statutory requirements. Psychiatrists may reasonably question the need for disclosure or may argue for limited disclosure, namely of only that information they regard as relevant. Disclosure is, however, mandatory under legal compulsion and psychiatrists, as well as their clinical records, are compellable witnesses and in the statutory context, subject to legislative requirements (for example reporting of child abuse or unfitness to drive a motor vehicle).

6   Psychiatrists may be released from their duty to maintain confidentiality if they become aware of, and are unable to influence, their patient's intention to seriously harm an identified person or group of persons. In these circumstances, psychiatrists may have an overriding duty to the public interest by informing either the intended victim(s), the relevant authorities, or both, about the threat.

7   In situations where psychiatrists do breach confidentiality and disclose information about their patients, they have an obligation to justify their actions.

8   If required to disclose information, psychiatrists shall as far as possible divulge only that information relevant to the case at hand, avoid highly sensitive and personal speculation, and take care to separate factual information from opinion.

9   The principle of safeguarding patients' confidences applies regardless of whether the psychiatrist–patient relationship has ceased or the patient has died, except in specific circumstances such as a relative's need to identify an hereditary risk.

---

nature of psychiatry with its multidisciplinary approach, and the legal requirement from statutory and quasi-statutory bodies to breach confidentiality.

A code cannot satisfy all

It is unlikely that any code of ethics will be universally satisfactory or even
acceptable—as for instance in the dilemma of a psychiatrist operating under
archaic law and the issue of misuse of professional knowledge and skill, should
he have to participate in a procedure deemed cruel and degrading in other
cultures (Principle 5 Annotations 4 and 5 (see Table 6.2)). The issue also
arises as to the applicability of a national code to members practising in
another country with, perhaps, an entirely distinctive culture and legal
framework.

Table 6.2   Principle five

Psychiatrists shall not allow the misuse of their professional knowledge and skills.

4   Whatever the legal circumstances, psychiatrists shall not participate, either directly
    or indirectly, in the practice of torture or other forms of cruel, inhuman or degrading
    punishment (see *Declaration of Tokyo*, 1975).

5   Psychiatrists shall not participate in executions.

The possible conflict between the disciplinary repercussions of a breach of
the Code and the doctrine of natural justice was at the seat of one of the
most controversial aspects of the Code. That is to what extent, if any, a code
should encroach upon the personal life of a person subject to that code.
The Code clearly does so in Principle 7, Annotations 1, 3, and 4 and Principle 1, Annotation 5 (see Table 6.3). These tensions arose because Principle 7
(and its annotations) is the most virtue-based of all, whereas others are more
duty-driven. Virtue here smacks of elitism which sits ill with the prevailing
ethos (at least in Western countries) of egalitarianism. Nevertheless, it is
difficult to gainsay the aphorism: 'Virtue is not defined by conformity to ethical
principles, but it is virtue that determines the goodness of the principles'.
Debate about the part personal values should play within a professional
context is unlikely to end, indeed it would be a matter of grave concern if it
did so.

Most doctors would accept that sanctions should apply to personal
behaviour which might impair patient care. There is less agreement in the
more hazy area of personal behaviour which might bring the profession into
disrepute. Obviously the moral obloquy of such behaviour will be determined
by the values and mores of the culture in which it occurs. These and other

Table 6.3 Principles seven and one

Principle seven

Psychiatrists shall share the responsibility of upholding the integrity of the medical profession.

1 Psychiatry as an integral part of the medical profession demands integrity, dedication for truth and service to mankind. Psychiatrists have a privileged position because of their calling and tradition. With such privilege they have an obligation to maintain appropriate personal and moral standards in their professional practice, and in those aspects of their personal life which may reflect upon the integrity of the medical profession.

3 Psychiatrists who become aware of a colleague's ill-health compromising the care of patients have an urgent duty to those patients and their colleague to see that the situation is appropriately dealt with. The necessary action may include an offer to assist the ill colleague and notification to relevant hospital authorities, employers and the medical registration body. It is advisable, when practicable, to consult with a senior colleague before deciding on the most appropriate action.

4 Psychiatrists who become aware of unprofessional conduct by a colleague shall take appropriate action; this may include a report to the relevant authorities.

Principle one

Psychiatrists shall have respect for the essential humanity and dignity of each of their patients.

5 Sexual relationships between psychiatrists and their patients are always unethical.

considerations acknowledge the fact that a code is a dynamic document and reinforces the imperative that it should be amended as necessary in the light of changes in the profession, society, and their interface. Mechanisms in the RANZCP ensure this occurs. A standing policy requires that all documents are periodically reviewed. In addition, to ensure the review is comprehensive and informed rather than a mere ritualistic exercise, the Ethics Committee has adopted a procedure whereby the Code's content is monitored regularly. At the time of writing, the Code is under revision, its completion scheduled for late 1998.

Second, the Ethics Committee in association with other committees promotes the established process of preparing specific ethical guidelines (six at the time of writing). Thus, whatever area of practice members are involved in, they have ready access to detailed, updated ethical guidelines.

Codes in practice

Since the introduction of the Code the Ethics Committee has applied its principles regularly, in the context of opinions it has been called upon to prepare by the College. Moreover, the Code's availability has facilitated the committee's judgements most effectively; indeed, members have wondered how they ever managed without it. The committee's reports cite particular principles and annotations as the representative summarized examples below demonstrate. They deal with issues in the three identifiable spheres of the committee's deliberations, namely ethical dimensions of clinical practice, forensic psychiatry, and teaching and supervision.

1. The administration of the atypical antipsychotic drug, clozapine, to involuntary patients serves well to illustrate the sphere of clinical practice. The issue here was the conflict between overriding a detained patient's refusal to provide consent to a treatment of proven value but with a small but definite lethal risk. The inquiring clinician, unable to obtain a clear answer from other professional sources, turned to the committee who responded within the framework of the Code. First invoked was Principle 1 ('Psychiatrists shall have respect for the essential humanity and dignity of each of their patients') whose relevant annotation deals with psychiatrists' statutory role in compulsory treatment and associated responsibility to relieve suffering of those whose autonomy is impaired. The second principle, that psychiatrists 'shall provide the best possible care for their patients', focused on its annotation of an obligation to consider the relative benefits and risks of all available treatments.

The fourth principle, dealing with informed consent, covers an incompetent patient's inability to give it and allowance for the substitution of a statutory agent, in this case a consultant psychiatrist. Furthermore, psychiatrists are enjoined in another annotation to exercise great care when there are questions of consent to a hazardous procedure or treatment. A final pertinent annotation outlines the circumstances in which consent can be waived, particularly when the patient is incompetent to judge.

Indeed, with these significant annotations in mind, the committee concluded that it would be unethical not to consider using what appeared to be the best possible treatment in the clinical circumstance.

2. Another issue requiring an opinion was the controversial one of a psychiatrist's participation in a judicial process which could lead to execution. The statements in the code that 'Psychiatrists shall not participate in executions' and 'Psychiatrists shall not allow the misuse of their professional knowledge and skills' were cited, although the ambiguity of the notion of 'participation' was acknowledged. Contribution by way of pre-trial assessment and providing evidence was ethically acceptable given all the above safeguards. But once an offender had been sentenced to death and then became mentally ill the dilemma was obvious, and its remedy elusive; however, this was dealt with, at least in part, by the principle that 'Psychiatrists shall have respect for the essential humanity and dignity of their patients'.

3. The potential for exploitation in a teaching situation was raised by a College training committee, the gist being whether the then more clearly defined nature of boundary violations between psychiatrists and patients should be applied when a supervisor and trainee entered into an intimate relationship. Although the Code did not refer to the dilemma, its seventh principle, that 'Psychiatrists shall share the responsibility of upholding the integrity of the medical profession', was pertinent. Moreover, two annotations enlarged on that duty by enjoining psychiatrists to 'maintain appropriate

personal and moral standards in those aspects of their personal life which may reflect upon the medical profession'. The other referred to the need to foster a sense of trust and mutual responsibility between colleagues. Although supervisor and trainee might be mature professionals, and no overt sexual harassment had occurred, the association could never be one between equals; there was always a potential for exploitation which could jeopardize the relationship. That such an association would be unethical was determined on three grounds: betrayal of a fiduciary (i.e. trustworthy), relationship, bringing the profession into disrepute, and being inimical to good patient care.

Given these principles the committee advised that the relationship described by the training committee was unethical. Moreover, it recommended that the attention of supervisor and trainee be drawn, through a process of counselling, to their obligations to adhere to the Code of Ethics.

Conclusion

The above illustrations,[42] three of dozens from which we could select, point to the utility of a code of ethics, at least for a professional body like the RANZCP. This chapter would be incomplete without at least a brief comment on a dissenting viewpoint which asserts that a code of ethics is a contradiction in terms. John Ladd[43], a notable proponent of this position, argues that ethics 'presumes that persons are autonomous moral agents' and, as such, their moral behaviour cannot be proscribed by an external agent.

Judith Lichtenberg[44] responds to Ladd in a balanced way conceding that it is reasonable to identify the ethical with autonomous action but it is equally reasonable to assume that 'codes of ethics can increase the likelihood that people will behave in certain ways', in part by making them more aware of the nature of their actions and also by 'getting [them] to behave in ways that have been determined ... to be morally desirable'.

A second line of argument relates to the obvious fact that codes of ethics are devised and applied by a *group* of people in order to pursue shared goals, determined by that group to be worthy of attainment. Thus, as we noted earlier, the psychiatric profession as a corporate entity may elaborate ethical standards which its members judge to be contributory to the common good— by fostering desired moral actions in relating to the patients they try to help, to the collegiateship in which they participate, and to the society they serve.

Lichtenberg's espousal of codes of ethics echoes our own conclusion that they can no longer be relegated to a footnote in the exercise of a profession. This is especially the case in psychiatry. Fullinwider[45] highlights the essence of a profession as a group having a body of special knowledge and training which renders a service to a vulnerable or dependent clientele. Mentally ill people are by virtue of their emotional distress and dysfunction among the most vulnerable of any group. A code of ethics cannot in and of itself guarantee that their interests will be safeguarded but it can certainly contribute to such a desirable goal.

References

1. Foucault, M.: *Madness and civilization: a history of insanity in the age of reason*. New York, Random House, 1965.
2. Temkin, O. and Temkin, C. (ed.) *Ancient medicine: selected papers of Ludwig Edelstein. Baltimore*. Johns Hopkins University Press, 1967.
3. Marketos, S., Diamandopoulos, A., Bartsocas, C., Poulakou-Rebelakou, E., and Koutras, D.: The Hippocratic oath. *Lancet* **347**:101–2, 1996.
4. Veatch, R.: Medical codes and oaths.1. History, in *Encyclopedia of bioethics*, ed. W. Reich. New York, Macmillan, 1995, vol. 3, pp. 1419–20.
5. Rosner, F. and Muntner, S.: The Oath of Asaph. *Annals of Internal Medicine* **63**: 317–20, 1965.
6. *Encyclopedia of bioethics*, ed. W. Reich. New York, Free Press, 1978, 1734–5.
7. Unschuld, P.: *Medical ethics in Imperial China: a study in historical anthropology*. Berkeley, University of California Press, 1979.
8. *Encyclopedia of bioethics*, ed. W. Reich. New York, Free Press, 1978, pp. 1736–7.
9. Percival, T.: *Codes of institutes and precepts adapted to the professional conduct of physicians and surgeons*. Birmingham, Alabama, Classics of Medicine Library, 1985.
10. Pellegrino, E.: *Thomas Percival's ethics: The ethics beneath the etiquette. Introduction to Percival*, see reference 9.
11. Katz, J.: *The silent world of doctor and patient*. New York, Free Press, 1975.
12. Veatch, R.: *A Theory of medical ethics*. New York, Basic Books, 1981.
13. Veatch, R.: Medical codes and ethics. 1. History, in *Encyclopedia of bioethics*, ed. W. Reich. New York, Macmillan, 1995, vol. 3, pp. 1423–4.
14. See Annas, G. and Grodin, M. (ed). *The Nazi doctors and the Nuremberg codes*. New York, Oxford University Press, 1992.
15. Katz, J.: The Nuremberg code and the Nuremburg trial: A reappraisal. *Journal of the American Medical Association* **276**:1662–6, 1996.
16. *The principles of medical ethics with annotations especially applicable to psychiatry*. Washington, DC, American Psychiatric Association, 1989.
17. The Canadian Medical Association codes of ethics annotated for psychiatrists. *Canadian Journal of Psychiatry* **25**:432–8, 1980.
18. Blomquist C. : From the Oath of Hippocrates to the Declaration of Hawaii. Paper presented to World Psychiatric Association Conference, London, June, 1976.
19. Bloch, S. and Reddaway, P.: *Russia's political hospitals*. London, Gollanz, 1977; Bloch, S. and Reddaway, P.: *Soviet psychiatric abuse*. London, Gollancz, 1984.
20. Pargiter, R. and Bloch, S.: Developing a code of ethics for psychiatry: the Australian experience. *Australian and New Zealand Journal of Psychiatry* **28**:188–96, 1994.
21. Polubinskaya, S. and Bonnie, R.: The code of professional ethics of the Russian Society of Psychiatrists. *International Journal of Law and Psychiatry* **19**:143–72, 1996.
22. Hughes, E.: Professions. *Daedalus* **92**:655–68, 1963.
23. Stone, A.: Law science and psychiatric malpractice: a response to Klerman's indictment of psychoanalytic psychiatry. *American Journal of Psychiatry* **147**:419–27, 1990.
24. Bloch, S. and Brown, P.: Can there be a right to effective treatment in psychiatry? *Changes* **9**:101–12, 1991.
25. Skene, L.: A legal perspective on codes of ethics, in *Codes of ethics and the professions*, eds. M. Coady and S. Bloch. Melbourne, Melbourne University Press, 1996.

26. Pellegrino, E.: The virtuous physician, and the ethics of medicine, in *Contemporary issues in bioethics*, 3rd edn, ed. T. L., Beauchamp and L. Walters. Belmont, CA, Wadsworth, pp. 316–22, 1982.
27. *Plato, Dialogues* ed. B. Jowett. Oxford, Oxford University Press, 1953.
28. Clouser, K. I.: Medical ethics: some uses, abuses and limitations. *New England Journal of Medicine* **293**:384–7, 1975.
29. Bloch, S.: Teaching psychiatric ethics. *Medical Education* **22**:550–3, 1988.
30. Thompson, I.: Letter to the Editor. *British Journal of Psychiatry* **137**:302, 1980.
31. Rest, R. J.: A psychologist looks at the teaching of ethics *Hastings Center Report* **12**:29–36, 1982.
32. Pond Report: *On the teaching of medical ethics*. London, Institute of Medical Ethics, 1987.
33. Calman, K. and Downie, R.: Practical problems in the teaching of ethics to medical students. *Journal of Medical Ethics* **13**:153–6, 1987.
34. Gillon, R.: *Philosophical medical ethics*. Chichester, Wiley, 1985, p. 108.
35. *Codes of Practice, Discussion Paper No. 20*. Melbourne, Law Reform Commission of Victoria, 1990.
36. *Code of Practice*. Department of Health and Welsh Office, London, 1990. A revised version was published in 1993.
37. *Code of Professional Conduct*. Melbourne, Australian Psychological Society, 1994.
38. Paredes, J., Beyerstein, D., Ledwidge, B., and Kogan, C.: Psychiatric ethics and ethical psychiatry. *Canadian Journal of Psychiatry* **35**:600–3, 1990.
39. *Report of the Royal Commission into Deep Sleep Therapy (Slattery Royal Commission)*. Sydney, NSW Government Printer, 1990.
40. *Code of Conduct*. 9th edn. Sydney, Australian Pharmaceutical Manufacturers Association, 1990.
41. *Memorandum and Articles of Association*. Melbourne, Royal Australian and New Zealand College of Psychiatrists, 1991.
42. Pargiter, R. and Bloch, S.: The ethics committee of a psychiatric college: its procedures and themes. *Australian and New Zealand Journal of Psychiatry* **31**:76–82, 1997.
43. Ladd, J.: The quest for a code of professional ethics: an intellectual and moral confusion, in *Legal ethics*, ed. D. Rhode and D. Luban. St Paul, MN, Foundation Press, 1992.
44. Lichtenburg, J.: What are codes of ethics for? in *Codes of ethics and the professions*, ed. M. Coady and S. Bloch. Melbourne, Melbourne University Press, 1996.
45. Fullinwider, R.: Professional codes and moral understanding, in *Codes of ethics and the professions*, ed. M. Coady and S. Bloch. Melbourne, Melbourne University Press, 1996.

7

Confidentiality in psychiatry

David I. Joseph and Joseph Onek

Whatsoever I shall see or hear in the course of my profession ... if it be what should not be published abroad, I will never divulge, holding such things to be holy secrets.

(Hippocratic Oath)

Three people can keep a secret if two of them are dead.

(Benjamin Franklin, Poor Richard's Almanac)

Medicine has always stressed the importance of confidentiality, but the practice of psychiatry, even more than other branches of medicine, depends to a significant degree upon an understanding that confidentiality between patient and doctor will be maintained. *The principles of medical ethics with annotations especially applicable to psychiatry* state that each psychiatrist 'shall safeguard patient confidences within the constraints of the law'.[1] Confidentiality, which can be defined as entrusting information to another with the expectation that it will be kept private, is closely related to 'confidence, confession, trust, reliance, respect, security, intimacy, and privacy'.[2] Although doctors and their patients place a high value on the establishment and maintenance of the confidential relationship, confidentiality has been such a central aspect of the practice of medicine and psychiatry that its importance is often taken for granted, its maintenance frequently less than rigorous, and the degree of its erosion in recent years underestimated.

Confidentiality and the law

To a considerable degree the law regulates the extent to which information confided by a patient is actually non-disclosable. State privilege statutes establish when a psychiatrist must or must not testify concerning patient information in judicial or administrative proceedings. Reporting laws, such as those for child abuse, often require psychiatrists to disclose patient information to state officials. In many states there are statutes or judicial decisions regulating such areas as disclosure of patient information to insurance companies or collection agencies. The imposition of a duty to warn the potential victim of a dangerous patient represents a well-publicized example in which state tort (damage) law may regulate disclosure previously regulated by psychiatry's ethical standards regarding confidentiality.

Recent years have witnessed a range of challenges at the state level to the principle of psychotherapeutic privilege. Among these are the confidentiality of joint counseling sessions when a husband and wife undertake divorce (*Redding* v. *Virginia Mason Medical Center*, 878 P.2d 483, Washington Court of Appeals), and the disclosure of information regarding a husband's drug abuse which was confided to a psychologist whom the wife consulted (*Howes* v. *U.S.*, 887 F. 2d 729 {C.A. 6, Ohio, Oct. 19, 1989}). Leong and Silva[3] discuss a case in which the defense sought the records of a prosecution witness in order to assess her competence and credibility as a witness. After reviewing the records, the judge found very little of relevance, but did release 'sanitized' records to both prosecution and defense. Decrying this decision, the authors state 'The purpose of privilege is to protect information even when it is relevant. Relevance is a minimal protection against violating privacy when no privilege exists. If relevance always trumps confidentiality and privilege', this raises the question of whether the police should give Miranda-type warnings to potential prosecution witnesses. The widespread questioning of the principle of psychotherapeutic privilege makes it essential for psychiatrists to be knowledgeable about the laws in their states and active in their attempts to protect the confidentiality of their patients.[†]

There is a close relationship between the regulation of confidentiality required by the legal system and the regulation imposed by professional ethics. Whenever legal requirements such as those to report child abuse or undue familiarity override the principle of confidentiality, ethical norms are modified. At the same time, the ethical norms of psychiatry can constitute the basis for decisions regarding legal obligations. When considering whether the disclosure of patient information by a psychiatrist constitutes a breach of the psychiatrist's fiduciary duty or a breach of his implied contract with the patient, a court is very likely to accord great weight to the ethical norms of the profession. Even in this era of increased legislation regarding confidentiality there remains a need for a clear, comprehensive, code of psychiatric ethics.

The ethical aspects of confidentiality can be more clearly delineated by considering its relationship to privacy and privilege. Privacy can be narrowly defined as, 'the freedom of the individual to pick and choose for himself

---

[†] Countries have very different statutes regarding confidentiality. Weil[4] described the situation in Israel where everyone serves in the military and physicians 'must respond to requests of the military health services for information concerning specific cases. . .'.. In 1993 when this article was written, psychiatrists were attempting to have the law revised and the discussion limited to 'mentally ill persons presenting an actual potential danger which may be aggravated as a consequence of the condition of military service and specifically by the opportunity afforded of bearing arms'. In contrast, Weil noted the situation in France where the penal code 'establishes that confidentiality is absolute ... which means that a judge cannot order a therapist to testify and the patient can only obtain an attestation from his or her therapist and take advantage of it according to his or her own judgment'.

the time, circumstances and particularly the extent to which he wishes to withhold from others his attitudes, beliefs, behavior, and opinion',[5] or more broadly defined to encompass an individual's 'right to personal autonomy and freedom'.[2] If one uses the broader definition of privacy, then confidentiality can be considered to be one of many aspects of privacy. If one employs the narrower definition of privacy, then confidentiality becomes 'co-extensive'[2] with privacy.

Privilege is a legal concept which refers to the right of an individual to control which information, communicated in confidence, can be revealed in a judicial or administrative proceeding. Although the privilege protecting communications between priest and penitent, lawyer and client, and physician and patient has long been an integral aspect of our social structure, it is important to understand that the concept of privileged communications runs counter to the tradition of common law, which holds that the courts have access to all relevant information.[6] Privilege exists only when established by specific legal statute, and statutes, especially those pertaining to the practice of psychotherapy, differ considerably from one state to another. Although there have been legal challenges by psychiatrists[7] and recommendations to make it mutual,[8] the right to waive privilege belongs to the individual and not to the physician.

In 1995 the issue of psychotherapist–patient privilege was reviewed by the Supreme Court (*Jaffee* v. *Redmond*) which, in a 7–2 decision, ruled that such communication need not be disclosed in federal trials. The decision held that 'Like the spousal and attorney–client privileges, the psychotherapist–patient privilege is rooted in the imperative need for confidence and trust', and patients must be 'willing to make a frank and complete disclosure of acts, emotions, memories and fears'. While the majority opinion represented a strong endorsement of psychotherapeutic confidentiality, the dissenting opinion reflected an unsettling hostility to the principle of such confidentiality. Justice Scalia stated, 'Ask the average citizen: Would your mental health be more significantly impaired by preventing you from seeing a psychotherapist, or by preventing you from getting advice from your mom? I have little doubt what the answer would be. Yet there is no mother–child privilege'. It remains to be seen whether this denigration of psychotherapy will influence future judicial or legislative decisions.

Because of breaches of confidentiality by physicians, and because of 'the right of defendants to secure justice, the needs of insurers to guarantee equity and prevent fraud, and the desire of society to protect itself from future violent acts',[9] the legal system has devoted increased attention to the limits of confidentiality. Psychiatrists in turn have progressively looked to the law to provide guidelines for standards of conduct. Although thoroughly understandable, the wish for the law to answer most ethical questions is doomed to disappointment. Quen has noted that only non-lawyers believe that 'there is an abstraction called the law which is reliable, predictable, and standard. Actually, the law, even in statute, means only what the last judge who interpreted it said it means'.[10] Although overstated, this point of view correctly emphasizes that there are limits to how much guidance can be expected from the law. Moreover, the legal system is unlikely to consider even a small fraction of the many situations in which the disclosure of confidential information may occur. The *Guidelines on Confidentiality* of the American Psychiatric Association[11] delineate many situations in which psychiatrists will need to use ethical principles in reaching decisions about patient care. The management of confidentiality on a day-to-day basis is much more a matter of professional ethics than of legal requirements. It is precisely for this reason that psychiatrists and mental health professionals need to re-evaluate and reassert ethical norms.

The necessity of confidentiality in a psychotherapeutic relationship was initially based on theoretical assumptions, but research[12–18] has confirmed the importance of confidentiality to patients and their therapists. The shared value of confidentiality notwithstanding, given the realities of modern medical practice, and especially of hospital medicine, confidentiality has been considered, a 'decrepit concept'.[19] The importance of health-care teams, increasing subspecialization with multiple consultations, the role of third-party payers, and the rapid domination of the delivery of medical and psychiatric services by managed care companies have contributed to an increased tension between the patient's wish to maintain maximum confidentiality and his desire to receive the best possible care.[17,19] These factors, in concert with the legal obligations imposed on psychiatrists in such areas as commitment and child-abuse,[20] have resulted in what Stoller[21] has aptly called 'relative confidentiality'. Lindenthal and Thomas[22] support the establishment of some limits on confidentiality to enable enable psychiatrists to play a role in controlling deviant behavior.

In response to this gradual erosion of confidentiality, others[22–25] have argued passionately for the establishment of absolute confidentiality. Kottow[25] views confidentiality not as 'an invaluable moral value ... but as an interpersonal communications strategy that ceases to function unless strictly adhered to'. He reminds us that while one may break confidentiality to avoid a potential harm, the break, itself, always harms the 'confidant, the practice of confidentiality, and the honesty of clinical relationships'. To preserve the absolute confidentiality which they consider essential to the conduct of psychoanalysis and psychoanalytic psychotherapy, Bollas and Sundelson[26] recommend the adoption of the following:

The contents of a psychoanalysis are strictly confidential and any and all disclosures by the psychoanalyst—such as discussing the patient with colleagues, arranging for a hospitalization, acting in the interests of a child patient—must be given in the understanding that confidentiality is maintained and that in all circumstances privilege is retained by the psychoanalyst. (ref. 26 p. 156)

To protect its citizens from harms, they envisage society looking to others (social workers, teachers, etc.) and 'social therapists (as opposed to psychotherapists) who would have an 'advocacy partnership' with the client.

Although psychiatrists and mental health professionals are well aware that absolute confidentiality is a fiction, patients are strikingly uninformed about the circumstances under which confidentiality can and cannot be compromised.[15,18] Psychiatrists need to be expert about their professional discipline, but they also need to be knowledgeable about the laws regulating confidentiality. Where relevant, it is important at the outset of the initial consultation to inquire whether the patient is currently involved in a contested will, custody proceeding, or personal injury suits and to inform him about the possibility of compelled disclosure in a legal proceeding. It may also be clinically appropriate to make him aware of the legal and ethical requirements under which the psychiatrist is required to disclose information in instances of imminent harm to self or others, including child-abuse. When appropriate, the psychiatrist may suggest that the patient consult a lawyer to determine the likelihood that information confided to the psychiatrist may have to be disclosed in court. An early emphasis on this aspect of confidentiality underscores the seriousness which is accorded confidentiality and strengthens the therapeutic alliance.

When considering confidentiality psychiatrists must be aware that, by virtue of involvement in a personal injury suit or other litigation, any patient's records may be made public in a courtroom proceeding. Furthermore, patient records may have to be disclosed to insurance companies and other third parties, as well as to the patient himself. These ever-present possibilities routinely create difficult ethical considerations regarding which information to enter in the official patient record.

Throughout this chapter we will discuss a range of clinical situations, some in which the law requires disclosure of information, others in which the psychiatrist may favor disclosure which is not mandated by law. Regardless of the situation, the therapeutic alliance will be least undermined and may actually be strengthened if the psychiatrist can relate the issue of disclosure to the patient's internal conflicts. This perspective is clinically useful in dealing with suicidality (the patient's wish to live in conflict with the wish to die), the disclosure of information experienced as shameful (e.g. alcoholism) to a physician who has requested a psychiatric consultation, or informing an unknowing spouse about HIV positivity. When the psychiatrist discusses issues of disclosure from a clinical perspective, the patient is less likely to experience the psychiatrist's subsequent actions only as an instance of something being done to or forced on him and more likely to view them as a collaborative effort to deal with a difficult problem.

Confidentiality and office management

In the daily conduct of psychiatric practice, whether in a private office, psychiatric clinic, or hospital, psychiatrists affect patients' privacy and confidentiality by many subtle actions. Offices may be constructed with a separate entrance and exit to reduce the possibility that patients will see each other. If this is not the case or if the waiting-room is shared among several psychiatrists, a patient may habitually be late to protect his confidentiality (privacy) by time when architecture does not do it for him. Although a particularly significant concern for individuals well known to the public, this is more important to many patients than may be apparent. Psychiatrists have become so inured to the elimination of anonymity in shared waiting-rooms that the practice of announcing a patient's given name is rarely seen to be an unnecessary compromise of confidentiality. When seeing a patient for the first time, one can avoid this particular breach of confidentiality by announcing, 'I'm Dr Hamilton'; and for subsequent appointments one can enter the waiting-room without mentioning the name of the patient to be seen next.

The telephone, so integral a part of the psychiatrist's daily work, poses several serious threats to confidentiality. Telephoning a patient at work poses an immediate dilemma. Some, wishing to preserve as much of the patient's confidentiality as possible, will identify themselves as 'Michael Hamilton', concerned that 'Dr Hamilton' will arouse curiosity in the individual answering the phone. Patients may be hesitant to request that the psychiatrist calling at work should not identify himself by name, and it is useful to ask how the patient would prefer the situation to be handled. The telephone answering machine has created a new set of problems regarding confidentiality. A woman, whose family knew she was seeing a psychiatrist, was outraged when he left a message on her home answering machine regarding the proper dosage of medication, despite the fact that she had been urgently calling him for this information. She considered this to be confidential information, to which no one else should have been privy without her permission. When two psychiatrists share the same telephone number and answering machine, all messages are automatically shared. Although patients could leave a message such as 'Please have Dr. Hamilton call 244-5000', this seems unlikely to occur, in part because these subtle breaches in confidentiality have become so commonplace as to be overlooked and/or accepted by both patients and psychiatrists. Recent technology has developed 'voice mailboxes' which allow patients to leave a message at the psychiatrist's home without compromising their privacy and allow several psychiatrists to share the same telephone number and still maintain their patients' confidentiality.

Widespread use of the electronic transmission of medical and psychiatric information has resulted in a range of problems regarding the maintenance of confidentiality. In 1996, the American Psychiatric Association published a re-source document on *Preserving patient confidentiality in the era of information technology*[27] which emphasized the degree to which barriers that traditionally insured the privacy of medical information have been eroded by technological advances. In some settings, the distinctions between records kept in separate medical facilities have been largely erased. Coping with the dizzying rate of change in the storage and transmission of psychiatric data requires a constantly high level of vigilance on the part of all psychiatrists.

When data is transmitted though facsimile (fax), several potential threats to patient confidentiality arise. Immediate concern arises from uncertainty about who will receive the information. Whenever possible, the psychiatrist should be certain that the addressee is able to receive the fax personally. Given the very widespread access of a range of people to fax machines, especially in institutions, the possibility of unwarranted disclosure is greater than when material is mailed to a specific individual. There is also a risk that a fax will be sent to the wrong number. One report described an instance in which psychiatric information intended for an internist was mistakenly sent to the patient's employer, and a second in which the records of a woman in preterm labor were sent to a unit in hospital where she worked, thus allowing her colleagues access to the information that she had a history of herpes.[28] In addition to the proper education of personnel and inclusion of a cover sheet addressed to a named individual, we recommend that each institution develop a cover letter which includes a 'legal notice' regarding the confidential nature of medical records. One such notice[29] reads:

This message is intended only for the use of the individual or entity to which it is addressed and may contain information that is privileged, confidential and exempt from disclosure under applicable law. If the reader of this message is not the intended recipient, you are hereby notified that any dissemination, distribution, or copying of this communication and the attached is strictly prohibited. If you have received this communication in error, please notify us immediately by telephone and return the original message to us at the above address via the postal service.

Given these dangers, we recommend that psychiatrists avoid sending any patient information by fax and do so only in emergencies in which immediate communication is necessary.

Electronic mail (e-mail) creates a different set of threats to the maintenance of confidentiality. While the possibility of a wrong number is virtually eliminated, information transmitted electronically can be accessed by anyone with knowledge of the sender's storage code. Although technological advances have significantly improved the security of electronic mail and data retained in computers, 'many experts believe that privacy is jeopardized whenever sensitive information is maintained in a computer data base' (see ref. 27, p. 3). In addition, e-mail is likely to be discoverable in court proceedings in the same manner as written records. As with the use of the fax, we recommend that confidential information be sent by means of e-mail only if absolutely necessary and that any confidential e-mail messages, like other confidential communications, be stored only as long as necessary.

The development of the electronic patient record (epr) has created a new set of threats to confidentiality. Bengtsson[30] has noted that an epr must be accessible to the physician, must be accurate, and must be trusted. To insure trustworthiness and to insure confidentiality, he stresses the importance of reliable access control, an accurate logging system to create an audit trail, and the encryption of sensitive data. However, given that no system is immune to 'bribery and blackmail', complete confidentiality can never be totally protected. If it is essential to record certain highly sensitive information, a psychiatrist may want to keep it in a separate paper record and not include it in the epr.

Cellular telephones are always a risky means of conveying confidential information. Despite laws forbidding eavesdropping on such conversations, intercepting calls is relatively easy and may occur inadvertently. We recommend avoiding the use of the cellular telephone to convey confidential information. Even if the psychiatrist is not intending to discuss any confidential material on such a call, ethics dictate that the receiver of the call be informed that the call is being made on a cellular phone

Facsimile, the cellular telephone, and especially e-mail create a state of mind in the user that may lull one's vigilance about threats to confidentiality. Many individuals tend to be more 'loquocious' or less guarded when using these means of communication. The impact of this technology on the psychology of the psychiatrist increases the risk to the maintenance of confidentiality.

Careless storage of records commonly jeopardizes patients' confidentiality. Regardless of legal statutes, psychiatrists have an ethical obligation to ensure that patients' clinical and billing records, as well as appointment books, are securely stored. In hospitals and clinics where offices are cleaned at night, psychiatrists may forget that material left on desks or in unlocked drawers is readily available to unauthorized persons. The very need to keep so many routine behaviors in mind makes it surprisingly difficult to maintain the maximum degree of confidentiality. A more detailed discussion of privacy and the patient's record will occur later in this chapter.

Additional issues arise from the use of ancillary personnel such as secretaries, accountants, and bill-collection agencies. Patients who have little apparent concern over being seen by the secretary may be displeased should the secretary write the bill, even if it does not contain a diagnosis. Confidentiality is at greater risk when secretaries transcribe histories and process notes. This is especially troublesome in clinics and hospitals, where the individual psychiatrist may have little role in the selection of the secretary, and where the importance of confidentiality may not receive the formal emphasis and repeated reinforcement required for consistent maintenance. In such situations psychiatrists can easily ignore the ethical responsibility to ensure that ancillary personnel are thoroughly educated and trained in the importance of maintaining confidentiality, and that patients' names and identifying data are not revealed unnecessarily.

Depending upon the state, psychiatrists may be legally required to inform a patient in advance that an unpaid bill will be submitted to a collection agency or become the basis of a lawsuit. Regardless of legal requirements this course is consistent with ethical principles. In addition, the patient's confidentiality can be most effectively safeguarded by supplying the agency or court with the minimum amount of information necessary to secure payment, and by sanitizing billing records before they are given to an accountant.

Confidentiality and conversations about patients

Like other physicians, psychiatrists talk about their patients. In many instances such talk represents an informal consultation and is in the service of patient-care; in others it is more in the interest of relieving anger, guilt, or some other internal state, or achieving some personal end such as self-aggrandizement. However, questions may arise even in instances in which talking about a patient might appear to have no ethical dimension. As an example, a general practitioner who had referred a patient for a psychiatric evaluation met the psychiatrist at a party, and inquired about the patient. Some psychiatrists believe that unless express informed consent has been given, even to indicate whether or not the patient had been seen, violates the patient's confidentiality. Others take the position that such a response would reflect 'a misuse of confidentiality' that was 'absolutely discourteous'.[31] Given the actual way in which contemporary medicine is practiced, and in view of research regarding patients' attitudes toward confidentiality, it seems reasonable to assume that patients expect some discussion about them and trust that their physicians will exercise proper judgment regarding which information to convey and which to keep private. None the less, when a patient is referred by another professional, a routine request for permission to talk with the referring individual implicitly underscores the psychiatrist's commitment to confidentiality without interfering with the sharing of appropriate information.

Written reports to a referring physician, which will be included in a patient's permanent file and are likely to be read by others, raise ethical issues about which information to include. However, oral reports may also pose questions about confidentiality. For example, a man with headaches, splenic flexure syndrome, and depressed mood was referred by his general practitioner for a psychiatric consultation, which revealed a dysthymic disorder and a family history of depression, denied anger with his wife, alcohol abuse, and homosexual concerns. None of this material was known to the referring physician. If the patient gives general permission for the release of information, what should be conveyed in writing, what should only be conveyed orally, and what should not be shared at all? In addition to determining what is essential in assisting the referring physician to provide the best medical treatment, it is important to be clear that personal historical material belongs to the patient. If the patient does not wish the psychiatrist to reveal his alcoholism, a finding clearly of importance to his medical treatment, the psychiatrist can conduct a brief psychotherapeutic intervention with the goal of exploring the patient's refusal—a decision which may have been motivated by the avoidance of shame. From an ethical perspective, in the face of continued refusal, the final decision about what is conveyed belongs to the patient. By ensuring that the patient reads and approves any letter, both confidentiality and the therapeutic relationship can be protected.

When patients in psychotherapy are referred to a psychiatrist for a psycho-pharmacological or other consultation, a different ethical problem regarding confidentiality can arise. In one instance, a man in weekly psychotherapy with a psychologist for treatment of a depression which followed a mild left-sided cerebral infarction was referred for an evaluation of the advisability of anti-depressants. The referring psychologist spoke with the psychiatrist about the patient, and the patient, after getting a good response from an antidepressant, took 'a vacation' from psychotherapy. A month later he 'confessed' to the psychiatrist that one of the issues he had been dealing with in psychotherapy was a past incestuous relationship with his daughter. The psychologist and the patient had chosen to keep this information confidential, with the result that the psychiatrist's understanding of the case was significantly limited. If a patient refuses permission for certain important information to be shared with the consultant, the referring professional may decide not to proceed with the consultation.

Gossip is a more insidious, but no less serious threat to confidentiality. Gossip can be viewed as a 'triangular sociopsychological relationship in-volving the exchange of tales about others, fostering intimacy, discharg-ing hostility, and attended by a feeling of pleasure',[32] and the gossiping psychiatrist has been the focus of considerable attention.[33-36] The functions of gossip include a mastery of anxiety, a search for intimacy, the re-enactment of childhood sexual curiosity, titillation, self-aggrandizement of one's talents, or, by extension, the talents of one's children (patients), a search for admiration, and an attempt to manage envy. For psychiatrists, gossip also counteracts the profound psychological deprivation that is an inherent aspect of the professional requirement to keep so great a part of one's life private. From the perspective of confidentiality, when the psychiatrist gossips, internal conflicts have resulted in the unilateral breaking of the fiduciary trust with the patient. The compromise of confidentiality which occurs, regardless of whether the patient's identity is revealed, is likely to have subtle therapeutic as well as ethical ramifications. Such lapses by the psychiatrist should stimulate a serious self-inquiry to determine what motivated the seemingly trivial but important breach.

The maintenance of confidentiality can be especially difficult with regard to the psychiatrist's own family. When a psychiatrist is preoccupied with an anxiety-provoking case such as a suicidal patient, conflict exists between the wish to explain his preoccupation and the wish to protect the confidentiality of the patient, who may actually call and identify himself by name. Ethically, psychiatrists are obliged not to talk in any detail with their own families about any patients, especially those patients who may be identified by their family members in social or professional situations.

Confidentiality and patient records

When patients believe that their confidentiality is protected, they tell psychiatrists their most intimate thoughts, and physicians possess a natural inclination to include all relevant information in the patient's record. Psychiatrists need to exercise considerable discretion about entering private information in the official patient record. In clinics and hospitals it is obvious that many individuals have access to the records, but it is easy to overlook the fact that some staff may know the patient and that the seriousness with which confidentiality is maintained will vary greatly among them. Furthermore, any patient records may have to be turned over in the course of personal injury, child-custody cases, or other litigation, or at the request of insurance companies. On the other hand, in hospitals it is often essential that clinical staff have access to some very private information, and thorough records contribute to better patient care. Given the inherent tension between making information available to treating-staff and maintaining patient confidentiality, psychiatrists need to consider carefully just which personal data must be included in the record. Caution should be given to detailing marginally useful information about third parties, or descriptions of a patient's impulses and fantasies which have not resulted in overt behavior. If there is a necessity to record such information, it can be kept separate from the official patient chart, reviewed periodically, and, if appropriate, destroyed.

Particular care is necessary with respect to records that are likely to be the subject of litigation. For example, if a patient has been involved in an automobile or occupational accident, the record should not include the patient's thoughts about his blameworthiness—thoughts which may not be accurate. If, for some reason, these are included, the psychiatrist should clearly indicate any doubts about the accuracy of the speculations.

Not infrequently, situations will arise which require a creative, collaborative effort between psychiatrists and lawyers to protect patients' confidentiality while furthering the just efforts of law enforcement or other agencies. As an example, in June, 1990, a psychiatrist in Alexandria, Virginia was seriously injured by a pipe bomb that had been sent to his office. Law enforcement authorities understandably wanted to examine his records in hopes of discovering clues to the bomber's identity. The family (the psychiatrist was too badly injured to participate in the deliberations) objected, wishing to protect the patients' privacy. The judge ruled against the family, but he and lawyers for the family and the US attorney developed a plan in which both the government and the family would select a psychiatrist to review the record. Should either psychiatrist discover information that might be useful in determining the identity of the bomber, the information would be reviewed by the judge. Should he agree that the information was potentially important, the information would be released to those investigating the crime. This solution, to our mind respectful of both the needs of psychiatry and the law, was especially noteworthy given that the 'government did not have to agree to the unique review procedure and under federal law had the right to subpoena 'all of the psychiatist's records'.[37]

Perhaps because nearly everyone is somewhat intimidated by official communications from lawyers and the courts, psychiatrists often believe that they are legally obligated to comply with the demands of a subpoena. In fact, a subpoena, which means 'under pain' in Latin, is only a request by a lawyer, issued through the court, for information. The psychiatrist is obligated to respond to the subpoena, but not to turn over information. If the psychiatrist has reservations about disclosing the information, he can oppose the subpoena. The party seeking the information will then have to request the court to order the release of the information, and, in rendering its decision, the court will consider whether there are legal barriers to disclosure. If a psychiatrist or mental institutions disclose information in response to a subpoena as opposed to a court order, they may be held liable for breach of confidentiality. In a recent case,[38] the records of a woman who had charged a man with sexual battery were disclosed to the defendant, solely pursuant to a subpoena. The court initially held that the 'unauthorized reading and dissemination of a mental health record ... is a serious invasion of privacy', allowing for the injured party to seek damages. Although the court is rehearing the case, the risk of releasing information solely on the basis of a subpoena is clear. As discussed earlier, there may be instances in which the psychiatrist may believe that he has an ethical obligation not to testify even if compelled by the court to do so.

If a court is prepared to compel a psychiatrist to testify, and if the psychiatrist believes that the testimony will be damaging to the therapeutic relationship, the psychiatrist should explain this to the judge and request that the patient/litigant be evaluated by an independent psychiatrist. Courts are often amenable to such requests.

Under certain circumstances, psychiatrists have chosen to ignore court orders which they felt violated their obligations to their patients. In support of such a position, McConnell[39] has argued that breaking a patient's confidentiality simply because the law requires it is not justified. Noting that legislatures may pass immoral laws, he argues that 'the strength of the general obligation to obey the law is context dependent and cannot be divided from the particular statute's content'.

Finally, we draw attention to the question of how records are to be managed following a patient's death. In general, the confidentiality of the psychiatric record must be maintained after the patient's death. The fact that a patient's legal heirs request the release of clinical records should not lead to disclosure unless the law in that jurisdiction so requires. Many patients discuss information with a psychiatrist which they would not want family members to know about even after they are dead. The situation is more complex if the patient has consented to the release of information. One instance, which resulted in widespread discussion in the psychiatric literature, involved the decision of Dr Martin Orne to release audiotapes of his treatment of the poet, Anne Sexton, to Diane Wood Middlebrook, her biographer.[40–45] The patient had given the tapes to Dr Orne with a verbal request that he use them (as he saw fit) to help others. Despite the existence of very different standards of informed consent in the 1960s when the tapes were made, Orne was subjected to a long, arduous ethical investigation. As the controversy in the Orne case demonstrated, there will often be questions about the validity or the extent of the consent given by the deceased patient.

Confidentiality and requests for information from third parties

Since the importance of maintaining the confidentiality of patients' records is such a central tenet of psychiatry, it may come as a surprise that the peer-review process established between the American Psychiatric Association and the Aetna Insurance Company initially did not require that the patient provide consent before the treating psychiatrist filed the Mental Health Treatment Report.[46] It is also noteworthy that a recent Medicaid audit required that copies of patients' records be sent to a central agency.[47] And, according to Mosher,[48] current Medicare rules permit insurance carriers to 'inspect the records of all patients treated by an analyst who treats even one Medicare patient'. These occurrences underscore the serious difficulties regarding patient confidentiality which frequently result when a third party is involved.

Requests from third parties (insurers, employers, schools, licensing agencies, etc.) regularly pose conflicts regarding confidentiality. Chodoff[49] has elaborated upon the conflicts inherent in psychiatrist–patient–third-party relationships. With regard to the issue of confidentiality, additional difficulties stem from the fact that patients usually sign a general statement of consent for the release of information. Since patients are likely to believe that they have only agreed to the release of relevant information, it becomes the responsibility of the psychiatrist to clarify with the patient what information will be supplied. As Robitscher[50] has emphasized, the problem becomes especially thorny if the patient is no longer in treatment:

[The psychiatrist] does not feel he has the right not to release information after the patient has authorized the release, but he feels he is being forced into an unprofessional stance in retailing (detailing) confidences. It places the therapist at times in a position where he has to divulge information harmful to the patient—a violation of the Hippocratic injunction to do no harm—or alternatively, has to give a false picture of the patient to the inquirer. It raises a complicated informed consent question: if the patient had not been coerced, or if he knew what was going to be divulged, would he have signed the release of information form. It blackmails the therapist into giving information, because if he refuses as a matter of policy, discretion, or conscience to give information, he may be blocking the professional progress of his patient or at least it may lead to the inference that there is something to hide. (pp. 234–5)

By assisting patients to structure the consent, psychiatrists can protect them from acting in ways which might not be in their self-interest. Even when provided with a signed release which specifies the information to be revealed, psychiatrists should attempt to consult with former as well as current patients about what is going to be released. After such consultation, patients may choose to revoke their release. Some psychiatrists refuse, on principle, to provide information regarding current or former patients in situations such as government security clearances. If the government agency has resources to conduct an independent psychiatric examination, such a refusal may not be harmful to the patient, and protects the therapeutic relationship.

If the psychiatrist is planning to send a report to the institution or agency, this should be made absolutely clear at the outset. In general, patients should be informed about the specifics of the actual information that is being conveyed, and should be provided with an opportunity to discuss this information. In cases in which the psychiatrist believes that it would be harmful for the patient to know full details, discretion is both ethically and clinically indicated. Psychiatrists need to be aware that receiving institutions will manage clinical information with varying commitments to preserving confidentiality. A survey of state mental hospital directors and directors of mental health centers determined that identifying data were routinely reported to state offices in the following way: 30 per cent submitted names, 31 per cent addresses, and 25 per cent social security numbers; 51 per cent submitted one or more of these.[51] In contrast, a study of psychotherapists working in mental health facilities specifically for medical students found a strong reluctance to break confidentiality.[52] Given the disparity between the expectations of patients, the values of psychiatrists, and the procedures of institutions, the psychiatrist is ethically obliged to clarify what information will be conveyed, and seek assurances about the institution's handling of confidential material.

Confidentiality and managed care

Managed-care companies are simply another group of third parties which frequently request patient records. These requests do not raise conceptual issues different from those raised by other third parties. However, the rapid development of managed-care companies and their broad penetration of the marketplace has had a profound practical impact on the maintenance of confidentiality.

First, managed-care companies tend to ask for more information, more frequently than traditional insurance carriers. The greater the amount of information provided, the greater the likelihood of a disclosure of confidential information to an employer, life insurance company, or another physician.

This danger is heightened because managed-care companies often use reviewers who are not physicians and who may not have the same professional commitment to the maintenance of confidentiality. When managed-care companies require frequent reports, the presence of the third party in the consulting room inhibits, both consciously and unconsciously, the type of information the patient is willing to discuss.

Some managed-care companies (e.g. staff model health maintenance organizations (HMOs)) will often place psychiatric records along with all other medical records in a centralized location or system. This dramatically increases the number of people who have or who can gain access to the records. As a result, the records of outpatients become as accessible and potentially vulnerable to disclosure as inpatient records. This development underscores the need for psychiatrists to take extraordinary care in deciding what information to place in the patient's record. In general, information that is not directly related to specific decisions about diagnosis or treatment should not be included. In some circumstances a psychiatrist may wish to retain certain information in his own office rather than include it in a centralized system of records. Such information should not be retained any longer than absolutely necessary for the treatment of the patient.

When making reports or allowing access to records psychiatrists need be wary lest they respond with an unnecessary disclosure of information. In a front page article, *The New York Times* (22 May, 1996) described an instance in which a psychotherapist allowed the managed-care company to inspect a patient's records. They 'rifled through my files, made copies and went'. Not surprisingly, the patient whose files were inspected, terminated his treatment shortly afterwards. The compliance by the psychotherapist without apparently determining the intent of the inspection, attempting to limit the information released, and challenging the 'right' of the managed-care company to the record reflects the degree to which some in the profession may have surrendered confidentiality without a fight. Psychiatrists should discuss with managed-care companies precisely what information is sought and should provide the least information possible.

Confidentiality and disclosures in the public interest

Psychiatrists frequently become aware of information which, if disclosed in the proper manner, would benefit the public. A dramatic and not uncommon situation is created when a psychiatrist learns that his patient has had sexual relations with a previous therapist, but does not wish to bring charges or to bring the matter to the attention of the local ethics committee. When a patient reports sexual relations with a former therapist, psychiatrists should be aware that several state laws require the reporting of such information regardless of the patient's wishes. In the absence of such laws, psychiatrists are under no legal obligation to report the behavior. While exploration of the patient's reservations about reporting is therapeutically indicated, many considerations (not wishing the spouse or family to know, avoidance of a public investigation) might result in a decision to take no action. In such instances it would also be unethical for the psychiatrist to pressure the patient, directly or implicitly, to pursue a more aggressive course of action. If the patient gives consent for the psychiatrist to contact the former therapist or licensing board, the decision whether the psychiatrist should act on the information gained within the confidence of the therapeutic relationship poses an ethical problem. Of course, the patient herself can notify the appropriate authorities.

A different conflict regarding confidentiality and undue familiarity may be encountered in institutional settings. For example, a hospitalized patient told her psychiatrist that another psychiatrist on the ward had had sex with her. She refused to discuss the matter with the administrator of the ward and would not permit her psychiatrist to discuss it with anyone. In this instance the psychiatrist had an exceedingly difficult ethical dilemma—to protect his patient's confidentiality or to protect other patients for whom he had clinical responsibility, and with whom the psychiatrist might also be having sexual relations or might in the future. As an initial step, focused discussion and psychotherapy with the patient should be undertaken in the hopes that she will take action herself or will grant permission for the psychiatrist to pursue a specific course of action. *The principles of medical ethics*[1] state that a physician shall 'strive to expose those physicians deficient in character or competence who engage in fraud or deception'. *The APA annotations especially applicable to psychiatry* unequivocally state that sexual activity with a patient is unethical and that it is 'ethical, even encouraged for a psychiatrist to intercede'. If the patient continues to refuse to take any action herself or give permission to the psychiatrist, given the psychiatrist's responsibility for an identifiable group of patients, it is our opinion that some unilateral action by the psychiatrist is ethically permissible and is in accordance with the Principles. Speaking directly with the psychiatrist in question, informing the impaired physician's committee, consulting or filing a complaint with the hospital's ethics committee, or speaking with the hospital administrator are reasonable options. Regardless of which course of action is followed, ethics require that the patient should be fully informed of the psychiatrist's decision.

Not all conflicts regarding disclosure in the public interest concern undue familiarity. A less dramatic situation was created when the psychiatrist learned from his patient, a social worker in a psychiatric hospital, that the ward psychiatrist was billing insurance companies for time not actually spent with patients, information which the patient did not wish to report for fear of retaliation. In this instance, for the psychiatrist to institute any action based on his patient's report would violate the patient's right to keep this information confidential, and would constitute unethical behavior, even though it would protect the ethical standards of the profession. A unique situation was described by Chodoff (personal communication, 1988) who learned of an instance in which a psychiatrist became aware that his patient was considering politically defecting with sensitive material. In this instance a concern for national security was in conflict with the commitment to maintain the patient's confidentiality. Even in a case such as this, the question whether the danger posed to the public warrants disclosure is a difficult one.

Confidentiality with patients dangerous to themselves or others

Since the *Tarasoff* decision in 1974,[53] psychiatrists have been faced with the possibility of liability for the violent conduct of their patients towards third parties. One major problem inherent in the *Tarasoff* decision is the ascription to psychiatrists of an ability to predict future dangerousness which is greater than is justified by current knowledge. As a result of this decision, psychiatrists have been forced into a role strongly at odds with their therapeutic commitment to patients' confidentiality and their wish to avoid becoming involved in acts of social control. There are, none the less, circumstances in which the psychiatrist's conviction that a patient will carry out a dangerous act is strong enough to warrant breaking confidentiality. Four such situations involve suicide, homicide, child abuse, and AIDS.

Suicide and homicide

The ethical issues involved in cases of suicidal and homicidal patients have been discussed elsewhere in this volume. With specific regard to questions of confidentiality, psychiatric ethics do not preclude informing family members of a suicidal patient's intent, or notifying the potential victim of a homicidal patient. The degree of conviction necessary to justify disclosure will vary among psychiatrists, but if the data support it, the clinical decision to break confidentiality is justified. When such a decision has been reached, it is important to keep in mind that, in addition to safeguarding patients' confidentiality, psychiatrists also have the responsibility of informing patients when their own actions are jeopardizing their confidentiality. They have the additional ethical responsibility of attempting to develop with the patient a course of action so that the breaking of confidentiality, like its establishment, can be a mutual process. The thoughtful, creative interventions described by Roth and Meisel[54] in *Tarasoff*-type clinical situations can serve as a model for the management of potential homicidal and suicidal cases, as well as instances of child abuse and AIDS. Although the psychiatrist may ultimately have to act without the patient's participation or consent, efforts to involve the patient ensure the maintenance of ethical standards despite the breaking of confidentiality.

The pedophile: an example of child abuse

Although state law requires the reporting of child abuse, ethical issues regarding confidentiality can arise when the patient is not currently abusive or when, in the course of therapy, the psychiatrist learns that, in the past, the patient abused a child who is no longer a minor. To open an investigation of past abuse can be extremely stressful for the victim, regardless of the fact that the abuse occurred many years previously.[55] A similar dilemma is faced by the psychiatrist who learns that his adult patient was abused as a child. If the state reporting laws do not cover such instances, the decision regarding the reporting and investigation of the abuse belongs to the patient, provided, of course, there is no evidence to suggest current pedophile activity on the part of the alleged abuser. When a patient is a potential pedophile and a camp counselor, school-teacher, or youth-group leader, implementing the duty to warn can be difficult. In the absence of concern about a particular child, one must ascertain whether the duty to warn pertains to all the children, to the organization, or both. From an ethical perspective, unnecessarily alarming both parents and children is most certainly not a benign intervention. Informing the institution, rather than the class of individuals who might be affected, is a restrained but reasonable course of action.

AIDS

The current AIDS epidemic has given rise to many ethical issues.[56–58] In some states, psychiatrists are required to report all cases of HIV to public health authorities. But ethical issues involving confidentiality arise whenever people who are at high risk for AIDS or are HIV-positive are sexually involved with unknowing partners.[59] Guidelines pertaining to such situations have not been provided by statute or case law in most states. Although the American Psychiatric Association has developed a policy regarding confidentiality and disclosure for patients with AIDS,[60] at present a specific course of action will need to be evolved by psychiatrists in their own clinical settings. Absent state laws to the contrary, the American Psychiatric Association takes the position that it is ethically permissible for psychiatrists to warn partners or identifiable potential partners that a patient is HIV-positive, provided that the patient has been encouraged to provide the warning himself, has failed to do so, and is told what information will be shared and with whom. The issue, however, continues to be actively debated.[61–64] Since the 'duty to warn' put forth in the initial *Tarasoff* decision was superseded by the 'duty to protect',[65,66] informing the partner of the patient's positive HIV status should be accompanied by a recommendation that the partner obtain information and treatment. Boyd,[63] addressing the difficulty of developing a therapeutic alliance with some HIV-positive patients, stresses that 'mutual empowerment' of patient and physician in the context of AIDS serves both 'medical beneficience and patient autonomy'. At the same time he also notes that, to avoid being traced, many HIV-positive patients may give false names and addresses, a powerful indicator of the difficulty of developing a collaborative relationship with them.

Hospital psychiatrists are frequently confronted by complex problems regarding the confidentiality of a patient's HIV status.[67,68] Should a psychiatrist respect the wish for confidentiality of a non-psychotic, well-controlled man who does not wish other staff to be informed of his positive HIV status? How should a patient who is HIV-positive and sexually active on the ward be managed if he refuses to share this information with staff and patients? A depressed, HIV-positive man is to be transferred to another hospital for rehabilitation following a mild cerebral infarction, but will not consent to release of information regarding his HIV status. Can the psychiatrist ethically convey this knowledge without the patient's permission? A butcher is hospitalized for an acute adjustment reaction with depressed mood. He has used intravenous drugs in the past, and is HIV-positive. If he refuses to inform his employer, what is the psychiatrist's ethical responsibility? What is the ethical course of action for the psychiatrist whose HIV-positive patient refuses to inform his wife or to allow the psychiatrist to do so?

Although the ethical issues resulting from AIDS are serious and complicated, they are confronted more often by general practitioners than by psychiatrists. However, as many as 25 per cent of individuals in the early stages of HIV infection manifest subtle dementia on neuropsychological testing, and 33 per cent will show a mild to severe dementia during the course of their illness.[69] Because of this and because many other individuals at risk for AIDS are initially treated in mental health facilities, psychiatrists may be the first to test the patient for HIV infection. Both clinically and ethically, it is desirable prior to the testing to obtain the patient's consent and to elaborate the course of action resulting from a positive test. In addition, a careful assessment of organic impairment is an essential aspect of the evaluation of the AIDS patient, not only from the perspective of thoroughness, but also to assess the patient's ability fully to comprehend the implication of his illness and to give informed consent.

Confidentiality and psychiatric genetics

Some hereditary medical illnesses such as Huntington's disease and Wilson's disease may present with psychiatric symptoms and may confront the psychiatrist with a difficult ethical dilemma. A man sought psychiatric treatment for depression and was found to have Huntington's disease. Recently married, he refused to inform his wife, fearing that she would elect not to have children. In such cases, despite the pain that would be inflicted on the mother and child should offspring develop the disease, in the absence of an imminent and definite threat, any disclosure by the psychiatrist would, in our opinion, be difficult to justify. This position of non-disclosure reflects the high degree of restraint which is required to prevent concern and compassion from overriding the patient's fundamental right to regulate the disclosure of personal information.

Ethics, confidentiality, and the treatment of children

When working with children, the ethical principles which guide the psychiatrist's management of confidentiality in the treatment of adults need to be significantly modified.

Until they achieve a sense of themselves as separate, autonomous individuals, children do not develop a mature sense of confidentiality. Young children believe that parents know their private thoughts and feelings, and may be concerned that their secrets are revealed through their secretions (for example, nocturnal emissions, urine, feces).[35] Before the age of seven, children operate by pre-logical cognition, and cannot achieve the sense of personal responsibility essential to an understanding of confidentiality.[70] Even by the age of twelve, when children begin to think according to the principles of formal operations, that level of cognition may only be achieved in areas where they have regular practice. Erikson has stressed that 'morality, ideology and ethics must evolve in each person by a step by step development from less to more differentiated and insightful stages ... Developmentally speaking, we must ... differentiate between an earlier moral conscience and a later ethical one.'[71] Kolansky (personal communication, 1989) has noted that, if promised total confidentiality, a young child may actually become more rather than less anxious. This is especially true of pre-school and latency children, but may at times even be true of adolescents. Thus the point of view that confidentiality is an inherent good in therapeutic relationships cannot automatically be applied to work with children. Ethical behavior requires that the psychiatrist evaluate what, if anything, about confidentiality should be explained to the child, rather than pursue the abstract goal of promising total confidentiality. The decision of when to keep or when to break confidentiality must be reached anew not only with each child, but also in each instance in which the issue occurs with the same child.

In every treatment of a child, a thorough discussion with parents about the management of confidentiality is essential. In theory, the person who provides consent for the treatment has access to anything discussed between child and psychiatrist. In practice, however, therapeutic communications with the child are confidential, and the psychiatrist determines what, if any, information will be shared with parents. Clarification with the parents at the outset that the child's therapy is confidential and that the disclosure of information conveyed by the child will depend upon clinical judgment is not only ethical, but may eliminate a future conflict that might result in the parents' discontinuing the child's therapy abruptly and against the psychiatrist's advice. There are instances, as with a schizophrenic adolescent who wishes no information to be communicated to his parents, in which the ethical duty to provide optimum treatment overrides the duty to protect confidentiality and allows the psychiatrist to convey essential information to the parents. Psychiatrists need to keep in mind that the content of a child's therapy may be indirectly communicated. As Lipton[72] has noted, the nature of the questions which a child psychiatrist asks of parents during the course of therapy indirectly reveals some of the subjects discussed by the child.

Child psychiatrists take a range of positions with regard to the confidentiality of sessions with parents. Although a psychiatrist might promise to keep the material of parental sessions 'confidential', such information cannot be isolated from the psychiatrist's thinking. Family secrets are secrets only in the sense that they have not been explicitly divulged, and, in actuality, are 'known', and strongly influence family functioning and the experience of the child. Similarly, information which parents convey must influence the way the psychiatrist listens and responds to the child. Ethically, child psychiatrists who wish to keep private some information conveyed by parents need to explain that, regardless of whether it is directly communicated to the child, such information will have some impact upon treatment. It would seem prudent to emphasize that clinical judgment will determine what material from sessions with parents is directly discussed with the child.

Although legal issues are central in child-custody cases, ethical issues concerning confidentiality frequently arise. Control of all information about the child's treatment generally belongs to the parent who has the legal responsibility to give consent for the treatment. For example, the custodial parent may refuse permission for the psychiatrist to provide the non-custodial parent with any information regarding the child, even though the child might be spending the summer with that parent. The psychiatrist, believing that a consultation with the parent would benefit the child, is in the ethical dilemma of depriving the patient of the maximum therapeutic benefit in order to conform with the law. The problem is further compounded in work with young children, to whom it may be almost impossible to explain the situation adequately. Ethics dictate that the psychiatrist be prepared to work intensively with the custodial parent, and, if necessary, to request that the court intervene on the child's behalf and permit appropriate disclosures to the non-custodial parent.

Ethics, confidentiality, and adolescents

Nowhere are the issues of confidentiality more fluid and complex than in the psychiatric treatment of the adolescent, who may have the legal right (depending on the state) to be responsible for the decisions regarding the disclosure of confidential material, but whose psychological immaturity compromises his ability to make the best choices regarding its management.[73]

Although the child's ability to conceptualize confidentiality evolves gradually, by 12 to 15 years of age most children understand and value the concept.[74] By this age they have passed from Piaget's stage of moral realism to the stage of moral relativism, and have acquired the sense of personal responsibility essential to the development of ethical standards and full understanding of confidentiality. At this point they can also recognize its importance in psychotherapy.[68] While it has long been assumed that confidentiality is especially important to adolescents, a 1993 study[75] indicated that 58 per cent of adolescents had health concerns they wished to keep private from their parents, and 25 per cent would not seek health care if their parents 'might' find out. Only 33 per cent were aware of a right to confidentiality. Given these findings, it is especially important that confidentiality be discussed and boundaries defined at the very outset of the treatment.

In addition to the striking variability in the degree to which adolescents understand confidentiality, the kinds of issues which they bring to the psychiatrist are often much more serious than those brought by younger children. Assuming that an adolescent has the right to consent to treatment without parental permission and therefore has the right to control the maintenance of confidentiality, what ethical course of action shall the psychiatrist pursue if the child informs him of plans to run away; what is ethically indicated if he admits that he has moved from the occasional use of marijuana to the frequent use of cocaine, but refuses permission for the psychiatrist to discuss these issues with the parents? Should a psychiatrist maintain the confidentiality of a 13-year-old girl who plans to have sex with her 17-year-old boyfriend while the parents are away for the weekend? How shall one respond to reports of parental nudity if the patient refuses permission to raise the issue with them? How does one discuss confidentiality with a teenager who knows full well his legal rights at the outset of treatment? Given that the psychological development of adolescents may lag significantly behind the legal rights achieved by chronology alone, it seems prudent to be realistic regarding confidentiality. Frank explanation of the psychiatrist's wish to respect the patient's rights and at the same time protect the treatment and the patient's welfare will provide a framework for resolving issues of confidentiality should they arise. Crucial in such a dialogue is the complete assurance that confidentiality will not be broken without prior discussion with the patient.

Ethics, confidentiality, and group, family, and couples' therapy

Groups by their very nature are public, and group therapy can be conceptualized as 'a form of communal living where there is little privacy among its members, and privacy is not a value. Outside the group, however, isolation and privacy prevail'.[76] Additional problems with establishing and maintaining confidentiality result from the permeability of group boundaries, and the fact that the responsibility to maintain confidentiality is shared by all members, and therefore necessarily diluted.[36] To these problems are added the human proclivity to gossip and the fact that in most states the law has not definitively forbidden the breaking of confidentiality by group members. Given these obstacles to the maintenance of confidentiality, psychiatrists have employed a number of mechanisms. Among these are:

(1) using first names only;
(2) urging group members to see themselves as co-therapists, thereby increasing their sense of responsibility;
(3) discouraging or forbidding meetings of group members outside the psychotherapeutic setting;
(4) rigorous analysis of any breaks in confidentiality;
(5) terminating treatment of anyone who breaks confidentiality,[77] and
(6) the establishment of a contract regarding confidentiality.

In group settings no psychiatrist can assure the degree of confidentiality which can be maintained in work with a single person. The group psychotherapist, not his patients, has a professional code of ethics which is based on confidentiality.[78] Group members will need relatively frequent reminders of the importance of confidentiality,[78] especially given the multiplicity of forces which work to weaken it. This is true even for 'closed' groups in which no new members are added for the duration of the group. As discussed in the above consideration of the confidentiality of meetings with the parents of a child in psychotherapy, it is impossible for the psychiatrist to be unaffected by the information which a group (or family or couples') psychotherapy patient might discuss in an individual session.[79] We believe that ethical responsibility requires the psychiatrist to explain this clearly to the patient, emphasizing that while overt disclosure will not occur, unconscious communication reflecting the information confided is likely to occur to some degree. At the very least, the psychiatrist, knowing this 'confidential material', will listen differently to the patient and his responses will be subtly affected.

To a significant degree, these issues pertain to family therapy as well as to group therapy. Further difficulties arise in the treatment of families because the developmental maturities of the members are so disparate. Young children, for example, cannot be expected to maintain confidentiality over private matters (for example, alcoholism, violence, and infidelity), and it is therefore important to clarify this with the parents before the beginning of therapy. The therapist also has the responsibility of ensuring the confidentiality of the parents with respect to the children.[80]

Confidentiality when patients are seeing more than one therapist

In contemporary psychiatric practice it is not unusual for patients to be treated by more than one mental health professional. When a patient sees one person for psychotherapy and another for pharmacotherapy, the two treatments are somewhat discrete. By contrast, when a patient is seeing one person in individual psychotherapy and another in couples or group psychotherapy, the treatments clearly overlap. In both situations initial discussions between the two therapists are often indicated, and, depending upon the patient and the manner of practice of the therapist, ongoing communication may be desirable. Permission given for an initial sharing of information does not automatically pertain to future discussions. In one instance, a woman in individual psychotherapy entered a group specifically devoted to the treatment of adults who had been sexually abused as children. She freely gave permission for her therapists to consult prior to her entering the group. After several months, the group therapist called the individual therapist to convey some concern about the nature of the patient's participation in the group. The individual therapist asked whether the patient had given permission for the call, and, upon learning that she had not, ended the conversation. The patient, on learning of the group therapist's call, was angered, both because her permission had not been asked and because she had been unaware of the therapist's concern.

In general, this type of communication is best conceptualized as one would any other release of information. As such, it needs to be clearly structured with the patient beforehand. For example, a man in couples treatment had discussed his extramarital affair only with his individual therapist. The couple's therapist requested and was granted permission to speak with the individual therapist, who postponed the conversation until he had discussed what information the patient wished to be kept confidential. To avoid just such a dilemma many individual psychotherapists would refuse any discussion at all. Whether one takes this position, whenever possible, permission for discussion should be obtained in each instance, and the specific information to be disclosed should be clarified prior to each discussion. In addition, ethics dictate that the specifics of each discussion should be shared with the patient. This course of action is prudent, because the information belongs to the patient and because the information conveyed will affect the thinking and behavior of the therapist. Therefore, when discussing a patient with another therapist, one should share only those thoughts which one would not have any hesitation in discussing directly with the patient.

Confidentiality and writing and speaking

In a thoughtful paper, Davis[81] explores the ethics in medical writing of the 'thick description', a term drawn from anthropology. Arguing from specific case examples, she suggests that only thick descriptions allow consideration of universalizable ethical norms and of relationships that extend over time and 'avoid getting out of a case only what we put into it'. 'Thin cases' on the other hand, shut off the possibility of seeing new perspectives. Disguising a case so that the patient could not recognize himself compromises the integrity of the case, but writing thick case descriptions raises serious ethical issues.

Freud struggled with these issues in his introductory comments to the case of Dora.[82] Noting that there are those who would give 'first place to the duty of medical discretion', he concludes that:

in my opinion the physician has taken upon himself duties not only towards the individual patient but towards science as well; and his duties towards science mean ultimately nothing else than his duties toward the many other patients who are suffering or will some day suffer from the same disorder. Thus it becomes the physician's duty to publish what he believes he knows of the causes and structure of hysteria, and it becomes a disgraceful piece of cowardice on his part to neglect doing so, as long as he can avoid causing direct personal injury to the single patient concerned. [p. 8]

The inclusion of detailed clinical material in oral presentations and in the psychiatric literature presents the psychiatrist with the unavoidable ethical dilemma of protecting the patient's confidentiality while at the same time avoiding a reduction of the material's scientific merit by excessive disguise. Even if written with the utmost attention to the disguise of identifying data and with all due discretion, a detailed case-study raises 'serious questions about its effect on the patient in relation to his social milieu. Even if these can be discounted, we must still consider the implications with respect to persisting transferential attitudes towards his [former] analyst. We know that they do exist and they must be taken into account. To have one's analyst become one's biographer must acquire a significance difficult to define over the long run.'[85]

Stoller in a provocative, thoughtful discussion of this problem quotes a patient whose case-vignette had been published without her knowledge: ' "You said", she stated, "it hadn't hurt me, that you were justified because I couldn't be identified" (I recall that slightly differently: I believe I said it need not have hurt her because she could not be identified, thereby ignoring, in the comfort of proper ethics, her more complex experience...) "How could you know that by not informing or warning me or whatever that you were transgressing that sacred boundary, the infinite trust I placed in you." ' [p. 382][21]

Stoller, who allows patients to read and edit any detailed report, emphasizes the problem of obtaining truly 'informed consent' from a patient whose transference strongly influences the freedom to refuse. If the patient is currently in treatment, the ability to give informed consent is likely to be especially affected by the transference. In such a situation patients should be encouraged to consult with another psychiatrist regarding publication, and this consultation might be paid for by the author. When writing about patients in the mental health field whose friends and colleagues can be expected to read the psychiatric literature, the need for disguise is especially great. When the identity of the author will make identification of the patient more likely, the article might be published under a pen-name. Lipton[72] reported a situation indicative of the extreme caution that one must take in writing about patients. In the instance he described, an analyst in a study group presented a case. A member of the study group, without asking or informing the presenter, used the case in an article. The patient's father read the case, recognized his son as the patient, and informed him of the article. The patient was predictably furious with his analyst. It seems clear that a psychiatrist intending to publish a detailed case history must obtain the patient's consent. We believe that meaningful consent requires that the patient should read the actual material and then give permission for publication. If the psychiatrist thinks that it would be detrimental to the patient to read this material, ethics would indicate that it should be excluded from the publication.

Finally, we draw attention to the ethical issues involved in the large case conference in which patients agree to be interviewed and the issue of giving informed consent for taped sessions which are to be used in the future for 'educational purposes'. With regard to taping, the consent should be as specific as possible with respect to the circumstances in which the tape will be used. If the treating psychiatrist is seeking the consent, the patient should be encouraged to have a consultation with an independent psychiatrist which will maximize the likelihood that the consent is free and fully informed. Furthermore, the consent should be renewed on a periodic basis. As emphasized by Graham (see Chapter 14), this is especially important with regard to children and adolescents who may wish to prevent disclosure when they come of age. Since confidentiality is significantly compromised and devalued whenever patients are interviewed or tapes are played before large audiences, one needs to be certain that the information could not be effectively conveyed in a less revealing fashion. In addition, psychiatrists should remind members of the audience of their obligation to leave if they know the patient or anyone in his family.

Ethics, confidentiality, and psychiatric education

Psychiatric education invariably involves discussion of personal thoughts and feelings of trainees and medical students and the relationship between psychiatric supervisors and their students is likely to elicit stronger transference responses than between students and teachers in other medical or non-medical settings. Furthermore, members of the psychiatric faculty may be in possession of important information about residents, which they have acquired under confidential circumstances. These factors contribute to ethical issues regarding the maintenance of confidentiality which are encountered in procedures of admission, patient-care, supervision, and evaluation.

Admissions committees regularly face ethical choices regarding the confidentiality of material pertaining to applicants. In one instance, a committee member had treated an applicant for a serious depression on several occasions. He had significant reservations about the applicant, who had not informed any interviewers of the treatment. Concerned that the applicant, the applicant's patients, and the residency would be adversely affected should the applicant matriculate and later decompensate, he was faced with the ethical conflict between his responsibility to the patient (applicant), the residency program, and the community. He considered this information to be confidential, and ultimately chose to keep it private. Admissions committees must routinely decide whether to inquire about an applicant from a former therapist. Should such a request be made, it would be the responsibility of the therapist, in consultation with the applicant, to determine what, if any, information should be shared with the committee. From an ethical perspective, however, such a request places the committee in the position of asking the applicant to violate a basic tenet of the psychiatrist–patient relationship. Furthermore, since the committee has significant control over the applicant's future, it is questionable whether truly informed consent can be given.

There is considerable disagreement regarding the ethical obligation of psychiatric residents (or psychiatrists) to inform patients when their cases are being supervised. Medical and surgical patients receiving care in a teaching hospital expect their cases to be used for educational purposes; but psychiatric patients treated by residents or other students may not be aware that the details of psychotherapy sessions will be discussed with another person on a regular basis. Psychiatrists have taken broadly divergent positions on this topic,[84–86] ranging from the opinion that telling the patient about supervision represents an unanalyzable parameter which unnecessarily burdens him with the therapist's problems (for example, feelings about being in training) to the point of view that the supervisor should be present at the initial interview, and that the role of the supervisor should be clearly explained. Since a high value is placed on confidentiality in therapeutic relationships, and since decisions to break confidentiality are generally made by the patient or with his knowledge, a unilateral and ongoing compromise of confidentiality, such as is inherent in supervision, would seem to require prior discussion with the patient. Confidentiality, however, is not an end in itself; confidentiality is protected to enhance the efficacy of the treatment. With many patients, especially those who are suspicious or overtly psychotic, complete candor about supervision may sacrifice the therapeutic alliance on the altar of confidentiality. In arriving at what is ultimately a clinical decision, the psychiatrist must weigh the impact of disclosure. Should the psychiatrist elect to discuss the issue of supervision, patients may subsequently displace their mistrust from therapist to supervisor—a development requiring therapeutic exploration. Even in such circumstances, the candor of the therapist in informing the patient of the supervisor's role will underscore the seriousness with which the therapist views the subject of confidentiality, and will help to repair any rift in the therapeutic alliance. Should patients inquire whether their cases are supervised, ethics would dictate a frank and open discussion of the subject. Psychiatrists who are in psychotherapy themselves may often discuss patients with their therapists. However, to inform patients of this compromise of confidentiality would be honest, but almost always counter-therapeutic.

Additional issues of confidentiality are also inherent in the process of supervision. Psychiatric educators are so accustomed to the importance of supervision that 'it is difficult for them to see it as impinging on trainees' privacy and therefore on their security within the training program'.[87] Especially when exploring residents' personal reactions to their patients, supervisors will acquire considerable information which may be only marginally relevant to their evaluation, and which should therefore be kept confidential. Supervision, which can be considered to be the 'psychotherapy of work' (D. Scharff, personal communication, 1973), is rooted in education and in psychotherapy, thus creating the ethical issue of confidentiality for the supervisor and concerns about the degree of disclosure of personal information for the supervisee. Moreover, residents frequently experience significant conflict about how much of the patient's identifying data should be revealed to the supervisor—the patient's full name or the names of others mentioned by the patient, a particularly thorny problem when well-known people are involved. While each resident–supervisor pair must make its own decision regarding this matter, we consider the nature of supervision to be such that the resident is not required to maintain the confidentiality of material revealed in therapy. In fact, if the resident does not feel required to edit the patient's material, the supervision may be freer and more productive. As do psychotherapists, supervisors may have to discontinue supervision if they know the patient or someone important in the patient's life.

The evaluation of residents, and especially candidates in psychoanalytic institutes, poses difficult problems of confidentiality.[88-90] One analytic institute which adopted a principle of strict confidentiality, completely separating a candidate's analysis and evaluation, was unable to adhere to this principle, and broke confidentiality in a number of ways, some overt, others more subtle.[88,89] Although the maintenance of confidentiality may be more difficult in psychoanalytic institutes (it was broken by the institution when the analyst reported on the progress of the patient to the committee evaluating candidates' progress), it is not easy in psychiatric residencies, especially those in smaller communities where a member of the faculty may be treating one of the residents. Compromises of confidentiality are exemplified by the following:

1. Dr Smith, a member of the psychiatric faculty, hears from a patient that a resident exhibited immature and unprofessional behavior by mocking Dr Smith at a party. Without informing the resident in question, Dr Smith enters a note in the record which is not available for review by the resident.

2. An analyst hears from a psychoanalytic candidate in treatment some highly negative comments about another candidate; he participates in the second candidate's evaluation, introducing the material but protecting the source by invoking confidentiality.

3. A resident confides to a faculty member that he is seriously depressed, and clinically he appears quite paranoid. He is referred to a psychiatrist not associated with the residency, whom he can see for treatment. Although the resident's work is satisfactory, the degree of his paranoia gives the faculty member significant concern. Can he ethically discuss his concerns with the faculty without the resident's knowledge or permission?

4. A resident informs the director of residency training that a respected, long-time supervisor from the community has made repeated explicit sexual overtures. She wishes to be transferred to a different supervisor, and does not want the director to speak to the supervisor or to inform the faculty of the reasons for the change. The director, convinced of the accuracy of the report, accedes to her wishes and assigns her to a different supervisor. Ethically, what courses of action are open to him regarding the supervisor whose future absence from the list of supervising psychiatrists would be certain to attract attention?

While each of these situations is complicated by the involvement of a third party, the faculty, ethical principles dictate that confidentiality should be broken only if absolutely necessary, and only after discussion with the party conveying the confidential information. This approach seems applicable in institutional and educational situations, as well as in clinical work.

Responding to material heard in confidence from the patient

When psychiatrists hear certain material within the confidential boundaries of the therapeutic relationship, several ethical problems may be created. One category of situations concerns the degree to which psychiatrists can ethically use information which the patient conveys within the therapeutic setting; a second concerns possible actions which the psychiatrist might take in response to information about a patient from a third party.

Laws regulating insider-trading apply to information acquired in treatment. A psychiatrist who invests or makes other business deals on the basis of insider-information obtained through the psychotherapeutic relationship can be found guilty of insider-trading. Thus, when the president of a small firm whose stock is traded publicly informs his psychiatrist that his company is going to be bought out, the psychiatrist cannot act on this information himself, nor can he convey it to others. But laws regulating insider trading do not pertain to decisions which the psychiatrist might wish to make on the basis of a non-insider stock tip offered him by a patient who has had great success with investments. However, a psychiatric code of ethics might require that this information should not be used for any investment decisions by the psychiatrist. If conveyed to the patient, any investment decision will significantly alter the nature of the therapeutic relationship. If the recommendation proved successful, the patient might wish or feel obliged to offer other suggestions. It is not inconceivable that he could reasonably expect to be reimbursed for his professional advice by a fee reduction or 'free hour'. If unsuccessful, he might feel guilty and seek to make amends or avoid expressing hostility. Even if the psychiatrist never informs the patient that he acted on the investment suggestion, the relationship with his patient will be affected. Good advice might lead him unconsciously or even consciously to encourage the patient to provide other investment information. If the tip proved to be a poor one, the psychiatrist's disappointment and resentment would be likely to find a means of expression within the therapeutic relationship. As strictly as the psychiatric boundary is regulated by concern for privacy and confidentiality, so strictly is it governed by the implicit understanding that the psychiatrist's sole interest in the patient is to provide treatment and to further the achievement of therapeutic goals. Using information acquired in the therapeutic relationship to make specific investment decisions cannot help but alter the nature of the psychiatrist–patient relationship, and therefore has ethical ramifications.

Based on what their patients tell them, psychiatrists inevitably do engage in a wide range of extratherapeutic actions which are within the boundaries of ethical behavior. In the field of finance, for example, a psychiatrist cannot be expected to ignore general information regarding interest rates which his banker-patient tells him in the hopes of earning the psychiatrist's admiration or affection. Similarly. attending a movie, reading a book, or eating at a restaurant on the suggestion of a patient do not cross the line separating ethical from unethical action. But psychiatrists need to keep in mind that every such action may have an impact, even if minor, on the relationship between them and their patients.

Responding to confidential material heard in another setting of relevance to the patient

Numerous situations occur in which the psychiatrist learns in a confidential relationship of information of significant importance to a patient. We believe that these instances of 'reverse confidentiality' merit serious consideration. In smaller communities, for example, or in psychoanalytic institutes in which a limited number of psychiatrists are available to treat the same population, the psychiatrist is routinely faced with the ethical problem of how to handle material about one patient which is conveyed to him by another. How should a psychiatrist respond to the report from Mr A that Mr B (another patient) is abusing drugs if Mr A is unwilling to inform Mr B that he has told the psychiatrist, and is also unwilling to be identified as a source of information.

Unless the danger to the patient is considered to be extremely severe, unilateral breaking of Mr A's confidentiality seems unwarranted, and the psychiatrist and Mr A must attempt to resolve the issue therapeutically. A different type of problem is presented by participation in the activities of professional ethics committees. A psychiatrist, who was a member of the local psychiatric ethics committee, learned that his patient's daughter is about to enter treatment with a psychiatrist whom he knows will definitely be expelled from the local psychiatric society for having had sexual relationships with a patient. In this instance the psychiatrist had conflicting fiduciary responsibilities—one to maintain the confidentiality of the proceedings of the ethics committee, the other to protect his patient's daughter. An ethical (and legal) solution to this situation might be to express serious reservations about the daughter's psychiatrist, without identifying the specifics or the source of one's doubts.

Another situation, also more common in small or circumscribed communities. but not infrequent in any psychiatric practice, is created when a patient describes intimate details of the life of someone whom the psychiatrist knows well. While it is an everyday occurrence for a psychiatrist to hear confidential material about named third parties, there is an inherent ethical conflict if the third party is the psychiatrist's close friend. In such instances, professional ethics dictate that the psychiatrist consider referring the patient to someone else—a step which, from a therapeutic perspective, will allow the treatment to proceed without the difficulties inevitably faced by the psychiatrist who is forced to listen to material which the friend might wish to keep private.

Informing patients about the limits of confidentiality

As we have discussed throughout this chapter, absolute confidentiality cannot be assured. Psychiatrists may be understandably reluctant to begin a consultation with a discussion of the limitations of confidentiality. On the other hand, if the psychiatrist delays such a discussion for only a brief time he may learn damaging information about the patient that he will be required to disclose in a custody case, or other proceeding. There may be an inherent conflict between a psychiatrist's responsibility to provide the patient immediately with all the knowledge relevant to a patient's decision to initiate treatment and disclose confidential information and the psychiatrist's ability to establish an enduring and effective therapeutic alliance. Such decisions require considerable reflection and yet, the psychiatrist must often make rapid decisions without the time for reaching a decision more deliberately. We believe that the profession needs to address this issue and to develop techniques for reducing this conflict.

Conclusions

In psychoanalysis and in most psychiatric treatments, 'one of the understandings about confidentiality is that the analyst wields no power in the life of the patient other than the power of psychoanalysis itself'. Confidentiality embodies the recognition of a power never to be used.[50] Although confidentiality has been shown to be highly valued by psychiatrists and patients, its boundaries are assaulted from without by changes in the health-care system, electronic communication of confidential information, and changes in legal statutes, and threatened from within by the human urge to gossip, the therapeutic need for periodic consultation, the educational and scientific requirement that clinical case material be made available for discussion, and the need to protect against such potential harms as suicide, homicide, and child abuse. Current and future legal statutes and judicial decisions may provide some guidelines for psychiatrists. In most contexts, however, ethical norms rather than laws will be the primary source of guidance towards solutions which respond to the specific situation while maintaining the basic principle of compromising as little confidential material as possible.

Bollas and Sunderson,[26] in a sharp, incisive book, have taken the profession to task for its largely silent compliance with the widespread erosion of the absolute confidentiality of the psychiatric consulting room. In labeling psychotherapists as the 'new informants', they document numerous instances in which they believe that our patients have been betrayed. Their book poses a challenge which the profession and the society as a whole must grapple with.

The *Oxford English Dictionary* gives four definitions of 'confidence':

- 'the mental attitude of trusting or relying';
- 'the feeling sure or certain of a fact or issue';
- 'assurance ... arising from reliance on oneself';
- as an adjective 'a method of professional swindling in which the victim is induced to hand over money or other valuables as a token of "confidence"'
  A confidence man is 'one who practices the confidence trick; a professional swindler of respectable appearance and address'.

Etymology can tell us much about the kind of environment which nurtures human development and personal growth in psychiatric treatment. For children, the mental attitude of trusting in another contributes greatly to an enduring sense of self-reliance which grows from an internalization of the relationship and an ability to assess the external world for trustworthiness. For our patients, the establishment of an environment of trust and reliance is at the core of the psychotherapeutic process. Given all the developments that jeopardize confidentiality, we must be vigilant lest we become psychiatric confidence men and women, inducing our patients to hand over to us their intimate thoughts and life stories which we then fail to protect.

We are only too aware of the effort required, and, in the case of writing and speaking, of the sacrifice which may be entailed in the ethical maintenance of confidentiality. However, the psychiatrist's primary responsibility to the welfare of his or her patients merits this degree of vigilance and care.

References

1. *The principles of medical ethics with annotations especially applicable to psychiatry.* Washington DC, American Psychiatric Association, 1995.
2. Winslade, W. J.: Confidentiality, in *Encyclopedia of bioethics*, ed. W. T. Reich. New York, Free Press, 1978, pp. 184–200.
3. Leong, G. B. and Silva, J. A.: Another courtroom assault on the confidentiality of the psychotherapist–patient relationship. *Journal of Forensic Sciences* **40**:862–4, 1995.
4. Weil, F.: Releasing the treating psychiatrist from confidentiality. *Medicine and Law* **12**:249–55, 1993.
5. Shah, S. T.: Privileged communications, confidentiality and privacy. *Professional Psychology* **1**:56–69, 1969.
6. Knapp, S. and Vandecreek, L.: *Privileged communications in the mental health professions.* New York, Van Nostrand Reinhold, 1987.
7. In *re Lifschutz*. 85 Cal. Rptr 829, 476 P.2d 557 Cal. Sup. Ct 9 (1970).
8. Everstine, L., Everstine, D. S., Heymann, G. M., et al.: Privacy and confidentiality in psychotherapy *American Psychologist* **35**:828–40, 1980.
9. Applebaum, P. S.: Confidentiality in psychiatric treatment, in *The American annual psychiatric review*, ed. L. Grinspoon. Washington, DC, American Psychiatric Press, pp. 327–34, 1982.
10. Gilmore, M. and Shear, K.: Ethical and legal considerations of confidentiality in the treatment of hospitalized health professionals. *Psychiatric Quarterly* **50**:237–45, 1978.
11. American Psychiatric Association: guidelines on confidentiality. *American Journal of Psychiatry* **144**:1522–6, 1987.
12. Jagim, R. D., Wittman, W. D., and Noll, J. O.: Mental health professionals' attitudes toward confidentiality, privilege and third-party disclosures. *Professional Psychology* **9**:458–66, 1978.
13. Lindenthal, J. J. and Thomas, C. S.: Consumers, clinicians and confidentiality. *Social Service and Medicine* **16**:333–5, 1982.
14. Lindenthal, J. J. and Thomas, C. S.: Psychiatrists, the public and confidentiality. *Journal of Nervous and Mental Disease* **170**:319–23, 1982.
15. Schmid, D., Appelbaum, P. S., Roth, L. H., and Lidz, L.: Confidentiality in psychiatry: a study of the patient's view. *Hospital and Community Psychiatry* **34**:353–5, 1983.
16. Appelbaum, P. S., Kappen, G., Waiters, B. Lidz, C., and Roth, L. H.: Confidentiality: an empirical test of the utilitarian perspective. *Bulletin of the American Academy of Psychiatry and The Law* **12**:109–16, 1984.
17. Lindenthal, J. J., Thomas, C. S., and Ghali, A.Y.: A cross cultural study of confidentiality. *Social Psychiatry* **20**:140–44, 1985.
18. McGuire, J. M., Toai, P., and Biau, B.: The adult client's conception of confidentiality in the therapeutic relationship. *Professional Psychology* **16**:375–84, 1985.
19. Siegler, M.: Confidentiality in medicine–a decrepit concept. *New England Journal of Medicine* **307**:1518–21, 1982.
20. Slovenko, R. and Usdin, G. L.: The psychiatrist and privileged communication. *Archives of General Psychiatry* **4**:431–44, 1961.
21. Stoller, R. J..: Patients' responses to their case reports. *Journal of the American Psychoanalytic Association* **36**:371–92, 1988.

22. Lindenthal, J. J. and Thomas, C. S.: Confidentiality in clinical psychiatry. *Medicine and Law* **11**:119–25, 1992.
23. Dubey, J.: Confidentiality as a requirement of the therapist: technical necessities for absolute privilege in psychotherapy. *American Journal of Psychiatry* **131**:1093–6, 1974.
24. Plaut, E. A.: A perspective on confidentiality. *American Journal of Psychiatry* **131**:1021–4, 1974.
25. Kottow, M. H.: Medical confidentiality: an intransigent and absolute obligation. *Journal of Medical Ethics* **12**: 117–22, 1986.
26. Bollas, C and Sundelson, D.: *The new informants: the betrayal of confidentiality in psychoanalysis and psychotherapy*. New Jersey, Jason Aronson, 1995.
27. American Psychiatric Association: state update. December, 1996.
28. Genensen, C., Sharp, H., and Genensen, M.: Faxing medical records: another threat to confidentiality in medicine. *Journal of the American Medical Association* **271**:1401–2, 1994.
29. Schetky, D. H.: The confidentiality of electronic communication. *American Association of Child and Adolescent Psychiatry News* September/October, 1996.
30. Bengtsson, S.: Clinical requirements for the security of the electronic patient record. *International Journal of Bio-medical Computing* **35** (Supplement), 29–31, 1994.
31. Fink, R.: Viewpoint. *Psychiatric News*, p. 18, 3 Feb. 1989.
32. Rosenbaum, J. E. and Subrin. M.: The psychology of gossip. *Journal of the American Psychoanalytic Association* **11**:817–31, 1963.
33. Medini, G. and Rosenberg, E. H.: Gossip and psychotherapy. *American Journal of Psychotherapy* **30**:452–6, 1976.
34. Olinick, S. L.: The gossiping psychoanalyst. *International Review of Psychoanalysis* **7**:439–45, 1986.
35. Caruth, E. G.: Secret bearer or secret barer? *Contemporary Psychoanalysis* **4**: 548–62, 1985.
36. Lakin, M.: *Ethical issues in the psychotherapies*. New York, Oxford University Press, 1988.
37. American Psychiatric Association: *Psychiatric News* **25**, p. 1, July 6, 1990.
38. *Psychiatric Times* **14**, p. 1, February, 1997.
39. McConnell, T.: Confidentiality and the law. *Journal of Medical Ethics* **20**:47–9, 1994.
40. Chodoff, P.: The Anne Sexton biography: the limits of confidentiality. *Journal of the American Academy of Psychoanalysis* **20**:639–44, 1992.
41. Joseph, D. I.: Discussion of the panel: Anne Sexton and the ethics of psychotherapy. ibid. 665–70,
42. Onek, J. N.: Legal issues in the Anne Sexton Case. ibid. 655–8.
43. Viorst, J.: Listening at the keyhole: the Anne Sexton Case. ibid. 645–54.
44. Weissberg, J. H.: Therapeutic responsibility in the case of Anne Sexton. ibid. 633–8.
45. Weissman, S. M.: Discussion of the panel: Anne Sexton and the ethics of psychotherapy. ibid. 659–64.
46. Rosner, B. L.: Psychiatrists, confidentiality and insurance claims. *Hastings Center Report* **10**:5–7, 1980.
47. Schwed, H. J., Kuvin, S. F., and Baliga, R. K.: Medicaid audit: crisis in confidentiality and the patient–psychiatrist relationship. *American Journal of Psychiatry* **136**:447–50, 1979.
48. Mosher, P. W.: A disturbing trend: defining confidentiality down. *American Psychoanalyst* **29**:10, 1995.

49. Chodoff, P.: The effects of the new economic climate on therapeutic practice. *American Journal of Psychiatry* **144**:1293–7, 1987.
50. Robitscher, J.: *The powers of psychiatry.* Boston, Houghton Mifflin, 1980.
51. Noll, J. O. and Hanlon, M. J.: Patient privacy and confidentiality at Mental Health Centers. *American Journal of Psychiatry* **133**:1286–8, 1976.
52. Lindenthal, J. J., Amaranto, E. A., Jordan, T. J., and Wepman, B. J.: Decisions about confidentiality in medical student mental health settings. *Journal of Counseling Psychology* **31**:572–5, 1984.
53. *Tarasoff* v *Regents of the University of California* 529 P.2d 553 (1974).
54. Roth, L. H. and Meisel, A.: Dangerousness, confidentiality and the duty to warn. *American Journal of Psychiatry* **134**:508–11, 1977.
55. Kelly, R. J.: Limited confidentiality and the pedophile. *Hospital and Community Psychiatry* **38**:1046–8, 1987.
56. Ginzburg, H. M. and Gostin, L.: Legal and ethical issues associated with HTLV-III diseases. *Psychiatric Annals* **16**:180–5, 1986.
57. Kelly, K.: AIDS and ethics: an overview. *General Hospital Psychiatry* **9**:331–40, 1987.
58. Dyer, A. R.: AIDS, ethics and psychiatry. *Psychiatric Annals* **18**:557–61, 1988.
59. Eth, S.: The sexually active, HIV infected patient: confidentiality versus the duty to protect. *Psychiatric Annals* **18**:571–6, 1988.
60. American Psychiatric Association: AIDS policy: confidentiality and disclosure. *American Journal of Psychiatry* **145**:541–2, 1988.
61. Perry, S.: Warning third parties at risk of AIDS: APA's policy is a barrier to treatment. *Hospital and Community Psychiatry* **40**:158–61, 1984.
62. Zonana, H.: Warning third parties at risk of AIDS: APA's policy is a reasonable approach. *Hospital and Community Psychiatry* **40**:162–4, 1984.
63. Boyd, K. M.: HIV infection and AIDS: the ethics of medical confidentiality. *Journal of Medical Ethics* **18**:173–9, 1992.
64. Seawright, H. R. and Pound, P.: The HIV positive patient and the duty to protect: ethical and legal issues. *International Journal of Psychiatry in Medicine* **24**:259–70, 1994.
65. *Tarasoff* v. *Regents of the University of California.* 131 Cal. Rptr 14, 17 Cal. 3d 425, 551 P.2d 334 (1976).
66. Weinstock, R.: Confidentiality and the new duty to protect: the therapist's dilemma. *Hospital and Community Psychiatry* **39**:607–9, 1988.
67. Carlson, G. A., Greeman, M. and McClellan, T. A.: Management of HIV-positive psychiatric patients who fail to reduce high risk behaviors. *Hospital and Community Psychiatry* **40**:511–14, 1989.
68. Zonana, H., Norko, M., and Stier, D.: The AIDS patient on the psychiatric unit: ethical and legal issues. *Psychiatric Annals* **18**:587–93, 1988.
69. Price, R. W., Sidtis, J. J., and Navia, B. A.: The AIDS-generation complex, in *AIDS and the nervous system*, ed. M. G. Rosenblum. New York, Raven, 1988.
70. Green, J. and Stewart, A.: Ethical issues in child and adolescent psychiatry. *Journal of Medical Ethics* **13**:5–11, 1987.
71. Erikson. E.: Psychoanalysis and ethics—avowed and unavowed. *International Review of Psychoanalysis* **13**:409–15, 1986.
72. Lipton, E. L.: Considerations concerning discussions and publication of case histories. Delivered at the meeting of the American Psychoanalytic Association, New York, 17 December, 1988.
73. Pert, I. N.: Confidentiality and consent in psychiatric treatment of minors. *Journal of Legal Medicine* **4**:9–13, 1976.

74. Kobocow, B., McGuire, J. M., and Blau, B. I.: The influence of confidentiality conditions on self disclosure of early adolescents. *Professional Psychology* **14**: 435–43, 1983.
75. Cheng, T. L., Savageau, J. A., Sattler, A. L., and De Witt, T. G.: Confidentiality in health care: a survey of knowledge, perceptions, and attitudes among high school students. *Journal of the American Medical Association* **269**:1404–7, 1993.
76. Slovenko, R.: Group psychotherapy: privileged communication and confidentiality. *Journal of Psychiatry and Law* **5**:405–66, 1977.
77. Gutheil, T. G. and Appelbaum, P. S.: *Clinical handbook of psychiatry and law*. New York, McGraw-Hill, 1982, Chapter 1.
78. Davis, K. L.: Is confidentiality in group counseling realistic? *Personnel and Guidance Journal* **58**:197–201, 1980.
79. Hines, P. M. and Hare-Muslin: Ethical concerns in family therapy. *Professional Psychology* **9**:165–71, 1978.
80. Margolin, G.: Ethical and legal considerations in marital and family therapy. *American Psychologist* **37**:788–801, 1982.
81. Davis, D. S.: Rich cases: the ethics of thick description. *Hastings Center Report* **21**12–17, 1991.
82. Freud, S.: *Fragment of an analysis of a case of hysteria*. Standard edn, vol. 7, pp. 7–122, 1901–1905. Hogarth Press, London.
83. Stein, M. H.: Writing about psychoanalysis. *Journal of the American Psychoanalytic Association* **36**:105–24, 1988.
84. DeBell, D. E.: A critical digest of the literature on psychoanalytic supervision. *Journal of the American Psychoanalytic Association* **11**:546–75, 1963.
85. Cavenar, J. O., Rhoades, E. J., and Sullivan, J. L.: Ethical and legal aspects of supervision. *Bulletin of the Menninger Clinic* **44**:15–22, 1980.
86. Hassenfeld, I. N.: Ethics and the role of the supervision of psychotherapy. *Journal of Psychiatric Education* **11**:73–7, 1987.
87. Betcher, R. W. and Zinberg, N. E.: Supervision and privacy in psychotherapy training. *American Journal of Psychiatry* **145**:796-803, 1988.
88. Dulchin, J. and Segal, A. J.: The ambiguity of confidentiality in a psychoanalytic institute. *Psychiatry* **45**:13–25, 1982.
89. Dulchin, J. and Segal, A. J.: Third party confidences: the uses of information in a psychoanalytic institute. *Psychiatry* **45**:27–37, 1982.
90. Kernberg, O. F.: Institutional problems of psychoanalytic education. *Journal of the American Psychoanalytic Association* **34**:799–834, 1986.

8

Boundary violations

Glen O. Gabbard

The notion of professional boundaries is a rather recent development in the history of psychiatry. While the Hippocratic Oath had long proscribed sexual relations between physician and patient, the early history of psychoanalysis was replete with sexual boundary violations.[1] Ernest Jones indicated in a letter to Freud that his common-law wife, Loë Kann, had been a patient of his. Sàndor Ferenczi was analyzing Elma Palos, the daughter of his mistress Gisela Palos, and fell in love with her. Although it is not entirely clear that he had sexual relations with her, he professed his love for her and certainly was physically affectionate with her.[2] Carl Jung was clearly overinvolved with Sabina Spielrein, and Wilhem Stekel was well known as a seducer of women. Otto Gross, another disciple of Freud's, engaged in group orgies to try to help neurotic patients overcome their sexual inhibitions.

Although Freud, as far as we know, was never sexually involved with his patients, he confessed in a letter to Jung that 'I have come very close to it a number of times and had a *narrow escape*'.[3] He was sufficiently concerned about the devastating impact of transference and countertransference that he was observing all around him in his disciples, that at times his 1912 technique papers sound like a version of the Ten Commandments designed to keep his students in line. One might consider these efforts as the beginning of what we now regard as professional boundaries within the field of psychiatry. For example, note the following passage in Freud's 1912 paper, 'Recommendations to physicians practising psycho-analysis': 'I cannot advise my colleagues too urgently to model themselves during psycho-analytic treatment on the surgeon, who puts aside all his feelings, even his human sympathy, and concentrates his mental forces on the single aim of performing the operation as skillfully as possible'.[4]

This quotation is of particular interest, because it represents a radical departure from Freud's actual behavior during analytic sessions, according to accounts from his patients who have reported their experiences.[5] Freud was anything but an anonymous or neutral figure. His personal presence was very much in evidence to his patients, and he made no effort to disguise his own personal judgments about issues that arose. Nevertheless, his concern that wild countertransference acting-out might sink his fledgling profession made him sound quite stern in some of his early technique papers.

Another example occurs in his 1915 paper, 'Observations on transference love':

If the patient's advances were returned it would be a great triumph for her, but a complete defeat for the treatment. She would have succeeded in what all patients strive for in analysis—she would have succeeded in acting out, in repeating in real life, what she ought only to have remembered, to have reproduced as psychical material and to have kept within the sphere of psychical events. [p. 166]

Despite these injunctions, psychoanalysts and other psychiatrists continued to become sexually involved with their patients both in Freud's time and since. Only in recent years, perhaps because of the rise of feminism and the courage of women who have felt empowered to make complaints to licensing boards and ethics committees, has the problem received the attention it deserves. Along with the recent burgeoning literature on sexual boundary violations, the profession has developed a heightened awareness of a number of other violations that do not involve sexual contact. Both will be considered in this chapter.

Definitions

Professional boundaries

A simple and succinct definition of professional boundaries would be to describe them as the 'edge' or limit of appropriate behavior by the psychiatrist in the clinical setting.[6] The fundamental idea is that attention to the basic aspects of the professional—as opposed to personal—nature of the relationship will serve to create an atmosphere of safety and predictability that facilitates the patient's ability to use the treatment. First and foremost, the psychiatrist is a professional being paid for a service, which places the interaction in the context of a *fiduciary* relationship. The awareness that the clinician is being enlisted as a professional to assist in the treatment of certain difficulties establishes a power differential. Other significant boundaries would include the absence of physical contact (other than a handshake), except in extraordinary circumstances; a circumscribed length to the appointments; confidentiality; declining lavish gifts; the avoidance of social or financial relationships with the patient that might interfere with the doctor–patient relationship; a relative asymmetry of self-disclosure, particularly regarding the personal problems of the clinician; and a specific location, such as an office or hospital, where the clinical contacts take place. When these parameters are considered *in toto*, they are often referred to as the *therapeutic frame*.[6–8] This frame is generally regarded as comprising more than just the sum total of the professional boundaries employed in treatment. In addition, certain human qualities that define the interaction are part of the frame as well. Clinicians attempt to be helpful and non–judgmental, understanding rather than critical, and willing to forego their own gratification in the interests of assisting their patients with the problems that brought them to treatment.

Unfortunately, some contemporary clinicians have misconstrued the concept of professional boundaries to suggest rigidity and remoteness in the relationship between the clinician and patient. This interpretation is a serious misreading of the role of boundaries in practice. The frame must be sufficiently flexible that it accommodates individual differences among patients and among clinicians. Similarly, it in no way implies coldness or aloofness. Rather, the boundaries are structural characteristics of the relationship that allow the therapist to interact with warmth, empathy, and spontaneity within certain conditions that create a climate of safety. One might say that the external boundaries of the treatment are established so that the psychological boundaries between patient and therapist can be crossed through a number of means that are common to psychotherapeutic experience. These would include identification, empathy, projection, introjection, and projective identification.[7,9]

Inherent in this understanding is that each therapist–patient dyad creates its own particular way of interacting with one another through a negotiation process. The degree of gratification versus frustration, the extent of self-disclosure versus discretion, and even flexibility involving the rescheduling of sessions or the length of sessions are all determined by the two subjectivities of the members of the therapeutic dyad.[7,10,11]

Professional boundaries also vary depending on the nature of the treatment itself. Most of the writing on boundaries has evolved from psychoanalysis and psychodynamic psychotherapy practice.[6,7,12–16] However, psychiatrists functioning in other roles may define somewhat different boundaries. For example, while a dynamic psychotherapist would not take a patient to a shopping mall in the therapist's personal automobile, a behavior therapist engaged in systematic desensitization might well drive an agoraphobic patient to the shopping mall for *in-vivo* exposure to a feared situation. In the latter case, the behavior therapist is functioning within the professional boundaries that are associated with the community standards of that treatment modality. A psychiatrist doing 'case management' in the community mental health center might have occasion to go to a chronic patient's apartment and assist with cleaning the apartment and getting the patient to an appointment on time. Psychopharmacologists have a set of boundaries more closely related to those of general physicians,[17] which include occasional physical examinations for tardive dyskinesia or other syndromes. Nevertheless, the basic principles of placing the patient's needs ahead of the clinician's needs are inherent in all treatment relationships. Moreover, an overarching principle is that whatever the clinician is doing should be part of a carefully organized treatment plan.

Boundary violations

Boundary violations involve transgressions that are *potentially* harmful to or exploitative of the patient. These may be sexual or non-sexual in nature. The 'potential' harm of the boundary violation is emphasized because one often cannot assess by the immediate impact whether harm has occurred. A clinical example will illustrate the complexity of determining whether or not harm has taken place:

Case 1

A 45-year-old male therapist told a 29-year-old female patient at the end of the hour that he was sorry he hadn't been listening more attentively. When the patient asked him what was the matter, he responded that his wife had left him for another man, and he was crying himself to sleep every night. He also explained that his youngest son was in trouble with the juvenile court for delinquent behavior. The patient's response to this self-disclosure was quite appreciative: 'I feel closer to you than I've ever been. It's so nice to know that you, too, have problems. I feel like I can tell you things more openly than I ever have because it feels more like an equal relationship now'. One year later, the same patient was ventilating in a written ethics complaint about how the therapist had misused her time and her fee to tell her about his personal problems.

As this vignette demonstrates, the impact of a boundary violation may take time to become apparent to the patient. The idea of focusing on *potential* harm also recognizes the fact that the therapist can never know the ultimate impact a boundary transgression will have on the patient. There may be other subtle breaks in the professional boundaries that appear to have no harm. For example, a therapist may gossip about a piece of information learned in therapy, thus breaking confidentiality. This break may never get back to the patient and overtly harm the treatment, but there is certainly potential harm in violating confidentiality because it alters the basic privacy of the therapeutic relationship.

Sexual boundary violations, of course, involve oral or genital contact, fondling of breasts or genitals, or sensual kissing. Non-sexual boundary violations can range widely from using the patient as a babysitter for the therapist's children to role-reversals in which the therapist talks to the patient at length about personal problems. Not all non-sexual boundary violations lead to sexual misconduct, but there is a well-known phenomenon, often referred to as the 'slippery slope', that involves the gradual progression of boundary violations from the most subtle and non-sexual to frank sexual involvement.[6,7,18]

Boundary crossings

Gutheil and I[6,9] have differentiated boundary violations from *boundary crossings*. In our view, a boundary crossing is a non-sexual boundary transgression in which the ultimate effect is positive in that it advances the therapy constructively. Subtle boundary crossings of this nature are inevitable in the course of the psychotherapy process or in an ongoing clinical relationship. Many involve human responses to unusual events.

Case 2

A 35-year-old patient with chronic paranoid schizophrenia came regularly for a medication appointment but was highly reserved, guarded, and hypervigilant in her interaction with her psychiatrist. She would answer questions tersely, but would hesitate to talk about any of the delusional material she was thinking about during the sessions. After a period of time, she began to develop more of a sense that she might be able to trust her psychiatrist. A breakthrough occurred when she came to a session and announced that she had been to a local fast-food restaurant. She explained to her psychiatrist that she had stopped for lunch and had purchased a cookie for dessert. She was unable to finish her lunch, and she asked if the psychiatrist would like the cookie. He accepted it graciously and thanked her for her generosity. Following this incident, the patient seemed more at ease with her doctor and was able to talk more openly about her psychotic thoughts.

In this vignette the psychiatrist transgressed a common boundary involving gifts. Nevertheless, accepting the patient's cookie promoted a trusting therapeutic alliance so that the treatment ultimately advanced. To have declined the gift might have been a devastating error, in that the patient's paranoia might have increased, and her perception of the psychiatrist as a malevolent individual might have caused her to disrupt the treatment and never return.

In expressive psychotherapy, a boundary crossing may be difficult to differentiate at times from a boundary violation. Often the fact that it can be discussed beneficially between therapist and patient may be the primary differentiating factor. The previous vignette also illustrates how boundaries must be considered as something more than simply a list of 'ethics rules' that must be obeyed to deliver effective treatment. Many ethical transgressions also involve errors in clinical judgment. Conversely, one could adhere to boundaries but make serious mistakes in clinical judgment.

Sexual boundary violations

Prevalence

The true prevalence of sexual misconduct in the mental health professions is unknown. Most of the estimates have been derived from self-report questionnaire surveys, which have notorious methodological problems. Many individuals do not return questionnaires. Other subjects will not feel assured of anonymity and answer questions dishonestly. The surveys that have been done suggest a prevalence among male therapists of somewhere between 1 per cent and 12 per cent and female therapists between 0 and 3.1 per cent.[19–26] The prevalence appears to decline when the later studies are compared with the earlier studies, but this apparent trend may relate more to the national trend towards criminalizing therapist–patient sex, which may lead some respondents to fear answering the questions truthfully. Most of the studies have focused on psychologists, but those that have surveyed psychologists, psychiatrists, and social workers[26] have found no difference in prevalence among the three major mental health disciplines.

Although by far the most common gender constellation in clinician–patient sexual misconduct is a male treater and a female patient, other combinations are not at all rare. In a large sample of 2000 therapists who were seen at the Walk-In Counseling Center in Minneapolis, Schoener *et al.* estimated that 20 per cent of cases involved a female therapist and 20 per cent of cases involved same-sex dyads.[27]

Several surveys have involved other medical specialties besides psychiatry.[28–32] These surveys have suggested that the prevalence among non-psychiatric medical specialties is roughly the same as it is among psychiatrists.

Profiles of clinicians

One of the major barriers to dealing with the problem of sexual boundary violations has come from the psychiatric profession itself. In some quarters there is an insistence on viewing the problem as one involving a handful of ethically corrupt predatory male clinicians who systematically prey on female patients. In this formulation no preventive measures are necessary for the rest of the practitioners in the field. The only step that is required is the identification of the 'bad apples', who can then be extruded from the profession, leaving only ethical practitioners to see patients. This kind of defensive disavowal of one's own vulnerability to boundary transgressions can lead the clinician to have a *laissez-faire* attitude about monitoring his or her own countertransference.

A much more sensible approach to prevention is to assume that all clinicians are potentially at risk of violating boundaries, especially given certain forms of life stress, such as divorce, death of a family member, malpractice litigation, or profound dissatisfaction in one's marriage or partnership. The various typologies that have been developed in the examination of large numbers of clinicians who have been involved in boundary violations bear out this notion that vulnerability is not limited to a few antisocial individuals.

Schoener and Gonsiorek[33] classified the therapist accused of sexual boundary violations into six categories or clusters: (1) uninformed and naïve; (2) healthy or mildly neurotic; (3) severely neurotic and socially isolated; (4) impulsive character disorder; (5) sociopathic or narcissistic character disorder; and (6) psychotic or borderline personality. They stressed that the first two groups respond well to education, treatment, and supervision in terms of their potential for rehabilitation, while the other four groups have a much worse prognosis.

Simon[34] broke the group into five clusters: (1) therapists with a character disorder such as antisocial, borderline, or narcissistic; (2) therapists with paraphilias or sexual disorders; (3) poorly trained and incompetent therapists; (4) therapists who are impaired by alcohol, drug addiction, or major mental illness; and (5) individuals who are reacting to a situation such as marital discord or the loss of a personal relationship.

These groupings can be subsumed under four psychodynamically based categories that I have found useful in my own work.[7,35]

Psychotic disorders

This group is by far the smallest and represents the occasional clinician whose sexual behavior towards the patient grows directly out of a psychotic process. One therapist in a manic episode, for example, began to believe that he was able to cure his patients through the act of intercourse. When the manic episode subsided, and he became euthymic, he recognized the absurdity of his delusional thinking. These conditions so rarely figure in sexual misconduct that a more detailed discussion will be omitted here.

Predatory psychopathy and paraphilias

In this category clinicians who meet DSM-IV criteria for antisocial personality disorder may be included, but many other individuals who would be regarded as having severe narcissistic personality disorders are also subsumed by this classification. The common theme is a sadistic and exploitative abuse of power in which the clinician has no remorse or guilt for what was done to the patient. Paraphilias are included in this category not because all clinicians with sexual perversions are predatory psychopaths, but because in my experience those who enact their perversions with patients they are treating tend to have the same underlying character pathology and superego problems that typify the predatory psychopathy group. Almost always male, clinicians in this group view their patients as 'easy targets' whom they can manipulate because of their position of power and because of their role as a transference object to the patient. They often have histories of corrupt and unethical behavior in other areas as well. They may have mishandled funds as a treasurer of an organization. They may have been caught cheating while in medical school or residency. They also may demonstrate predatory sexual behavior in their personal lives. There is generally a profound inability to empathize and a consequent use of other people as nothing more than objects of gratification.

Lovesickness

This group includes a range of diagnostic categories. What they all have in common is the subjective experience of being infatuated or 'madly in love' with their patients. This group may involve neurotically organized practitioners, many with mild narcissistic disturbances, and often those in a state of personal and professional crisis. This category is the one most common among *female* therapists. Psychodynamic issues include a desperate need to be validated, loved, and idealized by patients as a way of regulating the clinician's own self-esteem. There is also a failure in specific ego functions, such as judgment, as manifested by the inability to anticipate the consequences of one's actions, and a failure in reality testing, in which there is a circumscribed loss of the 'as if' quality of the ordinary experience of countertransference. In other words, the clinician cannot see that something from the patient's and/or the therapist's past is being repeated in the present and that understanding is necessary to make sense of it. Whereas the predatory psychopaths frequently have many victims, this group ordinarily falls in love with one particular patient while conducting competent treatments of their other patients.

These relationships often involve re-enactments of incestuous longings or actual incestuous relationships from the past of either therapist or patient. The clinicians who are lovesick often mistake their own needs for the patient's needs, and feel they are providing love for the patient while actually trying to obtain love for themselves. There also may be a desperate effort to fend off aggression and frustration with the patient by attempting to 'love' the patient back to health. When the clinician is female, she may be attracted to a charming young male with a personality disorder and substance abuse. She may view him as only 'a baby' and think that she can 'settle him down' by providing love for him.

Masochistic surrender

These clinicians often take special pride in treating 'impossible' or 'difficult' patients. In these treatment relationships they may be repeating an object relationship from the past in which they allowed themselves to be intimidated and controlled by a demanding and tormenting object, such as a parent. In some circumstances, these therapists believe that by sacrificing themselves, they are somehow saving a patient from suicide. Unable to set limits on the patient or confront the patient's aggression, they repeatedly give in to the patient's demands. In a typical scenario, the therapist first stops charging the patient because the patient insists he or she cannot afford the fee. Then phone calls are accepted at all hours of the night to try to save the patient from suicide. Eventually, the therapist responds to the patient's demands to be held by embracing or holding the patient during the hours. None of these extraordinary measures seem to work, so finally the boundary violations escalate to frank sexual contact. Psychodynamic treatment of these therapists frequently reveals a secret fantasy that they might yet be loved by tormenting parents if they were merely sufficiently submissive.

Post-termination relationships

All mental health professionals generally agree that sexual contact between a clinician and patient is unethical. Such behavior is unethical for the following reasons:

1. The clinician is equated with a parent in the transference and the relationship is symbolically incestuous.

2. It is an abuse of power because the professional is being paid to help the patient with psychological difficulties.

3. It is a frank exploitation in the sense that the clinician's needs are placed ahead of the patient's needs.

4. It is a failure to provide the service for which the patient has contracted the clinician.

However, the situation is more controversial with sexual relationships following the termination of treatment. While some organizations, such as the American Psychiatric Association, consider sexual contact with *any* former patients to be unethical, other groups, such as the American Psychological Association, have enacted a prohibition that applies for a two-year period after termination. Some advocates for a time limit suggest that one cannot infringe on constitutional rights of privacy and freedom of association by enacting a permanent ban on future relationships.[36] Others argue that if therapist and patient marry, exploitation is very difficult to substantiate.

Those on the other side of the argument point out that all studies of transference following termination show that it is instantly re-established years after termination if the therapist and patient meet again.[37] Another compelling argument is that as long as there is a possibility of a future romantic or sexual relationship, the therapy itself is profoundly contaminated. Neither party could speak freely about their observations if they wanted to preserve a positive image in the eyes of the other. It is only by virtue of the fact that the therapist–patient relationship will never be anything *but* professional that the patient can speak freely about all of his or her problems. Yet another reason for imposing a permanent ban on post-termination relationships is that many patients recontact the therapist for further consultation or treatment in the years following the end of the formal treatment. Ethics codes commonly implement policies that are more restrictive than what the Constitution provides, because they are established in the service of standards of professional conduct rather than constitutional protections. Finally, marriage in no way sanctifies the relationship as non-exploitative. History has shown that marriage has been used as an excuse for rape, assault, and a host of other sins. Just as love is irrelevant to considerations of ethics, so is marriage.

Assessment and rehabilitation of accused clinicians

Most clinicians who have been involved in sexual boundary violations come to the attention of impaired physicians' organizations, state licensing boards, or ethics committees of professional organizations when a complaint has been filed by the patient or other interested party. In other cases the clinician is wracked with guilt and comes forward on his or her own volition. At any rate, two separate but related processes are set in motion by reports to such a body. First of all, discipline or punishment is determined after an investigation of allegations in which each member of the dyad is given a fair hearing. Second, in parallel with such hearings, or sometimes after them, the clinician should be evaluated regarding whether he or she is suitable for rehabilitation. A central principle is that a thorough psychiatric evaluation, preferably by a disinterested party, must *precede* the determination of amenability to rehabilitation and the design of an individually tailored plan.[7,27] In the course of this psychiatric evaluation, the presence of collateral information about the accused psychiatrist must be available so that the evaluator does not rely exclusively on the psychiatrist's own self-report. Investigatory reports from licensing boards or ethics committees may be used to provide this separate perspective. Alternatives include a patient's written account of the transgression or a personal or telephone interview of the patient. In the course of the evaluation the examining psychiatrist must assess the causes, the character of the accused clinician, and the basic psychodynamic conflicts within that clinician. Often projective psychological testing is of extraordinary value in making such an assessment.

In most cases, those clinicians who fit the category of predatory psychopathy and paraphilias are not suited for rehabilitation plans. Those who fall into a lovesick or masochistic surrender category are often, but not always, amenable to rehabilitation, depending on the extent of their remorse, their motivation to avoid future transgressions, and the characteristics of their superego or conscience. After an assessment has been made, the findings should be reviewed with both the accused psychiatrist and the requesting agency or ethics committee.[27] The rehabilitation plan should be implemented only when there is agreement by all parties. Typical components of a rehabilitation plan include some or all of the following.[27,38,39]

1. Mediation: although in most cases the patient who has filed a complaint will be referred to another psychotherapist to deal with the trauma from the sexual boundary violation, mediation may be of extraordinary healing value for the patient as well as rehabilitative value for the therapist.[7,27,40] In this form of intervention the patient and accused clinician sit down together with a third party present, usually another psychiatrist or other mental health professional trained in mediation. This arrangement allows the patient to express how he or she felt about the therapist's sexual violation. When the therapist presents rationalizations or justifications for his or her behavior, the patient can confront the therapist's denial, often with the assistance of the mediator. Mediation also provides an opportunity for the therapist to apologize to the patient for his or her behavior. Victims of clinician–patient sexual misconduct maintain that it is exceedingly important to receive an apology from the boundary transgressor.[41] In addition, some form of restitution, such as refunding the money paid for the treatment, can be arranged under the circumstances of mediation. Anywhere from three to five sessions may provide rather remarkable results if both parties are willing to participate in mediation.

2. Personal psychotherapy: psychotherapy is indicated in most cases of sexual boundary violations when the therapist is deemed suitable for rehabilitation. Obviously, motivation on the part of the accused therapist is essential. Psychotherapy will prove to be a waste of time for accused clinicians who deny any sexual misconduct or deny having any psychological problems that require help. The psychodynamic conflicts that led to the sexual misconduct could be addressed, and the meanings of the transgression can be understood within the context of psychotherapy or psychoanalysis. In most rehabilitation plans, someone other than the accused therapist should select the professional who will conduct the psychotherapy so that no collusion occurs between the accused professional and the therapist based on friendship or feelings of obligation.

Psychotherapists of accused clinicians will face considerable countertransference difficulty as they deal with their own contempt and feelings of moral superiority. They must also carefully monitor the boundaries and frame of the psychotherapy, as many clinicians who have committed sexual boundary violations will also test the boundaries of their treatment when they are in the role of patient. The psychotherapist must try to avoid policing the accusing clinician and instead seek to understand the main psychological themes that led to the transgression.

3. Assignment of a rehabilitation coordinator: the individual selected for the role of rehabilitation coordinator is in charge of the overall rehabilitation plan. Usually a psychiatrist or other experienced mental health professional, the coordinator meets regularly with the accused clinician and makes reports to the licensing board. The rehabilitation coordinator should not be the same person as the psychotherapist so that the confidentiality of the psychotherapy can be preserved. Without confidentiality assured, a clinician in the process of rehabilitation may feel that he or she cannot speak openly to the therapist for fear of being reported. In some arrangements the rehabilitation coordinator is given periodic reports from the therapist that may involve a minimum of information, such as regular attendance or a brief comment about the patient's progress.

4. Practice limitations: various kinds of stipulations on an accused clinician's license may be part of the rehabilitation arrangement. For example, the clinician's practice may be limited to hospital treatment or treatment of only male patients. In other cases the practice limitations may include avoidance of patients with specific diagnoses or limitations to one type of treatment modality, such as pharmacotherapy.

5. Supervision: almost all rehabilitation plans require weekly supervision to be built in to the accused clinician's schedule. The supervisor should be fully informed about the nature of the sexual boundary violation, and the clinician undergoing rehabilitation must be willing to speak openly about countertransference temptations that arise in the course of clinical work. The

supervisor may report either to the rehabilitation coordinator or to the responsible agency.

6. Continuing education: many psychiatrists have had limited training in how to handle erotic transference or countertransference as it emerges in the process of treatment. Similarly, professional boundaries may not have been a part of their training curriculum. As a result, workshops and readings on these subjects may be extremely useful as part of an overall rehabilitation plan.

Most rehabilitation plans last for 3 to 5 years, with yearly assessments of how the clinician is progressing. In the course of a rehabilitation plan, other measures may be necessary. For example, a clinician who becomes suicidal may require pharmacotherapy or hospitalization. Before re-entry into unsupervised practice, the clinician should be assessed by all parties involved in the rehabilitation plan as to the advisability of that course of action.

Non-sexual boundary violations

Compared with sexual boundary violations, non-sexual boundary violations have been studied much less systematically. No typology of therapist profiles has been developed for non-sexual boundary violations. Nevertheless, the last 10 years have produced a growing literature on this subject.[7,9,16,18,26,34,42–44] This literature has evolved from several directions. First, the study of cases of sexual misconduct has led to an appreciation of the slippery slope phenomena involving non-sexual boundary violations that *precede* overt sexual contact. In the process, it has become clear that considerable harm may be experienced by the patient even when the descent down the slope stops short of sexual involvement.

Another source of interest in non-sexual boundary violations has grown out of malpractice litigation. Many malpractice insurance carriers no longer will insure psychiatrists against claims involving sexual misconduct. Hence plaintiffs' attorneys have realized that to collect damages for their clients, they must focus instead on the non-sexual boundary violations and demonstrate that harm resulted from them.

A third source of interest in non-sexual boundary violations has been the increasing focus on countertransference enactments in the psychoanalytic literature.[45–49] With the recognition that psychoanalytic therapy is fundamentally a two-person endeavor in which passionate feelings of hate and love arise in both members as a result of mutual influence, the old view of the therapist as a dispassionate 'blank screen' is no longer viable. Therapists cannot avoid introducing their subjectivity into the process spontaneously. In fact, the analyst is inevitably 'sucked in' to the patient's internal world through a variety of enactments that dislodge the therapist from the classic posture of a quiet, reflective listener. With the widespread consensus that certain kinds of spontaneous enactments that depart from standard technique may be useful in advancing psychoanalytic therapy in a positive direction, the determination of whether a particular enactment is a boundary crossing or a boundary violation is often unclear initially and may depend on how the incident is handled by the therapist and how the process eventually reveals its meaning. Waldinger[50] observed that 'the intrapsychic meanings of a boundary crossing may be the only clues to understand whether a violation has occurred' [p. 226]. In making such determinations, the context plays a critical role in understanding whether a transgression is a violation or crossing.[9] For example, hearing that a psychodynamic therapist drove a patient home from his therapy session may raise questions if no context is provided. When it becomes clear that the context was a raging blizzard that had brought public transportation to a halt and the patient's car would not start, the therapist's behavior makes more sense. As Karl Menninger was fond of saying, 'When in doubt, be human'.

A number of guidelines can assist a psychotherapist or members of an investigating ethics committee in differentiating how a boundary crossing differs from a boundary violation.[7] In addition to examining the context, therapists who catch themselves in the midst of an emerging enactment may prevent a crossing from becoming a violation. Similarly, the capacity of both therapist and patient to discuss and analyze an incident may prevent it from becoming a destructive and harmful boundary violation. The opposite is also true—if an incident cannot be discussed for one reason or another, it may grow in its significance and ultimately be harmful to the patient. A third guideline involves whether the enactment is repetitive and unresponsive to the therapist's own efforts at self-monitoring. An example may illustrate some of these principles:

Case 3
A 45-year-old divorced female therapist was seeing a 42-year-old male patient who continued to profess his love for the therapist. At one point near the end of a therapy hour, the man leaned forward and held the therapist's hand. He said that he greatly appreciated all her help. The therapist reached with her other hand so that she was clasping his hand in both her hands. The patient seemed deeply moved by her gesture, and he said, 'I love you.' After he left, she recognized that she was becoming over-involved with the man because of her own needs. She 'phoned a colleague and used him as a consultant. She explained to the colleague that she was divorced and had no one to go home to at night. She said it felt wonderful to have a man say 'I love you' to her. She also recognized that it was not helpful to subtly encourage his acting on his feelings with her in the therapy rather than talking about them. The consultant urged her to bring up the incident first thing in the next session.

When the patient arrived, the therapist informed him that she thought it would be a good idea to discuss what had happened at the end of the last session. As he talked about the incident, he said he was somewhat worried that the therapist might be losing control by clasping his hand in that way. The therapist encouraged further exploration of his concern. He said it reminded him of how his mother turned to him rather than father when she had emotional problems, and he felt that something like that was being repeated with him and the therapist. The therapist acknowledged that it probably wasn't a good idea for them to hold hands because it involved taking something into action that should be discussed and understood between them. Further discussion led to an awareness of other ways in which the patient's relationship with his mother was being repeated in the transference–countertransference dimensions of the treatment.

This vignette is illustrative of how these guidelines can be usefully applied. The therapist caught herself as the enactment was developing and sought consultation to figure out what was going on. She also discussed it openly with the patient and connected it with important therapeutic goals. Finally, the enactment was not repetitive but was a one-time-only event. The vignette also demonstrates the great value of seeking consultation from a colleague when boundary difficulties begin to emerge. The incident seemed to involve issues from the therapist's own personal life as well as a re-creation of an old object relationship from the patient's past. In this regard, countertransference enactments can generally be considered some form of a *joint creation* involving the therapist's own conflicts as well as the evocation of certain responses in the therapist that reflect the patient's internal object world.[46]

These considerations about boundary crossings and boundary violations, of course, assume an average, well-intentioned therapist who may be under the influence of countertransference. Some non-sexual boundary violations are promulgated by unscrupulous and exploitative therapists similar to the psychopathic predators already described. These clinicians may use the power derived from the patient's transference to enlist the patient as an investor in a financial scheme, arrange for the patient to donate money to an organization from which the therapist will directly profit, or use the patient as someone who will run errands or do chores for the therapist.

For the most part, however, non-sexual boundary violations involve a confluence of clinical error and ethical misconduct rather than deliberate and corrupt exploitation of the patient. The boundary involving sexual contact between clinician and patient is an inflexible one because sexual activity between clinician and patient is never acceptable. The non-sexual boundaries require more flexibility, but guidelines can be developed around a number of specific boundary issues.

Time

The limits of the clinical session should be clearly defined from the beginning of the treatment. If clinicians find themselves regularly extending the session well beyond the time, this should raise questions about possible countertransference issues. Similarly, sessions scheduled late in the evening, after office personnel have gone home and the building is more or less deserted except for therapist and patient, may be viewed as problematic by investigating ethics committees. While some patients will require late sessions, those patients who have erotic transferences or who are extraordinarily demanding are probably best seen during high traffic times in the middle of the day.[5]

Location of contact

Most psychiatric treatment takes place in the context of a hospital unit or in a professional office. Scheduling a session in other than one of those locations may raise questions in the patient's mind about the purpose. Certainly, there are circumstances where different meeting places are necessary. The reason for meeting in another location can be documented in the chart and supported as part of community standards for such treatment. Home visits are occasionally necessary for bedridden patients or those who are chronically mentally ill. The ideal arrangement is for more than one treater to go to the patient's home, and certainly documentation of the reason is also important.

Money and gifts

The fact that the patient must pay the clinician for the treatment underscores that psychiatric treatment is work. Clinicians who allow the bill to mount without asking for payment or who discontinue charging a fee send a problematic message to the patient. 'Why am I getting this for free?'; the patient may think, 'Maybe I'm expected to be giving the therapist something in return.' The patient may also feel that he or she has no right to express anger or dissatisfaction when the treatment is free or at such a low fee that the patient feels guilty about it.

Gifts may also be problematic. A large gift of money or an extremely expensive gift may be meant as an unconscious bribe. The patient who gives such a gift may be expecting the therapist to avoid confronting the patient about some unpleasant aspect of the patient's psychopathology. Expensive gifts may also be a way of trying to suppress anger or aggression in the therapeutic dyad. Therapists who give gifts to their patients may send the same message in the reverse direction. On the other hand, small gifts that the patient has made, such as artwork or a ceramic bowl, may be accepted graciously by the therapist, who may wish to discuss the meaning of the gift with the patient. The previous example of the woman with paranoid schizophrenia who was able to present a gift of a cookie demonstrates that certain kinds of gifts may signal a turning point in the treatment and that to decline the gifts can be a devastating technical error.

Self-disclosure

Every time psychotherapists speak, they disclose something about themselves, even if only an opinion or judgment about an aspect of the patient's behavior. They also have information about themselves on display around their offices in their choice of artwork, photographs, and so forth. Rigid guidelines on how much to disclose are not particularly helpful. In general, therapists should avoid burdening the patient with their own problems. Short of this kind of role reversal, it is primarily a matter of clinical judgment. Certain kinds of counter-transference feelings in the 'here and now' may be usefully explored. If a borderline patient, for example, asks an obviously angry therapist if he or she is upset, the therapist may validate the patient's observation and try to explore it with the patient to figure out what sort of interaction is irritating the therapist. On the other hand, when a therapist reveals having sexual feelings for the patient, such information can be overwhelming and experienced as a boundary violation in and of itself.[50] In the same vein, it would be ill-advised to say to a patient, 'I hate you', or 'You are boring me'.

Some information about the therapist's private life may be useful at times in developing a therapeutic alliance with the patient. For example, when treating a teenager who does not want to talk to the therapist, a common area of interest, such as sports, may open up pathways of communication between therapist and patient. Similarly, talking about movies that have recently been seen may lead to further exploration of psychological themes that are useful for the therapy.

Non-sexual physical contact

While in some forms of psychiatric practice, physical examinations will be routine and within the community standard, in many cases they will not. In office psychotherapy, the extent of physical contact should probably be limited to handshakes. However, it would be hard to generalize and say that a hug is *never* acceptable within the framework of psychotherapy. One can think of situations, such as a grieving mother who enters the therapist's office and announces that her son has just died. If that patient then puts her arms around the therapist while sobbing, a therapist who fails to return the hug may wound the patient to the extent that she never returns to his office again. On the other hand, it is hard to imagine situations in which the therapist should initiate hugs because of the great risk that the impact on the patient will be different from the therapist's intent.[51] Therapists can never be certain of their unconscious wishes and intent when initiating a hug, and even if the intent was above reproach, the patient may experience such a hug as an intrusion or an assault. With patients who have been sexually violated in the past, a non-sexual touch or a hug can be re-experienced as assaultive.

Preventive strategies

In considering measures to prevent boundary violations, we must first acknowledge that the radical privacy of psychiatric treatment is such that we can never completely eradicate boundary violations. What we can do is educate psychiatrists beginning in their residency with courses on ethics, boundaries, and the management of erotic transference and countertransfer-ence, so they have a conceptual framework within which to think about the problems. We should also educate psychiatrists to monitor carefully their countertransference and their deviations from standard boundary guidelines. When these deviations occur, psychiatrists should be trained to seek consultation from a colleague.

Education will not, of course, stop unscrupulous individuals who have antisocial tendencies, and we must do what we can to screen such individuals out of medical schools and psychiatric residencies when their dishonest behavior is encountered. For those individuals who aspire to do intensive psychotherapy, a personal treatment experience is a must. Personal analysis or therapy will assist the future therapist or analyst in gaining familiarity with his or her own internal world and the specific countertransference vulnerabilities that can be expected with certain kinds of patients. Even a personal treatment experience, however, cannot be expected to prevent boundary violations many years in the future.

Isolation is one of the most important factors in the development of boundary violations, and any organizational efforts to deal with that isolation may go a long way to prevent boundary violations. For example, peer supervision groups are springing up in many parts of the country. In this context therapists get to know one another well and present their struggles with countertransference difficulties as they develop. Whenever intense sexual feelings are developing in either patient or therapist, routine consultation is probably a good idea for most therapists.

Psychiatric institutions can also take a number of measures to prevent boundary violations. Each applicant for a position should have a careful screening of any history of criminal behavior. Personal contact with previous employers over the telephone is also essential. Each psychiatric hospital or clinical department should have clearly written policies that prohibit all sexual contact between staff and patients. Other boundaries, such as those involving financial dealings with patients, should also be spelled out. Annual educational meetings should take place for employees working within psychiatric hospitals so that sample situations involving boundary issues are brought up and discussed openly. In psychiatric hospitals, team leaders should encourage the open sharing of countertransference feelings and regard them as a useful part of the treatment.

In many states risk management laws require certain procedures, such as reporting and investigating allegations of boundary violations or other substandard or unethical behavior. In the absence of such laws, institutions should create them so that there is a standard method of reporting to supervisors or risk managers any behavior that appears to be unethical or substandard. Complaints then can be investigated by standing committees so that a swift decision is reached, taking both the staff member's and the patient's interests and concerns into account. Institutions should also establish peer review and supervision as a structured part of the working week so that no practitioner becomes completely isolated. Patient education can be helpful.

Some clinics distribute brochures that clearly state that certain behaviors by a mental health professional should raise questions in the patient's mind.

Perhaps one of the most effective preventive measures—one that cannot easily be legislated—is for every mental health professional to nurture close personal relationships. If one's emotional and sexual needs are met in gratifying personal relationships, there is much less risk that one's needs will be acted out with patients.

References

1. Gabbard, G. O.: The early history of boundary violations in psychoanalysis. *Journal of the American Psychoanalytic Association* **43**:1115–36, 1995.
2. Dupont, J.: The story of a transgression. *Journal of the American Psychoanalytic Association* **43**:823–34, 1995.
3. McGuire, W. (ed.): *The Freud/Jung letters: the correspondence between Sigmund Freud and C. G. Jung.* Princeton, NJ, Princeton University Press.
4 Freud, S.: Recommendations to physicians practising psycho-analysis, in *The complete psychological works of Sigmund Freud*, vol. 12 (1912). London, Hogarth Press, 1958.
5. Lohser, B. and Newton, P. M.: *Unorthodox Freud: the view from the couch.* New York, Guilford, 1996.
6. Gutheil, T. H. amd Gabbard, G. O.: The concept of boundaries in clinical practice: theoretical and risk-management dimensions. *American Journal of Psychiatry* **150**: 188–96, 1993.
7. Gabbard, G. O. and Lester, E. P.: *Boundaries and boundary violations in psychoanalysis.* New York, Basic Books, 1995.
8. Langs, R.: *The therapeutic interaction: a synthesis.* New York, Aronson, 1977.
9. Gutheil, T. H. and Gabbard, G. O.: Misuses and misunderstandings of boundary theory in clinical and regulatory settings. *American Journal of Psychiatry* **155**: 409–14, 1998.
10. Greenberg, J. R.: Psychoanalytic technique and the interactive matrix. *Psychoanalytic Quarterly* **64**:122, 1995.
11. Mitchell, S. A.: *Hope and dread in psychoanalysis.* New York, Basic Books, 1993.
12. Gutheil, T. G.: Borderline personality disorder, boundary violations, and patient–therapist sex: medicolegal pitfalls. *American Journal of Psychiatry* **146**:597–602, 1989.
13. Epstein, R. S. and Simon, R. I.: The exploitation index: an early warning indicator of boundary violations in psychotherapy. *Bulletin of the Menninger Clinic* **54**: 450–65, 1990.
14. Gabbard, G. O.: Lessons to be learned from the study of sexual boundary violations. *American Journal of Psychotherapy* **50**:311–22, 1996.
15. Langs, R.: *Psychotherapy: a basic text.* New York, Aronson, 1982.
16. Epstein, R.: *Keeping boundaries: maintaining safety and integrity in the psychotherapeutic process.* Washington, DC, American Psychiatric Press, 1994.
17. Gabbard, G. O. and Nadelson, C.: Professional boundaries in the physician-patient relationship. *Journal of the American Medical Association* **273**:1445–9, 1995.
18. Strasburger, L. H., Jorgenson, L., and Sutherland, P.: The prevention of psychotherapist sexual misconduct: avoiding the slippery slope. *American Journal of Psychotherapy* **46**:545–55, 1992.

19. Holroyd, J. C. and Brodsky, A. M.: Psychologists' attitudes and practices regarding erotic and nonerotic physical contact with patients. *American Psychologist* **23**: 843–9,1977.

20. Pope, K. S., Levenson, H., and Schover, L. R.: Sexual intimacy in psychology training: results and implications of a national survey. *American Psychologist* **34**:682–9, 1979.

21. Pope, K. S., Keith-Spiegel, P., and Tabachnick, B. G.: Sexual attraction to clients: the human therapist and the (sometimes) inhuman training system. *American Psychologist* **41**:147–58, 1986.

22. Pope, K. S., Tabachnick, B. G., and Keith-Spiegel, P.: Ethics of practice: the beliefs and behaviors of psychologists as therapists. *American Psychologist* **42**:993–1006, 1987.

23. Gartrell, N., Herman, J., Olarte, S., *et al.*: Psychiatrist–patient sexual contact: results of a national survey, I: prevalence. *American Journal of Psychiatry* **143**:1126–31, 1986.

24. Akamatsu, T. J.: Intimate relationships with former clients: national survey of attitudes and behavior among practitioners. *Professional Psychology: Research and Practice* **19**:454–58, 1988.

25. Gechtman, L.: Sexual contact between social workers and their clients, in *Sexual exploitation in professional relationships* (eds. G. O. Gabbard). Washington, DC, American Psychiatric Press, 1989, pp. 27–38.

26. Borys, D. S. and Pope, K. S.: Dual relationships between therapist and client: a national study of psychologists, psychiatrists, and social workers. *Professional Psychology: Research and Practice* **20**:283–93, 1989.

27. Schoener, G. R., Milgrom, J. H., and Gonsiorek, J. C., *et al.*: *Psychotherapists' sexual involvement with clients: intervention and prevention.* Minneapolis, MN, Walk-In Counseling Center, 1989.

28. Kardener, S. H., Fuller, M., and Mensh, I. N.: A survey of physicians' attitudes and practices regarding erotic and nonerotic contact with patients. *American Journal of Psychiatry* **130**:1077–81, 1973.

29. Gartrell, N. K., Milliken, N., Goodson, W. H., *et al.*: Physician–patient sexual contact: prevalence and problems. *Western Journal of Medicine* **157**:139–43, 1992.

30. Committee on Physician Sexual Misconduct. *Crossing the boundaries: the report of the Committee on Physician Sexual Misconduct.* Vancouver, College of Physicians and Surgeons of British Columbia, 1992.

31. Wilbers, D., Veensstra, G., van d Wiel, H. B. M., *et al.*: Sexual contact in the doctor–patient relationship in the Netherlands. *British Medical Journal* **304**:1531–4, 1992.

32. Lamont, J. A. and Woodward, C.: Patient–physician sexual involvement: a Canadian survey of obstetrician–gynecologists. *Canadian Medical Association Journal* **150**:1433–9, 1994.

33. Schoener, G. R. and Gonsiorek, J. C.: Assessment and development of rehabilitation plans for the therapist, in *Psychotherapists' sexual involvement with clients: intervention and prevention* (eds. G. R. Schoener *et al.*). Minneapolis, MN, Walk-In Counseling Center, 1989, pp. 401–20.

34. Simon, R. I.: *Clinical psychiatry and the law*, 2nd edn. Washington, DC, American Psychiatric Press, 1992.

35. Gabbard, G. O.: Psychotherapists who transgress sexual boundaries with patients. *Bulletin of the Menninger Clinic* **58**:124–35, 1994a.

36. Appelbaum, P. S. and Jorgenson, L.: Psychotherapistpaitent sexual contact after termination of treatment: an analysis and a proposal. *American Journal of Psychiatry* 148:14661473, 1991.
37. Gabbard, G. O.: Reconsidering the American Psychological Association's policy on sex with former patients: is it justifiable? *Professional Psychology: Research and Practice* **25**:329–55, 1994.
38. Gabbard, G. O.: Sexual misconduct, in *Review of psychiatry* (eds. J. Oldham and M. Riba), vol. 13. Washington, DC, American Psychiatric Press, 1994, pp. 433–56.
39. Pope, K. S. and Gabbard, G. O.: Individual psychotherapy for victims of therapist–patient sexual intimacy, in *Sexual exploitation in professional relationships*. Washington DC, American Psychiatric Press, 1989.
40. Margolis, M.: Analyst–patient sexual involvement: clinical experiences and institutional responses. *Psychoanalytic Inquiry* 17:349–70, 1997.
41. Wohlberg, J.: Sexual abuse in the therapeutic setting: What do victims really want? *Psychoanalytic Inquiry* 17:329–48, 1997.
42. Epstein, R. S., Simon, R. I., and Kay, G. G.: Assessing boundary violations in psychotherapy: survey results with the Exploitation Index. *Bulletin of the Menninger Clinic* 56:150–66, 1992.
43. Frick, D. E.: Non-sexual boundary violations in psychiatric treatment, in *Review of psychiatry* (eds. J. Oldham and M. Riba), vol. 13. Washington, DC, American Psychiatric Press, 1994.
44. Lamb, D. H., Strand, K. K., Woodburn, J. R., *et al.*: Sexual and business relationships between therapists and former clients. *Psychotherapy* 31:270–8, 1994.
45. Chused, J. F.: The evocative power of enactments. *Journal of the American Psychoanalytic Association* **39**:615–39, 1991.
46. Gabbard, G. O.: Countertransference: the emerging common ground. *International Journal of Psycho-Analysis* 76:475–85, 1995.
47. Jacobs, T. J.: On countertransference enactments. *Journal of the American Psychoanalytic Association* **34**:289–307, 1986.
48. McLaughlin, J. T.: Clinical and theoretical aspects of enactment. *Journal of the American Psychoanalytic Association* **39**:595–614, 1991.
49. Renik, O.: Analytic interaction: conceptualizing technique in light of the analyst's irreducible subjectivity. *Psychoanalytic Quarterly* 62:553–71, 1993.
50. Waldinger, R. J.: Boundary crossings and boundary violations: thoughts on navigating a slippery slope. *Harvard Review of Psychiatry* **2**:225–7, 1994.
51. Gabbard, G. O.: The analyst's contribution to the erotic transference. *Contemporary Psychoanalysis* **32**:249–73, 1996a.

9

Analytic philosophy, brain science, and the concept of disorder

K. W. M. Fulford

Like biomedicine, bioethics has traditionally neglected psychiatry in favour of the high-profile problems of 'high-tech' medicine.[1] Why should this be so? Ethical problems, after all, as this book amply demonstrates, are more pervasive here than in other areas of medicine. They are also, as we will see in this chapter, deeper problems—deeper practically and deeper philosophically.

The explanation for the neglect of psychiatry by bioethics, to anticipate a little, is that bioethics has adopted the same biomedical model of disease as biomedicine. This has been a case of bioethics taking on the colours of its enemy. Bioethics developed as a direct response to the ethical challenges raised by the explosive advances in 'high-tech' scientific medicine after the Second World War. In this environment, medicine was assumed to be essentially a branch of biology, in which disease theories were developed scientifically by the accumulation of facts about disturbances of the functioning of bodily parts and systems (hearts, livers, etc.). Ethics was important, but only to the *appliance* of the new medical sciences, to controlling such areas as treatment choice, research, and the distribution of resources. Small wonder, then, that psychiatry, with its relatively undeveloped scientific base, should have been assumed to be correspondingly unproblematic ethically.[2]

In this chapter we will be turning this traditional picture upside down, psychiatry emerging as more, rather than less, problematic ethically than other areas of medicine. Starting from a case history, the case of Mr AB, we will find that the biomedical model of disease, and with it traditional bioethics, is incomplete. The ethical dilemmas presented by Mr AB require a model of disease (or, more generally, of disorder) in which facts and values are on an equal footing. Analytic philosophy, drawing particularly on value theory, gives us the required fact-plus-value model. This model is not anti-scientific, however. It really does add values to the facts of the biomedical model; and this turns out to be important across a wide range of practical applications, including the newly developing brain sciences. This, then, is the A, B, C of a bioethics (we should call it rather a philosophical ethics) fit for psychiatry:

*A*nalytic philosophy combined with the *B*rain sciences to give an understanding of the *C*oncept of disorder which is sufficiently rich and subtle to encompass the ethical dilemmas presented by clinical work and research in this
most difficult of health-care disciplines.

Mr AB—a suitable case for bioethics?

Mr AB's story illustrates the usefulness but also the limitations for psychiatry
of a bioethics based on the biomedical model of disease.[3]

The Case of Mr AB

Mr AB, a 48-year-old bank manager, was brought to the casualty department of his
local hospital by his wife. He had burning pains in his face and head but his general
practitioner's referral letter said she thought Mr AB was seriously depressed. Over the
last three to four weeks he had become gloomy and preoccupied and had lost interest in
his work. He had been waking earlier than usual and had lost weight. Normally he was a
hard-working, cheerful extrovert. However, he had had periods of depression before,
and during the last of these (when he had complained similarly of head and facial pains)
he had made a sudden and nearly fatal suicide attempt. Mr AB had become angry at his
general practitioner's suggestion that he see a psychiatrist but had agreed to come to
casualty for further investigation of his head pains.

The casualty officer found Mr AB to be morose and unsmiling. He gave a clear and
consistent description of his pain, but was guarded and suspicious when asked about his
health generally. The casualty officer then talked to Mr AB's wife. She confirmed the
recent changes in his mood and said that he was behaving very much as he had before
his suicide attempt. The duty psychiatrist was called. In the course of a careful physical
and neurological examination he was able to question Mr AB further about his health.
Mr AB now admitted that he believed he had 'advanced brain cancer'. However, at the
suggestion that he stay in hospital, he again became angry, saying that there was 'no
point any more', and that all he needed was 'something for the pain'. The psychiatrist
explained that he found no signs whatsoever of brain cancer and that he thought in
fact Mr AB had become depressed again. He said that further tests were needed—skull
X-ray, electroencephalogram, and so on—but that the burning pains were almost
certainly due to depression. Mr AB, however, refused even to consider this possibility,
saying that brain cancer did not always 'show itself', and that anyone with brain cancer
would be likely to feel as he had been feeling.

At this stage the psychiatrist decided that in view of the high suicide risk, Mr AB's
protestations notwithstanding, he had no option but to consider compulsory treatment under the Mental Health Act, 1983. In his view, as required by the Act, Mr AB
was suffering from a mental illness, which, in the interests of his own safety, warranted
detention in hospital for further assessment and treatment. He discussed this with
Mr AB's wife and with his general practitioner, both of whom agreed. A Section-2
order was accordingly made, and Mr AB was admitted to the psychiatric ward. There,
on antidepressant drug therapy, he made a full recovery over the next eight weeks.
At his first outpatient follow-up he admitted to the psychiatrist that he had agreed
to attend casualty originally only because he thought he would be given something

stronger than aspirin for his pains, and that he had been planning to use this to kill himself. Now, far from wanting to kill himself, he was concerned about the risks of a further relapse. In addition to routine follow-up, therefore, which would continue for some time, he agreed that he or his wife should contact either his general practitioner or the psychiatrist immediately if his head pains or gloomy mood returned.

The first point about psychiatric ethics to take from Mr AB's story, is that it is an *everyday* story. This is an aspect of the pervasiveness of ethical problems in psychiatry. Many of the ethical problems of high-tech medicine arise with novel techniques (like organ transplantation) at the margins of practice. But the problem of involuntary psychiatric treatment, as in Mr AB's case, is a problem for *everyone*. Nor is it a merely theoretical problem. Mr AB's case may seem fairly straightforward ethically. He was mentally ill (suffering from major depression), and at serious risk of suicide. Hence as described more fully in Chapter 20 of this book, he satisfied both limbs of the Mental Health Act, 1983 (the relevant legislation in his case; but there is similar legislation in many parts of the world). Mr AB's is just the kind of case, indeed, in which a failure to use involuntary treatment could be held to be negligent. Yet in a case vignette study, Mr AB's case was one of those over which clinicians were split 50:50 about whether involuntary treatment would be appropriate.[4] Moreover the misuse of involuntary treatment, notoriously in the former USSR, but also sporadically throughout psychiatry, is the basis of some of the worst abuses of psychiatric care.[5]

As well as being a pervasive problem, however, a problem for everyone in psychiatry, involuntary psychiatric treatment is also a *deeper* ethical problem than those arising typically in high-tech medicine. This is the second point about psychiatric ethics illustrated by Mr AB and it takes us directly to the practical significance for psychiatry of the concept of disorder. At one level, the ethical issue presented by Mr AB is the familiar bioethical problem of involuntary treatment. Medical treatment, according to current norms, should normally be given only with consent. There are exceptions of course: a child, or an unconscious adult, or someone with severe learning difficulties, may sometimes be treated without consent in their best interests; and someone who is a threat to others (a typhoid carrier, say) may be treated without consent in the interests of third parties. It is only in psychiatry, however, as in Mr AB's case, that a fully conscious adult patient of normal intelligence may be treated without consent not (just) for the protection of others but in their own interests.

So there is something ethically special about *mental* illness, something which justifies involuntary *psychiatric* treatment in circumstances in which involuntary treatment for a physical condition would *not* be justified. The importance of the concept of disorder in cases like Mr AB's is evident in a number of ways. As just noted, all Mental Health legislation includes mental disorder as a condition of involuntary treatment.[6] This indeed reflects a widespread ethical intuition. In many cultures, and going back historically to classical times, it has been taken to be self-evident that involuntary *medical* intervention, to prevent, say, suicide, requires that the sadness and distress of the person concerned are not merely sadness and distress but symptoms of a *medical* condition. There may be other grounds for intervening to prevent someone who is not ill from killing themselves (humanitarian or religious grounds, say). But *medical* interventions require *medical* grounds. Moreover, there must be something special about *psychiatric* medical grounds, for it is precisely on this point that in physical medicine the patient's wishes (in the case of a fully conscious adult of normal intelligence) normally prevail over those of the doctor. As noted a moment ago, this is the well-recognized principle of autonomy of patient choice, the principle that a patient is normally free to choose or to reject treatment (even where the treatment concerned is potentially life-saving).

Bioethics has not been wholly blind to this problem, of course. A particularly careful analysis of the ethical importance of the concept of mental disorder in justifying involuntary psychiatric treatment is given by the American philosophers T. L. Beauchamp and J. F. Childress, in their foundational *Principles of biomedical ethics* (see also Chapter 3).[7] Like many others who have written on this topic they treat psychiatry derivatively, as a special case of the general problem of involuntary treatment. Unlike most other authors, however, they take the special case of psychiatry seriously, examining it in detail and discussing a clinical example, a patient with dementia. As is well known, Beauchamp and Childress analyse involuntary treatment in terms of two of their four prima facie principles, as reflecting a balance between (patient) autonomy and (professional) beneficence. Beauchamp and Childress are the first to point out that there is more to ethical reasoning in medicine than, just, principles. But the principles, in cases like Mr AB's, are clearly relevant. Moreover they suggest a direct link between the general ethical issue of involuntary treatment and the concept of mental disorder. For autonomy, so Beauchamp and Childress suggest, means not just free choice but *rational* free choice; rationality, in turn, depends on certain *competencies,* such as coherence, understanding, and deliberation; and these competences *are undermined or lacking altogether* in the case of dementia. Hence the mental disorder, dementia, involving as it does a disturbance of rationality in which coherence, understanding, and deliberation are impaired, undermines the capacity for autonomous patient choice; and, autonomy being so undermined, involuntary treatment in cases of dementia is justified on grounds of beneficence, of the clinician's duty to act according to the patient's best interests.

So far so good. But does this help with Mr AB's case? Mr AB was suffering from depression rather than dementia. He was entirely coherent and he had clear deliberative capacity (it was his capacity for carrying through his intention to kill himself that put him at risk of suicide). On these grounds alone, therefore, he could not be said to lack the competencies necessary for rational, and hence for autonomous, choice. What about understanding, though? Mr AB was, after all, deluded (he had a delusion of brain cancer). So could he be said to lack understanding? The defect in understanding in depression is different from dementia, certainly. In dementia there is a plain lack of understanding; whereas in depression understanding is, somehow, distorted (everything looks gloomy; the opposite of rose-tinted spectacles). In the extreme this depressive distortion of thinking can result in delusions, as in Mr AB's case. Delusions, moreover, so defined, have the advantage from the point of view of the bio-medical model of being, in principle, defined objectively. It was not obvious that Mr AB's belief was wrong (brain tumours presenting with depression may be small and deeply placed and hence difficult to detect); but, in fact, his belief that he had brain cancer *was* wrong. Anthony Flew, writing on *Crime or Disease*,[8] identified the objectivity of delusion as 'the one sure defence against the abuse of psychiatry'. Here then, at least, is an objective symptom of mental illness, one consistent with the scientific expertise of doctors, placing judge-ments of rationality beyond the vagaries of human values.

QED, then, for bioethics, for biomedicine, and for the biomedical model of disease? Well, this whole system of ideas is helpful up to a point. It is, perhaps, sufficient for cases of dementia, and for cases in physical medicine, such as patients who are unconscious. In such cases the absence of well-defined functional competencies can be established by straightforward empirical means. But is this true of delusion? At first glance, it may appear that it is. And as we have seen, ethicists and philosophers no less than doctors have assumed that it is. They have assumed that the *falsity* of delusions shows, in an ethically relevant sense, lack of understanding; and hence impairments of the competencies required for autonomous choice. Of course, *mere* false belief is not pathological; and the medical textbooks seek to cover this by adding to the definition of delusion some caveat such as that delusions are culturally atypical, and/or based on false inferences or inadequate evidence.[9] These additional criteria, it is well recognized, are not wholly satisfactory even in everyday cases like Mr AB's—his belief was not culturally atypical; and as we have seen, he *could* have had a brain tumour. As it turned out, he did *not* have a brain tumour. His original belief, therefore, *was* false, reassuringly for Flew and others who have taken the falsity of delusions as the key to their ethical significance.[10] But, and this is the crucial 'but', delusions, although commonly false, and often bizarrely so, *may not be false at all.*

That delusions are not necessarily false beliefs has been recognized for some time. Shepherd, for example, pointed this out in his early paper on the Othello syndrome.[11] The beliefs of the patient with Othello syndrome about the infidelity of their sexual partner are irrational; but whatever the irrationality of their beliefs consists in, it cannot be falsity of belief as such, since their beliefs may be *concordant* rather than *discordant* with the facts. The same point is made by the occasional patient with hypochondriacal delusions based on the idea that they are mentally ill: if delusions really were, essentially, false factual beliefs, then the delusion of mental illness would be paradoxical—if false, it would be true (i.e. if the patient's belief that he is mentally ill is a false belief, then he *could* be deluded according to the standard definition): but if his belief is true (i.e. if he *is* mentally ill), then his belief could not be a delusion after all; so it would be a false belief. The hypochondriacal delusion of mental illness, then, if the standard definition of delusion were correct, would be a belief which if true would be false and if false would be true.[12]

Cases such as these are relatively unusual (though no less significant logically for that). Hence one response of the biomedical model to such cases has been to substitute for 'false belief' in the definition of delusion, 'unfounded belief'; the implication being that delusion arises from some putative disturbance of cognitive functioning, and hence that although normally false, delusions will occasionally express true beliefs just by chance.[13] We will return in the final section of this chapter to the significance of the fact that the required disturbance of cognitive functioning has not yet been identified. For the moment, though, there is a clear difficulty with this approach arising from the psychopathology of delusions themselves. This difficulty is that delusions may not be beliefs about matters of fact at all, either true or false, but *value judgements*.[14] Evaluative delusions, moreover, far from being unusual, are clinically commonplace. Delusions of guilt, common in depression for example, provide a clear illustration of the point. A patient with depression may believe, say, that he or she has started a nuclear war; this is something (a matter of fact) about which anyone might reasonably feel guilty. Equally, though, in such a case the patient may evaluate something trivial which they have actually done, as deeply wicked or evil. In other words, what is delusional in the latter case is not the patient's belief as to the *facts* but the way they *evaluate* the facts. Similar cases with positive rather than negative evaluations, occur in hypomania. Delusions of grandeur, for example, commonly take the form of unreasonable evaluations of the patient's abilities or achievements.

Delusional thinking, therefore, which is central to cases like Mr AB's, is not readily reducible either to the functional capacities relied on by Beauchamp and Childress or to the false beliefs relied on by Flew, in order to give an account of the special ethical status of mental disorder which is consistent with the biomedical model. Delusions are not the false beliefs of the textbook definitions; they are not identifiable with any well-defined impairment of cognitive functioning; and they may, indeed commonly do, appear to involve judgements of value. Of course, philosophers working outside bioethics have consistently emphasized the value-laden nature of rationality. In general philosophy, therefore, it comes as no surprise to find that *ir*rationality, too, should be a value-laden notion. But this is no help to the biomedical model of disease. For the whole point of this model is to give us a value-free scientific concept of disease. Indeed Beauchamp and Childress themselves, acknowledging that judgements of rationality involve value judgements, then go on to conclude, consistently with the medical model that a judgement of rationality amounts to a 'moral *not a medical* problem' (see ref. 15, emphasis added).

Mr AB's case has thus illustrated: (1) that ethical problems in psychiatry are more pervasive than in other areas of medicine (the problems being endemic in all aspects of *everyday* psychiatric practice); (2) that these problems, although not different in kind from those arising in other areas of medicine, are deeper practically; and (3) that they are also deeper philosophically. To understand Mr AB's case we have had to move from issues of autonomy and beneficence (the tools of traditional bioethics) into the nature of rationality, and of rationality specifically as impaired in the case of delusion. Rationality of this kind, we have found preliminary reason to believe, involves value judgements as well as facts. This, according to the standard bioethical model, reflecting the scientific focus of the biomedical model, makes delusion a 'moral not medical' problem (in Beauchamp and Childress' words). But delusion is the central symptom of mental illness. Hence if Beauchamp and Childress are right, mental illness (and with it psychiatry) is properly located not in the scientific world of medicine but in the human world of morals. This is an unfortunate result for bioethics and for the biomedical model, then, for it seems to play directly into the hands of the opponents of psychiatry, the 'anti-psychiatrists', who, in the debate about mental illness, have consistently argued that mental illness is indeed a moral not a medical concept.

The debate about mental illness and the biomedical model of disease

If delusion, as a symptom at the centre of psychiatry, can be shown to be an evaluative concept, there are other more peripherally placed disorders which are transparently so. This is illustrated by Fig. 9.1 which shows a conceptual 'map' of mental disorders.[16] As the map shows, mental disorders in effect form a bridge between physical illness (on the right of the map) and moral problems (on the left). Some mental disorders, such as dementia, are conceptually close to physical disease—they are straightforwardly thought of as being defined by scientifically described facts of disturbed functioning. At the other extreme, though, are conditions like psychopathy, sexual disorders, and alcoholism, the very differential diagnoses of which include moral categories (delinquency, perversion, and drunkenness, respectively).

As is well known, the equivocal status of mental disorder, stretched as it is between medicine and moral, has generated a wide-ranging debate about the validity of the concept of mental illness.[17] A variety of alternatives to the biomedical model have been described (psychological, sociological, etc.), many of which can be associated with particular areas of the map (the psychological model is associated particularly with anxiety and depressive disorders, for example). More radically, though, there have been those, like Thomas Szasz, who have rejected the idea that mental disorders are properly thought of as illnesses at all.[18] This more radical debate has thus taken the form of a tug-of-

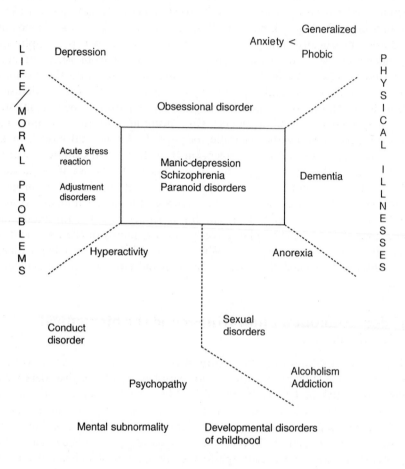

Fig. 1 A conceptual map of psychiatry. Some mental disorders (such as dementia) are conceptually close to physical illness, while others (like conduct disorder) are conceptually close to moral problems. The wide variety of mental disorders thus forms a bridge between the medical and moral worlds (see text).

war between anti-psychiatrists, like Thomas Szasz, seeking to pull all mental disorders to the left of the map, into the world of morals (for Szasz, mental illnesses are 'problems of living'), and psychiatrists, like R. E. Kendell,[19] trying to pull all mental disorder to the right, arguing that mental disorders are really no different from physical disorders.

Closer inspection of this debate shows, however, that what the two sides are really in conflict over is not the meaning of mental illness at all, but that of physical disease.[20] This perhaps rather surprising conclusion becomes clear if we stand back for a moment from the details of the claims of those on the two sides in this debate, and look at the close parallels between them in the forms of argument that they adopt. First, both authors assume that mental illness is the target problem: Szasz wants to 'raise the question, is there such a thing as mental illness'? Kendell, similarly, seeks to 'decide whether mental illnesses are legitimately so-called'. Both then turn to the concept of physical illness, acknowledging certain difficulties of definition, but suggesting criteria which they take to be self-evidently essential to its meaning: Szasz's criterion is 'deviation from the clearly defined norms of the structural and functional integrity of the human body'. Kendell's is 'biological disadvantage, which must embrace both increased mortality and reduced fertility'. Finally, both return to mental illness. Szasz points out that for mental illnesses, the relevant norms of bodily structure and functioning are not available: on the contrary, he argues, the norms of mental illness are 'ethical, legal and social'. Kendell, on the other hand, draws on epidemiological and statistical data to show that many mental illnesses are biologically disadvantageous in his sense, being associated with reduced life and/or reproductive expectations. Hence, by Szasz's criteria of physical illness, mental illness is a myth, whereas by Kendell's it is not.

It will be clear from this summary of their arguments that neither author's proposed criteria of physical illness are wholly satisfactory: among other problems, Szasz's is too restrictive, Kendell's is over-inclusive. However, what is important to us here is to see that the debate itself, although starting out as a debate about mental illness, ends up as a debate about physical illness. The debate could have come out differently. Szasz and Kendell could have ended up agreeing about the criteria for physical illness but disagreeing about the application these criteria to (putative) mental illness. Instead, they disagreed *about the criteria by which physical illness itself is defined* (and a wide variety of other criteria have been suggested by other authors—for a review article, see note 17).

Why should this be so? Why should a debate which starts out as a debate about mental illness turn out to be, really, a debate about physical illness? To understand this we need to adopt a distinction from linguistic analytic philosophy, that between the 'use' and 'definition' of concepts.[21] We normally assume that the meaning, use, and definition of concepts all run together. Often they do: problems in the *use* of the concept of schizophrenia, for example, were shown to be due to psychiatrists in different parts of the world using it with different *meanings*; and these have been greatly reduced by the introduction of clear, explicit *definitions* (as in the DSM for example).[22] But meaning, use, and definition do not always go together in this way. The concept of time, for example, is largely problem-free in *use* (outside theoretical physics). In this sense, then, we could all be said to know what it *means* (we know how to use the concept). But just try *defining* time! Unlike the concept of schizophrenia, the concept of time is largely problem-free in use *despite* the fact that we are unable to give it a clear explicit definition.

The way that the debate about mental illness comes out, therefore, as being a debate about physical illness, shows that the concept of physical illness is more like the concept of time than the concept of schizophrenia. It is one of those concepts that we are better at using than defining. And once we recognize this, it gives a wholly different spin to the debate about mental illness. We have still to explain why mental illness is more problematic in use than physical illness (we will find that this is connected with its more value-laden nature). But we have now to explain as well, why physical illness is *less* problematic in use *despite* being equally obscure in meaning. In the debate as recast, then, physical illness and mental illness are seen to be on a par, the problem-*free* use of the concept of physical illness being as much a matter for explanation as the problem-*laden* use of that of mental illness. Far from arguing the pros and cons of mental illness by reference to physical illness, therefore, the first step in the debate about mental illness must be a more careful analysis of the meaning of physical illness.

The American philosopher, Christopher Boorse, is among those who, though concerned with the problems associated with the concept of mental illness, tackles the concept of physical illness head-on.[23] His argument, although not presented in this way, can be understood as seeking to reconcile the points of view illustrated here by Szasz and Kendell. Much of the difficulty about mental illness, he suggests, goes back to a misunderstanding about the nature of health, namely that it is an essentially evaluative concept. This misunderstanding has arisen from a failure to distinguish between illness and disease, the terms which he appropriates to the practical and theoretical aspects of medicine, respectively. In its practical aspects, Boorse suggests, health is indeed a value-laden concept; hence illness is too. Szasz would therefore be right according to Boorse's argument, in pointing to ethical norms as criteria of mental illness (as distinct from disease), though wrong in failing to recognize that ethical norms are also criteria of physical illness. However, at the theoretical heart of medicine, Boorse continues, there is a body of objective knowledge which is 'continuous with theory in biology and the other basic sciences'. It is in terms of this scientific knowledge that diseases are defined, and the concept of disease is thus value-free. If Boorse is right, therefore, then Kendell is right in pointing to value-free norms as criteria of physical disease (Kendell's norms and Boorse's are in fact essentially the same): though in extending these norms to the area of mental health, Kendell (on Boorse's view) should have restricted their application to mental *disease* as distinct from mental illness.

Boorse's analysis is detailed and subtle and it has rightly been widely influential. He shares with Szasz and Kendell, a biomedical model of disease: but the model is now presented in a form that accords well with modern medical thinking. Most doctors nowadays acknowledge that value-judgements come into the practice of medicine; not just ethical judgements, but also aesthetic, prudential and legal judgements, among others. Illness, furthermore, in so far as it is a concept distinct from disease, is indeed relatively prominent in this area. It is associated naturally with the patient's experience of ill-health: it is subjective and value-laden, a matter of feelings and sensations, of complaints, and of symptoms. Yet all this, according to the biomedical model is peripheral to the area of technical scientific knowledge to which doctors, as specialists, are truly expert. It is in the area of *disease,* defined by scientific knowledge of structure and function, that medical theory, and hence the doctor's particular skill in the diagnosis and treatment of illness, resides. Boorse's analysis, furthermore, provides at least a partial explanation for the relatively problem-free use of the medical concepts in physical medicine as compared with psychiatry. Boorse focuses here on the concept of illness. But even at the level of disease it can be seen that the relatively undeveloped state of the 'mental' sciences makes mental conditions, on his analysis, more likely to be problematic practically; and this is indeed what he suggests.

Despite its attractions however, there are a number of objections to Boorse's analysis. Some of these are technical. Illness, for example, is marked out by Boorse as 'serious' disease; and while this certainly brings into the concept of illness the required logical element of evaluation, it conflicts with our ordinary usage of these concepts—ordinarily we use both disease and illness equally readily of serious and of minor conditions. Similarly, the idea that illness should be understood as a subcategory of disease at all (i.e. the subcategory of serious diseases) has to be understood stipulatively, since it conflicts with the fact that the experience of illness ordinarily *precedes* knowledge of the particular disease from which one is suffering—just as historically there were illnesses long before the development of scientific disease theories in terms of abnormal structure and functioning.[24]

A more fundamental objection to Boorse's analysis, however, is that its main practical effect is to marginalize medical ethics. This is built right into the structure of his theory. Ethical considerations are shifted to the periphery, outside the supposed value-free theoretical heart of medicine. This marginalizing effect comes out clearly when Boorse applies his analysis to some of the practical problems with which, at the start of his paper, he says he is concerned. His solution to what he takes to be the controversial diagnosis of homosexuality, for example, amounts to no more than a solution by exclusion.[25] Doctors, he argues in effect, should confine themselves to understanding the *biology* of sexuality rather than being concerned with whether homosexuality is a disease. We may or may not agree with this. But when Boorse considers the concept of psychosis—the key concept it will be recalled in relation to compulsory psychiatric treatment, as in Mr AB's case—his analysis gives entirely the wrong result. In this connection Boorse discusses the closely related issue of responsibility in law. But his analysis leads to the counterintuitive result that psychotic disorders should be peripheral rather than (as they are) central, to the status of mental illness as an excuse.[26]

It could be said that these objections to Boorse's theory are beside the point. After all, if there are points of conflict between Boorse's analysis of the medical concepts and ordinary usage, perhaps it is ordinary usage which is wrong. Boorse himself says as much at one point, suggesting that certain features of ordinary usage are 'two thousand years out of date'. This *could* be said, however, were it not for the fact that there is a philosophically central difficulty with his theory, namely that when Boorse himself shifts from defining disease to *using* the concept, he slips straight back into giving it clear evaluative meaning. For example, having defined disease in value-free terms as a 'deviation' from the normal functional organization of the species, he uses it only two lines later to mean a 'deficiency' in functional efficiency. Similarly, a little further on, the evaluatively neutral 'environmental causes' (as an element in the further elaboration of his definition of disease) becomes the value-laden 'hostile environment'.

This is highly significant for our understanding of the meaning of the concept of disease. The marginalizing of medical ethics in Boorse's version of the medical model, and indeed (many of) the more technical objections to his analysis, arise from his central contention that disease can be defined without reference to values. The issues surrounding this contention are many: indeed, they include all the issues involved in the 'is–ought' debate in general ethical theory. But it is crucial that even Boorse, although defining disease without reference to values, continues to use it (in flat contradiction to his own definition) with clear evaluative force. This is no mere oversight. Coming as it does at the very heart of Boorse's theory, it shows that while disease may be defined (stipulatively) in value-free terms, it cannot actually be used without value-judgements slipping back in. As a feature, then, even of Boorse's use of the concept of disease, this strongly suggests, contrary to the biomedical model, that disease as well as illness, and hence the theoretical centre as well as the practical periphery of medicine, are essentially value-laden rather than value-free.[27]

Philosophical value theory and a fact-plus-value model of disease

In the first part of this chapter Mr AB's case history showed the central importance of concepts of mental disorder, and of psychotic mental disorder in particular, for psychiatric ethics. In the second part of the chapter we explored two ways of trying to get to a clearer understanding of the ethical importance of mental disorder, via bioethics in the form of Beauchamp and Childress' analysis, and via the debate about mental illness in the form of Boorse's attempt to reconcile the poles of the traditional psychiatry and anti-psychiatry positions. The arguments of both these authors led to values, though in both cases in a marginal position, located at the periphery of an essentially science-based biomedical model. However, Boorse's continued use of disease with evaluative force suggested that even this most scientific of medical terms is, really, not value-free at all. This now begs the question of why disease (and physical disorder generally), at least as used in 'high-tech' areas of medicine, *appear* to be value-free, compared with mental illness, and mental disorder generally, the appearances of which are more overtly value-laden.

To answer this question we will need to make a further borrowing from linguistic analytical philosophy. In the last section we adopted the distinction between use and definition of concepts to explain the way in which the debate about mental illness turned out to be a debate about physical illness. In this section we will be using some observations about the way in which value terms are used in order to explain the relatively value-free appearance of physical illness. This section will be fairly theoretical, but the insights of analytic philosophy into the concept of disease lead to a whole series of important practical results for psychiatry, and for psychiatric ethics in particular, to which we will come in the next section.

The borrowing from analytic philosophy that we need to understand the more value-laden nature of mental illness, comes from the work of the Oxford philosophers, R. M. Hare,[28] Geoffrey Warnock,[29] J. O. Urmson[30] and others, on the logical properties of value terms. Working in the 1950s to 1970s, these authors were very much in the linguistic analytical tradition in philosophy. Although not very fashionable at present, this is a practically useful approach to philosophy in that it encourages us to make observations, to look carefully at the way words are actually used.[31]

The key observation about the way words are used for understanding the relatively value-free appearance of physical illness, is that *all* value terms may under certain circumstances, be used with clear factual meaning. Notice that this is not, as such, anything special to medicine. It is a general property (a logical, or conceptual, property) of *all* value terms. Thus, even the most general value terms, good and bad, may be used with factual meaning in certain contexts. Used of, say, pictures, 'good' and 'bad' are clearly evaluative in meaning. But if you go into a shop to buy eating apples, for example, and are offered some with pulpy flesh and brown skins, you will say 'these are no good, they are bad'. So clear, indeed, are the descriptive (or factual) criteria for 'good apples' that we can look them up in the Ministry of Agriculture regulations. Urmson[30] gives an example of a government classification of apples into 'good', 'fine' and 'superfine' according to the descriptive characteristics of the apples in question. So with apples 'good' and 'bad' have clear factual meaning, even though, in other contexts (as used of pictures) their meaning is more as we should expect, largely evaluative.

As a point about the logic of value terms this observation already looks promising for helping us to understand the medical concepts. If *all* value terms may sometimes look like factual terms (as in the case of apples), then in principle there is no reason why 'disease' and 'physical illness', although used with largely factual meaning, should not be value terms. And the explanation for this property of value terms, their property of looking like factual terms, shows that this is indeed the case. We need to look briefly at this explanation, and apply it to the medical concepts, before coming back to the practical implications of all this in the next section.

So, why should value terms sometimes be used with mainly factual meaning? The key point is that value-judgements are made by reference to *factual* criteria, and that where these criteria are more or less stable they become *attached by association* to the value term in question. Thus, the factual criteria for 'bad' use of apples—brown skin, pulpy flesh, and so on—are relatively stable. That is to say, most people most of the time use the term 'bad' of apples with brown skin and pulpy flesh. They do not *have* to do so. 'Bad' used of apples (except where it is used as a synonym for 'decomposing') does not always mean brown skin, pulpy flesh, and so on. In the context of cider-making, indeed, such apples are judged good. All the same, the fact that most people most of the time use 'bad' of apples with brown skin and pulpy flesh has the result that 'bad' used of apples normally implies that the apples in question have, as a *matter of fact,* brown skins and pulpy flesh. Used of pictures, on the other hand, 'good' and 'bad' have no such stable factual criteria. People disagree widely over the features of pictures that make them good or bad. Hence 'good picture' and 'bad picture' retain overtly evaluative meaning.

The difference, then, between value expressions which carry factual meanings and those which do not, is in the extent to which the factual criteria for the value judgements they express are settled or agreed upon. If the factual criteria are widely agreed then the value term in question (as in 'bad apple') will come to carry factual meaning; if the factual criteria vary widely then the value term in question (as in 'bad picture') will remain overtly evaluative in meaning.

We are now in a position to apply this idea to the medical concepts. If as we have come to suspect, not only 'illness' but also 'disease', and not only 'physical illness' but also 'mental illness', are all value terms, then the general point made by Hare, Urmson, Warnock and others about the logical properties of all value terms, should apply equally to the medical value terms as to the all-purpose value terms, like 'good' and 'bad', with which these authors were concerned.

This is indeed what we find. 'Disease' is the more complex case because it is used in both symptomatic and causal senses (see note 24). But the basic point is that the more strongly factual connotations of 'disease' compared with 'illness' arise from the term tending to be used of those conditions that are widely (by most people most of the time) negatively evaluated as illnesses. One consequence of this is that, in contrast to the biomedical model, disease turns out to be a subcategory of illness. According to philosophical value theory, 'illness' is used of *any* condition that may be negatively evaluated as illness (i.e. rather than as any other kind of negatively evaluated condition, such as, say, ugliness or wickedness—see also below, pp. 182–185), while 'disease' is used only of those conditions that most people most of the time negatively evaluate in this way. This has the virtue of explaining the factual connotations of disease while avoiding the contradictions inherent in the biomedical model. For instead of making disease a factual term, this formulation preserves its status as a value term, thus leaving open the possibility of its continued use with evaluative connotations. Hence, on this view, the continued use (even by Boorse) of disease with evaluative force, far from being an embarrassment to the theory, is actually to be expected.

Philosophical value theory thus gives a more self-consistent account of the concept of disease. But the same point about the logic of value terms also gives a more convincing and practically fruitful account of the more value-laden nature of 'mental illness' compared with 'physical illness'.[32] Thus, given that mental illness is more overtly evaluative than physical illness, we should expect to find that the criteria by which the symptoms of mental illness are evaluated are more variable—from person to person and for a given person on different occasions—than the corresponding criteria for the symptoms of physical illness. And this is what is found. For example, the criteria by which we evaluate anxiety, a typical symptom of mental illness, are more variable—in the sense defined here—than the corresponding criteria for, say, physical pain. Pain is at best a 'necessary evil' for almost everyone: but anxiety, though widely negatively evaluated, may be positively sought out—in horror films, for example, or through participation in dangerous sports such as hang-gliding. And if this is true for anxiety, as one of the less complex phenomena (evaluatively speaking) with which psychiatry is concerned, it is even more true of the higher functions, such as desire, affect, belief, volition and motivation. Individual variation in what we judge to be good or bad of phenomena such as these, is wide indeed. Hence, for this reason alone, i.e. for reason of the natural differences in individual human values, mental illness will be a more overtly value-laden concept than physical illness. As Fig. 9.2 illustrates, 'mental illness', being in this respect like 'good picture', will carry clearly evaluative meaning, while 'physical illness', being more like 'good apple', will carry mainly factual meaning.

We now have a basis for understanding the medical concepts which is radically different from that offered by the biomedical model. Where the biomedical model can be characterized as a fact-centred model, the model that is derived from the linguistic-analytical work of Hare, Urmson, Warnock and others, is a fact-plus-value model.

A fact-plus-value model thus gives us an account of the value-ladenness of mental illness which is quite different from that offered by Boorse in his version of the biomedical model. Boorse identified the more value-laden nature of mental illness with the underdeveloped state of psychiatric science: 'mental illness', according to Boorse, is a legitimate medical concept but only to the extent that it is a subcategory of a (putative) value-free concept of 'mental disease'. In a fact-plus-value model, by contrast, the more value-laden nature

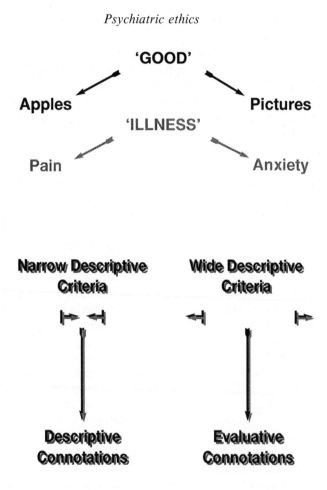

Fig. 9.2 The parallels between the value terms good and illness. All value terms (including such general value terms as 'good' and 'bad') may have factual connotations where the criteria for the value judgements they express are largely agreed upon. This property of value terms explains why 'physical illness' has largely factual connotations, while 'mental illness' is more overtly evaluative (see text).

of 'mental illness' has nothing (directly) to do with science. It is explained, straightforwardly, by a logical property of value terms combined with the natural variability of our values as individual human beings. A fact-plus-value model is thus essentially neutral in respect of psychiatry. The biomedical model, even in the sophisticated philosophical form developed by Boorse, is inherently prejudicial to psychiatry—the legitimacy of the concept of mental illness is dependent on advances in the brain sciences establishing a value-free theory of 'mental disease' equivalent in scientific status to the value-free disease theories of physical medicine. In a fact-plus-value model, as Fig. 9.2 illustrates, the more value-laden nature of 'mental illness' is no less, and no more, legitimate than the more fact-laden nature of 'physical illness'. Both arise from the same logical property of value terms combined with the same fact of human nature, that our values differ more widely over anxiety, belief, etc. (as built into 'mental illness') than over pain, nausea, etc. (as built into 'physical illness').

This in turn gives us a quite different understanding of the debate about mental illness. In the biomedical model, you will recall, mental illness was torn between anti-psychiatry (pulling it into the human world of moral problems) and psychiatry (pulling it into the scientific world of disease). A fact-plus-value model reconciles these extremes. To the extent that it endorses the legitimacy of the concept of mental illness, it is consistent with the pro-psychiatry side in the debate. To the extent, though, that a fact-plus-value model traces the value-ladenness of 'mental illness' to the diversity of our values as individual human beings, it is also consistent with the anti-psychiatry side. For it shows that 'mental illness' is, inherently and irreducibly, more problematic ethically than 'physical illness'. It is from this insight of a fact-plus-value model that many of the practical consequences of the model for psychiatric ethics are derived.

Turning philosophical theory into practice

A fact-plus-value model has a number of direct implications for practice: (1) it raises the profile of ethics in psychiatry, making ethical considerations (or more broadly questions of value) central, while, at the same time, (2) not displacing science. In making values central (alongside facts), a fact-plus-value model also, (3) extends the scope of traditional psychiatric ethics, to include questions of psychopathology and diagnosis as well as treatment. This in turn has implications for, (4) the organization of services (in particular the role of patients and of multidisciplinary terms), (5) education, and (6) research. We will consider each of these briefly.

1. *Raising the profile of ethics*: a fact-plus-value model makes ethics unavoidable. It increases the visibility of the logical element of evaluation in medicine; and greater awareness of this element, as the editors of this book point out (p. 1), is essential if ethical standards in medicine are to be maintained and improved. In this, however, it is in principle no different from the conventional approach, at least as developed by authors like Boorse. Where it differs radically from the biomedical model is in showing the logical element of evaluation to be *central* in medicine. Boorse, as we saw earlier, regarded the theoretical heart of medicine as being value-free, and his theory thus marginalized medical ethics, making it so far as medical theory is concerned, an optional extra. This corresponds broadly with the way many doctors still view

the place of medical ethics. A fact-plus-value model, on the other hand, has the opposite effect, placing the logical element of evaluation, and with it medical ethics, uncompromisingly at the theoretical heart of the subject.

It is important to add that on this model, ethics cannot be displaced from its central place by future developments in medical (including brain) science. This is implicit in what was said earlier about the relationship between illness and disease. Boorse's theory, reflecting biomedical thinking generally, anticipates that the value-ladenness of psychiatry (and, hence, the practical importance of ethics), will shrink as brain science expands. This is because on the biomedical model the value-ladenness of psychiatry arises from the underdeveloped state of psychiatric science. In a fact-plus-value model, the value-ladenness of psychiatry arises from legitimate differences between us in our values as human beings. Science, therefore, can no more displace ethics from its centrally important place in psychiatry, than it can displace values from their centrally important place in our uniqueness as individual human beings.

2. *Not displacing science*: a fact-plus-value model, though, is just that, a fact-*plus*-value model. It is not a value-centred model aiming to displace the fact-centred biomedical model.

A fact-plus-value model makes science and ethics equal partners in medicine: it reconciles the 'what *can* be done' questions of medical practice with the 'what *ought* to be done' questions. It is thus not anti-scientific. On the contrary it makes it easier to pursue the advancement of what Boorse calls a value-free science of health. For in place of the value-excluding strategy of the biomedical model—which as we saw is essentially a strategy of *denial*—a fact-plus-value model offers a strategy of *clarification*. Some have argued that a value-free science of any subject may be an illusion. But a fact-plus-value model actually advances the possibility of a value-free science of health by making explicit, and hence helping to clarify, the relationship between fact and value as twin and equally vital logical elements in the conceptual structure of medicine.

3. *Extending the scope of psychiatric ethics to include psychopathology and diagnosis*: Bioethics, consistently with the biomedical model, has traditionally focused on issues of treatment choice (including the control of patient involvement in research). A fact-plus-value model has the direct consequence that values will be important practically in classification and diagnosis in psychiatry as well as in treatment. According to this model, values are present in principle in diagnosis and classification in all areas of medicine. But they are (largely) unimportant practically in physical medicine because the relevant values are (largely) shared. The key difference, though, between psychiatry and physical medicine, according to a fact-plus-value model, is that in the area of mental health there will be significant and legitimate *variation* in values. Hence values, as well as facts, will be important in practice as well as in principle to the classificatory concepts we employ in psychiatry and in psychiatric diagnosis.[33]

The importance of values in psychiatric classification can be shown directly by inspection of the language used in our current classifications of mental disorders. Even DSM, with its self-proclaimed scientific status, relies on value judgements, not only in the way it defines mental disorder but even in the criteria for some of its specific categories: a paraphilia, for example, is defined by reference to social value norms. These are not one-offs, moreover. In a study of the problems identified by the authors of the DSM-IV themselves, questions of value (although not recognized by the authors as such) were shown to be important in over half the cases.[33]

A particularly clear illustration of the importance of values in psychiatric disorders is provided by the psychotic disorders. This is surprising from the point of view of the biomedical model, these disorders being intuitively the closest counterparts among mental disorders of physical diseases. Yet in a study of religious experience and psychopathology, the differential diagnosis between schizophrenia was shown to turn, crucially, on questions of value.[34] In this study, a number of subjects were identified whose spiritual experiences had the phenomenological features of first-rank symptoms of schizophrenia (including primary delusion and thought insertion). According to the diagnostic criteria in ICD, these subjects should therefore have had schizophrenia. But by any common-sense criteria they were not even ill, their experiences being life-enhancing and enabling. The DSM does make the required differential diagnosis possible, by adding to the traditional first-rank symptoms an additional criterion of 'social/occupational/*dys*function' (DSM, p. 285, emphasis added) (see note 22). But this criterion, as the italicized prefix indicates, has the form, essentially, of a value judgement: it requires that the 'symptoms' be associated not just with a change in occupational or social functioning, but with a change for the *worse*. This indeed is made explicit in the further definition of the criterion, which speaks of functioning being *'markedly below'* the standard previously achieved, or, in the case of a child or adolescent of a *'failure* to achieve expected levels' (emphases added).

Critical, therefore, to the differential diagnosis of a condition at the heart of psychiatric pathology, is a value judgement. There are other more theoretical indications that value judgements are important to the diagnosis of psychiatric disorders: delusions themselves, as we saw earlier, although often defined as false beliefs, and hence sometimes considered as providing an objective measure of genuine mental illness, commonly take the form of value judgements—our earlier examples were delusions of guilt in depression and grandiose delusions in hypomania, both of which are commonly evaluative rather than factual in form.

Equally important, though, is practical experience of the way in which the neglect of values in psychiatric diagnosis leads to poor standards of practice. There is good evidence from sociological and ethnographic studies of an important mismatch between professionals and patients in the process of diagnosis, not only of spiritual and religious experiences, but also more generally in cross-cultural aspects of psychiatric care.[35] Neglect of values may be important, too, in making psychiatry vulnerable to the more gross forms of abuse, for example in the former USSR. As is well known, for many years towards the end of the communist era, political dissidents were increasingly diagnosed as psychotic and treated with neuroleptics. This had been widely assumed to reflect lax scientific standards. However, a study of the Russian-language medical literature produced at the time, showed clearly that the diagnostic concepts employed were even more firmly driven by a value-free biomedical model than their counterparts in Britain and America. Other factors (legal, professional training, etc.) were important in the processes by which abuse of psychiatry became widespread in the USSR. But the essential vulnerability of psychiatry to abuse was shown to be due to political values driving judgements of rationality behind a mask of value-free science (see note 5).

The case therefore, for values being important in diagnosis and classification in psychiatry, as well as in treatment, is persuasive. Theoretical work in philosophy on the logic of values suggests that values *should* be important to psychiatric classification and diagnosis; practical experience shows that they *are*. It is sometimes felt that to acknowledge this, to depart from the biomedical ideal of value-free disease concepts, is to open up a Pandora's box of value-relativism, of 'anything goes'. This is quite wrong. Law, for example, and aesthetics, or for that matter traditional medical ethics, are all value-driven; but in none of these areas could it be said that anything goes. Human values, after all, if diverse, are not random.

On the other hand, a fact-plus-value model does make it inescapable that the evaluative (as well as factual) elements in psychiatric diagnosis are and will continue to be important practically. In other words, we have to face up to values, and this has implications for the organisation of services, for education and research.

4. *The organization of services*: A fact-plus-value model shifts the organization of services away from a doctor-centred model to one in which both patients (and carers) and the multidisciplinary team have more important roles.[36] Both these shifts arise directly from the displacement of a (supposedly) value-free scientific theory of disease from the centre of the medical concepts and its replacement by a structure of facts plus values.

Thus, on the biomedical model, a doctor decides what is or is not disease by reference as an expert to scientifically defined concepts of disease. The doctor thus sets the agenda for everything else that may happen. But in a fact-plus-value model, values weigh equally with facts. As noted earlier, this is not anti-scientific. Everything that is important in the genuinely scientific part of medicine on the biomedical model (identifying symptoms, knowledge of syndromes, causation, etc.) remains equally important in a fact-plus-value model. Indeed it has been shown recently that ideologically driven attempts to jettison the more traditional aspects of psychiatric diagnosis have thrown out the baby with the bath water, leaving the seriously mentally ill without proper treatment.[37] So a fact-plus-value model aims to make psychiatric services, not less scientific, but more humanistic. The model aims to bring the patient's values, as well as the doctor's facts, firmly into the frame.

Just as a fact-plus-value model is not anti-science, so it is not anti-doctor. Bringing the patient's values into the frame, is not to displace the doctor's values; it is not to substitute for the doctor-led biomedical model a patient-led consumer model. What is needed, rather, is a balance of values. It is this that a well-functioning, multidisciplinary team can help to supply. In the biomedical model, the multidisciplinary team provides a range of skills which are important for treatment. In a fact-plus-value model the multidisciplinary team has an important additional role. For the different perspectives of nurse, psychiatrist, social worker, and so on, and in some circumstances also of carers and relatives, can all help to provide a balance of evaluative considerations. This is no guarantee of good practice, of course. But it is at least a step towards avoiding the more severe forms of abuse, whether institutionalized (as in the former USSR) or sporadic, many of which arise through the unbalanced exercise of the values of any one group or individual, whether these values be political, ideological, commercial, managerial, or indeed professional.

5. *Education and training*: a fact-plus-value model, with its implications for the organization of services, clearly has implications also for education and training in health care. Here too, though, it is important to keep a balance. The old model of medical education, with its exclusive focus on scientific facts (anatomy, physiology etc.) is not sufficient. Equally, though, we cannot do without a really firm grounding in the sciences basic to healthcare.

One way to strike the required balance is by focusing on the idea of medical education as learning to solve clinical problems.[38] A number of medical schools in Europe and America are moving in this direction. Sometimes their conception of problem solving is still exclusively scientific. But in other cases it includes attention to ethical, legal, and communication aspects of clinical problem solving. These are increasingly important in all aspects of health care, but in psychiatry, on a fact-plus-value model, they are essential. At a postgraduate level, furthermore, as well as medical schools moving towards philosophy, philosophy departments are increasingly moving towards psychiatry— Oxford, Southampton, and Durham in the UK, for example, now include courses on abnormal psychology and psychiatry in their undergraduate courses, while other universities offer full Masters and PhD programmes in philosophy and mental health (e.g. Sheffield, Warwick, and Kings College, London).

6. *Research*: as has several times been emphasized, a fact-plus-value model is not anti-scientific. It adds values to, rather than displacing science from, medicine. It is important to add, though, that in psychiatry a fact-plus-value

model offers a more appropriate framework than the biomedical model for science itself.

The reason for this is the greater importance of values in psychiatry. In the more 'high-tech' areas of acute physical medicine, the values involved in diagnosis can be thought of as a constant (to the extent that they vary relatively little from person to person). In psychiatry, by contrast, the corresponding values involved in diagnosis are a *variable,* and, as the differential diagnosis of schizophrenia and religious experience illustrated, often a *critical* variable at that (see note 34). This is important in epidemiological research, for example, in which studies based on first-rank symptoms alone will conflate schizophrenia and religious experience. But the same conflation could also be crucial in neuroscience. The results of brain-imaging studies, for example, however detailed a picture they give of the functioning of the brain, would be fatally prejudiced by a failure to distinguish between the two quite different phenomena of genuine psychopathology and genuine religious experience.

Mad or bad? Mad or sad?

Philosophical value theory thus offers a rich return for psychiatry in the form of a fact-plus-value model of the medical concepts. Value theory itself, however, is not sufficient to ground psychiatric ethics. This is because the problems with which psychiatric ethics is concerned are often not simply problems of evaluation but of specifically *medical* evaluation. With compulsory treatment, for example, as we saw with Mr AB's case at the start of this chapter, what is at issue, generally speaking, is not simply whether the person's condition (of sadness, distress, etc.) is a bad condition. The question is whether it is a bad condition of the specifically *medical* kind required to justify specifically medical means of intervention. And in forensic psychiatry, similarly, there are the closely related issues raised by mental illness as an excuse: 'Mad or bad?' is the slogan here, corresponding with the 'Mad or sad?' questions of involuntary treatment. In forensic psychiatry the question is whether the accused was suffering from an illness and was therefore not responsible, or whether he or she as a free agent was capable of choosing right from wrong, and hence bad (i.e., immoral, foolish, criminal, etc.) rather than mad (i.e. mentally ill).

In the biomedical model, as both Beauchamp and Childress's and Boorse's accounts showed, the demarcation between pathological and healthy (whether good or bad) conditions is taken to be a matter for science to decide. Diseases are marked out from other kinds of negatively evaluated conditions by scientifically defined disturbances of bodily or mental functioning. In a fact-plus-value model, by contrast, 'disturbance of functioning', no less than 'disease', is taken to be a value-concept. Hence some other criterion for dermarcating 'mad from bad', connected with the evaluative element in the meanings of the medical concepts, is required.

A full account of the demarcation criterion in a fact-plus-value model of the medical concepts is beyond the scope of this chapter. It is important, though, to see broadly how this can be derived. The key step is that, just as in this chapter we have added value to fact, so now we need to add action to function. The difference between action and function, as these terms are used here, is the difference between actions as characteristic of *persons*, and functions as characteristics of the *parts* of persons, of bodily or mentally parts and systems.[39] Thus if I pick up my pen this is a (simple) *action* of mine even though a neurologist, say, might speak of my hand, arm, etc. as *functioning*. (Note that when we speak of people having functions it is as parts of society— e.g. as policemen, or as parents, etc.) Action and function, so differentiated, map naturally on to the medical concepts. For just as disturbance of function is the obvious way to analyse medical knowledge of disease (liver disease, Alzheimer's disease, etc.), so disturbance of agency is the obvious way to analyse the patient's experience of illness, i.e. as failure of action: the core feature of the experience of illness is incapacity, a failure to do the things we can ordinarily do; when we are ill, as Toulmin has pointed out, we are literally patients not agents.[40]

As with philosophical value theory this is another of those seemingly simple ideas which offers a rich return for our understanding of the medical concepts and of their importance in psychiatric ethics. In the first place, it explains why these concepts are indeed value concepts. This is an important technical point. In the biomedical model, values were added to a value-free concept of disease to generate a value-laden concept of illness with relevant applications to practice. In a fact-plus-value model, you will recall, instead of illness being derived in this way from disease, disease is derived from illness. Hence the evaluative element in the meaning of disease (or dysfunction) must be derived from an evaluative element in the meaning of illness (or failure of action). On an action-failure model the required evaluative element is provided by the notion of intention (this being a central component of action). For intention, as the Oxford philosopher Elizabeth Anscombe pointed out,[41] is an inherently evaluative concept; that is to say, it is a positive evaluative concept in the sense that to claim something to be one's intention while at the same time, and other things being equal, denying that one evaluates it positively, is self-contradictory: like saying both that I want and (in the same sense of 'want') do not want something—a psychological, but not a logical, possibility! Therefore, *failure* of intention is, correspondingly, an inherently *negative* evaluative concept. Therefore, the experience of a particular kind of failure of intentional action could be the origin of the particular kind of negative evaluation that is expressed by illness, and hence by its derivative disease.

All the implications, therefore, of a fact-plus-value model of the medical concepts apply equally to the model upgraded, as it were, to a function-plus-action model. This includes the recognition that the diversity of human values, and hence the importance of values in psychiatry, will not be reduced by future developments in brain science. A function-plus-action model, though, offers additional resources for understanding the medical concepts arising from the complexity of what J. L. Austin called the 'machinery of action' (see note 21). The Swedish philosopher, Lennart Nordenfelt, has shown how action theory can illuminate problems in medical ethics.[42] Crucially, though, from the point of view of *psychiatric* ethics, action theory explains, where the biomedical model as we saw earlier fails to explain, the central place of psychotic disorder in the 'map' of psychiatry.

The idea, essentially, is this. On a function-plus-action model, the experience of illness in general is to be interpreted in terms of disturbance in the machinery of action. Hence, on this model, the variety especially of mental illness experiences (i.e. of psychopathology) can be interpreted as disturbances of different kinds and in different parts of this machinery. There is good evidence, as with values, that we draw on notions of agency even in our scientific classifications of mental disorder.[43] Reasons, however, have a central place in this machinery. Sensation, movement, volition, memory, perception, etc. are all executive—they are all necessary to the *carrying out* of an action. But reasons *define the action itself*: a standard philosophical example is the different actions performed in waving one's arm—signalling, bidding, etc. These different actions are differentiated not by the movement as such (which is the same in each case), but by the reasons for which the movement is performed. If, therefore, reasons (of this reasons-for-action kind), are a central rather than merely executive component of action, psychotic illness as a *disturbance* of reasons-for-action, emerges quite naturally in an action-failure account of psychopathology, as the central kind of mental illness.

Reasoning of the reasons-for-action kind is often called practical reasoning. The evidence that psychotic illness really is a disturbance of practical reason is partly negative, partly positive. The negative evidence has to do with a difference between reason as studied by philosophers and reason as studied by scientists. Practical reasoning, being the reasoning of agents (of whole persons), has been studied mainly by philosophers, notably in moral philosophy, in the philosophy of law, and, more recently, in the philosophy of mind. Scientists, by contrast, and consistently with the biomedical model, have studied specific subcomponents or elements of reasoning, i.e. particular cognitive functions. And the negative evidence for psychotic disorder being a disturbance of practical reasoning rather than of cognitive functioning, is simply that the scientific paradigm has so far failed to identify a disturbance of cognitive functioning specific to the key psychotic symptom, delusion.[44]

Of course, such a discovery may be around the corner. But in the meantime the positive evidence linking delusions with reasons for action, is that delusions share with reasons for action the remarkable phenomenological feature of taking the form of fact or value. We noted earlier that delusions may take the form of factual beliefs (e.g. the delusion of guilt that I started the war in

Yugoslavia) or of value judgements (e.g. the delusion of guilt that my forgetting to give my children their pocket money was the worst sin in the world).
We can now see that the same is true of reasons: if you ask why I am waving
my arm, for example, the reason could be a fact (e.g. 'I am making a bid') or
a value (e.g. 'the picture is worth going higher for'). This is remarkable
philosophically, because facts and values are like logical chalk and cheese. It is
also remarkable psychiatrically, because, as we saw earlier, although evaluative
delusions are commonplace clinically, delusions are defined in the textbooks,
consistently with the biomedical model of a value-free psychopathology, as
false factual beliefs. Yet the parallel in this respect, between delusions and
reasons for action, is wholly *un*remarkable, indeed it is entirely *consistent* with
a function-plus-action (and hence with a fact-plus-value) model of the medical
concepts.[45]

Conclusions

In this chapter, starting from a case history, the case of Mr AB, an outline has
been given of a model of the medical concepts in which fact and value, disease
and illness, function and action, all play equal roles. This model, called a
fact-plus-value model for short, has been contrasted with the standard biomedical model, in which facts, disease and dysfunction have a central place,
while values, illness and failure of action (or incapacity) come in only at the
periphery (see Fig. 9.3).

It has been argued that the biomedical model, although assumed equally by
bioethics as by biomedicine, fails to meet the challenge of psychiatric ethics. It
works for the more high-tech areas of physical medicine but only because
these are simpler, evaluatively speaking, than psychiatry. In high-tech areas
of physical medicine the evaluative element in the meanings of the medical
concepts can be ignored because, although this element is still there, the values
involved are by and large *shared* values (physical pain is at best a necessary evil
for everyone), and hence they are unproblematic practically. In psychiatry,
though, the relevant values, concerned as they are with the higher functions of
wish, desire, belief, and the like, are highly variable, from person to person,
from culture to culture, and from one time to another. This is no artefact of
brain science being at an early stage of development. On the contrary, it
is a direct reflection of the diversity of human values, which in turn is a key
aspect of our uniqueness as individual human beings. Hence in psychiatry
the evaluative element in the meanings of the medical concepts cannot be
ignored but has to be faced as a key aspect of the problematic nature of mental
illness.

This had a number of important practical implications: it raised the profile
of ethics in psychiatry, though without in any way reducing that of science; it
extended the scope of ethics from treatment to classification and diagnosis (in
the biomedical model these are the preserve of science alone); it showed the

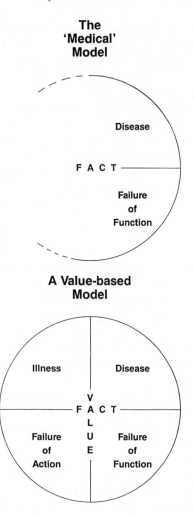

Fig. 3 Diagrammatic representation of the relationship between the medical model and a value-based analysis of the medical concepts An analysis of the medical concepts as value concepts is not antiscientific. It adds value to fact, the patient's experience of illness to medical knowledge of disease, and the analysis of illness in terms of failure of action (incapacity) to the analysis of disease in terms of failure of function (see text).

importance of the patients' values and of the values of the multidisciplinary team in the organization of services; and it had a range of implications for training and research. A deeper theoretical account of the key practical problem from which we started, involuntary psychiatric treatment, illustrated by the case of Mr AB, required that we considered briefly the particular kind of value expressed by the medical concepts, i.e. medical as opposed to moral, aesthetic, prudential or other values. This took us from value theory into the philosophy of action from which we derived a potentially fruitful way of understanding delusion, not (as in the biomedical model) as a disturbance of cognitive functioning, but as a disturbance of reasons for action.

For all this, we should not expect the biomedical model to fade away. Too many, in biomedicine and in bioethics, are too deeply invested for that! And a fact-plus-value model does indeed challenge the established biomedical order. In the biomedical model, psychiatry is an add-on, a scientific poor relation of technological medicine. This is the basis of the remarkable neglect of psychiatry by biomedicine and bioethics alike. Once, though, the central place of values in the medical concepts is recognized, it is psychiatry which moves to the central place. For in psychiatry, as we have seen, issues of value (as well as of fact) are inescapable, both clinically and in research. In a fact-plus-value model, then, psychiatry is no longer the soft end of scientific medicine. It is at the cutting edge of a medicine in which science and the humanities are equally essential to good clinical care.

References and notes

1. Fulford K. W. M. and Hope R. A. Psychiatric ethics: a bioethical ugly duckling? Chapter 58 in Gillon, R. and Lloyd, A. (ed.) *Principles of health care ethics.* Chichester, Wiley, 1993.
2. It might be thought that I overstate the extent to which doctors take medicine to be a science, and the medical concepts to be correspondingly value-free. However, aside from a minority of philosophically minded doctors, there is a widespread view that medicine is at heart, in its technical aspects, a science like any other. Furthermore, as Boorse's theory illustrates, it is possible to give cogent philosophical shape to this view, drawing on what I suggest in Chapter 3 of my book (see note 12) is a form of moral descriptivism. G. J. Warnock in his *Contemporary Moral Philosophy* (1967), London, Macmillan, gives a concise introduction to descriptivist and non-descriptivist moral theories, and to the wider philosophical debate about whether value judgements can be derived from factual statements alone (the 'is–ought' debate). The sociologist, Peter Sedgwick (Illness—mental and otherwise. *Hastings Center Report*, **1**, 3:19-40, 1973) gave an early account of the view that disease concepts are essentially evaluative in nature.
3. Mr AB is based on real case material, but with all biographical or other individually identifying personal information altered to ensure confidentiality.
4. This study is described in Fulford, K. W. M. Thought insertion and insight: disease and illness paradigms of psychotic disorder, in Spitzer M., Uehlein F., Schwartz M A., and Mundt C. (ed.), *Phenomenology, language and schizophrenia*, pp. 355–71. Springer, New York, 1993.
5. Fulford, K. W. M., Smirnoff, A. Y. U., and Snow, E. Concepts of disease and the abuse of psychiatry in the USSR. *British Journal of Psychiatry* **162**, 801–10, 1993.

6. This was borne out recently by the results of a survey carried out in a number of European countries under the Biomed 1 programme of the European Community—see Fulford, K. W. M. and Hope, T. Informed consent in psychiatry: comparative assessment of Section 5 of the National Reports—control and practical experience. Report for Biomed 1 Project: Biomedical ethics in Europe—control and practical experience, published as pp. 31–66, in Koch, H.-G., Reiter-Theil, S., and Helmchen, H. (ed.), *Informed consent in psychiatry: European perspectives on ethics, law and clinical practice*. Nomos Verlagsgesellschaft, Baden-Baden, 1996.
7. Beauchamp, T. L. and Childress, J. F. *Principles of biomedical ethics*. 4th edn. Oxford University Press: Oxford, 1994.
8. Flew, A. *Crime or disease?* Barnes and Noble, New York, 1973.
9. See for example, the definition of delusion in Harre, R. and Lamb, D. (ed.). *Dictionary of philosophy and psychology*. Blackwells, Oxford, 1987.
10. For example, Glover, J. *Responsibility*. London, Routledge & Kegan Paul, 1970; and Quinton, A. Madness. Chapter 2 in Griffiths, A. P. (ed.) *Philosophy and practice*. Cambridge University Press, Cambridge, 1985.
11. Shepherd, M. Morbid jealousy: some clinical and social aspects of a psychiatric syndrome. *Journal of Mental Science*, **107**:687–704, 1961.
12. A case of the paradoxical delusion of mental illness is described in Chapter 10 of Fulford, K. W. M. *Moral theory and medical practice*. Cambridge University Press, Cambridge, 1989; reprinted in paperback 1995.
13. For example, in Gelder, M. G., Gath, D., and Mayou, R. *Oxford textbook of psychiatry*, 2nd edn. Oxford University Press, Oxford, 1989.
14. Evaluative delusions are described in Chapter 10 of Fulford, K. W. M. (1989). (see note 12); and in Fulford, K. W. M. Evaluative delusions: their significance for philosophy and psychiatry. *British Journal of Psychiatry* **159**:108–12 (Suppl. 14, Delusions and awareness of reality), 1991.
15. Beauchamp, T. L. and Childress, J. F. (1989). (see note 7), page 84.
16. A version of this map was published in Fulford, K. W. M. Value, action, mental illness and the law, in Shute, S., Gardner, J., and Horder, J. (ed.), *Action and value in criminal law*, pp.279–310. Oxford University Press, Oxford, 1993.
17. A still valuable review is, Clare, A. (1979). The disease concept in psychiatry, in Hill, P., Murray, R., and Thorley, A. (ed.), *Essentials of postgraduate psychiatry*. Academic Press, New York. An important collection of original papers is Caplan, A. L., Englehardt, T., and McCartney J. J. (ed.), *Concepts of health and disease: interdisciplinary perspectives*. Addision-Wesley, Reading, Mass., 1981. A more recent review is Fulford, K. W. M. Mental Illness: long entry in Chadwick, R. (ed.), *Encyclopaedia of applied ethics*, Academic Press, San Diego, 1998.
18. Szasz, T. S. The myth of mental illness. *American Psychologists* **15**:113–18, 1960. Among the very large number of contributions to the debate about mental illness, those of T. Szasz, R. E. Kendell (note 19), and C. Boorse (note 23) considered here represent particularly clear expressions of well-defined views.
19. Kendell, R. E. The concept of disease and its implications for psychiatry. *British Journal of Psychiatry* **127**:305–15, 1975.
20. See Chapter 1 of Fulford, K. W. M. (1989) (ref. 12 above).
21. A particularly clear exposition of this approach is Austin, J. L. (1956–7). A plea for excuses. *Proceedings of the Aristotelian Society* **57**:1–30. Reprinted in White, A. R. (ed.) *The philosophy of action*. Oxford University Press, Oxford, 1968.
22. *Diagnostic and statistical manual of mental disorders* (4th edn). American Psychiatric Association, Washington, DC, 1994.

23. See Boorse, C. On the distinction between disease and illness. *Philosophy and Public Affairs* **5**:49–68, 1975. Boorse, C. What a theory of mental health should be. *Journal of Theory and Social Behaviour* **6**:61–84, 1976.
24. See Fulford, K. W. M. (1989). (ref. 12 above). Chapters 2 and 4. Philosophical value theory suggests that the relationship between illness and disease can be visualized in terms of a Venn diagram. The universal set is made up of any condition that may be construed as an illness. This construal is according to complex criteria, one element of which (according to the theory suggested here) is a negative value judgement. But people vary in their value judgements. Hence, within the set of conditions that may be negatively evaluated as illnesses, there will be a subset of conditions that most people most of the time negatively evaluate in this way. One sense of the term 'disease', roughly corresponding with symptomatically defined diseases, is thus identified with this subset, other senses (for example, those causally defined) being derived from it. Of course, in ordinary usage the terms illness and disease, let alone different senses of disease, are not sharply differentiated in this way. An analysis of the kind proposed here seeks, however, to identify those conceptual elements which, when added together, reproduce the appearance of ordinary usage as a whole.
25. By Boorse's criteria, homosexuality must be a disease, since it involves species-atypical desires which are associated with reduced fertility. But, he says, provided it is possible 'to maximise intrinsic goods such as happiness ... it is hard to see what practical significance [this] theoretical judgement of unhealthiness would have'. In other words, according to Boorse's theory, the dispute about the status of homosexuality lies outside the scope of medical theory, for it involves an attempt 'to justify the value of health *in other terms'* [italics mine—see Boorse, 1975, section III].
26. Boorse (1975, section III) suggests that the loss of responsibility associated with mental illness might be explained by the relevant mental functions being un-conscious, and hence outside our control, rather as digestive functions (such as peristalsis) are outside our control. However, as Boorse indicates, there are many problems with this account. In particular, there is not the same sharp distinction between a person and their psychological functions as there is between a person and their physiological functions. Psychotic illness, and delusional thinking in particular, is peculiarly difficult to analyse in functional terms. Yet the psychoses provide the clearest cases of loss of responsibility due to mental illness. Hence, on this important point for psychiatric ethics, Boorse's theory fails to give the (intuitively) right result.
27. For a more detailed discussion of Boorse's argument, see Chapter 3 of Fulford, K. W. M. (1989) (ref. 12 above).
28. Hare, R. M. Descriptivism. *Proceedings of the British Academy* **49**:115–34, 1963. (reprinted in Hare, R. M. (1972). *Essays on the moral concepts.* Macmillan, London.)
29. Warnock, G. J. *The Object of morality.* Methuen, London, 1971.
30. Urmson, J. O. On grading. *Mind* **59**:145–69, 1950.
31. The practical value of this approach to philosophy is discussed in Fulford, K. W. M. Philosophy and medicine: the Oxford connection. *British Journal of Psychiatry* **157**:111–15, 1990.
32. The details of this are given in Chapter 5 of Fulford, K. W. M. (1989). (ref. 12 above).
33. See Fulford, K. W. M. Closet logics: hidden conceptual elements in the DSM and ICD classifications of mental disorders. Chapter 9 in Sadler, J. Z., Wiggins, O. P.,

and Schwartz, M. A. (ed.). *Philosophical perspectives on psychiatric diagnostic classification*. Johns Hopkins University Press, Baltimore, 1994.

34. Jackson, M. and Fulford, K. W. M. Spiritual experience and psychopathology. *Philosophy, Psychiatry and Psychology*, 4, pp. 41–66 (commentaries by Littlewood, R.; Lu, F. G., *et al.*; Sims, A.; and Storr, L. A., with response by authors, pp. 67–90), 1997.

35. See several chapters in Bhui, K. and Olajide, J. (ed.), *Studies in cross-cultural psychiatry*. W. B. Saunders, London, 1998.

36. Fulford, K. W. M. Concepts of disease and the meaning of patient-centred care. Chapter 1 in Fulford, K. W. M., Ersser, S., and Hope, T. (ed.), *Essential practice in patient-centred care*. Blackwell Science, Oxford, 1995.

37. Clinical Standards Advisory Group. *Schizophrenia*. Vol. 1. HMSO, London, 1995.

38. See Hope, R. A. and Fulford, K. W. M. (1993) Medical education: patients, principles and practice skills. Chapter 59 in Gillon, R. (ed.). *Principles of health care ethics*. Wiley, Chichester; and Hope, T., Fulford, K. W. M., and Yates, A. *The Oxford practice skills course: ethics, law and communication in health care education*. Oxford University Press, Oxford, 1996.

39. Fulford, K. W. M. (1989) (ref. 12), Chapters 5 and 6. Function and action, although distinct concepts, are of course not unrelated. One aspect of their relationship is shown by the senses of 'do' in which people do things. These can be arranged in an approximate spectrum from more or less pure functioning (for example, biochemical processing) through to full-blown intentional actions. Somewhere in the middle of this spectrum there are things that, although capable of being done as full-blown intentional actions (*viz* with one's intentions more or less consciously before one's mind), we ordinarily 'just get on and do' (J. L. Austin's phrase in: A plea for excuses, in White, A. R. (ed.). *The philosophy of action*. Oxford University Press, Oxford, 1968). Here, in this middle ground of 'ordinary' doing, function may actually be equivocal: lifting my coffee cup can be construed either as me lifting my coffee cup (something that I 'ordinarily' do), or as my arm/hand functioning. The conventional approach to understanding the medical concepts concentrates on analysing them from the function side of this equivocation. My suggestion is that we may be able to achieve a richer and more self-consistent understanding if we are prepared to explore them from its action side as well—see, for example, note 26 on the analysis of delusions. (It should be added that implicit in the equivocal relationship of function and action is the idea that function, as well as intention, is an inherently evaluative concept. In my book I argue that this is indeed so, the evaluative element in function being derived from that of intention, Fulford 1989, Chapter 6 (ref. 12 above).

40. Toulmin, S. Agent and patient in psychiatry. *International Journal of Law and Psychiatry* 3:267–78, 1980.

41. Anscombe, G. E. M. (1959). Intention. *Proceedings of the Aristotelian Society* **57**: 321–32. Reprinted in White, A. R. (ed.) *The philosophy of action*. Oxford University Press, Oxford, 1968.

42. Nordenfelt, L. *On the nature of health: an action-theoretic approach*. D. Reidel, Dordrecht, Holland, 1987.

43. ICD-9—*Mental disorders: glossary and guide to their classification in accordance with the ninth revision of the International Classification of Diseases*. Geneva, World Health Organization, 1978. Addictions and obsessive–compulsive disorders, for example, are among the most transparent of mental illnesses in this respect. The notion of action-failure is similarly transparent in certain areas of physical

medicine, for example with neurological disorders, such as paralysis, chorea, and epilepsy. It is less transparent in other areas, mental as well as physical, for example in relation to sensations (such as pain) and emotions (such as anxiety). It is still there, however, essentially because sensations and emotions, although not things that we do, are none the less things that we do things about (withdraw from pain, escape from anxiety). Action-failure is less transparent in relation to what is perhaps the central symptom of mental illness, namely delusion. Yet it is here, above all, that if the analysis presented here is right, action-failure (as distinct from failure of function) becomes essential to a satisfactory understanding of the medical concepts (see Fulford, K. W. M. (1989) (ref. 12 above), Section III.

44. Garety, P. A. and Freedman, D., Cognitive approaches to delusions: a critical review of themes and evidence. *Journal of Abnormal Psychology*, in press.
45. See Chapter 5 of Fulford, K. W. M. (1989) (ref. 12 above).

10

Psychiatric diagnosis as an ethical problem

Walter Reich

Institutions, professions, and technologies pose ethical challenges because they are controlled by human beings and are capable of causing good or harm to other human beings. Accidents of nature, such as fetal malformations, do not in themselves pose ethical problems, even if they cause harm, because they are not under human control. But when they come under such control—for example, through the creation of a technology, such as amniocentesis—then what once may have been an accident becomes, as a result of the possibility of human intervention, preventable, and what was once ethically neutral therefore becomes ethically charged.

In psychiatry, powers, institutions, and technologies exist that, through their acts, systems, and techniques, have the potential for causing good as well as harm. And, as the profession's practitioners, psychiatrists have the freedom to act within it. Clearly, then, psychiatry's practices, as well as those who carry out those practices, inhabit an arena of ethical concern.

Ever since psychiatry emerged as a separate discipline it has been criticized for ethical abuses in every sphere of its activity. Its ability summarily to cancel a person's freedom through its power to commit that person, against his or her will, to a psychiatric hospital probably has been the subject of most such criticism: psychiatrists have been accused of forcibly hospitalizing persons who have not required it—indeed, persons who have not even been mentally ill. Other aspects of the profession have also been criticized on ethical grounds. Psychiatric institutions have often been accused of demeaning patients, and the technologies of electroconvulsive therapy, behaviour-modification, medication, psychosurgery, and psychotherapy have raised vexing and abiding issues regarding the control of behaviour.

Common to all these activities is one psychiatric act: diagnosis. It is the prerogative to diagnose that enables psychiatrists to commit patients against their wills, that delineates the populations subjected to their care, and that sets in motion the methods they will use for treatment. And it is therefore this prerogative that should provoke perhaps the most fundamental—and, consequently, the most serious—ethical examination.

Of course, the ethical problem of diagnosis stems from its capacity for misuse—that is, the knowing misapplication of diagnostic categories to persons to whom they do not apply, a misapplication that may place those individuals at risk for the harmful effects of psychiatric diagnosis. These effects include not only the loss of personal freedom, and not only the subjection to noxious psychiatric environments and treatments, but also the possibility of life-long labelling,[1-3] as well as a variety of legal and social disadvantages ranging from declarations of non-responsibility in family and financial affairs to, under the most extreme circumstances, under Nazi rule, the deprivation of life.[4-23]

In general, misdiagnoses may be said to originate in two ways. The first way is *purposeful*: the psychiatrist applies a standard psychiatric diagnosis to a person for whom he or she knows it to be inappropriate in order to achieve some end that is not, by common definition, medical. That end may vary from instance to instance. For example, the psychiatrist may be under direct and obvious pressure from a family to hospitalize a troublesome member of that family, or from political authorities to hospitalize a troublesome dissident. On the other hand, the psychiatrist may also issue a purposeful misdiagnosis at the person's own request. For example, a diagnosis resulting in hospitalization may be a protection against a worse fate, such as jail in the case of a criminal offender, the military draft in the case of a war-resister, or the birth of an unwanted child in the case of a woman seeking an abortion in a place where the procedure is available only to those who can show medical need. In both types of cases of purposeful misdiagnosis, harm may be said to result. In the first type the harm is obviously to the person. In the second, it is to the integrity of the profession. One's concern should certainly be for the first type of harm; but the second, largely overlooked as a sort of victimless crime, also requires attention.

But though purposeful misdiagnoses should be a serious concern, it is the *other* kind—misdiagnoses that result not from the wilful misapplication of psychiatric categories, but from the primarily *non-purposeful* causes—that deserve the greatest scrutiny. They deserve it because most misdiagnoses belong in this category. And they deserve it because purposeful misdiagnoses are in general clear and usually understood as unethical, while those that are non-purposeful are much more subtle and insidious, much more a part of the fabric of the field itself, and much more difficult to identify and stop.

To be sure, there is a sense in which it could be argued that non-purposeful misdiagnoses do not constitute a true ethical problem: after all, if such diagnoses are not purposefully carried out then they do not involve knowledge or free will on the part of psychiatrists and are beyond their control. But that is not quite the case. The mere fact that something is not completely purposeful does not entail that it is completely non-purposeful. This category involves, in the main, non-medical needs, pressures, and compromises that affect the diagnostic process but enter the psychiatrist's awareness to only a partial degree. The fact that psychiatrists allow themselves, for their own comfort, to ignore this awareness, or their responsibility to strengthen it, raises this category of misdiagnosis to the highest level of ethical concern.

Non-purposeful misdiagnoses, it should be stressed, are different from *mistakes* in diagnosis. Mistakes in diagnosis result from a process in which, for want of adequate information about the patient or the illness, or lack of proper training, the psychiatrist issues a diagnosis to a person whose clinical state should be categorized differently. Non-purposeful misdiagnoses by contrast, result from a process in which a psychiatrist has both adequate information about the patient and the illness and proper training, but issues an incorrect diagnosis because of factors extrinsic to the patient—and does so without being aware, or fully aware, that he or she is doing so. Sometimes, such awareness is altogether absent: the misdiagnosis is non-purposeful in the fullest sense. Sometimes, however, awareness would be present were it not for the efforts of the psychiatrist, through the use of various techniques of denial and self-delusion, to escape the moral self-condemnation that would result from such awareness. At this most extreme end of the spectrum of non-purposefulness, the veneer of non-awareness may be so thin as to allow awareness, and there-fore purposefulness, to emerge in such a manner as to make it difficult to distinguish from the purposefulness present in clear-cut cases of conscious, fully purposeful, misdiagnosis. In the main non-purposeful misdiagnosis can be traced to at least three sources. It will be to these sources that the remainder of this discussion will be devoted.

The inherent limitations of the diagnostic process

Certainly the simplest source of non-purposeful misdiagnosis lies in the vul-nerability of the diagnostic process to error. Over the years it has been shown that the process can have poor or questionable reliability;[24-26] may be subject to inconsistency and change; may suffer from bias;[27-32] and tends to rely on subjective criteria (such as, in the case of the diagnosis of schizophrenia, the psychiatrist's impression of the patient's 'understandability',[33-35] or 'peculiar behaviour',[36] his assessment of 'the feel of the case',[37] or his development, during the interview with the patient, of a 'praecox feeling'.[38] In addition, psychiatrists may diagnose health rather than illness because, as Scheff has observed, physicians as a group feel that a 'type-2 error' (accepting a hypo-thesis that is false) is less dangerous than a 'type-1 error' (rejecting a hypothesis that is true).[39]

Many of these limitations have been eased considerably by the introduc-tion of diagnostic classification systems and manuals that employ relatively objective criteria for the diagnosis of mental illnesses, particularly the American Psychiatric Association's *Diagnostic and statistical manual of mental disorders*.[40] This manual is constructed in a fashion that tends to reduce significantly the effects of those aspects of the diagnostic process that are influenced by subjective factors or ideologically based theories regarding the aetiologies of mental illnesses. In the absence of clear, conclusive, and universally accepted criteria, such as physical evidence for the presence of, say, one or another type of schizophrenia or affective disorder, such diagnostic approaches as the one taken by this manual provide important, though by no means certain, safeguards against diagnostic error.[41-49] Nevertheless, psychiatric diagnosis, though increasingly rooted in scientific research, remains a process that is vulnerable to error; and it is the responsibility of the diagnosing psychiatrist to remember its limitations with humility, and to maintain a willingness to review diagnostic decisions and admit fallibility. At best, psychiatrists are no better than their tools; and they must acknowledge the limitations of those tools as the starting-points of their own.

The power of diagnostic theory to shape psychiatric vision

But vulnerable as the diagnostic process in psychiatry is to its own limitations, likely as those limitations may be to lead psychiatrists to a misdiagnosis, and hard as they must try to guard against them, psychiatric diagnosis has yet other vulnerabilities that are even more subtle, more pervasive, and more difficult to recognize—and that, therefore, demand even greater vigilance. Again, the danger is misdiagnosis—non-purposeful but still damaging—and the ethical problem is the degree to which psychiatrists allow themselves to ignore the forces and circumstances that lead to, and make use of, such misdiagnosis.

In large measure diagnosis is a social act. It takes place in a social context. The psychiatrist observes behaviour and judges it against a social—often local —norm. This is not necessarily inappropriate. Psychiatric illnesses, particularly those characterized by psychosis, often affect persons in ways that lead them to ignore social norms and transgress generally accepted verbal and behavioural boundaries; and such trespasses may, in fact, be the most sensitive and early indicators of possible illness. To be sure, the social basis of diagnosis is itself a problem, since the psychiatrist must know precisely where the social boundaries should be drawn, and which trespasses are the result not of illness but of some other cause—such as, for example, social activism, artistic style, mere eccentricity or, for that matter, a rearing in another culture. But psychiatrists are, in the main, at least dimly aware of these problems, having been apprised of them during training or, failing that, in the course of ongoing practice.

Another basis for diagnostic judgement—one that shapes the diagnostic vision of the psychiatrist no less powerfully than the social one, but is, nevertheless, generally unrecognized—is the diagnostic theory itself. In most countries psychiatrists are guided by one or more theories of mental illness; and often those theories are associated with diagnostic systems that are their functional and practical expressions. And, depending on the specificity of the system to which he or she subscribes, the ways in which a psychiatrist assesses a person's behaviour, draws conclusions about it, weighs the variance between the person and the social norm—indeed, *sees* the person—may be heavily influenced by the assumptions underlying the system and the approach that system takes to recognizing and identifying mental illness. The system, after all, delineates categories of illness and identifies the criteria by which behaviours and the persons who exhibit them deserve to be placed in those categories; and every time such a placement is made the categories, as well as the system itself, are reified. To the psychiatrist who accepts the system as real, this occasions no concern: the reality of the system has merely found a correspondence in the reality of the patient's illness. To one who finds the categories mistaken, however, or the criteria too narrowly or too broadly defined, such reification may be simply self-deceptive and false, and may result in misdiagnoses that are as systematic as only a system can make them.

In many countries this danger, though important, has been limited in recent years. In the United States, for example, the most recent editions of the official diagnostic manual have shifted to a descriptive, atheoretical approach to the diagnosis of mental illnesses, the aetiologies of most of which have not been established using commonly accepted scientific methods. In the main, the American Psychiatric Association's *Diagnostic and statistical manual* (DSM) defines mental illnesses by describing their clinical features, which are generally easily identifiable behavioural signs or symptoms. Moreover, these manuals have classified those mental illnesses not according to aetiologies they are presumed (but have not necessarily been proved) to share, but rather according to the clinical features they share. In addition, they have listed specific diagnostic criteria for making diagnoses, the use of which increases diagnostic reliability. As a result of all this, clinicians have been more successful than in the past in agreeing on the diagnoses of mental illnesses characterized by features that are easily described and recognized, such as the psychoses; in the cases of other disorders, particularly the personality disorders, the criteria for which are more unclear, there has been less consensual reliability.

In other countries the World Health Organization's *International classification of diseases* (ICD) has been widely used. The ICD provides less detail in its descriptions of mental illnesses than does the *Diagnostic and statistical manual*; but it, too, provides a basis for relatively good reliability in diagnosis, particularly in the diagnosis of the major mental disorders.

In the former Soviet Union, however, a diagnostic system was put in place in the 1960s through the 1980s that, though in many ways highly descriptive, was, unlike the *Diagnostic and statistical manual*, not based on research that meets commonly accepted scientific standards. In its definitions of the schizophrenic disorders this system employed such broad and loose criteria that it permitted the diagnosis of schizophrenia in cases in which, in the West, there would be no finding of any mental illness. As a result, Soviet psychiatrists who used this diagnostic system systematically tended to diagnose as ill—and, often, genuinely to *see* as ill—persons who would not be diagnosed as ill anywhere else.

This Soviet diagnostic system was developed during the 1960s by Andrei V. Snezhnevsky, the founder of what came to be called the Moscow School of Psychiatry and, until his death in 1987, the head of the Institute of Psychiatry of the USSR Academy of Medical Sciences (renamed in 1983 the All-Union Centre for Psychiatry and Mental Health), the central psychiatric research institution in that country. During the 1940s and 1950s Snezhnevsky worked at, and then became chairman of, the Department of Psychiatry of the Central Postgraduate Medical Institute, probably the most prestigious institute in the Soviet Union for advanced training and degrees. Upon his ascension to the directorship of the Institute of Psychiatry in 1962 Snezhnevsky dedicated the institute and its resources to the problem of schizophrenia, which was the focus of his central theory and of his diagnostic approach. Over the next decade, he and his staff continued to refine the system, doing clinical research designed to elaborate its details. By the early 1970s many of his former students and trainees were in charge of the nation's academic psychiatric centres; the journal he edited, the *Korsakov Journal of Neuropathology and Psychiatry*, was the only psychiatric periodical in the USSR and regularly carried news of his school's research and of the fine points of its diagnostic system. The pattern of psychiatric teaching and research in centres far from Moscow felt the effect of his guidance and views, exerted through his role as an influential member of review committees for government ministries responsible for the approval of research and training grants. By the middle and late 1970s the hegemony of the Moscow School in the realm of psychiatric theory and practice, particularly diagnostic theory and practice, was almost complete: it was clearly the dominant force in Soviet psychiatry, and its diagnostic system was the standard Soviet approach to the diagnosis of mental illness. This dominance continued for some time even after Snezhnevsky's death, despite criticisms of Soviet psychiatry in general and Soviet diagnostic methods in particular.[50–53]

Following the collapse of the Soviet Union the Moscow School ceased being an institutional force, though its teachings continued to influence the persons who had been trained by it. Nevertheless, its experience is very telling. The Moscow School's diagnostic system focused particularly on schizophrenia; but because its definition of schizophrenia was so extraordinarily broad, that definition took in vast sectors of non-schizophrenic psychopathology—sectors that, grouped together, encompass much of the territory of mental illness. The theory behind the system was based on the assumption that schizophrenia has three different forms; that these forms vary from each other not so much in their symptoms, as traditionally has been assumed in the West since Kraepelin, but in their course; and that a particular schizophrenic patient's course-form may be identified on the basis of a retrospective analysis of the development of his or her illness.[54–57]

A schematic rendering of the characteristics distinguishing the three course-forms of schizophrenia is presented in Fig. 10.1.

1. The 'continuous form' is characterized by the development of symptoms early in life, usually by late adolescence or early adulthood, with a general worsening as life progresses. Patients falling into this category do not, as a rule, improve.

2. The 'periodic form' is characterized by periods of acute illness, interspersed with periods of remission during which the patient regains health.

3. The 'shift-like form' is a mixture of the other two. As in the periodic form there are acute attacks; however, each attack leaves the patient more ill than he or she was prior to that attack, so that, overall, as in the continuous form, there is a general worsening of the illness during the course of the patient's life.

What is so unique—and, in the end, so problematic—about this system is the fact that *two of the course-forms have subtypes ranging from mild to severe, and that in those two, the continuous and the shift-like, the mild subtypes are characterized by symptoms that are not psychotic.* In almost all countries psychiatrists would probably agree that persons who satisfy the Moscow School's criteria for the moderate and severe subtypes of each of these course-forms really are, by their criteria as well, schizophrenic. But they would probably disagree about the Moscow School's criteria for the mild subtypes, and would judge the persons who satisfy them to be neurotic, rather than schizophrenic, suffering from a personality disorder, or even mentally well. Fig. 10.1 notes the characteristics attributed by the Moscow School to persons grouped according to these subtypes.

The other feature of the system that adds to its potential danger—indeed, multiplies it—is the Moscow School's assumption that *each of the course-forms represents, in essence, a separate illness, one that has its own biological basis, which is, in turn, genetically determined.* This implies that a person categorized

	Course forms						
	Continuous			Periodic	Shift-like		
Life course of the illness							
Subtypes	Sluggish (mild)	Paranoid (moderate)	Malignant (severe)		Mild	Moderate	Severe
Some characteristics	Neuroticism; self-consciousness; introspectiveness; obsessive doubts; conflicts with parental and other authorities; 'reformism'	Paranoid; delusions; hallucinations; 'parasitic life-style'	Early onset; unremitting; overwhelming	Acute attacks; fluctuations in mood; confusion	Neurotic, with affective colouring; social contentiousness; philosophical concerns; self-absorption	Acute paranoid	Catatonia; delusions; prominent mood-changes

Fig. 10.1   Features of the Snezhnevsky course-forms

as belonging in, say, the sluggish (mild) subtype of the continuous form has the same illness as anyone else in that form, including someone belonging in the malignant (severe) subtype; and, though he or she has a more mildly expressed version of that illness, he or she has it nevertheless—and for life. Such a person may therefore be subject to many of the disadvantages, social and personal, as the person who is much more severely ill.

What is so troubling about this is that the criteria given for the mild subtypes of schizophrenia apply to many persons who clearly would be seen by most psychiatrists in the West as not schizophrenic. In fact, it could be predicted that, applied to a broad population, this system would draw into the schizophrenic fold precisely such persons—persons, that is, with neuroses, personality disorders, affective illnesses, or no mental illnesses at all. There is evidence that this has indeed occurred. Some of the evidence is impressionistic. Rollins, for example, reported in her book on child psychiatry in the Soviet Union that patients with primarily neurotic or psychopathic-like symptoms were typically given diagnoses by Soviet psychiatrists in the schizophrenic range.[58] More directly, Holland reported, after a sojourn in Moscow's Institute of Psychiatry, that Soviet patients could be diagnosed as schizophrenic even if they exhibited no signs of the illness, and that once the diagnosis was given, even if it were further subtyped as being of the mild variety, it continued to be used on the assumption that the patient had a lifelong, genetically based condition.[59–62]

But the most telling evidence came from the International Pilot Study of Schizophrenia (IPSS). During the late 1960s and early 1970s nine centres around the world, including centres located in Washington, DC, and Moscow, evaluated patients for schizophrenia and collected data about them. The centre in Moscow was Snezhnevsky's Institute of Psychiatry. As part of the study, a computer was programmed by John K. Wing to re-diagnose the patients originally diagnosed as schizophrenic using data regarding the patients' symptoms that were gathered by the various centres; the computer used strict criteria for its own re-diagnoses, notably those formulated by Kurt Schneider.[63] While most centres did 'well'—that is, while the computer 'agreed' with most of the diagnoses of schizophrenia rendered at those centres—two centres did poorly.

One of these, Washington DC, did poorly primarily because its diagnosticians followed the rules of their own diagnostic system, and, unlike the computer, tended not to differentiate between schizophrenia, schizophrenia-like psychoses, and paranoid psychoses. The computer gave them low marks because it found their schizophrenic patients to be, by its criteria, psychotic in other ways, though agreement as to psychosis was high. The other centre that did poorly was Moscow's Institute of Psychiatry; however, the reasons were different. A larger percentage of its diagnosed schizophrenics were reassigned by the computer not to the psychotic, but rather to the depressive and neurotic categories. Table 10.1 shows the computer classification (i.e. re-diagnosis) of

Table 10.1 IPSS computer classifications of schizophrenia subtype diagnoses

IPSS Centre	Schizophrenia subtype diagnoses	No. of patients	Computer classifications (%)				
			Schizophrenic similar psychoses	Paranoid psychoses	Manic psychoses	Depressive psychoses	Depressive neuroses
Washington	Simple Latent	4 2	50	33	17	0	0
Moscow	Sluggish	12	0	0	33	8	58
7 remaining centres	Simple Latent	27 8	71	9	6	0	14

patients who were originally diagnosed at the nine centres as belonging to those subtypes most likely to contain patients who would be considered by psychiatrists in many countries to be 'borderline schizophrenic', or merely 'borderline'. For eight of the centres these subtypes were identified as 'simple' and 'latent,' for Moscow, it was 'sluggish' (the mild subtype of the Moscow School's continuous form). Although the numbers are small the difference seems striking. The patients classified as belonging in these subtypes in eight of the centres, including Washington DC but not Moscow, were classified by the computer as overwhelmingly schizophrenic or as having paranoid or schizophrenia-like psychoses, while the patients classified in the mild subtype by the Moscow diagnosticians, following the rules of the Moscow School, were classified by the computer as being primarily affectively ill or depressed, just as one might have predicted from an inspection of the system's broad diagnostic criteria.[64]

A final confirmation of the tendency of the Moscow School's diagnostic system to overdiagnose schizophrenia came from a Soviet psychiatrist, one working at Moscow's Serbsky Institute of Forensic Psychiatry. In an unprecedented article in a Western psychiatric journal, E. P. Kazanetz used his own computer exercise to show that the Moscow School's system tended to overdiagnose as endogenous schizophrenics persons who were only exogenously ill—that is, it tended to diagnose, as chronically ill, persons whose illnesses were primarily of an acute, externally caused type. Furthermore, Kazanetz added the observation that such overdiagnosis could be harmful to persons with acute illnesses assigned irrevocably to psychiatric registers of the chronically ill. Together with the evidence from the IPSS, Kazanetz's study reveals the degree to which an overbroad diagnostic scheme can result in overbroad diagnostic practice.[65]

What is so extraordinary, and so ethically significant, about the Soviet experience is that patients who were misdiagnosed in the IPSS and in the population studied by Kazanetz were misdiagnosed—that is, diagnosed as schizophrenic despite the fact that almost all other psychiatrists would diagnose them as belonging in less severe categories of mental illness—*only because of the dictates of the diagnostic system that was then officially in place.* Those Soviet psychiatrists really *saw* the patients as schizophrenic; or, to put it another way, *the system created a category, first on paper and then, through training, in the minds of Soviet psychiatrists, which was eventually assumed to represent a real class of patients and which was inevitably filled by real persons.* Those diagnosticians came to see schizophrenic pathology as including very mild forms and diagnosed accordingly. Persons who should not have received those diagnoses did, to their detriment; and psychiatrists who should not have given them did, in apparent full faith. Had those psychiatrists been sensitive to the capacity of diagnostic systems to shape the way psychiatrists understand, categorize, and perceive psychopathology, they might have been able, one hopes, to avert this result.

It would be valuable to examine briefly, in this context, the role played by the Moscow School of Psychiatry's diagnostic system in the diagnosis of Soviet dissidents during the quarter-century before the collapse of the Soviet Union. The purposeful misdiagnosis of Soviet dissidents will be noted at the end of this essay. A number of dissidents, however, were probably not misdiagnosed purposefully. Rather, they were probably misdiagnosed because their behaviour was socially odd, a kind of oddness for which there is a diagnostic niche in the Moscow School's broad definitions of schizophrenia. For, as it happens, many of the ways in which Soviet dissidents behaved, often in response to the governmental pressures brought to bear on them, were precisely the same, almost uncannily so, as the behaviours and characteristics said by the Moscow School to be common among mild schizophrenics, sluggish or otherwise. Table 10.2 contains a list of characteristics that were cited by Soviet psychiatrists in the case histories of certain dissidents in order to buttress their findings that those dissidents were ill. To be sure, those characteristics are typical of the ones that were often cited as signs of illness by the Moscow School's theoreticians. But they are also very typical of dissidents, particularly those who had to live the kinds of lives lived by dissidents in the Soviet Union. For example: fear, suspiciousness, and depression (hardly unexpected feelings among persons being hounded by the state); poor adaptation to the social environment (something without which you wouldn't *be* a dissident); and 'reformism' (which is another way of describing the tendency to dissent, at least before the advent of *perestroika*).

Table 10.2   Vulnerable styles

Overlap of common dissident styles and schizophrenic symptoms as described by the Moscow School of Psychiatry

- Originality
- Ideological formulations
- Fear and suspiciousness
- Religiosity
- Depression
- Ambivalence, guilt, internal conflicts, and behavioural disorganization
- Intensity
- Attention to detail
- Poor adaptation to the social environment
- Shift of interests
- Reformism

The result of all this was devastating for dissidents during the quarter-century before the end of the Soviet Union. Dissidents were, of course, routinely arrested. Some of them were then sent by the KGB, quite cynically, to psychiatrists, even though the KGB had no reason to think they were ill. These psychiatrists, learning of the KGB's wish that the dissidents be found mentally ill, did indeed find them ill, often giving them as a diagnosis one of the categories of mild schizophrenia. The dissidents' trials could then be held without them, they could be sent for indeterminate amounts of time to hospitals for the criminally insane, and their views could be depicted as the sick products of sick minds. Such unethical behaviour by psychiatrists will be discussed later in this chapter.

But in other cases another process sometimes also occurred—a process involving different motivations but ending with the same results. In those instances the KGB, encountering dissidents, saw before them persons who were, in a few striking ways, very different from nearly everyone else in Soviet society: in the name of goals (e.g. democratization or freedom of speech) that were, by all rational standards of the time, hopelessly elusive, they were willing to court inevitable and overwhelming punishment. Moreover, they were extra-ordinarily committed to those goals, and sometimes even chastised their inter-rogating officials for transgressing the Soviet constitution. Those investigators, struck by the apparent inability of these dissidents to appreciate reality, sometimes interpreted their behaviours as odd and a sign that something might not be quite right with them—that they were, perhaps, mentally ill. They then asked psychiatrists to examine these dissidents. But the psychiatrists were themselves the products of the same societies as the officials, were also struck by the same self-endangering and, by ordinary Soviet standards, apparently irrational behaviour, and were left with the same doubts about the dissidents' mental health. They knew, however, that it was precisely such behaviours that were said to be characteristic of the mild schizophrenias described by the Moscow School. And, resolving their doubts, they issued that diagnosis, thereby beginning the process that resulted in court-ordered hospitalizations on the grounds that, having committed socially dangerous crimes as a result of mental illness, they must be socially dangerous and, therefore, separated from society.

That this latter path to hospitalization actually took place appears to have been supported by the findings of delegation of American psychiatrists who visited the Soviet Union in 1989.[69] In that visit about half the Soviet patients who were re-diagnosed by the American psychiatrists were found not to be mentally ill by Western standards. Of these, a number had been hospitalized in 1987 or later and others, who had been hospitalized earlier, remained in hospital in 1987 and 1988—during the period, that is, after Gorbachev's 'new thinking' on human rights had hit its stride. One could reasonably assume that during those two years the KGB and the psychiatrists who had so willingly served them would have been expected *not* to purposefully hospitalize dissidents they knew to be mentally well; after all, each such hospitalization could have seriously undermined the effort of the Soviet Union to improve its human-rights image abroad, an effort that was necessary if the Soviets were to achieve a number of their goals in the international arena. That psychiatrists nevertheless diagnosed such people as ill suggests, to this writer at least, the likelihood (at least some cases) that they really thought the dissidents were ill. To be sure, some of these cases could also have been, and probably were, a result of the persistence of cynical habits among officials and psychiatrists who just couldn't change their ways; but the other explanation seems at least as compelling (and, to me, more so).[67–70]

Although the consequences of an unusually broad and vulnerable psychiatric diagnostic system have been particularly painful and destructive in the Soviet context, that context should not be considered the only one in which such damage could be wreaked. The Soviet diagnostic scheme represents an extreme spectrum system—a system that posits a spectrum of schizophrenic illness ranging in severity from the most mild to the most severe, and caused by a genetic deficit of variable clinical expression. Such diagnostic schemes have, in fact, been considered in some form in the West.[71–81] To be sure, they have not been introduced into formal diagnostic systems; however, given the Soviet experience, it would be valuable to weigh the potential of such systems for similar overdiagnoses.

The beauty of diagnosis as a solution to human problems

A third source of non-purposeful psychiatric misdiagnoses, and probably the most significant, is the attractiveness of the diagnostic process as a means of solving or avoiding complex human problems. With remarkable ease diagnoses can turn the fright of chaos into the comfort of the known; the burden of doubt into the pleasure of certainty; the shame of hurting others into the pride of helping them; and the dilemma of moral judgement into the clarity of medical truth. Because of their nature, functions, and meanings, diagnoses can do such things in efficient and powerful ways; and the fact that they can makes their use by psychiatrists for such ends remarkably irresistible, enormously unrecognizable, and, in the final analysis, utterly human.[82]

Diagnosis as explanation, mitigation, and exculpation

Perhaps the most fetching beauty of diagnosis is its capacity to instantly explain: behaviour that is odd, objectionable, troublesome, or illegal, can be through the mediation of diagnosis, suddenly be understood, explained, and explained away. To be sure, such behaviour may indeed be the product of diagnosable mental illness. But the capacity of a diagnosis to perform this function makes its use a temptation even in cases in which such illness does not exist or, at best, is only marginally present.

The arena in which this diagnostic temptation has been most evident has been the law. For years psychiatrists have been asked to testify as witnesses in cases of persons accused of various crimes. Often the prosecution and defence have called upon such witnesses who, in turn, have presented conflicting testimony about whether or not the actions carried out by the accused were a product of mental illness. While such conflicts have occasionally embarrassed the profession by suggesting that either side in a case can get psychiatric testimony in support of any diagnosis it wishes, at least they have been straightforward. Generally, the clinical questions have had to do with the presence or absence of some kind of psychosis, a group of mental conditions that can render a defendant legally not responsible for his or her actions; and the testimony has usually involved judgements about whether or not the defendant's behaviour and history met certain widely-accepted criteria for these, the most agreed-upon areas of psychopathology.

Naturally, defendants and defence counsels have often sought findings of 'not guilty by reason of insanity', even when they have suspected or known insanity not to have played a role, because of their belief that, at least in cases of such serious crimes as murder or rape, confinement in a hospital may be shorter than the sentence that would be likely to be imposed should the defendant be found guilty and not insane. Still, some persons *do* commit crimes because they are insane: the law recognizes that insanity compromises free will, and classifies someone without free will as legally not responsible for his or her actions; it is the right of defendants to use that defense; and psychiatrists have a role, as a result of their expertise in recognizing such mental illness, in testifying on the substance of that defence.

The trouble is that attempts have been made to expand that role into realms in which psychiatrists do not have expertise. The pressure for that expansion has been the wish to explain diagnostically—and explain away legally—criminal behaviours that do not involve classical psychotic states. Instead of insanity the clinical questions have involved issues about which psychiatry has almost no validated knowledge: questions primarily of coercion, persuasion, and influence. In a series of cases defence lawyers have turned to psychiatrists to testify about the effects of certain environmental pressures on individual development and judgement, and on the role these factors played in the genesis of the criminal behaviour. The defence argument has usually been that these factors created a diagnosable mental condition, one that explained the behaviour and, in a legal sense, either mitigated or totally exculpated it.

A well-known case of this sort is the 1976 bank-robbery trial of Patricia Hearst, in which the defendant was said to have been incapable of criminal intent because she had undergone a process of 'coercive persuasion', a process that had affected her capacity for free will. Not only the defense, but also many observers, favoured such a diagnostic exculpation: it made it possible to understand how such an ordinary, peaceful, apolitical, and utterly American young woman could have turned so suddenly into such an extraordinary, violent, ideological, and anti-American revolutionary. The court allowed the novel defence—novel because it stepped beyond the traditional realm of insanity into the broader arena of persuasion—and a battery of psychiatrists supported it with their testimony. The jury, however, rejected it, despite its attractive advantages: it did not accept diagnostic explanation as a basis for legal exculpation.[83,84]

The attractiveness of the diagnostic process as a means of explanation and exculpation has revealed itself in the legal arena a number of times since the Hearst trial. In each instance the defence contended that environmental factors had influenced or determined the criminal act; and, in each instance, psychiatrists took the stand to issue their supporting diagnostic opinions. In a celebrated Florida case, a young boy who was accused of having killed an old woman was defended with the explanation that his mind had been affected by television violence. As in the Hearst trial, the jury found such use of diagnosis inadequate to the task of explaining away the defendant's behaviour.

Despite these setbacks it seems likely that the beauty of diagnosis will continue to be appreciated in the legal arena, and that psychiatrists will continue to expand the ambit of their diagnostic expertise into realms about which almost nothing certain is known. It seems possible that in time psychiatric testimony will offer itself in support of psychological defences of all kinds—defences, for example, that attribute criminal actions to the defendant's early childhood rearing or to the pressures of his or her adolescent peers. While such influences undoubtedly exist, almost nothing is known about how they affect the capacity for individual judgement and the existence of free will. That some psychiatrists are willing to testify on these matters in the belief that they have such knowledge demonstrates not only the settled habit of such psychiatrists to opine on issues beyond their scientific domain, but also, it seems, the satisfaction gained from finding in the storehouse of the profession some explanation that will transform a person's criminal act into a symptomatic one, and that will turn a painful moral question into a painless medical one.

Nor should the turn to diagnosis in such cases on the part of psychiatrists occasion any wonder. It is a natural turn when an explanation for unwanted behaviour is needed, and is accomplished every day, outside the arena of the law, by non-psychiatric laymen as well. For example, journalists and other observers turn to it for simplifying explanations when political figures engage in behaviour that is inexplicable in ordinary political terms.[85-89] Still others call upon diagnostic explanations to justify forgiveness or elicit sympathy in situations ranging from breaches of airline etiquette[90] to more serious transgressions of industrial ethics[91] and literary propriety.[92] That psychiatrists similarly turn to diagnoses in the search for satisfying explanatory simplification, ones that substitute medicine for morals, is therefore not surprising; the satisfactions and advantages are the same, except that in the hands of the psychiatrists diagnoses achieve official status and recognition, and result in lasting effects which are not always, even in these cases, salutary.

Diagnosis as reassurance

A second beauty of diagnosis is its power to reassure. When acts are committed whose implications are disturbing—acts that suggest vulnerabilities in ourselves, our institutions, or our communal beliefs—diagnoses often come to mind, both in the layman and psychiatrist, which serve to shift the frame of the behaviour from the threatening personal or social arena to a safer medical one.

In one widely publicized case this shift was effected toward its reassuring end through the cooperation of all concerned, psychiatrist and laymen alike. In 1974, Dr William T. Summerlin, a young researcher hired by the Memorial Sloan-Kettering Cancer Center on the basis of his promising work in transplantation immunology, reported that he had been successful in grafting skin from genetically unrelated animals. When other researchers were unable to confirm these astonishing results Summerlin, in response, repeated his experiments, reportedly inking in the skins of his mice to make it appear as if the grafts had taken. When this was revealed by Summerlin's research assistant, a special in-house committee was constituted to investigate the matter. The major threat posed by the Summerlin affair was the possibility that the American public might conclude that not only that researcher, but research itself, was suspect. To a community that depended on the magnificent largess of its various constituents and supporters—a largess that from US government sources alone approached more than two billion dollars a year at the time (and is about six times that figure now)—such a prospect was indeed distressing. Moreover, there were other concerns. Summerlin's story, after all, did violence to the new American dream: he was a young man from the country's heartland who had been embraced by the Eastern scientific establishment only to prove himself, if the allegations were true, shamefully unreliable. What of that dream? And, besides, what was to become of young Summerlin himself?

The solution to all these distressing concerns was quick in coming. First, the investigating committee issued its findings: Summerlin's 'unusual behavior involved at least a measure of self-deception, or some other aberration, which hindered him from adequately gauging the impact and eventual results of his conduct'.[93] Then, at a press conference, the cancer centre's president, Dr Lewis Thomas, a researcher and physician himself, went on to elaborate. 'The fraud in this work,' Dr Thomas informed the assembled reporters, was 'a result of mental illness'.[94]

In one stroke, all concerns were eased. Summerlin's actions were the result not of a vulnerability in research, nor of the habits of researchers, but, rather, of a fault in the man. Moreover, that fault was not moral, but, rather, medical. And, besides that, it was short-lived. At his own news conference, four days later, Summerlin volunteered that he had been suffering from an acute depression, a condition that accounted for his 'irrational act', and for which he had already begun psychiatric treatment. The psychiatrist, Summerlin explained, had prescribed rest and physical exercise, and he was already feeling much better. And so, indeed, did those who had been so distressed by the implications of Summerlin's act: the diagnosis preserved not only the good name of science, and not only the integrity of the scientific community, but also Summerlin, who could now be seen in more reassuring terms, not as a person who would be forever morally tainted, but rather as one whose treatment would leave him clean, whole, and good, and ready to resume his professional life.

Whether Summerlin's behaviour was or was not, in fact, the result of an acute depression cannot, of course, be confirmed here; but the case is important because it illustrates the ease with which a turn to diagnosis can, at the same time, allay multiple concerns. When a psychiatrist is faced by such a case, when a means—the diagnostic process—is available that can accomplish so much, and when others are themselves inclined to think that mental illness can or should be used to explain the behaviour, it is hard to imagine that the psychiatrist will not look seriously at that option, and even find himself or herself considering it with greater favour than ordinarily he or she might in other cases involving similar behaviours—even when those cases pose no threat or raise no concerns.

Diagnosis as the humane transformation of social deviance into medical illness

Another beauty of diagnosis is its power to reclassify whole categories of socially unacceptable behaviour as the products of psychiatrically diagnosable conditions. This kind of reclassification derives, in essence, from a liberal utopian impulse: people are naturally good, and if someone acts to the detriment of society he must be ill. Hence, the social response should aim not at punishment, and not merely at control, but rather at treatment. If this approach is taken, presumably everyone benefits: the deviant, the 'root causes' of whose transgressions are thereby recognized and cured; society and its authorities, which are no longer in the position of exacting harsh punishments; and psychiatrists, whose redefinitions make all this possible, and who can feel themselves in the noble position of healing where others would have only hurt.

Probably the most striking examples of such reclassification may be found in connection with sexual behaviours that have traditionally been classified as socially undesirable. As a result of developments in medical technology, as well as shifts in popular views, some of these behaviours have been reclassified in psychiatric—and, therefore, diagnostic—terms. One such development, the synthesis of drugs that reduce sexual drive, has resulted in calls for their use in cases involving sexual offenders. Some years ago, for example, one drug company advertised in the *British Journal of Psychiatry* that its product 'had proven to be of value in treating men who have been guilty of sexual offences such as exhibitionism; paedophilia; indecent assault; rape; incest; voyeurism; bestiality and paederasty'. In addition, the company pointed out that other types of 'aberrant' sexual behaviours, even those not considered illegal, may also be 'controlled', including 'homosexual activities; fetishism; transvestism; compulsive masturbation; and sexual aggression in senile or mentally defective hospital patients'. In the United States, prisoners serving jail sentences for rape have gone to court demanding that they be treated with similar agents.[95] Other technological developments, those of a surgical type, have made still other 'treatment' options available, with individuals and their doctors rushing in to re-classify the aberrancy or malady in medical terms that have been tailored to fit the new treatments—and the increasing demands.

The danger here is that despite their humanitarian goal, it is not at all clear that such re-classifications serve that end. Attributing to an exhibitionist, or rapist, or a voyeur an underlying diagnosable psychiatric condition—hyper-sexualism—and then treating that condition by pharmacological or surgical means is not necessarily humane—and, in fact, has not yet been proved to work. Indeed, the surgical approach to transsexualism, a darling of 1960s medical technology, has been shown to be seriously questionable.[96] Certainly it is not at all clear that such redefinitions have improved the lots of the persons redefined.

Analogous attempts at reclassification have also occurred in other areas of psychiatry, with equally questionable results for both the professionals and their newly classified patients. Young offenders, for example, have been told by courts and other authorities that they would not be punished for their drug-taking or other social trespasses if they submitted to psychiatric treatment; and psychiatrists and psychiatric hospitals sometimes have acquiesced in this process by making their practices, facilities, and diagnoses available to this population, usually in good faith and full belief. Instead of being recorded as criminals such persons have been hospitalized as sociopaths or, sometimes, as persons with borderline personality disorders, or even one or another form of schizophrenia—with the result that they have been labelled and treated as such, with inadvertently worse effects for the individuals than would have resulted from their original designations as deviants or criminals.

Diagnosis as exclusion and dehumanization

So far we have examined the beauty of diagnosis as a means of accomplishing ends that in some sense reflect the universal wish to be or do good. From time to time we all have an urge to exculpate, to reassure, and to turn deviance into illness; diagnosis does these things, does them magically and utterly; and, in turning to it, whether as laymen or as psychiatrists, we have what we think are the diagnosee's interests at heart. However, the diagnostic process has a beauty that leads us well beyond the realm of generous human interest. We also use it because it helps us do things we otherwise could not bring ourselves to do.

The roots of this tendency are primitive, powerful, and universal. When we want to do unto others as we would not have them do unto ourselves, we find some way of turning them into others. We usually do that by labelling them, by excluding them from our own group, and by dehumanizing them—by defining their status as less than ours and, therefore, less human. Stalin knew that, and did it on a national scale when he wanted to turn popular opinion against those who disagreed with him. Khrushchev, in his 1956 Twentieth Party Congress speech, described the process well. Stalin, he said:

originated the concept of 'enemy of the people'. This term automatically rendered it unnecessary that the ideological errors of man or men engaged in a controversy be proven; this term made possible the usage of the most cruel repression, violating all norms of revolutionary legality, against anyone who in any way disagreed with Stalin...[97]

Stalin understood that a person labelled 'an enemy of the people' would be seen by a wary and besieged population as a dangerous outsider who must be excluded from Soviet society. So seen, the outsider would be suddenly transformed into someone who is different, not truly a member of society, not truly a man—and, therefore, into someone who could and should be imprisoned, shot, or otherwise silenced without the sympathy that ordinarily would be accorded a non-labelled fellow comrade. In her remarkable memoir of her life with Osip Mandelstam, *Hope against hope*, Nadezhda Mandelstam, the poet's widow, located the origin of the Soviet tendency to distinguish between 'one of us' and 'not one of us' (the second group commonly being known as 'alien elements') in Lenin himself. Lenin, she points out, established that distinction during the Civil War with his 'Who whom', the phrase he used to summarize the difference between the Bolsheviks and their enemies.[98] In the same memoir she also showed how widespread was the tendency under Stalin, even among the intelligentsia, to exclude and dehumanize those officially cast out. Thus, when an acquaintance was arrested on unknown and usually arbitrary charges, people would tell each other—probably to reassure themselves that they would not be next—that 'he isn't one of us'. It was, for many, necessary 'to avoid those stricken by the plague'.[99]

Even more graphic examples of the dehumanizing power of labelling, and the universal tendency to use it, can be drawn from the context of war. In the First World War both sides had ways of turning each other into objects whose deaths would be less than tragic, somehow almost deserved. In the Second World War the Nazis pushed this strategem to the limits, using labelling to transform various groups, especially Jews, into 'vermin' whose extermination would be a blessing.

Diagnosis is perfectly suited to label, exclude, and dehumanize in both its informal and formal usages. Informally, the terms 'crazy', 'mad', and even 'schizophrenic' often serve as exclusionary labels that are used in everyday language to identify others who are annoying, discomfiting, and different.

Formally applied—that is, by psychiatrists—diagnoses can make a person into someone who seems wholly other, and who *requires* exclusion. Depending on the severity of the diagnosis, he or she may be seen as disordered, polluted, and dangerous. In short, a diagnosis can turn him or her into another kind of human being, perhaps less than human, certainly not a fellow human being; and he or she not only has a need to be put away—he or she *needs* to be put away. Such diagnostic transformations can serve the needs of psychiatric systems under certain conditions in exactly the same way that it can serve the needs of family and social systems when their peace and tranquillity are disturbed by the symptoms of the mentally ill.

Psychiatric systems can benefit from the process of diagnostic exclusion and dehumanization, because those systems subject individuals to experiences and conditions that would be difficult to impose without the advantage that such diagnostic transformation affords. Psychiatric hospitals, especially of the public variety, may be unpleasant places; and some psychiatric techniques, such as the use of drugs, electric shock, restraints, and confinement to seclusion rooms, may be experienced by patients as highly noxious. Psychiatrists know that in hospitalizing patients they may be, in the service of treatment, also causing them a certain degree of harm. The awareness of possible harm is compounded if the patient is an involuntary one, if the most invasive or liberty-depriving techniques are used, and if the patient responds to those conditions and techniques with the insistence that he is not sick and with a plea that they should be altered or stopped and that he should be released. At such times the psychiatrists must harden their hearts. And what facilitates this process is, among other things, the diagnosis. With it, the psychiatrist can see the person as a patient, one whose pleas are not simple, soulful, human importunings, but rather the routine and expected reactions of ill patients to the illnesses that have possessed them and to the treatments to which they have been subjected. With such a diagnosis, psychiatrists can proceed, and not have to see themselves as violators of human freedom and dignity. In fact, they can see themselves as helping, through the hospitalization and the use of such interventions, to transform a psychiatric case back into a human being, back into someone like themselves: they can, in good conscience, allow themselves to do unto the patient that which they would not have others do unto them.

The advantage to the psychiatrist of diagnostic dehumanization is only a special instance of that disadvantage in everyday life. After all, psychiatric patients carry on the largest portions of their lives outside the psychiatric system, and place non-psychiatrists in similar, even more vexing dilemmas. The behaviours of such patients may be extremely distressing to friends, neighbours, and relatives, who, in turn, seek help for themselves by persuading the individual to consult mental health authorities, by coercing him to do so in some way, or by enlisting others, such as the police, to carry out such coercion. Sometimes, having been successful, these friends, neighbours, or relatives may recognize that their wish to be rid of the individual, and their actions to accomplish that end, were in part in the service of their own comfort; and, realizing the unpleasantness that may result to the patient because of their actions, they may feel some shame. That shame, however, can be dissipated if they remind themselves that the person is, in fact, mentally ill, that his objectionable behaviours are caused not by him but by a disease, and that their purpose in bringing him to the attention of civil and mental health authorities was related not to their own needs but to the needs of a person temporarily beset by a disease. This disease, they may reassure themselves, has obscured his usual humanity, and makes it necessary to carry out acts that, in the cases of healthy people, would constitute transgressions of their civil liberties, but that, in his case, represent only kindness, concern, and the desire to restore him to the normal community of man.

Of course, people do become psychotic, and do, in their psychoses, sometimes require interventions that we would not want inflicted upon ourselves. What is important here, though, is the capacity of diagnosis to enable persons who respect and even love such individuals to suspend their ordinary tendency to honour these individuals' stated wishes—to reverse, that is, the usual meaning of compassion, so that what the person wants is precisely the opposite of what he or she is given.

If diagnosis enables us to do that in such cases, then it has a great capacity to do it in other cases as well, ones that involve no respect or love. For example, in cases of marginal illness, when persons annoy others by their socially unacceptable behaviour, it may become too easy to enlist the aid of diagnosis in response. In that circumstance civil authorities can turn to the psychiatric system in the hope that it will aid them in removing the disturbance and in making them feel, through the issuance of a diagnosis, that they had been right in making that resort; and it may become too easy for those in the psychiatric system to acquiesce and issue a diagnosis—even when such a diagnosis may be somewhat doubtful, and even when the consequences may be unpleasant—on the basis of the self-deceptive rationale that a diagnosed person is not quite a person, and probably needs to undergo this kind of treatment, at least until it has its effect, exorcizes the disease, and brings him back to a fully human state.

Diagnosis as self-confirming hypothesis

Perhaps the most remarkable property of diagnosis, and sometimes the most enraging for the diagnosed patient, is its capacity for inevitable self-confirmation. That property is used in everyday life by persons who call others 'crazy' or 'weird': once they do so, everything that the receivers of such lay diagnoses do can be attributed to, and dismissed as a result of, those or similar psychopatholizing epithets. In fact, everything they do subsequently can become a proof that the original assessment was correct. This 'catch-22' quality of the pathological naming therefore functions with even greater efficiency and inevitability within psychiatry itself. An actual clinical case observed by this author illustrates this well.

Case 1
The chief psychiatrist at a medical-school teaching hospital was asked to see a 65-year-old woman by the woman's son, a medical-school faculty member, and by her husband, a physician in a nearby community. The woman, they explained, had become 'negative' at home, disagreeable, more insistent than she previously had been about her views, and, in other ways as well, had undergone changes of personality. The chief psychiatrist, who tended to interpret behaviour and its aberrations as direct products of brain-functioning or malfunctioning, concluded that, in the case of this woman, such a malfunctioning had taken place. He diagnosed an organic brain syndrome, one probably caused by the ageing process, and admitted her to the hospital to confirm the diagnosis. The resident psychiatrist assigned to the case, however, could find no objective evidence of such malfunctioning. Meanwhile, the patient—finding herself in the strange circumstances of a therapeutic community, in which staff and patients were expected to aid each other in recognizing illness and in promoting health—became extremely distressed. She repeatedly insisted, to all who would hear, and in every community or group meeting, that she was not ill and should not be a patient. The response she received was consistent: she would certainly not have been admitted to the hospital had she not been ill, and the only way for her to achieve health was to acknowledge her illness. At first she quietly tried to accept the ward routines in the hope that she would be discharged rapidly. When this failed she complained loudly, angrily, and at length. The senior medical and nursing staff, observing her behaviour, cited it to the resident psychiatrist as a 'catastrophic reaction', typical of persons with her diagnosis who are challenged by tasks they can no longer master. Given fluphenazine, she quieted; and the drug-induced response was then cited as an improvement that further demonstrated the validity of the original diagnosis.

Of course the diagnosis may indeed have been correct: the resident psychiatrist may have been wrong and the chief right. But, given the authority structure of the ward, and the nature and effects of diagnoses, particularly those issued in such settings, it became almost inevitable that the chief's clinical pronouncement would confirm itself no matter what occurred. In the absence of objective, physically based criteria, many psychiatric diagnoses are capable of such self-confirmation whether they derive from a psychoanalytic orientation or, as in this case, an organic one. Indeed, even in this case in which a psychiatric diagnosis was issued that is more susceptible to physical confirmation than most, the lack of such confirmation failed to derail the inevitable train of events. In such a climate it becomes simply too easy to diagnose: one is rarely proved wrong, and the penchant for rapid assessment, valued so highly in general medical settings (especially academic ones) as an emblem of knowledge and expertise, has few means of objective checks in the psychiatric arena, and can result in too cavalier an issuance of diagnoses—diagnoses that, because they may be wrong, and because they have so pronounced a tendency to persist, can be highly distressing and, ultimately, damaging. Of course, this dilemma is made still worse under circumstances in which the diagnoses are issued not in the spirit of academic showmanship, or as an expression of ideological bias, but, rather, as a result of hasty or uncaring judgements. But whatever the spirit, the results to the patient are the same.

Diagnosis as discreditation and punishment

One particularly destructive function of diagnosis evident in everyday life is its capacity to discredit by attributing a person's views, politics, actions, or conclusions to a mind gone sick: diagnosis as a weapon.

We see this everywhere. In the Middle East, for example, the Shah of Iran, before losing power, identified Libya's Colonel Qadaffi as a 'crazy fellow'.[100] In turn, Ahmed Zaki Yamani, then the Saudi oil minister, described the Shah as 'highly unstable mentally'.[101] Egypt's President Anwar Sadat diagnosed Iran's Ayatollah Ruhollah Khomeini 'a lunatic',[102] a compliment the ayatollah then passed on to President Carter.[103] In Israel, the Labour opposition had similar views about Prime Minister Begin,[104] while, on the West Bank, Ali Jabari, the Palestinian mayor of Hebron, campaigned to have the leaders of the PLO locked up in insane asylums.[105]

And elsewhere, at other times. Thus Lenin, in 1919, said of the poet Maxim Gorky: 'all of your impressions are totally sick ... your nerves have obviously broken down ... Just as your conversation, your letter is the sum total of sick impressions carrying you to sick conclusions. This is all a pure sick psyche ... It is clear that you have worked yourself up into sickness'[106] The Soviet press, in 1977, criticized the dissident physicist Andrei Sakharov for 'pathological individualism'.[107] A West German political leader described the Carter administration's reported plan to produce a neutron bomb: 'a symbol of mental perversion'.[108] And, after learning of his shift from black radical militant to capitalist religious conservative, Eldridge Cleaver's friends called him 'schizophrenic'.[109]

Within psychiatry diagnosis has also surfaced as a weapon. In 1964 American psychiatrists were polled, and diagnosed the presidential candidate, Barry Goldwater, with whose views many of them disagreed, as mentally ill. A decade earlier, members of the profession, supporting the Alger Hiss defence, diagnosed Hiss's accuser, Whittaker Chambers, as a psychopath without ever having examined him. And the CIA, understanding the power of diagnosis to discredit, made plans in 1954 to use it in its covert operations.[110] Its hopes were to administer LSD to those it wished to make mad—or, more to the point, to those it wished to be diagnosed by others as mad. Under the influence of the drug these enemies of the United States would seem psychotic, with the anticipated result that their own people, having come to that diagnostic conclusion, would reject or depose them.

But the most flagrant setting for the raw use of psychiatry to discredit—and, indeed, to intimidate and punish—has been the former Soviet Union. And it is here that the category of *non-purposeful* misdiagnoses that was defined earlier in this chapter, and to which most of the chapter has been devoted, begins to merge with, and seems at times indistinguishable from, the category of *purposeful* misdiagnoses.

During the last quarter-century of the former Soviet Union several hundred dissidents were arrested for political trespasses and, as noted earlier, sent to psychiatrists, found mentally ill, and committed for involuntary stays at psychiatric hospitals for the criminally insane.[111–120] Of these a number have been truly ill.[121] A number almost surely have not.[122] To the extent that they have not, and to the extent that the diagnoses in those cases were rendered at the direct or indirect request of governmental authorities, these actions represent the worst expression of *purposeful* misdiagnoses—that is, purposeful psychiatric abuse. In many cases, however, the misdiagnoses were probably issued in full or partial sincerity;[123–126] as noted earlier in this chapter, at least some of these misdiagnoses having been the result of the influence of the Moscow School's overbroad and overinclusive criteria for the diagnosis of schizophrenia that reigned in Soviet psychiatry during the period between the 1960s and the end of the Soviet era.

Whatever the motivations behind the particular misdiagnoses may have been—whether they were issued purposefully or non-purposefully, in full awareness of their inaccuracy or in non-awareness (or only partial awareness)—the very fact that psychiatrists were asked to examine the dissidents in the first place illustrates the beauty of diagnosis in all its array—not only as a means to discredit, and not only as a means to punish, but also as a means to dehumanize, to transform social deviance into medical illness, as well as a means to reassure and to explain.

Diagnosis as the reflection of social trends

One use of diagnosis that has been particularly problematic has involved the diagnosis of 'recovered' or 'repressed' memory. This diagnosis was made with particular frequency in the United States during the early 1990s by mental-health practitioners (especially psychologists and social workers, but also a number of psychiatrists) who attributed certain symptoms they believed persons had, or certain of their behaviours, to experiences that they were assumed to have had during their childhoods but could not remember because memories of those experiences had been 'repressed'. These experiences were generally assumed to have involved sexual abuse, often said to have been carried out by a parent. In some cases the abuses were believed to have involved bizarre, sometimes satanic, rituals. On occasion, as a result of these diagnoses, parents or others, such as persons in charge of schools, would be subjected to criminal charges and punishments.[127–132]

The great frequency of such diagnoses diminished rapidly after a number of celebrated cases resulted in lawsuits against therapists making such diagnoses. Some of them were found to be baseless when it became apparent that therapists, believing in the diagnosis, suggested it in various ways to patients who then 'produced' memories 'documenting' the diagnosis.[133] In reaction, the phenomenon produced an organization, the False Memory Syndrome Foundation, founded in significant measure by parents who had been accused of such abuse and supported by a number of prominent psychiatrists. A number of professional organizations, including the American Psychiatric Association and the American Psychological Association, issued statements warning against the possible dangers related to such diagnoses.[134] In addition, medical malpractice insurance companies provided guidelines to psychiatrists on how to minimize the likelihood of lawsuits related to such diagnoses.[135]

To some extent the growth of the tendency to expect—and to 'recover'—'repressed memories' was a product of trends in the general culture, especially in the United States, related to a focus on victimization and concerns particularly regarding women. Such victimization, as well as childhood abuse, obviously occurs. But when the search for such abuse becomes part of the diagnostic enterprise, and especially when psychiatric 'symptoms' said to be the products of such abuse are identified that are ambiguous and could be the result of numerous factors, what can follow is considerable harm not only to the families of patients but also to the patients themselves—and, not least, to the mental health professions and the diagnostic enterprise. It is not surprising, given the vulnerabilities of the latter, that diagnosis was turned to in the effort to condemn reprehensible practices that take place; but it was unfortunate that diagnostic procedures were distorted in the process.

Conclusion

If we turn to diagnosis because of its non-medical beauty we are at risk, whether we are laymen or psychiatrists, of being injured by that beauty. For years people have been coming to psychiatrists to circumvent the law: they have sought diagnoses to help them get abortions or evade the military draft. Psychiatrists often saw little danger in such humanitarian deeds, and responded to the requests willingly. But the danger was there, and we need only look to the former Soviet Union to appreciate its extreme potential. Things went awry in that country because a powerful tool was just too attractive and too capable of misuse to be protected from it; the fear of governmental power was too great, the respect for the law too weak, the diagnostic scheme too broad, and the opportunities for self-deception on the part of both ordinary bureaucrats and well-trained psychiatrists too available. But the same attraction to diagnosis, the same appreciation of its multiple beauties, exists in the West; and though our laws have protected us from succumbing to a similar fate, the law itself has a certain weakness for diagnosis, tends to be partial to its charms, and is exquisitely susceptible to its inroads. Psychiatrists have to understand that diagnosis plays a powerful, varied, and unrecognized role in the lives of all persons; that that role is equally powerful and no less varied and unrecognized in the lives of psychiatrists; and that all abuses of diagnoses are a psychiatric problem in considerable measure because they are a *human* problem, and probably stem less from the corruption of the profession than from the needs and vulnerabilities of us all.

Naturally, psychiatrists must be expected not to misdiagnose knowingly. But in order to avert non-purposeful misdiagnoses, psychiatrists must come to appreciate the limitations of the diagnostic process itself, the capacity of diagnostic theories and schools to influence and shape psychiatric perceptions of behaviour, and the inherent beauties of diagnosis that make it so enticing to use that only the most stringent efforts on the part of psychiatrists, and the most serious attention on the part of their teachers, will keep that them from yielding unknowingly to those beauties—indeed, will keep psychiatrists from failing to recognize that they even exist.

References

1. Balint, M.: *The doctor, his patient, and the illness*. New York. International Universities Press, 1957.
2. Scheff, T.: *Being mentally ill: a sociological theory*. Chicago, Aldine, 1966.
3. Levene, H. I.: Acute schizophrenia: clinical effects of the labeling process. *Archives of General Psychiatry* **25**:215–22, 1971.
4. Friedlander, Henry.: *The origins of Nazi genocide: from euthanasia to the final solution*. Chapel Hill, University of North Carolina Press, 1995.
5. Mendelsohn, John (ed.): *The Holocaust: selected documents*, 18 vols. New York, Garland, 1982.
6. Kintner, Earl W. (ed.): *The Hadamar trial: trial of Alfons Klein, Adolf Wahlman, Heinrich Ruoff, Karl Willig, Adolf Merkle, Irmgard Huber, and Phillipp Blum*. London, William Hodge, 1949.
7. *Trials of war criminals before the Nuremberg military tribunals under control council law no. 20 (green series)*, 14 vols. Washington, DC, Government Printing Office, 1950–52.
8. Alexander, Leo.: Medical science under dictatorship. *New England Journal of Medicine* **241**:39–47, 1949.
9. Breitman, Richard.: *The architect of genocide: Himmler and the final solution*. New York, Alfred A. Knopf, 1991.
10. Browning, Christopher R.: *The path to genocide: essays on the launching of the final solution*. New York, Cambridge University Press, 1992.
11. Cocks, Geoffrey.: *Psychotherapy in the Third Reich: The Göring Institute*. New York, Oxford University Press, 1985.
12. Hilberg, Raul.: *The destruction of the European Jews*. Rev. edn, 3 vols., New York, Holmes and Meier, 1985.
13. Kater, Michael H.: *Doctors under Hitler*. Chapel Hill, University of North Carolina Press, 1989.

14. Mosse, George L.: *The crisis of German ideology: intellectual origins of the Third Reich*. New York, Grosset and Dunlap, 1964.
15. Weindling, Paul.: *Health, race, and German politics between national unification and Nazism, 1870–1945*. Cambridge, Cambridge University Press, 1989.
16. Annas, George J. and Michael A. Grodin.: *The Nazi doctors and the Nuremberg code*. New York, Oxford University Press, 1992.
17. Lifton, Robert Jay: *The Nazi doctors: medical killings and the psychology of genocide*. New York, Basic Books, 1968.
18. Mitscherlich, A. and Mielke, F.: *The death doctors*. London, Elek, 1949.
19. Mitscherlich, A. and Mielke, F.: *Doctors of infamy: the story of the Nazi medical crimes*. New York, Henry Schumann, 1949.
20. Ternon, Y. and Helman, S.: *Le massacre des aliénés: des theoriciens nazis aux praticiens SS*. Paris, Casterman, 1971.
21. Kogon, E.: *The theory and practice of hell*. New York, Berkley, 1980.
22. International Auschwitz Committee: *Anthology*, 3 vols in 7 parts. Warsaw, 1971–4 [Articles published originally in 1961–7 in the Polish medical journal *Przeglad Lekarski*]
23. Muller-Hegemann, D.: Psychotherapy in the German Democratic Republic, in *Psychiatry in the Communist world*, ed. A. Kiev. New York, Science House, 1968, pp. 51–70.
24. Mehlman, P.: The reliability of psychiatric diagnoses. *Journal of Abnormal and Social Psychology* **47**:577–8, 1952.
25. Overall, J. E. and Hollister, L. E.: Comparative evaluation of research diagnostic criteria for schizophrenia. *Archives of General Psychiatry* **36**:1198–205, 1979.
26. Cantwell, D. P., Russell, A. T., Mattison, R., *et al*.: A comparison of DSM-II and DSM-III in the diagnosis of childhood psychiatric disorders. I. Agreement with expected diagnosis. *Archives of General Psychiatry* **36**:1208–13, 1979.
27. Babigian, H. M., Gardner, E. A., Miles, H. C., *et al*.: Diagnostic consistency and change in a follow-up study of 1,215 patients. *American Journal of Psychiatry* **121**:895–901, 1965.
28. Babigan, H. M., Gardner, E. A., Miles, H. C., *et al*.: ibid.
29. Pasamanick, B., Dinitz, S., and Lefton, L.: Psychiatric orientation in relation to diagnosis and treatment. *American Journal of Psychiatry* **116**:127–32, 1959.
30. Katz, M. M., Cole, J. O., and Lowery, H. A.: Studies of the diagnostic process: the influence of symptom perception, past experience, and ethnic background on diagnostic decisions. *American Journal of Psychiatry* **125**:937–47, 1969.
31. Temerlin, M. K.: Diagnostic bias in community mental health. *Community Mental Health Journal* **6**:110–17, 1970.
32. Plutchik, R., Conte, H., and Landau, H.: A comparison of symptom evaluations by psychiatrists and social workers. *Hospital and Community Psychiatry* **23**:13–14, 1972.
33. Jaspers, K.: Eifersuchtswahn: Ein Beitrag zur Frage 'Entwicklung einer Personlichkeit oder Prozess'. *Zeitschrift fur Gesamte Neurologie und Psychiatrie* **1**:567, 1910.
34. Fish, F.: *Schizophrenia*. Bristol, John Wright,1962.
35. Astrup, C. and Odegard, O.: Continued experiments in psychiatric diagnosis. *Acta Psychiatrica Scandinavica* **46**:180–212, 1970.
36. Langfeldt, G.: Diagnosis and prognosis of schizophrenia. *Proceedings of the Royal Society of Medicine* **53**:1047–52, 1960.
37. Zigler, E. and Phillips, L.: Psychiatric diagnosis and symptomatology. *Journal of Abnormal and Social Psychology* **63**:69–75, 1961.

38. Rumke, H. C.: Signification de la phenomenologie dans l'etude clinique des delirants. *Psychopathologie Generale* **1**:125, 1950.
39. Scheff, T.: *Being mentally ill: a sociological theory*. Chicago, Aldine, 1966.
40. *Diagnostic and statistical manual of mental disorders*, 4th edn. Washington, DC, American Psychiatric Association, 1994.
41. Baldessarnini, R. J., Finkelstein, S., and Arana, G. W.: The predictive power of diagnostic tests and the effect of prevalence of illness. *Archives of General Psychiatry* **40**:569–73, 1983.
42. Boyd, J. H., Burke, J. D., Gruenberg, E., *et al.*: Exclusion criteria of DSM-III: a study of co-occurrence of hierarchy-free syndromes. *Archives of General Psychiatry* **41**:983–9, 1984.
43. Helzer, J. E., Brockington, I. F., and Kendell, R. E.: Predictive validity of DSM-III and Feighner definitions of schizophrenia: a comparison with Research Diagnostic Criteria and CATEGO. *Archives of General Psychiatry* **38**:791–7, 1981.
44. Hyler, S. E., Williams, J. B. W., and Spitzer, R. L.: Reliability in the DSM-III field trials: interview vs case summary. *Archives of General Psychiatry* **39**:1275–8, 1982.
45. Kass, F., Skodol, A. E., Charles, E., *et al.*: Scaled ratings of DSM-III personality disorders. American *Journal of Psychiatry* **142**:627–30, 1985.
46. Leckman, J. F., Merikangas, K. R., Pauls, D. L., *et al.*: Anxiety disorders and depression: contradictions between family study data and DSM-III conventions. *American Journal of Psychiatry* **140**:880–2, 1983.
47. Spitzer, R. L. and Fleiss, J. L.: A re-analysis of the reliability of psychiatric diagnosis. *British Journal of Psychiatry* **125**:341–7, 1974.
48. Spitzer, R. L., Endicott, J., and Robins, E.: Research diagnostic criteria: rationale and reliability. *Archives of General Psychiatry* **23**:41–55, 1978.
49. Spitzer, R. L., Endicott, J., and Robins, E.: Reliability of clinical criteria for psychiatric diagnosis, in *Psychiatric diagnosis: exploration of biological predictors*, ed. J. Akiskal and W. Webb. New York, Spectrum Publications, 1978, pp. 61-73.
50. Buyanov, M. I.: Heal thyself, medicine. *Uchitel'skaya gazeta*, 19 November 1988.
51. Churkin, A.: Interview in 'Psychiatry and Politics'. *New Times*, No. 43, October 1988, pp. 41–3.
52. Novikov, A., Razin, S. and Mishin, M.: Does Soviet psychiatry need a tighter rein? *Komsomolskaya pravda*, 11 November 1987, p. 4.
53. Reddaway, P.: Should world psychiatry readmit the Soviets? *New York Review of Books*, 12 October 1989, pp. 54–8.
54. Snezhnevsky, A. V. and Vartanyan, M.: The forms of schizophrenia and their biological correlates, in *Biochemistry, schizophrenia, and affective illness*, ed. H. E. Himwich. Baltimore, William and Wilkins, 1970, pp. 1–28.
55. Snezhnevsky, A. V.: Symptom, syndrome, disease: a clinical method in psychiatry, in *The world biennial of psychiatry and psychotherapy*, ed. S. Arieti, vol. 1, 1971, pp. 151–64.
56. Snezhnevsky, A. V.: The symptomatology, clinical forms and nosology of schizophrenia, in *Modern perspectives in world psychiatry*, ed. J. G. Howells. New York, Brunner-Mazel, 1971, pp. 423–47.
57. Nadzharov, R. A.: Course forms, in *Schizophrenia*, ed. A. V. Snezhnevsky. Moscow, Meditsina, 1972, pp. 16–76.
58. Rollins, N.: *Child psychiatry in the Soviet Union*. Cambridge, Mass., Harvard University Press, 1972.
59. Holland, J. and Shakhmatova-Pavlova, I. V.: Concept and classification of schizophrenia in the Soviet Union. Unpublished, 1974.

60. Holland, J.: Draft of pilot study of joint classification of schizophrenia. Psychiatric Research Institute USSR/Academy of Medical Sciences and NIMH (USA). Unpublished, 1975.
61. Holland, J.: 'State' hospitals in the USSR: a model of governmental psychiatric care, *in Future roles of state hospitals*, ed. J. Zusman and B. Bertsen. Toronto, Lexington (D. C. Heath), 1977, pp. 373–85.
62. Holland, J.: Schizophrenia in the Soviet Union, in *Annual review of research in schizophrenia*, ed. R. Cancro. New York, 1977.
63. World Health Organization: *Report of the International Pilot Study of Schizophrenia*, vol. 1. Geneva, WHO, 1973.
64. Reich, W.: The spectrum concept of schizophrenia: problems for diagnostic practice. *Archives of General Psychiatry* **32**:489–98, 1975.
65. Reich, W.: Kazanetz, schizophrenia and Soviet psychiatry. *Archives of General Psychiatry* **36**:1029–30, 1979.
66. *Report of the US Delegation to Assess Recent Changes in Soviet Psychiatry to the Assistant Secretary of State for Human Rights and Humanitarian Affairs, US Department of State*, 12 July 1989. Washington, DC, US Department of State, 1989. [Reprinted as Supplement of *Schizophrenia Bulletin*, vol. 15, no. 4, 1989.]
67. Reich, W.: Glasnost in psychiatry: Soviets still see dissidence as an aberration. *Los Angeles Times*, 23 September 1989, II8.
68. Reich, W.: The spectrum concept of schizophrenia: problems for diagnostic practice. *Archives of General Psychiatry* **32**:489–98, 1975.
69. Reich, W.: The world of Soviet psychiatry. *New York Times Magazine*, 30 January 1983, pp. 21–6 and 51.
70. Reich, W.: The theories and leadership of Soviet psychiatry. In *US and USSR psychiatric care practices. Hearing before the subcommittee on health and the environment, committee on energy and commerce, House of Representives*, 2 October 1989. Washington, DC, US Government Printing Office, 1989 Serial No.101-82. [Note: portions of this chapter were presented in testimony at this hearing.]
71. Rosenthal, D.: *The Genain quadruplets*. New York, Basic Books, 1963.
72. Kety, S. S., Rosenthal, D., Wender, P. H., *et al.*: The types and prevalence of mental illness in the biological adoptive families of adopted schizophrenics, *in The transmission of schizophrenia*, ed. D. Rosenthal and S.S. Kety. Oxford, Pergamon, 1968, pp. 345–62.
73. Rosenthal, D., Wender, P. H., Kety, S. S., *et al.*: Schizophrenic's offspring reared in adoptive homes, in *The transmission of schizophrenia*, ed. S. S. Kety, D. Rosenthal, and P. H. Wender. Oxford, Pergamon, 1968, pp. 377–91.
74. Rosenthal, D., Wender, P. H., and Kety, S. S., *et al.*: The adopted away offspring of schizophrenics. *American Journal of Psychiatry* **128**:302–6, 1971.
75. Wender, P. H., Rosenthal, D., Kety, S. S., *et al.*: Crossfostering: research strategy for clarifying the role of genetic and experimental factors in the etiology of schizophrenia. *Archives of General Psychiatry* **30**:1218, 1974.
76. Kety, S. S., Rosenthal, D., Wender, P. H., *et al.*: Mental illness in the biological and adoptive families of adopted individuals who have become schizophrenic: a preliminary report based upon psychiatric interviews, in *Genetic research in psychiatry*, ed. R. Fieve, D. Rosenthal, and H. Brill. Baltimore, Johns Hopkins University Press, 1975, pp. 147–65.
77. Fowler, R. C., Tsuang, M. T., Cadoret, R. J., *et al.*: Non-psychotic disorders in the families of process schizophrenics. *Acta Psychiatrica Scandinavica* **51**:153–60, 1975.

78. Reich, W.: The schizophrenia spectrum: a genetic concept. *Journal of Nervous and Mental Diseases* **162**:3–12, 1976.
79. Rieder, R. O.: The schizophrenia spectrum. Presented at the 131st Annual Meeting of the American Psychiatric Association, May 8–12, 1978.
80. Kety, S. S., Rosenthal, D., Wender, P. H., *et al.*: The biologic and adoptive families of adopted individuals who became schizophrenic: prevalence of mental illness and other characteristics, in *The nature of schizophrenia*, ed. L. C. Wynne, R. L. Cromwell, and S. Matthysse. New York, Wiley, 1978, pp. 25–37.
81. Kety, S. S., Wender, P. H., and Rosenthal, D.: Genetic relationships within the schizophrenia spectrum: evidence from adoption studies, in *Critical issues in psychiatric diagnosis*, ed. R. L. Spitzer and D. F. Klein. New York, Raven Press, 1978, pp. 213–23.
82. Reich, W.: The diagnosis of everyday life. *Harper's Magazine*, February 1980.
83. Reich, W.: Brainwashing, psychiatry and the law. *New York Times*, 29 May 1976, p. 23.
84. Reich, W.: Brainwashing, psychiatry and the law. *Psychiatry* **39**:400–3, 1976.
85. Sinclair, W.: After the upheaval: who's running what? *The Washington Post*, 21 July 1979, p. A-1; also Weicker suggests Carter not run. *The Washington Post*, 22 July 1979, A6.
86. Quinn, S.: Rosalynn's journey. *The Washington Post*, 25 July 1979, B1.
87. Schram, M.: The troubled times of a different Billy Carter. *The Washington Post*, 25 February 1979, A1.
88. Gup, T.: Brooding replaces clowning. *The Washington Post*, 25 February 1979, A1.
89. Evans, R. and Novak, R.: Brother Billy: political blunders. *The Washington Post*, 2 March 1979.
90. The stewardess and the 'witch'. *Newsweek*, 30 April 1979, p. 31.
91. Berry, J. D. and Egan, J.: Alleged embezzling, maneuvering in moviedom. *The Washington Post*, 25 December 1977, A1.
92. Mitgang, H.: Greene calls profile of him in *New Yorker* inaccurate. *New York Times*, 12 May 1979.
93. Brody, J. E.: Inquiry at cancer center finds fraud in research. *New York Times*, 25 May 1974.
94. Brody, J. E.: Scientist denies cancer research fraud. *New York Times*, 29 May 1974.
95. Colen, D.: Drug for sex offenders called success. *The Washington Post*, December 1975.
96. Myer, J. K. and Reter, D. J.: Sex reassignment: follow-up. *Archives of General Psychiatry* **36**:1010–15, 1979.
97. Khrushchev, N.: *Khrushchev remembers*, trans. and ed. S. Talbott. Boston, Little, Brown, 1970, p. 566.
98. Mandelstam, N.: *Hope against hope*. New York, Atheneum, 1970, p. 28.
99. Mandelstam, N.: *Hope against hope*. New York, Atheneum, 1970, p. 26.
100. Libya helping terrorists with arms and training. *New York Times*, 16 July 1976.
101. Anderson, J. and Whitten, L.: Saudis suspect an Iran–US plot. *The Washington Post*, 17 September 1976.
102. *New York Times*, 10 November 1979, A8.
103. Khomeini, R.: The world is not on your side. *The Washington Post*, 22 November 1979, A23.
104. Farrell, W.: The furor surrounding Begin: he fights harder and doesn't budge. *New York Times*, 25 July 1978.

105. Randal, J. C.: Role in UN session builds confidence among Palestinians. *The Washington Post*, 12 January 1979.
106. Lenin, V. I.: Letter to Gorky of 31 July 1919. *Sochineniya* (Works), 4th edn. Moscow State Political Literature Publishing House, 1951-67. [Quoted in Lev Navrozov, *The education of Lev Navrozov.* New York, Harper's, 1975, p. 164.]
107. Mrs Sakharov flies home. *The Washington Post*, 24 November 1977, A39.
108. Getler, M.: Bonn party aide calls US bomb a 'perversion'. *The Washington Post*, 18 July 1977, A1.
109. Allman, T. D.: The 'rebirth' of Eldridge Cleaver. *New York Times Magazine*, 16 January 1977, p. 10.
110. Horrock, N. M.: Drug tested by C.I.A. on mental patients. *New York Times*, 3 August 1977, A1.
111. Committee on the Judiciary: *Abuse of psychiatry for political repression in the Soviet Union.* Hearing before the subcommittee to investigate the administration of the internal security act and other internal security laws of the committee on the judiciary, United States Senate, ninety-second Congress, second session. Washington, DC, US Government Printing Office, 26 December 1972.
112. Stone, I. F.: Betrayal by psychiatry. *New York Review of Books*, 10 February 1972, pp. 7–14.
113. Chodoff, P.: Involuntary hospitalization of political dissenters in the Soviet Union. *Psychiatric Opinion* 11:5–19, 1974; also Amnesty International: *Prisoners of conscience in the USSR: their treatment and conditions.* London, Amnesty International, 1975.
114. Grigorenko, P.: *The Grigorenko papers: writings by General P. G. Grigorenko and documents on his case.* London, C. Hurst; Boulder, Colorado, Westview Press, 1976.
115. Yeo, C.: The abuse of psychiatry in the USSR: the evidence. *Index on Censorship*: **4**, No.2 (Summer 1975).
116. Bloch, S. and Reddaway, P.: *Psychiatric terror: the abuse of psychiatry in the Soviet Union.* New York, Basic Books, 1977.
117. Bloch, S. and Reddaway, P.: *Soviet psychiatric abuse: The shadow over world psychiatry.* Boulder, Colorado, Westview Press, 1985.
118. Lader, M.: *Psychiatry on trial.* Harmondsworth, Penguin, 1977.
119. Plyushch, L.: *History's carnival*, with a contribution by Tatyana Plyushch, ed. and trans. Marco Carynnyk. New York, Harcourt Brace Jovanovich, 1979.
120. Bukovsky, V.: *To build a castle: my life as a dissenter*, trans. M. Scammell. New York, Viking Press, 1979.
121. Reich, W.: Diagnosing Soviet dissidents. *Harper's Magazine*, August 1978. pp. 31–7.
122. Reich, W.: Grigorenko gets a second opinion. *New York Times Magazine*, 13 May 1979, pp. 18ff.
123. Reich, W.: Diagnosing Soviet dissidents. *Harper's*, August 1978, pp. 31–7.
124. Reich, W.: Soviet psychiatry on trial. *Commentary*, January 1978, pp. 40–8.
125. Reich, W.: The world of Soviet psychiatry. *New York Times Magazine*, 30 January 1983, pp. 21–6, 51.
126. Reich, W.: Glasnost in psychiatry: Soviets still see dissidence as an aberration. *Los Angeles Times*, 23 September 1989, II8.
127. Wright, Lawrence. *Remembering Satan.* New York, Alfred A. Knopf, 1994.
128. Yapko, Michael D. *Suggestions of abuse.* New York, Simon and Schuster, 1994.

129. Terr, Lenore: *Unchained memories: true stories of traumatic memories, lost and found*. New York, Basic Books, 1994.
130. Loftus, Elizabeth and Ketcham, Katherine: *The myth of repressed memory: false memories and allegations of sexual abuse.* New York, St Martin's, 1995.
131. Ofshe, Richard and Watters, Ethan: *Making monsters: false memories, psychotherapy and sexual hysteria.* New York, Scribners, 1995.
132. Rubin, Bonnie Miller: Presumed guilty: when allegations of abuse surface after many years, is society too quick to believe them?, *Chicago Tribune*, May 30, 1993, A1.
133. Reich, Walter: The monster in the mists. *New York Times Book Review*, May 15, 1994, pp. 1; 33–38.
134. Psychologists release statement on abuse memories, *Psychiatric News*, December 18, 1994, p. 4.
135. Managing the risks involved in cases of recovered memories of abuse, *Rx for Risk*, vol. 3, No. 10, November/December, 1994, p. 4f.

11

Ethical aspects of the psychotherapies

Jeremy Holmes

As in individual development, ethical awareness in psychotherapy has emerged rather late in its maturational process. Self-awareness is a fundamental principle in psychotherapy—and yet until the 1990s practitioners could be forgiven for ignoring the ethical dimension of the subject. But after a century of evolution, ethics are increasingly central to the organization, practice, and intellectual life of psychotherapy.

The guiding values underlying bioethics have been summarized by Beauchamp[1] under the rubric of the 'four principles' of respect for autonomy, beneficence, nonmaleficence, and justice. In this chapter I shall discuss the extent to which these principles apply to psychotherapy. Thus, for example, under the principle of beneficence we may consider whether it is ethical to offer patients therapies which are not of proven efficacy, or ask whether the fact that ethnic minorities are under-represented both as patients and practitioners contravenes the principle of justice.

Ethics impacts on practice in several distinct ways which correspond, schematically with the psychoanalytic tripartite model of the mind: ego, id, and superego. In day-to-day practice therapists and therapy organizations must negotiate the interface between therapy and the real world. Therapists should respect the need for informed consent, and the therapeutic contract, and justify their handling of these issues with patients. Equally, it is essential that practitioners understand the nature of and need for boundaries—especially in relation to confidentiality and sexual transgression. Psychotherapeutic ethics safeguards patients against exploitation, and this exploitation is often best understood as a transgression of the boundary between patient and therapist.

Second, there is growing recognition of the way values underpin therapy—operating as unexamined basic assumptions influencing practice just as many of our choices and preferences are unconsciously determined. Becoming aware of these and how they influence practice, for good or for ill, is a further task for the ethically responsible practitioner.

Third, with the move towards the formation of a psychotherapy 'profession', psychotherapy organizations have been compelled to draw up 'superego-type' guidelines, and to consider how ethical practice may be encouraged and transgressions punished.

After presenting brief clinical examples, I will consider each of these aspects in turn.

Ethical aspects of psychotherapeutic practice

Consider the following vignettes, all derived from clinical experience, which illustrate the ways in which ethical issues arise in the course of practice.

Case 1
A patient consults a therapist in his office. She has chosen him on the recommendation of a friend. The patient describes her problem. The therapist listens carefully and suggests at the end of the session that the patient needs therapy, that he has a vacancy, and that they start the following week with twice-weekly sessions. The patient has only the vaguest idea about the arrangements of the therapy and when after a few weeks she announces that she will be away on holiday for a fortnight, is staggered to hear the therapist tell her that he expects payment for the missed sessions.

Case 2
A trainee counsellor consults a new therapist, Dr X, about the possibility of therapy. A few days later she bumps into a friend, also a counsellor, who informs her, 'I hear you are going into therapy with Dr X; I believe he's very good'. [Not so good at keeping confidences!]

Case 3
A young man suffering from repetitive hand-washing and other typical obsessive–compulsive symptoms refers himself to a hypnotherapist who teaches him relaxation and then embarks on a course of 'regression' therapy to uncover traumatic events in his childhood. After 3 months he feels generally better but his symptoms have not improved. He then has a period of analytic counselling with another therapist, again without change. Having run out of money, he consults his general practitioner who refers him to the psychotherapy unit at the local general hospital where, following a comprehensive assessment, he is offered and pursues a course of behaviour therapy, with moderately good results.

Case 4
A consultant psychotherapist sees a patient in supportive therapy over many years. The patient, who has extreme difficulty in trusting people, eventually comes to rely on him, bringing him jottings and pictures on a regular basis. One day, browsing through a medical magazine, she stumbles on an article by him containing a case history, clearly about her, albeit thinly disguised, and quoting verbatim from some of her writings.

Case 5
An unhappy young woman, sexually abused in childhood by her stepfather, becomes increasingly fond of her male therapist, and begins to realize that what she wants more than anything from him is warmth and comfort. He in turn desperately wants to help

her, but finds that he is beginning to have sexual fantasies about her. His marriage is in difficulty, and he is exasperated by his apparent inability to help the client. Although the sessions go well, her sadness and vulnerability seem more evident than at the start of therapy. He begins to lend her books which have meant a lot to him. When she complains that he is merely a remote professional, he impulsively suggests that they might meet for a drink sometime. Suddenly at the end of a session she stands up and says, 'Hold me!'. Before he has time to think he is embracing her. They arrange to meet the next evening, and end up in bed together.

Ethics and evidence-based practice

Ethical practice of psychotherapy requires that it be beneficial, and not harm the recipient—or perhaps the other way round, given the principle of *primum non nocere*. Thus ethics abuts the vast and complex field of psychotherapy research, an area outside the traditional concerns of psychotherapeutic ethics (but see ref. 2). *Is* psychotherapy beneficial, and for whom? Does it matter what kind of psychotherapy is offered, or are all types equally effective, and, if so, is it not (on the principle of justice) ethically correct to prescribe the most cost-effective, thereby freeing resources for other potential beneficiaries? Or might this contravene the principle of respect for autonomy since the patient, if properly informed, should be free to choose (or 'consent to') the form of treatment she feels suits her best? Are some forms of psychotherapy more effective for some kinds of difficulty, and, if so, is it unethical not to offer them? Can psychotherapy be harmful, and if so, under what circumstances?

Psychotherapy research is beginning to provide answers to these questions,[3] but the central ethical issue to which psychotherapy research can contribute is that of informed consent: potential patients and third-party funders need to know what they are letting themselves in for when a course of therapy is prescribed. This needs to be differentiated from exploitation of patients by therapists—for instance a patient might be offered an inappropriate form of psychotherapy in good faith—and also takes on a different hue depending on whether the context is private practice or third-party funding.

In an attempt to address these quasi-political questions, the UK Department of Health commissioned two studies, one a Cochrane-style summary of the evidence for the effectiveness of psychotherapy,[4] the other a survey of public, health service-funded psychotherapy services.[5] Taken together, these documents provide a basis for ethically sound, publicly funded psychotherapy, in contrast to 'poorly targeted, inappropriate interventions and ineffective organisation and delivery of services'[5] which they found to be widespread.

The Cochrane-oriented document[4] covers six features of good psychotherapy services; they should be comprehensive, coordinated, user-friendly, safe, clinically effective, and cost-effective.

Comprehensive services, ranging from general practice-based counselling to specialized psychotherapy as part of secondary or tertiary health-care provision, are required if the full range of difficulties which present are to be adequately treated. It is inappropriate—and ultimately unethical—to offer, say, brief counselling to a person suffering from a severe personality disorder whose only hope of recovery depends on long-term therapy delivered by a well-trained and well-supervised experienced practitioner.

Similarly, the need for cost-effective therapy flows from the principle of justice which suggests that in publicly funded therapy 'psychotherapeutic intervention should be at the least complex, costly and intrusive level consistent with effective treatment'.[5] This sensible injunction is contentious however given the lack of consensus about how to measure outcome, and the position that symptomatic measures alone are inadequate to assess the aims of many therapies, especially the psychodynamic. For example, some damaged patients become dependent on treatment, and, if it ends prematurely, relapse. This may 'cost' the exchequer far more than the price of therapy itself. Interminable therapy may contravene the principle of justice, but it is equally 'unfair' to offer chronically ill patients brief 'packages' when evidence suggests that only long-term therapy is likely to help.

Ethical practice is based around triage. Patients with minor disorders should be offered time-limited treatment whereas those with intractable conditions should be given supportive psychotherapy, a form of treatment in which the patient is seen infrequently but indefinitely,[6] backed up by befriending, day-centre attendance, and other less costly forms of support.[7] The ethical/technical issue is to do with how frequently patients need to be seen, and whether they require the skills of a highly trained therapist as opposed, say, to a well-supervised 'befriender'.

Between those with disorders suitable for brief interventions, and those needing supportive therapy, there is a middle group who are often severely ill, yet have sufficient motivation, ego strength, and maturity of defences to benefit from intensive psychotherapy. Critics of psychotherapy complain that this is offered only to the 'worried well', with the implication that in ethical terms it is unjust to devote scarce resources to people who have little wrong with them in the first place. However, this view is apt to be prejudicial rather than evidence-based, since studies have shown that, if anything, patients attending psychotherapy departments are *more* disturbed than comparable attenders at general psychiatric outpatient clinics.[8]

Informed consent in psychotherapy

So far we have discussed psychotherapeutic ethics at an organizational level. When we consider the individual, as opposed to the corporate contract between therapist and patient, many of the same principles apply, both in third-party funded and in self-financed treatments. Thus, in principle, the therapist should be well trained for the type of therapy offered, should not offer treatment that is unlikely to benefit the particular patient, and should certainly avoid doing harm. The patient must provide informed consent to therapy, and should therefore be aware of the therapist's qualifications, what is involved in treatment, how long it is likely to take, what alternative treatments might be considered, and what adverse outcomes might arise.

As with all medical ethics, these are counsels of perfection; the reality of practice is different. A fundamental aspect is inherent in the nature of psychotherapy itself. Most treatments in medicine aim to relieve pain or discomfort; in this psychiatry is similar. The purpose of antidepressant or antipsychotic or anxiolytic medications is to relieve emotional pain. But in significant ways psychotherapy works differently. Here the aim is not so much alleviation of pain as enhancement of autonomy and integration (see below), based on self-knowledge. To know oneself inevitably means getting in touch with painful aspects of oneself. In psychotherapy it is often considered that the patient's difficulties arise precisely because he has adopted strategies *not* to feel pain, and the aim is to encourage him to experience rather than avoid, deny, split off, project, or repress unpleasant emotions—for example, that associated with being sexually abused as a child.

To warn the patient that he may feel distressed as a result of treatment—and that distress may also arise in those to whom he is close, with, for example, possible repercussions on a marriage—is desirable. Yet it is tempting to gloss over these for the sake of a positive therapeutic alliance, often with a difficult patient whose commitment is fragile, where good feelings towards the therapist is a major determinant of outcome. Nevertheless, these dangers *should* be pointed out. At least the patient will feel that the therapist is being honest, and that he is free to choose whether to embark on therapy in full possession of the facts; both will pay dividends in the long run. This is an example of a general point—ethical and technically correct practice usually coincide.

Three further difficulties illustrate the limitations of a conventional approach to informed consent when applied to psychotherapy. In medicine it is possible to separate the relationship with the practitioner from the procedure to which the patient needs to consent. But in psychotherapy the relationship is a key therapeutic agent. If the therapist points out the difficulties which may lie ahead, this can act as a powerful *suggestion* about what is to happen, and thus become a self-fulfilling prophesy.

In addition, because psychotherapy involves a relationship to which both patient and therapist contribute, it will be impossible for the therapist to inform the patient what he is letting himself in for since this will depend largely on the patient himself, about whom the therapist has limited knowledge at this stage. It is nevertheless part of the skill of assessment to be able to predict what difficulties this particular patient is likely to encounter.

Third, analytic therapists specifically eschew suggestion and try to keep their own opinions, predictions, and expectations out of sight, the better to foster transference, and to allow free, self-exploration. For them to enter into long explanations about the hazards of therapy might jeopardize the engine of change upon which they rely—here technique and ethics appear to be in conflict.

In practice, this conflict is usually resolvable. First, there is a clear distinction between assessment and treatment. At the end of the assessment there should be a frank discussion about options, and possible benefits and risks.[9] At this stage the therapist can be more forthcoming than he would be once treatment is under way. This window of judicious self-revelation may well stimulate transferential projections which form part of the material for treatment; it may turn out that the patient saw the therapist as harsh, seductive, brutally frank, coy, or whatever.

A second way round these dilemmas of informed consent is the use of an *evolving contract*. The therapist may suggest to the patient that they meet for a limited number of sessions and then decide whether or not to proceed. By the time that milestone has been reached, the patient will have a clearer understanding of what is involved, and thus be better placed to give informed consent. This arrangement is not unlike engagement prior to marriage, or, in house purchase, exchange of contracts as a preliminary to completion. It is as though the patient puts a deposit on therapy, following which he can decide whether or not to complete the purchase.

Although I have implied that informed consent in psychotherapy has distinct features, a surgical analogy serves to make the point that there are also similarities with routine medical practice. Psychotherapy can be likened to an orthopaedic intervention in which a broken bone has spontaneously knitted together but in a way that is misaligned, and reduces mobility. The surgeon's task is to break the bone again and reposition it so that a more functional limb will result. In doing so he will cause pain, and a plaster cast will be applied which holds the new bone in place, protects it, and allows healing to take place. The ultimate result will be less discomfort and restriction, and greater autonomy. All this needs to be explained before proceeding; the patient might otherwise expect a painfree operation, and be surprised to learn that he himself is ultimately responsible for his own healing, rather than the surgeon's prowess whose function is as much to support as it is to undertake operational pyrotechnics.

Exploitation in psychotherapy

To exploit people is to use them exclusively as a means to an end rather than as ends in themselves (the Kantian principle). Although most people are trustworthy most of the time, we have it within us to cheat, lie, steal, sexually use, deceive, injure, and harm others for our own ends. Non-exploitative interchange between people is regulated by rules of reciprocity, which arise implicitly out of a sense of 'fairness', and explicitly through the rule of law. Many patients presenting for psychotherapy have been exploited, for example, as sexual objects for abusive adults or objects of parental narcissism. Their own needs have been ignored, overridden, or turned against them. They in turn may have learned to live as victim, a role they exploit in the search for crumbs of gratification in a world in which, for them, exploitation appears the norm. The normal developmental pathways from the infant's egoism to a capacity to see the other's point of view, to share, to delay gratification, and to treat others with respect has often been perverted. Equally, some therapists have themselves had troubled childhoods, which they have turned to advantage, with varying degrees of success, in their chosen task of helping others.

A professional relationship is based on trust—both of the individual and of the professional organization which has trained and licensed them. We expect architects, lawyers, teachers, doctors, and retailers to deal fairly with us, and that we will only complain or litigate in extreme circumstances. But we also recognize that professionals are 'only human' and that at times they will take advantage of us; hence the legal safeguards to protect us, and to deter those who think of doing harm.

Exploitation in psychotherapy is in some ways no different from other professions, for example overcharging or failing to deliver what has been undertaken. But there are aspects of psychotherapeutic exploitation which needs to be specifically highlighted. First, psychotherapy patients may be especially vulnerable because of their histories; it is this background of exploitation that leads to their need for help. Second, the inherent intimacy and dependency of the therapeutic relationship makes it more difficult to scrutinize transgression, and more likely that the injured patient will remain silent or blame himself for wrongs that are being perpetrated against him. Third, psychotherapy goes beyond rational accounts of exploitation, recognizing that there may be unconscious wishes in the patient to be used (e.g. as the only means to achieve attachment), or, on the therapist's side, to exploit patients in the guise of 'helping' them. Let us consider the commoner forms of exploitation in therapy; sexual exploitation is however fully covered in Glen Gabbard's chapter (see Chapter 8).

'Information exploitation'

Confidentiality is inherent in the 'Hippocratic contract' between patient and doctor. No doubt this had something to do with preserving the mystique of medical practice. More importantly, if we are to confide in people we must feel secure that they will respect our privacy and treat our confidences as privileged information. People, especially if they are strangers, approach one another warily, seeking and offering information as they get to know one another, while at the same time holding back as they evaluate the progress of the encounter. Reciprocity is the usual safeguard against exploitation. 'If you use your knowledge of me to gain advantage I can retaliate in kind'. Obvious exceptions to this are kinship relationships where an information imbalance prevails between adults and children, but under ordinary circumstances this is balanced by the safeguard of a shared biology.

The patient–therapist relationship is also asymmetrical. The development of trust is a stepwise process. That trust rests partly on social approval and regulation of therapy (hence the need for professionalism), partly on the therapist's ability to keep confidences—to 'earn' the patient's trust. Clearly circumstances arise in which trust can be betrayed. The most common form is gossip, as in the example given earlier. For the world to know that a person is in therapy is to disadvantage him, since, however much we may deplore this, it is commonly seen as a manifestation of weakness. More fundamentally, people can only act autonomously if *they* and no-one else decide what information about themselves they wish to reveal. More rarely, and more spectacularly, for a therapist to reveal facts about someone for pecuniary gain (say in the tabloid press) is to do that person a wrong.

Are there circumstances in which it is *not* unethical to breach confidentiality? Two aspects are commonly highlighted. The first concerns the 'scientific' need for therapists to communicate with their peers, in order to improve under-standing and technique, perhaps to benefit future patients. Here there may be a conflict of interest between an individual patient's need for confidentiality, and the generality of patients' need for scientific advances. Thus most patients demur when asked if they mind a medical student attending an assessment ('No, they have got to learn'). However, people are more reticent about exposing their psyche than their body. Presumably this is because, for the reasons discussed already, a person *is* his or her psyche, whereas we merely 'own' our bodies. There is no psychic equivalent of the strip over the eyes that preserved the anonymity of the body's owner in old textbooks.

This raises tricky questions for psychotherapists. Their work cannot be 'crunched' into anonymous statistics, nor glossed into generalizations. The lifeblood of psychotherapy is the specificity and uniqueness of the case history. There are three ways round this problem, each of which has advantages and drawbacks.[10] The first is to alter details of the case to preserve confidentiality, while retaining enough of the truth for the scientific issues to be revealed. This is a time-honoured method, but weak in that the patient's permission is not usually obtained, and many cases are so thinly veiled that only lip service to confidentiality is observed. One patient who found to her horror that her case had been described in a journal complained that not only had the therapist not sought her permission, but that he had got the details of her life wrong, and was clearly inattentive!

The second method is to show the patient material which the therapist wishes to publish, and obtain written consent. Many journals now make this a condition of publication; book publishers seem less vigilant. However, this is not an easy task for therapists or patients and it can have a major impact on the transference.[11] The problem of informed consent where unconscious motivations are in question remains, since a patient might, for example, agree to publication in order to placate her therapist when her interests would be better served by refusal. A patient in the US successfully sued a therapist for breach of confidentiality, even though she had given signed permission to publish, on the grounds that the transference was so powerful at the time that she was unable to make an unbiased decision.

A safer strategy is for the therapist who wishes to write about his work to invent prototypical patients. This *can* be done successfully (see ref. 12 for a good example), but there is still a danger (one shared with novelists) of the *roman-a-clef* in which the unconscious of the therapist unwittingly describes aspects of a real patient whom he has 'forgotten'. Another drawback of fictionalization is that it lacks the verisimilitude and colour of the case history.

The second situation where confidentiality may have to be breached is in those cases where *not* to do so might jeopardize a person's welfare, or even their life. In the *Tarasoff* case (see refs 2, 13, and 14 for discussion of this case) a psychotherapist was sued by the bereaved parents of a young woman, Tatiana Tarasoff, who had been murdered by her ex-lover. He had announced his intention to kill to his therapist. The therapist discussed the case with two colleagues, and then informed the police. The patient was briefly placed in custody, but soon released, whereupon he broke off treatment. Two months later he committed the murder. The judges found that the therapist had failed in his 'duty to warn' the young woman and her parents, and pronounced the dictum: 'protective privilege ends where public peril begins'.

From a forensic perspective, psychotherapeutic confidentiality is a privilege, not a right, and when in doubt should be overridden by considerations of safety. The 'duty to warn' applies in the US, but there is no legal equivalent elsewhere.[15] However, in the current climate, if a psychotherapist is worried about harm to others (or to the patient herself), he should ask the patient's permission to speak to relevant people (those in danger, the police, psychiatric authorities). If consent is not forthcoming, he then may feel compelled to do so anyway.

Similar considerations apply to psychotherapeutic notes (or electronic recordings) which often contain personal and sensitive information. Most psychotherapy units which are part of institutions, such as hospitals, keep separate notes (but in the UK the courts do not consider any written material to be privileged to the extent of being inadmissible). Here too therapists may feel caught in a dilemma in which they wish and are trained to make extensive notes for purposes of supervision and good care but risk disadvantaging their patient in the rare circumstances of those notes being subpoenaed.

A different aspect of this situation arises when the therapist has reason to believe that a patient is abusing, or likely to abuse children, or if a child in treatment is suspected of being the victim of abuse. Clearly in the first case the therapist will urge the patient to seek specific help. Further, in either situation, if the therapist is a social worker he has a statutory obligation in several countries to inform the authorities about his suspicions. If the therapist is a medical practitioner he will in almost all circumstances wish to do so, but under law has the discretion not to, should he consider this to represent the greater good of the children and if his behaviour is thought to be within the boundaries of responsible practice.

Financial exploitation

Private psychotherapists are like small traders, working in a market economy. Fees and length of therapy vary depending on the model of therapy and type of training the therapist has received. A degree of price-fixing probably goes on, since therapists tend to know what their colleagues charge, and it is not easy for patients to 'shop around'. The possibility of financial exploitation is greatest among those offering long-term therapy, although among brief therapists exorbitant assessment charges are not unknown. Orlinsky *et al.*'s[16] 'dose-response curve' suggests that, up to a limit, the longer the therapy the greater the patient's gain, so that brief treatments might be a false economy for patients or third-party payers, the latter none the less being understandably wary of indefinite therapy.

Among long-term therapists it is standard to charge for missed sessions, to insist that patients take holidays at the same time as the therapist, and to charge if they choose to be away during therapy 'terms'. None of this can be deemed exploitative if the contract is explained at the start of treatment, although it might be argued that distressed people will agree to anything that promises to alleviate their unhappiness. Once therapy is established the patient becomes dependent on the therapist, and here the possibility of exploitation is greater, for example, raising fees in the knowledge that the patient is likely to want to remain in therapy at any price. Raising fees can be seen as an 'acting out' by the therapist (some argue that therapists should never raise their fees once treatment has begun, however long it lasts) which may well be influenced by the unconscious ambience of the therapy, and will have to be considered from a dynamic as well as a purely financial perspective.

Given the lack of publicly funded psychotherapy, especially for long-term treatment, therapists who both want to make a reasonable living, and to offer treatment to patients on the basis of need rather than ability to pay are in a dilemma. Some address this by a 'Robin Hood' arrangement, or a sliding scale, charging well-off patients a high fee, thereby subsidising poorer patients. This informal progressive taxation also needs to be considered in the context of the transference–countertransference matrix. If therapists charge low fees only to patients they find attractive, or who evoke their pity, or who are special in some way, that might compromise the therapy, for example by reinforcing the patient's narcissism or sense of victimization.[17]

Sexual exploitation

By far the most significant, well-publicized, and worrying malpractice among psychotherapists is sexual exploitation of patients. For this reason this topic is covered in a separate chapter (see Chapter 8 by Glenn Gabbard), and is mentioned here only for reasons of completeness.

Values in psychotherapy

Underpinning the ethical issues so far discussed is a deeper set of assumptions, goals, beliefs, attitudes, and values that inform practice, often in an implicit and unexamined way, and yet which profoundly influence practice and the ethos of therapy.

Autonomy and psychoanalysis

Psychoanalysis emerged at the end of a century of struggle between scientific rationality and romanticism. In the natural sciences reason, logic, and respect for observation and evidence triumphed. For Freud, born in the same year that Darwin published *The origin of species*, psychology was the last frontier; the psychoanalytic project was an attempt to encompass the irrational forces of the unconscious in a framework of analytic rationality. For Freud the values of psychoanalysis were identical with those of science: respect for truth, distrust of authority, humility, close observation, and a willingness to discard unsubstantiated theories.

Much has changed in the twentieth century. The absolutism of scientific knowledge has been questioned and its connections with historical and social forces established. The scientific basis of psychoanalysis has been challenged on many fronts, not least because of the inherent difficulty in establishing analytic 'facts', independent of the analyst's subjectivity. The therapist is no longer seen, as in Freud's early formulations, as a neutral screen on which the patient's unconscious is projected, but rather as an active participant in an intersubjective matrix or 'bipersonal field' to which analyst and patient contribute, albeit in different ways.

This does not mean that psychotherapy is not 'scientific' in the sense of being based on dispassionate inquiry and respect for truth, even if it fails to meet the narrow 'Popperian' criteria of refutation. It does suggest however that there is room for an ethical dimension to the process—which is hardly surprising given that it is essentially an encounter between two people struggling with the problem of how to live a more satisfying life.

Can the guiding principles of psychotherapy then be extended beyond Freud's starting point: a respect for truth, and belief that an honest facing of the worst aspects of human nature helps transcend them? He saw self-knowledge as crucial: the Delphic injunction 'know thyself' is central to the quest.[18] For Freud, self-knowledge is freedom—acknowledging the power of the unconscious, the paradoxical route to escaping its dominance.

Freud's emphasis on self-knowledge has been linked with the central liberal value of *autonomy*. As already discussed, in contrast to 'medical-model' psychiatry, psychotherapy offers autonomy—with its implications of wholeness, individuation, and freedom of choice—rather than absence of pain, or indeed the illusory search for happiness, as *the* goal worth striving for.

This emphasis on autonomy aligns psychotherapy with a general twentieth century movement towards political and personal liberation. Alongside the struggle for democratic political rights, sexual equality, freedom from discrimination and racism, there is a need for inner freedom, the domain of psychotherapy.

Successful therapy enhances the patient's autonomy, both subjectively and objectively. At the end of treatment people will say: 'I feel more in control of my own life'; or 'I have learned that I have the right to choose—to do what I want to do and not do what I don't want to do'; or 'I am no longer dependent on others for my security and sense of well-being'. This subjective sense of autonomy is accompanied by objective changes: people are better able to work or, for example, if suffering from phobias to travel more freely or to cope more effectively with social situations.

The idea of autonomy as a key goal has been questioned. Bowlby[19] (and others working in an attachment framework) are suspicious of the version of independence implicit in some accounts of autonomy. He argues that people remain *inter*-dependent throughout their lives, and that the isolation and ruthless economic self-serving implicit in the notion of autonomy is a pathological product of late capitalism. He distinguishes between immature and mature dependence, seeing the aim of psychotherapy as fostering the latter. Similarly, Holmes and Lindley[2] use the phrase 'emotional autonomy; to characterize the state of affective freedom—in contrast to heteronomy—that psychotherapy can produce, in which patients no longer feel they are 'passion's slave', and engage in more satisfying intimate relationships.

Using a Kleinian perspective, Hinshelwood[20] questions the notion of autonomy, arguing that it fails to take account of unconscious processes. In his view patients seek therapy in a state of dis-integration and unawareness, in which part of the self is 'spread' (his term to denote what is technically known as projective identification) to others in the person's environment. The aim of therapy is to help him become aware of this process, and so reintegrate projected parts of the self. Integration, not autonomy is the goal. However it could be argued that integration is subsumed under autonomy since the integrated person who uses less projective identification will depend less on others to contain his unwanted feelings and so be in an enhanced state of autonomy, which in turn will enable him to develop more satisfying and less unhealthily dependent relationships.[6]

Religion and psychotherapy—Bergin's bombshell

A bombshell hit the world of empirical psychotherapy research in 1980 when Bergin[21] argued that despite their reticence, psychotherapists had a set of values about a good life which could be called 'religious', and that such values correlated positively with mental health. Bergin's 'coming out'—religion being the 'last taboo', after sex and death, in psychotherapy—led, he claimed, to an explosion of requests for reprints, and initiated intense research activity in the field of values in psychotherapy.

Some important findings have emerged from this work. Strongly held religious beliefs are indeed protective against mental illness (for further discussion see ref. 22). Process researchers have investigated the question of whether congruence between the values held by patient and therapist are linked to a favourable outcome. Patients do assimilate their therapists' values—at least as perceived by therapists—but the best outcome arises when values shared between patient and therapist are moderately similar, neither too close nor too divergent.[23] This is consistent with viewing autonomy as a goal of therapy since to be autonomous is to discover one's own values, based neither on slavish adherence to, nor rebellious rejection of, authority.

Therapeutic neutrality

Perhaps the most contentious aspect of Bergin's broadside is his assault on the hallowed notion of therapeutic neutrality. Even the most 'non-directive' of therapists espouse firmly held values and that it helps if they are explicit about, for example, their judgement regarding: freedom, marital fidelity, work, truthfulness, and the spiritual dimension of life. Bergin's argument is however weakened by conflation of ethical *frameworks* with *techniques*, and by his failure to distinguish different *levels* of values.

Of course therapists operate within an implicit moral framework, but a key component is to suspend judgement through creating an atmosphere of tolerance. A balance has to be struck between facilitating a trusting relationship in which the therapist lets the patient know that they share values, and the need to be reticent if unconscious feelings are to surface in the service of fostering the patient's self-awareness and autonomy. People might, for different reasons, seek out Christian counselling, feminist psychoanalysis, or a therapist from the same ethnic group as themselves. Therapist and patient need to inhabit a similar overall moral universe and thus share 'higher level' moral assumptions. But at the level of specific beliefs—for example that abortion is always wrong, marriage invariably disadvantages women—the therapist's values, if they intrude, may hinder progress.

Values in practice

Bloch *et al.*[7] show how the therapist approaching a family is inescapably caught up in moral choices and has to maintain a delicate balance between his/ her personal moral framework and those of the family and the wider society. These choices exist on the fringes, a drumbeat that draws the therapy in one direction or another, and which arise out of the therapeutic context that is being created, but of which therapist and patient may be only dimly aware. For example, therapies with patients who have been abused can assume a flavour of righteous anger and blame, in which the patient is exclusively seen as a victim. Other approaches might examine the patient's contribution to their own continuing sense of victimhood and stress personal responsibility. Others might try to help the patient move from hatred and blame to understanding and acceptance. Whatever the approach, the ethical themes of suffering, retribution, forgiveness, justice, and responsibility are unavoidable.

If the unique feature of analytic psychotherapy as a system of expert knowledge is its emphasis on the workings of the unconscious, then therapists must strive to recognize out-of-awareness moral influences. Values operate mainly at an unconscious level and arise out of developmental experiences that precede rational thought. In his notion of reaction formation Freud saw that consciously held values may be defences against forces of envy, hate, and destructiveness, the very opposite of those that are overtly espoused. Therapists should make deliberate efforts to become aware of how their own values affect their work. 'Was I too encouraging when the patient announced that she intended to leave her husband?' 'Did I side too openly with the adolescent in his rebellion against his rigid, militaristic father?' 'Did I appear morally censorious, enthusiastic, or pruriently curious when a man boasted of his sexual conquests?' 'Was there an edge of aggression in my challenge to an agoraphobic patient's fears?' 'Was I impatient with the emotional withdrawal of a person suffering from schizophrenia?'

These everyday questions may be subsumed under the heading of 'examining the ethical countertransference'. Symington[24] sees the process of self-examination as based on the Socratic principle that one cannot do something vicious and know that one is doing it at the same time, which brings us back to what might be the most central psychotherapeutic value—the Delphic injunction to 'know yourself'.

Moral outcomes in psychotherapy are inherently subtle. For Bergin marital fidelity is an absolute value to which all therapists should aspire. But the *moral* quality of 'fidelity' is exactly what might be at stake in a therapy. Thus patients might enter therapy with sexual difficulties which mean they are 'unable' to be unfaithful to their partner but at termination have achieved the confidence to do so, but decide to opt for fidelity because their current relationship is now more satisfying, and they choose not to cause unhappiness, seeing that as a greater good than momentary pleasure. The key issue is not so much 'fidelity' in itself, as autonomy and the capacity for intimacy, the basis of mature fidelity.

Recovered memories and the 'ethical countertransference'

The confluence of ethics, values, and techniques is nowhere more apparent than in the heated debate about recovered memories in psychotherapy, and the so-called 'false memory syndrome'.[25–27] On the one side are those who see the ills of patients as springing from repressed abuse in childhood, and that the function of therapy is to bring forgotten memories into awareness and so, through catharsis, transcend them and their effects. On the other, are those who claim that these so-called memories are often implanted in the patient's mind by overenthusiastic therapists, determined to find a scapegoat for the ills of modern life and to produce a coherent story of neurosis. Families of 'victims' whose abuse has been 'discovered' in the course of therapy claim that they themselves have been victimized and have banded together into self-help organizations, mirroring those formed by abuse sufferers.

In this maelstrom, therapists are branded as either saviours or witch-hunters, diligent seekers after hidden truths, or malicious creators of hysteria and misery. In the face of this, a cool head and ethical probity are essential if psychotherapy is to retain balance and a good reputation. A starting point is the extensive cognitive and psychological research on the nature of memory and its failings.

Many therapists base their work around Freud's pre-1897 model of hysteria: symptoms equal repression equals abuse, ergo therapy equals remembering equals recovery. Some proceed as though unaware of the subsequent history and findings of psychoanalysis and cognitive psychology. There is undoubtedly truth in these original ideas, especially in relation to childhood abuse. Memories are often kept partially out of awareness. When they do surface they threaten to overwhelm the sufferer, who often develops symptoms (which in the nineteenth century were labelled as 'hysteria': feelings of panic, nausea, dizziness, sexual difficulties, and so on). The 'recovery' of memories often arises out of a contemporaneous trigger, such as a relationship difficulty or a child reaching the age the sufferer was when abused. Epidemiological evidence, however, suggests that *total* amnesia for abuse is rare, although amnesia for events before the age of two is universal (in any event abuse in that period is most unusual). In one study of women known to have been abused in childhood only 20 per cent could not recall it.[28] Much more common are patterns of unassimilated memory: facts are recalled but not feelings, or the individual develops trance-like states in which past and present are confused.

Prima facie evidence also exists that 'false memories' are possible, even if their prevalence is low. It is well established that the past takes on a negative colouring in depressed states, and that apparently robust memories of trauma are often questioned once the patient recovers. Similarly, depressed people regress to a paranoid–schizoid state in which, in Kleinian terms, there is a need to blame and which resolves when they feel better. There is also good data that memories can be 'created' through suggestion. Misrecall is enhanced in ways that is likely to occur in an intense therapeutic relationship: when the one who suggests is in a position of authority, the time between event and suggestion is long, the suggestions are frequently repeated, they are plausible, and when the 'suggestor' describes a possible scenario to which the subject is merely asked to give a yes or no answer—this then may lead to circumstantial elaboration.[28]

At worst, 'false memory' arises out of errors of logic. *Post hoc, propter hoc* bedevils discussion of causality in psychotherapy. Even if the simple recovery of memories did lead to cure —and there is little evidence that it does—that would not prove that forgetting trauma is pathogenic. Childhood trauma and abuse undoubtedly comprise significant vulnerability factors for adult disorder, but are not by themselves causes.[29] We need to know more about intervening variables, of which 'memory', in the sense of how the world is and was construed, is significant. A second error of logic is that of the 'undistributed middle'. Thus the argument: 'bulimic women have been sexually abused in childhood, you are bulimic, therefore you must have been sexually abused in childhood (even if you have no recall)' is logically unsound, although widely believed.[30]

In view of this confusing picture and of the confirmed effect of suggestion on vulnerable sufferers, it is crucial that therapists retain a position of neutrality so that the patient can use this space of creative uncertainty to explore the relative contributions of what might have happened in reality, what might have been repressed, and what might be a construction arising out of current need.[31] Livingstone-Smith has argued that Freud's 'seduction hypothesis' was a projection into the past of the current interaction between therapist and patient. In order to do this the therapist has to be self-reflective, monitoring her own thoughts, interpretations and actions as part of the interaction between herself and her patient.

The therapist has to steer a tricky course between helping the patient to face past harm and, on occasion, seek justice and retribution for it, while retaining objectivity to distinguish between wishes and feelings (her own and the patient's) as opposed to the factual truth. This position revolves around a version of psychotherapeutic ethics, in which self-reflection (the capacity to adopt a 'meta-perspective') is a core ingredient.

My own inclination is to view the therapist as predominantly an observer, referee and facilitator and only as an indirect agent of change. But in some forms of therapy the therapist is much more involved and collaborative, such as in behaviour therapy. But here too, although *techniques* may be active, the *stance* of the therapist is still one of concerned detachment, non-possessive warmth, or what I have called non-attachment,[22] even if to combine these ideals is challenging. This brings us, finally, to the topic of the regulation of therapists by the profession itself, and in society generally.

Codes of ethics and guidelines for good practice

The 1990s have seen a concerted effort towards the professionalization of psychotherapy. There may be a paradox in the attempt to institutionalize an activity, the practice of which requires a certain detachment from the prevailing mores of society. Even if that is not seen as a hindrance, regulating an activity as diverse of psychotherapy is daunting. Nevertheless, the ethical principles of good practice are common to all forms of therapy. For example, all member organizations of the United Kingdom Council for Psychotherapy are required to produce ethical guidelines together with codes of practice which interpret these principles in the light of the specific technical aspects of their approach. Codes of practice contain sections on the responsibility of practitioners to match therapy to patient need, to respect confidentiality, not to exploit patients sexually or financially, and to receive supervision and continuing education. Member organizations are required to have procedures to examine complaints against practitioners, and to discipline and, if necessary, expel errant therapists.

As well as benefiting the public, regulation has a self-serving aspect in lending respectability to the profession. It also has the advantage of taking contentious issues out of the consulting room and viewing them in the public arena, thereby enabling the practitioner to remain neutral. A good example is the question of whether homosexuality should be regarded as psychopathological. If the profession as a whole concludes that homosexuality is a variant of normal human behaviour, and is no more or less 'pathological' than aspects of heterosexuality, and declares that there should be no discrimination against homosexual applicants for psychotherapy training, this enables the specific problems associated with an individual's sexuality to be dealt with on its merits in the consulting room, without becoming politicized. Similarly, a statement about the reality of repressed memory *and* the risk of implanting memories with certain techniques can help take the heat out of cases arising in practice; the recovered memory debate does not have to be fought out with each patient.

Codes of practice create a 'Ten Commandments' of external principles against which the realities of practice can be judged, and justice disposed in the public interest. Psychotherapy is possibly unique as a profession in developing a nuanced stance on ethical practice. Psychotherapy is arguably the least technical of the professions, based as it is on a conversation between two people and the 'normal' things that go on in relationships—sexual feelings, differences in power, various forms of coercion, and so on. Psychotherapy is special because these are the focus of the therapy itself, not a by-product of the professional relationship.

Psychotherapy is also ethically special in that it differentiates between external prohibitions (represented by the 'superego'), and values in which the harshness of the superego is modified and incorporated into more mature ego functioning. With its emphasis on personal development for psychotherapists as well as patients, it can claim that to treat others as one would wish to be treated oneself, and to 'love one's patients', in the sense of approaching them with concern, tenderness and respect (and firmness when necessary, since limit-setting can be an aspect of love) are aspects of the maturity which training aims to foster. These are ambitious claims; whether they are achieved, and how this is evaluated, are matters for research.

Psychotherapy as an independent profession has emerged out of two parent disciplines, medicine and clinical psychology, each of which has its own set of ethical principles. Medical ethics has been forged over two millennia. Psychotherapeutic ethics is strongly based on medical ethics; the two professions are in a position to exert mutual influence. Medical practice aspires to be 'evidence-based', and this has clear ethical implications. To offer treatment for which no evidence of efficacy is available contravenes the principle of beneficence, although non-maleficence remains a prime responsibility (it is much worse to do harm than simply not to do any good). The need for evidence-based psychotherapy is increasingly recognised, a direct result of this principle. Conversely, psychotherapy's appreciation of transference and countertransference can help medicine to achieve a more mature appreciation of the doctor-patient relationship, and so promote understanding of its pitfalls and risks.

Conclusion

To conclude, I have argued that ethics and psychotherapy are inseparable. Technically good therapy will inevitably be ethically sound, and an ethically correct approach to patients will in itself be therapeutically beneficial. I have emphasized the need for psychotherapy research to underpin ethical practice, especially in the area of informed consent. I have suggested that exploitation in therapy can be understood in terms of boundary violation; supervision and self-awareness in therapist are the best safeguards against such infringement. Finally, I have argued for a balance between involvement and neutrality (or 'non-attachment') as the most desirable position from which to practise ethical psychotherapy.

References

1. Beauchamp, T.: The 'four principles' approach. In R. Gillon (ed.) *Principles of health care ethics*. Wiley, Chichester, pp. 3–12, 1994.
2. Holmes, J. and Lindley, R.: *The values of psychotherapy*. 2nd edn. Karnac, London, 1998.
3. Aveline, M. and Shapiro, D.: *Research foundations for psychotherapy practice*. Wiley, Chichester, 1995.
4. Roth, A. and Fonagy, P.: *What works for whom? A critical review of psychotherapy research*. Guilford Press, New York, 1996.
5. Parry, G. and Richardson, A.: *NHS services in England: review of strategic policy*. London, National Health Service, 1996.
6. Holmes, D.: Race and transference in psychoanalysis and psychotherapy. *International Journal of Psycho-Analysis*, **73**, 1–11, 1992.
7. Bloch, S., Hafner, J., Harari, E., and Szmukler, G.: *The family in clinical psychiatry*. Oxford University Press, Oxford, 1994.
8. Amies, P.: Psychotherapy patients: are they the 'worried well'? *Psychiatric Bulletin*, **20**, 153–6, 1996.
9. Mace, C. (ed.): *The art and science of assessment in psychotherapy*. Routledge, London, 1995.
10. Goldberg, A.: Writing case histories. *International Journal of Psycho-Analysis*, **78**, 435–8, 1997.

11. Stoller, R.: Patients' responses to their own case reports. *Journal of the American Psychoanalytic Association*, **36**, 371–92, 1988.
12. Malan, D.: *Individual psychotherapy and the science of psychodynamics*. 2nd edn. Butterworth, London, 1996.
13. Karasu, B.: Ethical issues in psychotherapy practice. In S. Bloch (ed.) *Introduction to the psychotherapies*. Oxford, Oxford University Press, 1996.
14. Leong, G., Eth, S., and Silvia, A.: The psychotherapist as witness for the prosecution: the criminalisation of Tarasoff. *American Journal of Psychiatry*, **149**, 1011–15, 1992.
15. Turner, M. and Kennedy, M.: Tarasoff and the duty to warn third parties. *Psychiatric Bulletin*, **21**, 465–6, 1997.
16. Orlinsky, D., Grawe, K., and Parks, B.: Process and outcome in psychotherapy. In ed. A. Bergin and S. Garfield. *Handbook of psychotherapy and behaviour change*. Wiley, New York, pp. 270–376, 1994.
17. Symington, N.: The analyst's act of freedom as an agent of therapeutic change. In G. Kohon (ed.) *The British school of psychoanalysis: the independent tradition*. Free Association, London, pp. 253–270, 1986.
18. Reiff, P.: *Freud: the mind of the moralist*. University of Chicago Press, Chicago, 1959.
19. Bowlby, J.: *A secure base: clinical applications of attachment theory*. Routledge, London, 1988.
20. Hinshelwood, R.: *Therapy or coercion? Does psychoanalysis differ from brainwashing?* Karnac, London, 1997.
21. Bergin, A.: Values and religious issues in psychotherapy and mental health. *American Psychologist*, **46**, 394–403, 1991.
22. Holmes, J.: Values in psychotherapy. *American Journal of Psychotherapy*, **50**, 259–73, 1996.
23. Bergin, A., Stinchfield, R., Gaskin, T., *et al.*: Religious life-styles and mental health: an exploratory study. *Journal of Consulting and Clinical Psychology*, **35**, 91–8 1988.
24. Symington, N.: *Emotion and spirit*. Karnac, London, 1994.
25. Loftus, E. and Ketcham, K.: *The myth of repressed memory*. St Martin's Press, New York, 1994.
26. Mollon, P.:. The memory debate: a consideration of clinical complexities and some suggested guidelines for psychoanalytic therapists. *British Journal of Psychotherapy*, **11**, 193–203, 1996
27. Holmes, J.: Psychotherapy and memory: an attachment perspective. *British Journal of Psychotherapy*, **13**, 204–19, 1996.
28. Lindsay, D. and Read, J.: Psychotherapy and memories of childhood sexual abuse: a cognitive perspective. *Applied Cognitive Psychology*, **8**, 281–338, 1994.
29. Mullen, P., Romans-Clarkson, S., Walton, V., and Herbison, P.: Impact of sexual and physical abuse on women's mental health. *Lancet*, **344**, 841–5, 1993.
30. Poole, D., Lindsay, D., Memon, S., and Bull, R.: Psychotherapy and the recovery of memories of childhood sexual abuse: US and British practitioners opinions, practices and experiences. *Journal of Counselling and Clinical Psychology*, **63**, 426–37, 1995.
31. Livingstone-Smith, D.: *Hidden conversations: Introduction to communicative psychoanalysis*. Routledge, London, 1991.
32. Holmes, J.: *Attachment, intimacy, autonomy: using attachment theory in adult psychotherapy*. Jason Aronson, New York, 1996.

12

Ethical aspects of drug treatment

Paul Brown and Christos Pantelis

Introduction

Contemporary approaches to drug treatment in psychiatry have been influenced by two parallel processes, one linear and scientific and the second cyclic and economic.

The scientific process, characterized as the psychotropic drug revolution, was inaugurated in 1952 with the discovery of chlorpromazine's efficacy in schizophrenia.[1] This was soon followed by the development of potent preparations for depression (imipramine, 1958[2]) and anxiety (librium/chlordiazepoxide, 1960[3]). Lithium, discovered in 1949, was not available until the 1960s because of fears of toxicity.[4] During this period clinicians optimistically believed that specific conditions could be managed with specific drugs, and saw a decline in the number of patients they treated in hospital. Claims of the proven effectiveness of these drugs ensued.[5] However, the context in which treatment was provided was largely ignored. Deinstitutionalization led to widespread therapeutic neglect, since community resources were inadequate to meet the needs of the chronically ill. This led not only to homelessness and rehospitalization but also to an unanticipated cost 'blow-out' in outpatient drug and other psychiatric treatments. The introduction of expensive novel drugs to treat schizophrenia and anxiety disorders exacerbated this problem. Drug treatment ethics initially centred on informed consent, risk–benefit analysis, professional accountability, and the Hippocratic Oath. A scientific and ethical backlash followed in the 1960s and 1970s. Challenges to perceived pharmacological scientism and paternalistic control came from across the spectrum of opinion, from radical psychiatrists[6,7] to moderate mental health professionals.[8] Clinical and ethical concerns then shifted to the public domain, with a focus on respect for patient autonomy and justice. A spate of actions in the US Federal Courts sought first to uphold a right to treatment and subsequently a right to refuse treatment. It became apparent that traditional systems and ethical guidelines based on autonomy, fidelity, and justice (which themselves could be reduced to beneficence and non-maleficence),[9] were too diffuse to deal with even in routine practice. Systems of meta-ethics or applied ethics were required to address specific ethical dilemmas, for instance to reconcile competing interests of patients (and their lobbies), clinicians (and their professional bodies), and society at large including those in the legal and political arenas. From the 1980s, professional standards were established on codes of practice, quality assurance and accountability, and the right to effective treatment.

At the fin de siècle, the downturn in the economic cycle and concomitant surge in costs threatened to oust decisions based solely on risk–benefit analysis and clinical science from centre stage. Restricted national budgets, substantially increased costs of community care, and the introduction of expensive novel drugs, shifted ethical concerns from those based on safety, standards, and rights, to those governed by budget restrictions. In short, governments and patients seek value for money, whereas business seeks a return on its investments. It is within this climate that we consider the ethics of drug treatment. We first consider risks and benefits of treatment and then the doctor–patient relationship in relation to drug prescription and informed consent. These issues lead to a discussion on doctors' duties and patients' rights. Finally, we deal with pharmacoeconomic issues. Ethical concerns affect not only patient and doctor but also other key players, such as the family, the media, the courts, drug companies, politicians, and third-party insurers.

Risks and benefits of drug treatment

The psychiatrist's decision to prescribe a drug is based on a scientifically—and consensually—informed consideration of risks and benefits. However, value judgements often influence the decision and, as we shall see, these can be politico-economic as much as professional.

Risks

The continuing development of new applications for existing drugs and of new psychotropic drugs—some even designated as 'designer drugs'—is associated with certain risks and benefits. The most notable developments have been the selective serotonin reuptake inhibitor group of antidepressants (e.g. fluoxetine and paroxetine), and the atypical anti-psychotics (e.g. clozapine, risperidone, and olanzapine). These drug advances, however, have not been matched by the elucidation of their mechanism of action. This has led to what has been called 'panacea therapy', the use of drugs for non-primary purposes, untested drug combinations, polypharmacy, and high- or mega-dosages with concomitant risk to the patient.

Scientific guidelines for drug treatment in psychiatry remain incomplete. Consider the benzodiazepines. Until the early 1990s, the clinical consensus was that injudicious use risked dependence.[10,11] However, scientific evidence then emerged that this problem had been exaggerated.[12,13] Ballenger[12] summarized the evidence as follows: 'most patients overcome withdrawal symptoms without much difficulty'. He further noted that the benzodiazepine, alprazolam, had been approved by the US Food and Drug Administration in 1992 for the treatment of panic disorder. Clearly, a decade of media and professional fears of dependence must take into account up-to-date scientific knowledge.

Another example where scientific guidelines have been in a state of flux is in the use of high-dose strategies to treat resistant schizophrenia (see ref. 14). There is no firm research evidence to support dose elevation; great care in the use of high doses is advocated,[15,16] particularly in the light of the potential for serious side-effects.[15] On the other hand, prescribing low doses of antipsychotics, as recommended by some clinicians (to reduce side-effects like tardive dyskinesia), significantly increases the risk of relapse.[17] Research helps to guide the clinician but it is often impossible to cover complex individual variations.

As advances in drug treatment levelled off in the 1980s, evidence for a vast undiagnosed reservoir of major mental illness in the community emerged. Notable were Goldberg and Huxley's[18] community surveys of depression, which revealed that overt mood disorder was but the tip of an iceberg. Traditional treatments reached only up to two-thirds of potential patients. A considerable need existed for potent new preparations. However, trazodone, a second-generation antidepressant, and zimelidine proved hazardous.

The introduction of the selective serotonin reuptake inhibitors (SSRIs) appeared to herald a second drug revolution. Extravagant claims were made, particularly in the light of an improved adverse-event profile, superior efficacy,[19,20] substantially fewer deaths in overdose than first-generation antidepressants,[21] and better compliance.[22] Indiscriminate use of SSRIs ensued with their inevitable application in non-depressed groups, for example in personality disordered patients. In addition, widespread advertising and 'media hype' also led to their popularity. At the height of the initial enthusiasm, SSRIs were given to enhance mood in non-clinical populations, and even to pets! When they proved ineffective, novel and risky drug combinations were tried. Behavioural reactions, particularly harm to oneself or to others were then ascribed to the SSRIs. There is, however, no evidence that they do trigger suicidal ideas above the usual rates encountered in depression. As competition between drug manufacturers escalated so did claims for a particular SSRI over the others. For example, a drug profile might emphasize relative absence of side-effects or greater potency. Companies also sought new applications for their product, for example for social phobia, dissociative identity disorder[23] and poor impulse control.[24] Mianserin has been recommended to treat sexual dysfunction caused by the SSRIs based on evidence from a single open study.[25] Potter *et al.*[26] have claimed that tricyclic antidepressants 'promise the surest response' in moderate to severe depression.

Drug companies have similarly highlighted the purported efficacy of the atypical antipsychotics in treating negative symptoms of schizophrenia, particularly poverty of speech, blunted affect, social withdrawal, and poor motivation. Given that these symptoms have proved resistant to treatment, manufacturers seek to exploit a 'niche' market. Evidence for their claims, however, are far from definitive[27-29] and few companies have specifically examined this question. Clearly, niche marketing is an ethical minefield, risking inappropriate application.

The traditional treatment of schizophrenia was hampered by motor side-effects, especially tardive dyskinesia and neuroleptic malignant syndrome. Previous evidence suggested that tardive dyskinesia was chronic, often progressive, and difficult to treat. However, evidence has emerged that it is more benign and less progressive following drug discontinuation.[30,31] Also, mortality from neuroleptic malignant syndrome has diminished.[32] The atypical neuroleptics, such as clozapine, act more specifically on mesolimbic than nigrostriatal structures.[33] They are characterized by minimal prolactin elevation, low incidence of extrapyramidal symptoms, and diminished dopaminergic activity in the limbic system.[34,35] Still the most effective of 'atypicals', clozapine, was developed in the 1960s,[33] used outside the US only in the 1970s,[36] and only obtained US Food and Drug Administration approval in 1990. Clozapine was recommended for refractory or medication-intolerant patients. It was thought to be effective against positive symptoms in non-responders to traditional medications. There were also claims for its efficacy in treating negative symptoms, though this remains controversial.[27] The atypical antipsychotics reduce the incidence of extrapyramidal (EP) side-effects; for instance there have been no reports of tardive dyskinesia (see ref. 14 for discussion), and clozapine may improve established tardive dyskinesia.[37] Further, the 'atypicals' improve cognitive deficits in schizophrenia.[38] While clozapine has doubtless improved the quality of life of countless intractable patients, it has not been without shortcomings or complications. From one-third to one-half of patients with treatment-resistant schizophrenia derive no benefit from clozapine.[39] Agranulocytosis, in 1–2 per cent of patients, is occasionally fatal. This has led to a strict protocol of initially weekly laboratory monitoring; mortality has dropped to 1 in 6000 in the US.[40] Other side-effects include seizures and cardiac complications, which may require monitoring. In this regard, Golden et al.[41] note our limited ability to recognize rare but potentially serious side-effects in new agents. This phenomenon has been observed with several drugs. For example, aplastic anaemia with use of the atypical antipsychotic, remoxipride, led to its removal from the market at the time of its launch, while identification of potentially serious cardiomyopathy and myocarditis with clozapine has only become apparent since the mid-1990s.[42]

Strategies to treat optimally and minimise risks from drug complications and toxicity remain disparate. The research literature is only a limited guide. Controversies impacting on clinical decisions include: length of washout period between treatments; use of combined therapy; regimens for initiation of treatments, particularly with newer drugs; optimal dosages; duration of treatment; target symptoms; and, last but by no means least, cost–benefit versus risk–benefit analyses. Resource issues equally affect clinical decisions, e.g. pressure to discharge patients promptly can prevent adequate evaluation of therapy.

A controversy in treating psychosis has centred on prescribing drugs for individuals at 'high-risk' for psychosis before the onset of illness. The argument that medication may prevent the onset of a serious psychiatric illness must be balanced against our inability to predict who will develop the illness and who will not. (Yung and McGorry[43] discuss relevant ethical issues with additional comment provided by Morice.[44])

Risky drug application must be weighed against the collective clinical sense of what is safe. These include use of placebos; combined therapy, for example tricyclics and SSRIs in treatment-resistant depression; polypharmacy, as in dissociative identity disorder with comorbid affective disorder, eating problems, and borderline personality disorder with transient psychosis; and drug-induced sleep therapy for alcoholism and schizophrenia. Preskorn[45] notes that the polypharmacy increases in the elderly, medically ill, and in those with complex, treatment-resistant psychiatric illness. Thus, up to two-thirds of depressed patients are prescribed two or more drugs in addition to their antidepressant, depending on the group studied.

There are ethical drawbacks in prescribing drugs directly from one's office, e.g. dispensing drug samples. As inpatient charts require full and correct labelling, so too must be the containers of outpatient prescribed drugs.

Ethical issues also arise as to whether psychiatrists should prescribe non-psychiatric drugs. The consensus is that specialist assistance is required for the management of ongoing and intercurrent medical conditions in both psychiatric in- and outpatients.

If psychiatric drugs like the antipsychotics are risky, prescribers can be no less-risk prone in their practice. Gullick and King[46] examined the appropriateness of drug treatment prescribed by general practitioners for patients with depression. General practitioners are particularly apt to make inappropriate drug and dose choices. Since the 1990s, growing community need and reduced specialist back-up has led to their greater participation in drug management of the mentally ill. Since the impetus for this is primarily politicoeconomic, risk–benefit must be balanced against cost–benefit. 'Pharmacoeconomic' issues will be discussed later in regard to social justice. Catalan and his colleagues[47] note difficulties in maintaining standards in the long-term treatment of patients with psychotropic drugs by GPs.

As metropolitan psychiatric services grow at the expense of peripheral and particularly rural services, telemedicine has been both advocated[48] and denigrated[49] in the distance-management of patients. Many clinicians acknowledge the increased risk in 'off-sight care' but these approaches will become an increasing reality in times of fiscal restraint.

Drugs and particular patient groups
The effect of both prescribed and illicit drugs on driving, with the potential to harm oneself or others, raises the question of medical responsibility to inform third parties such as police, licensing bodies, and families. Statutory guidelines

are in the offing in some countries but, in their absence, it is incumbent upon the therapist to discuss these matters with the patient and significant others and to mediate between the driver and third parties.

Drug use in pregnancy requires careful consideration. Illness relapse and its consequences must be weighed against the risk of harm by drugs to the fetus. Antenatal depression may be of such severity as to raise the issue of termination of pregnancy. The risk–benefit of medicating must then be carefully considered.

There is increasing awareness of the risk of self-harm, particularly with over-the-counter preparations. A significant proportion of cases involve large amounts and multiple substances often in people with personality disorders, and particularly in those who self-medicate repeatedly. Risk factors include less supervised programmes, and doctors with large numbers of complex patients.

Benefits

Psychotropic drugs are generally acclaimed by psychiatrists (and many patient-advocates) as bringing substantial benefits. They reduce symptoms and the rate of relapse, and extend the gap between illness episodes. However, when drug trials are scrutinized, benefits are much more qualified. Close examination of double-blind, controlled studies of antipsychotics[5] show a combined rate of placebo response and spontaneous remission of between 20 and 30 per cent, with up to a quarter of improved groups due to non-specific effects. Less than half the patients in these studies derive any direct benefit from the drug. Furthermore, trials tend to recruit cooperative patients, thereby introducing a bias; efficacy may be far less than the evidence suggests.

If drugs are less effective than claimed, comparative efficacy has yet to be established. Hope for a typology of antidepressants linking symptoms with receptor sensitivities has thus far proved unfounded. Drugs do differ in potency and side-effects, but there is frequently little to distinguish between them, or between drugs and alternative biological and psychological therapies,[50] thereby obscuring therapeutic guidelines. The usual strategy with antipsychotics following a poor response is to switch to a drug from another class (e.g. phenothiazine, thioxanthene, butyrophenone). With the introduction of drugs with greater specificity and more complex receptor activity, alternative strategies, such as trialing drugs with different receptor profiles, may prove more useful.[14] There is also encouraging evidence for specificity of new atypicals in ameliorating neuropsychological deficits,[38] suggesting that classical symptoms may not be the only target for therapeutic action.

How should we decide between various drugs? How should we evaluate evidence without prejudice? If science steps aside, the courts, governments, and industry step in to make their claims. Stockler and Coates[51] advocate a dispassionate approach based on scientific methods, in particular randomized, controlled clinical trials rather than reviews, consensus views, and medical authority. Since individual trials are too small to define therapeutic differences validly, statistical methods have evolved to evaluate series of trials. Meta-analysis integrates data from many studies to produce an estimate of the size of an effect—well-performed meta-analyses represent the highest level of scientific evidence.

This approach has been adopted on a large scale by the Cochrane collaboration which seeks to summarize available efficacy data from all well-designed, randomized controlled trials (including those unpublished).[52] However, this approach has its hazards, for example, there is an inherent bias in the type of patient recruited to trials, and it has been suggested that complementary naturalistic studies are needed.[53] Moreover, trials are commonly reported before all the data (often adverse) are finally in. It is the number of events, not the number of subjects, that determine a trial's power.[54] Both selection of trials and extraction of data are potential sources of bias. As Eysenck[55] once noted: 'garbage in, garbage out'. Meta-analyses using different inclusion criteria may come to opposite conclusions. However, although meta-analysis has its limits, it can provide compelling evidence for efficacy and guidelines for its critical appraisal are available.[56,57]

Collaboration of researchers, clinicians, journal editors and drug companies in drug evaluation is ethically fraught. Pressure may be brought to bear covertly on the researcher to suppress disclosure of negative and promote only positive findings. Negative results are less likely to reach publication since the researcher may lose interest in the study or find it difficult to publish negative results. An ethical duty demands that relevant parties disclose all findings, and above all negative outcomes. There have also been overt inducements to clinicians—some financial but mostly books, equipment, and travel—to prescribe through participation in 'pseudo-research', for example, sham, post-launch therapeutic studies.

In 1993, in the face of errant laboratories and doctors, legislation by the French Competition and Anti-Fraud Department—supported by the threat of severe financial penalties or incarceration—stipulated that written agreements with laboratories specifying 'the explicit purpose and real aim of the research or scientific evaluation' involved must be submitted for review by the local branch of the medical association.[58] Pharmaceutical and medical associations need to seek balanced rules with clear guidelines as to what is permitted and what is not. Ethics committees have a central role here and have become more sophisticated in evaluating drug study protocols and drug company participation.

Psychotropic drugs and the boundaries of mental illness

Although contemporary nosology, embracing the core disorders of schizophrenia, depression, and organic brain syndromes, is now well established (for example in DSM-IV[59]), there has been a parallel trend to broaden the definition of mental illness. This has resulted periodically in a risk of inappropriate medi-calization and associated abuse of treatment in order to exert social control.

Klerman and Schechter[60] proposed a triple diagnostic spectrum from core mental illness, to stress disorders, to mental health. Extended diagnostic definitions can occur in each category. The diagnosis of schizophrenia, for instance, has been malignantly applied to dissidents with all the risks alluded to earlier (see Chapter 10).

Included in the compendium of DSM-IV are stress disorders whose diagnostic status is still under investigation. Boon and Draijer[61] regard post-traumatic disorders as extending beyond post-traumatic stress disorder (PTSD) to multiple personality disorder and personality disorder associated with childhood sexual and physical abuse. While recognizing the psychiatric con-sequences of objective trauma, Ball[62] and Burges Watson[63] have cautioned against medicalization, and the drug treatment of what may be normal re-sponses to trauma. More contentious is the status of dissociative identity dis-order,[64] included in DSM-III[65] and DSM-IV,[59] but regarded by Kihlstrom[66] as an iatrogenic state and a manifestation of the 'false memory syndrome'. The psychotropic treatment of these disorders is notoriously difficult; no established guidelines for existing preparations, particularly combinations, are available. Nevertheless, Davidson and van der Kolk[67] have attempted to provide guidelines to treat target symptoms in PTSD, while Krystal *et al.*[68] have offered pointers to a rational approach to the pharmacological treatment of dissociative disorders.

Among stress responses closest to the border of mental illness are 'work stresses'. National Insurance for Worker's compensation was introduced in the UK in the 1880's[69] and since the late nineteenth century the borderlands between work stress and malingering or compensation neurosis in the indus-trial arena have been hotly and unceasingly debated in the Western World. Even when work stress is real, solutions may be only partially medical. The risk is to remove a person from the work arena and the domain of rehabilitation and establishing, maintaining, and 'chronifying' distress. Cases, which might otherwise be briefly treated medically as a prelude to rehabilitation, can be-come chronic while awaiting resolution of compensation claims.

Societal pressure, for example on harassed housewives (and exasperated executives), led to the demand for chemical relief and chemical enhancement of human potential with the use of 'designer drugs'. Fluoxetine has been promoted as a mood enhancer in normal people. Drugs to improve memory,[70] steroids and growth hormone derivatives to boost physical prowess in competitive sport, and vitamins and minerals and orthomolecular psychiatry to ensure *joie de vivre* are further illustrations. There have even been advocates for the use of hallucinogenic drugs in the quest for 'enlightenment'.[71] Massive promotional campaigns supported by media hype and quasi-documentaries have influenced the public to expect or even demand these drugs. Several books for the public have projected fluoxetine to the centre of populist therapeutics.

In child psychiatry, attention-deficit hyperactivity disorder (ADHD) was previously considered either as a condition requiring treatment or as an expedient term to disguise a social problem.[72] This controversy was compounded by treatment involving two potentially addictive drugs, methylphenidate and dextroamphetamine.[73] This controversy has not been fully resolved (see Chapter 14).

Similarly, drug management of behaviourally disturbed psychiatric patients or behaviourally disturbed, intellectually retarded people can come perilously close to restraint which serves the needs of the family or the institution rather than meeting the need for understanding and empathy. Most psychiatrists would agree that medication is warranted in cases of danger and emergency. The situation is more difficult to resolve when the underlying cause for the disturbed behaviour is not established, for example a legitimate protest quelled by the staff as a response to their own fears.[74] Analogous abuse of diagnosis and treatment by mental health professionals has been observed in the extreme political context of the Nazi and Soviet eras (see Chapter 4).[75] It is the responsibility of those dealing with the mentally ill to make an accurate assessment of the disturbed behaviour and its underlying significance, and to adopt an approach which considers sympathetically the interests of all concerned, particularly respect for patients' basic rights.

The treatment relationship and prescribing drugs

The doctor–patient relationship

The revolutionary contribution of psychoanalysis to the conceptualization and management of the doctor–patient relationship following World War II virtually passed psychopharmacology by. Psychiatrists with a biological orientation at times retreated into their traditional roles as arbiters of medical science, and subordinated the establishment of a treatment alliance promoting compliance. However, initial concerns regarding the detriment of informing patients about unwanted drug effects, and of involving them in treatment decisions, were overtaken by other concerns engendered by heightened public awareness of the risks of psychotropic drugs. This was particularly fostered by the electronic media, bolstered by the growth of consumerism and an energetic civil-rights movement.

If the substantive basis of ethical prescribing is a comprehensive knowledge of risks and benefits, the procedural basis for protecting patients and their rights is the doctor–patient relationship, particularly mediated by the doctrine of informed consent. Dyer and Bloch[76] have incorporated these ethical dimensions of the therapeutic relationship into the concept of the ethical alliance. Three principles compete for an ethical basis of the therapist–patient relationship: paternalism; respect for autonomy; and mutual trust (the fiduciary principle). Drawing on these, Dyer and Bloch[76] have described three *de facto* approaches to the therapist–patient relationship, ranging from complete ethical neutrality to total personal involvement. For example, a minimalist position favoured by Carl Rogers contrasts with that of Robert Jay Lifton who adopted a declarative stand and corresponding value transparency. Dyer and Bloch[76] proposed an intermediate, fiduciary approach based on therapeutic partnership and informed consent. The latter has three components: it must be informed, voluntary, and competent. In this context, information refers to ethical as much as substantive clinical data. Informed consent was further conceptualized as a dynamic, continuously evolving, interactional process. The therapist in recognition of his moral role acts as a so-called 'ethical interventionist'. Value testing occurs at all stages of treatment, the therapist monitoring his personal values so as not to burden the patient.

In the context of drug treatment the psychiatrist–patient relationship is fraught with difficulty. Lack of trust, inadequate communication, and manipulative and coercive tactics by therapist or patient can easily undermine the ethical basis of drug treatment as much as any drug hazards. And yet it is this very relationship which is necessary for the optimal application of informed consent.

Information

Psychiatrists have long sought to promote dissemination of accurate information over misinformation in the media. Since the 1990s, advances in communication technology have led to wider patient access to information, particularly through the internet. This ranges from access to the results of drug trials (sometimes pre-publication) to views on drugs offered on the homepages of an individual's and patient lobby groups. A need clearly exists to provide accurate and balanced information so as to minimize the risk of harm and enhance the process of informed consent.

Informed consent

Informed consent provides both an ethical and a legal framework for the therapist–patient relationship, and practical guidelines concerning the decision to treat. In this regard Winslade[77] advocates respect for persons over paternalism. Informed consent is often conceived of as a linear process: the therapist explains the risks and benefits of a treatment, the risks and benefits of therapeutic alternatives including no treatment, and the patient chooses one of the options. In a comprehensive meta-analysis of a variety of education strategies about medications, most proved beneficial producing gains in drug knowledge and a reduction in erroneous drug use.[78] However, there are obvious limitations with certain groups of the mentally ill.

Two contextual factors—patient freedom and patient competence to consent—render medical decision-making interactional and hence recursive, and much more than a mere paper exercise.[79] To ensure freely given consent, the therapist is required to discuss treatment recommendations thoroughly, objectively weighing up the patient's treatment requests. In non-urgent cases, the psychiatrist must be prepared to accede to drug refusal. However, each case must be evaluated by objective criteria.

Competence is defined as the patient's ability to understand, communicate, deliberate, and make rational choices.[80] Consent is adjudged to have occurred, not when patients have merely had the risks explained and have voluntarily accepted them, but only when they are also competent to do so. Belmaker *et al.*[80] argue that the patient's capacity to give truly informed consent varies with the diagnosis and the therapeutic context. Thus, medical and judicial consensus exists on the necessity to waive the process of informed consent in patients rendered incompetent through major mental illness, particularly psychotic disorders.

Appelbaum and Grisso[81] have explored patient decision-making in a large-scale, multicentre study. In this study, four abilities were evaluated: to make a choice; to understand information; to appreciate one's own situation; and to reason with information. The researchers concluded that patients are usually able to make competent decisions, thereby challenging stereotypic medical attitudes. The more rigorous the standards used in assessing competence, the more likely were patients to be deemed competent. These studies indicate that validity of assessment is a potential limiting factor, and greater credence must be granted to the consumer.

In the absence of firm guidelines on competence, and with an established civil-rights lobby, some American states have resorted to the legal doctrine of substituted judgement.[82] This requires that any treatment that the patient would have chosen, had he been able to choose, may be given. But who then should decide, and which procedures and criteria should be used. Suggested approaches range from judicial processes involving independent psychiatrists to informal review with the treating psychiatrist liasing with a legally appointed guardian.

Increasing empirical findings of deficiencies in the process of information delivery and patient retention have paralleled rising medico-legal expectations of the process of informed consent. Doctors cannot be perfect communicators, and patient retention rates are all too brief. In a study of hospital patients in the 1980s, only 18 per cent proved to be fully competent at initial assessment.[83] The remainder were ignorant of important side-effects such as tardive dyskinesia, and lacked a rational understanding of the relevance of medication. Only 36 per cent were able to demonstrate factual knowledge within 48 hours. These researchers then improved their methodology, and studied two groups of schizophrenic outpatients.[84] One group received a single information session on tardive dyskinesia while the other group had this session followed by a review meeting. Both groups demonstrated significantly improved knowledge of tardive dyskinesia. At two-year follow-up, the findings were confirmed.[85] Furthermore, while patients in these studies reported anxiety as a result of the information given there was no clinical deterioration or increase in compliance problems.

Prescription standards and guidelines

A controversial landmark case in Australia (*Rogers* v. *Whitaker*[86]) has focused attention on the relationship between the moral and legal ethics of medical treatment. Although the case related to a surgical intervention, the principles of the Australian High Court's judgement apply equally to drug treatment. The patient underwent cosmetic surgery to a blind eye and tragically suffered sympathetic ophthalmia in the unaffected eye with complete blindness the result. She had not been warned about this rare complication, despite requests for information on potential risks. The High Court dismissed Dr Roger's appeal, emphasizing the legal duty of doctors to provide adequate information about treatment options and material risks. It based its judgment on whether his conduct conformed to the standard of reasonable care demanded by the law rather than the standard in accord with mainstream medical opinion. Thus, information about risks and benefits must be dictated by individual patient expectations rather than by the norms of a professional peer group. Sexton[87] argues that *Rogers* v. *Whitaker*[86] implies that the medical profession failed to recognize that the standards of informed consent expected by the community no longer coincide with those of the profession. Nevertheless, he predicted that the courts would still be influenced by standards set by responsible professional bodies. He has recommended that we avoid arrogance or complacency, and monitor rigorously all standards and review processes. In other words, professional ethics requires an active reappraisal in order to remain in tune with both societal and legal expectations.

Liddel[88] has reviewed professional prescribing standards and related legal requirements. He noted that State Medical Board guidelines in Australia expect prescriptions to be written for specific, identifiable, and justifiable purposes, and warn of disciplinary action if these guidelines are breached. The Code of Ethics of the Australian Medical Association is vaguer, promoting patient autonomy. Neither body gives guidance on professional standards or advice regarding adherence to the law.

In 1989, the Australian Law Reform Commission recommended that the National Health and Medical Research Council (NH&MRC) formulate guidelines for the medical profession regarding the provision of information to patients about treatments and procedures. They also recommended that the common-law standard of reasonable care should not be replaced by statute, but in actions for professional negligence the guidelines would be admissible in evidence. As a result, guidelines were published in 1993. They cover the type of information to be given to patients, the manner of conveying it, and the circumstances for withholding information. The guidelines are based on the principle of self-determination, and expect patients to be given sufficient information to facilitate their own decisions about treatment. This shift to the patient-centred approach was also noted by Sexton.[87]

The Australian National Medicinal Drug Policy deals in part with methods to enhance the management of medications by patients and doctors. Over-prescribing (e.g. of benzodiazepines), drug underuse, polypharmacy, patients at increased risk of adverse drug reactions and compliance problems are examined, as is the need for good communication. Indeed, for the judicious, safe, and appropriate use of medications, better communication between patients and health-care providers must be developed.

Section 63 of the Australian Therapeutic Goods Act 1989 requires that printed consumer–patient information must be given with all new pharmaceutical products. Prescribers face problems with dissemination of such information since it is inordinately long. They may, however, face legal liabilities if they do not disseminate adequate information. The Psychiatric Division of the Victorian Government Department of Human Services subsequently produced a series of pamphlets for patients containing details on various psychotropic drugs (e.g. refs 89,90).

Evidence-based medicine

Guidelines can be provided applying diagnostic group or psychotropic class. Some, as in the psychotropic drug guidelines of the Victorian Postgraduate Medical Federation,[91] combine both. The Royal Australian and New Zealand College of Psychiatrists published *Guidelines for psychotropic drugs in psychiatric practice* in 1994.[92] Adapted from the American Psychiatric Association's *Manual of psychiatric quality assurance*, it is set out according to drug category rather than diagnostic condition. The *Australian psychotropic psychopharma-copoeia*[93] contains prescription guidelines and quality assurance procedures to audit medication use. The latter centres on 'clinical indicators', measures of clinical management, and outcome of care—introduced by the Australian Council of Healthcare Standards in 1996.

Patients' rights

Rights are the justified claims that individuals and groups can make on others and society. Patients are vulnerable to exploitation and require protection.[94] With respect to drug treatment, rights include: access to treatment; provision of necessary information; the freedom to accept or refuse treatment; and a voice in the selection of specific drugs and the conditions under which to take them. The civil liberties movement has promoted these rights since the 1960s. A complex dialectical interplay has ensued between assertion of rights and professional responses. This process was at first often mediated in the courts as much as the clinic or laboratory; only latterly has there been the evolution of clinicoethical responses based on empirically—validated and consensually —agreed guidelines.

We can discern three stages in the evolution of this dialectical process. The demand for the right of access to treatment was followed by the right to refuse treatment, even when it was considered to be optimal. Since the 1990s, there has been a move beyond litigation to promotion of standards and account-ability, and the right to receive effective treatment.

Patients and their advocates campaigned initially for the right to treatment. They called for an end to medical paternalism in the context of the demise of the psychiatric institution. Their aim was to press for better therapeutic conditions; advocacy extended well beyond the therapeutic milieu, in that the courts were widely used to promote patient rights. In a series of court deci-sions,[95,96] it was found to be contrary to due process to commit patients to hospital without adequate treatment.

The focus then shifted to the right to refuse treatment. Court actions rested primarily on arguments that involuntary administration of medication violates patients' somatic integrity and personal autonomy. Violations cited in the context of drug treatment included: polypharmacy; inattention to serious side-effects, particularly tardive dyskinesia; prescribing treatment with little medical justification or for inappropriate reasons; giving medications without the patient being seen by a psychiatrist; prescription by unlicensed psychiatrists; and using drugs coercively.

These issues have taken on a new poignant meaning in the context of deinstitutionalization and treating potentially behaviourally disturbed patients in the community. On the one hand, civil rights uphold patient autonomy, giving people a voice in their management of medication. On the other hand, both patient and the community must be protected. Patients' personal and legal rights must therefore be weighed against their medical needs and against community interests. This has been the basis for the involuntary admission of patients to hospital and the evolution of compulsory treatment orders in the community. The latter provide an alternative to admission when a less restrictive environment is considered desirable.

In summary, despite growing awareness of patients' rights, psychiatric institutions in their terminal phase and the community milieu into which patients are being integrated could still be portrayed as punitive, doctors as power-hungry and irresponsible, and drug treatment as a means of control.

Responding to these legal developments, Appelbaum and Gutheil[97] argued that the issue is not the right to refuse treatment but the right to receive 'good' treatment, to reject 'bad' treatment, and to have recourse to independent judgement. However, the political climate was not ready for the assertion of the right to effective treatment: patients and their advocates rejected what they felt to be covert paternalism, again avowing that the patient should not accept that the doctor knows best. The right to treatment refusal found support from prominent medical ethicists. Thus, Clayton[82] claimed that Applebaum and Gutheil's[97] argument failed to acknowledge the need to accommodate patients' values. The pivotal argument for her was not only whether patients should be able to reject bad treatment but also whether they could reasonably reject treatment known to be effective on clinical and scientific grounds, at least in competent, non-urgent cases. Arguing from first principles, she[82] demolished the notion of a general entitlement of doctors to intervene in the best interests of the patient, and further argued for the primacy of patients' rights to refuse treatment over any objective criteria as to what constitutes their best interests.

The pattern in the 1980s was, therefore, still away from informal medical ethics and resolution of conflicts of interest within the doctor–patient relationship. Instead, legal arbitration was frequently sought, based on the principle of rights. The clinical balance shifted from statutory support for the medical prerogative to prescribe to the enforcement of medical duties to acknowledge patient rights through the courts. Doctors were no longer free (if they ever were) to ignore patients' choices. Medication could no longer be prescribed without the patient's informed consent or, in the case of incompetent patients, through the application of the legal doctrine of substituted judgment. Further, it could only be enforced in cases of extreme emergency, particularly when doctors must protect themselves, other staff members, patients and their families or members of the public.

The right to drug treatment refusal in outpatients was considered by Geiselmann.[98] Preconditions for decision-making included: patient autonomy; the doctor's duty to inform and assessment of risks and benefits. Geiselmann[98] gave vivid case-examples illuminating the ethical dilemma between the patient's right to self-determination and the doctor's duty to choose the best treatment.

Court actions

Public and professional debate on patients' treatment rights was spurred by a series of court actions since the 1980s, particularly in the US. A New Jersey ruling[99] emphasized the potency and harsh side-effects of psychotropic drugs and accorded to the patient the right to exert control over their administration. The right was to be safeguarded by an independent psychiatrist at an informal hearing, and the patient could be represented by legal counsel.

The test case, however, was *Rogers* v. *Okin*[100] in which seven patients sued their psychiatrists and called for a ban on forced medication (and seclusion) for themselves and their fellows. The district court ruled in the patients' favour, concluding that involuntary commitment was not axiomatically a judgment of incompetence, and disagreed with the defendants' counter-argument that the state should act as *parens patriae*, guardians for the involuntarily committed. When a psychiatrist considered that medication should be enforced, it was the court's responsibility to judge the patient's ability to provide informed consent, or to appoint a guardian when incompetence had been established. Gutheil,[101] however, suggested that a guardianship approach is untenable in practice. Roth[102] offered an alternative means to serve the patient's interests:

an involuntary patient's right to refuse treatment should be determined at the point when the assessment for commitment was being considered. The commitment order could then permit the psychiatrist to treat the patient, if necessary without his consent.

The *Rogers* v. *Okin*[100] case did not end with the 1979 ruling and, over a period of six years, went to appeal. The Federal Court deferred to the State legislature on constitutional grounds;[103,104] but patients' rights to refuse treatment were confirmed. In giving its judgment,[105] the court took into consideration such factors as the level of intrusiveness of the treatment itself, the possibility of side-effects, the degree of emergency, the prognosis without treatment, the nature and extent of any prior judicial involvement, and the likelihood of conflicting interests. Patient-related factors, including personal preference, religious conviction, and family pressure, were particularly emphasized.

The *Rogers* v. *Okin*[100] case was soon followed by a spate of similar actions elsewhere in the US.[106] Outcomes included the appointment of patient advocates, the routine posting of drug side-effects in wards, and the ready availability of consent forms. The effects of these changes on the traditional psychiatric institutional ethos have been striking.

Psychiatric reactions to treatment refusal

Clinical and legal conceptions of patient autonomy differ considerably. Emphasizing patients' rights, the law places a higher value on the patient's stated wishes, either taking them at face value or applying the procedure of substituted judgment when incompetence can be demonstrated. Psychiatrists focus on actual intent, and argue that patients' stated wishes might be at odds with their clinical needs. They point to a number of possible detrimental consequences,[107] one of which is suboptimal patient care. There may be delays in drug treatment while doctors seek a court order to proceed.[108] As Roth[102] states, undertreatment is certainly no better than overtreatment.

Psychiatrists were also concerned about the trend away from therapeutic towards custodial functions.[109,110] Leong[111] cautioned against the expansion of psychiatric participation in social control, and Rodenhauser and Heller[112] drew attention to the potential role of forensic psychiatrists as law-enforcers, following a veritable pandemic of treatment-refusals. Finally, psychiatrists were worried about the erosion of their power to treat. Accustomed to having sole discretion over treatment, they saw the patient's refusal as a challenge to their professional authority and the exercise of their medical expertise.

Given these complications, research psychiatrists sought empirical elucidation of drug-refusal.[113,114] Research suggested that most cases of refusal were transient, and related to denial, grandiosity, psychotic perceptions, anger, ambivalence, negativism, and conflict with the family or with the treatment team. Refusal resulting from side-effects was remarkably uncommon.[115,116]

Refusal was regarded as ego-dystonic; in most cases patients eventually gave their free consent.[117,118]

In one illuminating study[113] 24 medication-refusers were interviewed after involuntary medication. A third initially manifested psychotic denial but, at discharge, 70 per cent felt that their refusal had been correctly overridden, and that they would wish to be treated against their will again if this proved necessary. Schwartz and his colleagues concluded that: 'treatment refusal should be considered primarily a psychotherapeutic issue and in most cases, should be subject to clinical rather than judicial review'.[113]

At first it seemed as if the legal view would predominate. Gutheil[101] warned: 'The way is paved for patients to rot with their rights on'. However, with decarceration and reorganization of mental health services, psychiatrists were able to relinquish any tendency to taking an adversarial stand and, as Ziegenfuss[119] recommended, increasingly recognized and accommodated patients' treatment rights into the newly changing services. At the clinical level this meant establishing drug treatment guidelines, elucidating drug refusal, and working alongside patient advocates to ensure that the necessary safeguards were in place. Through a process of mutual support, neither patient nor professional would then be victimized by 'the system'. Psychiatrists were, however, unprepared for the next challenge in the treatment rights arena—the claim for the right to effective treatment.

By the 1980s drug treatments had proliferated, but there were often insufficient scientific grounds for choosing between them. Drugs differed more in potency and side-effect profiles than in specificity of action. In the absence of scientific guidelines or consensus views, members of opposing camps had been able to make unsubstantiated claims for their preferred modes of treatment, while simultaneously alleging that rival approaches were unsafe, inefficient, or ineffective. Patients and their libertarian champions sought the establishment of treatment standards, and the right to effective treatment. Sider[120] wrote that value considerations are intrinsic to every choice of therapeutic modality and require more broadly based grounding than empirical findings or theory. He suggested that treatment goals should be based on a general understanding of the patient's clinical status, the patient's preferences, and the psychiatrist's own values. However, a landmark case pointed the way.

The right to effective treatment was enshrined in the case of Rafael Osheroff, a renal physician, who was unsuccessfully treated for depression in Chestnut Lodge, a noted psychoanalytic inpatient facility. He was subsequently transferred to a psychiatric unit where he recovered following the administration of psychotropic medications. The patient sued Chestnut Lodge for negligence and, following appeal, a settlement was reached out of court. Subsequent professional controversy revolved around the question of the patient's right to effective therapy.[121] Klerman[122] advocated prescription on the basis of the outcome findings of controlled trials, while Stone's[123] rebuttal argued for the priority of the 'collective sense of the profession' and the continuing contribution of a respectful minority.

In recognizing the shortcomings of the state of psychiatric treatment, Bloch and Brown[121] argued for an intermediate position, based on continuously evolving and interactionally based informed consent. If effective treatment for depression, a long-established disorder, is in doubt, how much more so for newer diagnostic entities such as post-traumatic stress disorder, where drug treatment trials are few and far between. The collective sense might favour more traditional treatments, but would the respectful minority extend to 'eye movement desensitization' or 'critical-incident stress debriefing'? Is informed consent an adequate safeguard when many treatments are relatively untried? In the event, the limit to the right to effective treatment proved to be fiscal rather than professional. Issues of cost–benefit have now come to the fore and will be considered in the next section.

Before turning to pharmacoeconomics, brief mention is made of patient rights operating outside the mainstream. Definitions of the psychiatrist's role have been challenged in regard to rights of persons seeking assisted suicide, sex offenders, and prisoners facing the death sentence. In a study exploring physician-assisted suicide in a sample of Dutch psychiatrists,[124] one-third were faced with a persistent request to assist in suicide, and two-thirds found such requests acceptable. In this regard, in a thoughtful paper, Block and Billings[125] examined the role of the psychiatrist in assessing those seeking assisted suicide or refusing further treatment.

Finally, it must be reiterated that rights are always associated with duties; this applies to doctors and patients alike. Osinga[126] draws attention, in a useful way, to the patient's duty to collaborate, from which can be derived preparedness to cooperate with the professional.

Pharmacoeconomics

Treatment provision always operates within budgetary constraints: potential benefit must be viewed not only in terms of associated risk, but also with respect to financial cost to patients, third-party payers, governments, and insurance companies. Guided by equal opportunity legislation and international conventions, the medical profession has to weigh up a complex web of factors in order to ensure equitable access to the highest possible standards of care, in the pursuit of social justice.

The psychotropic drug revolution following World War II has always been subject to the vicissitudes of the economic cycle. Postwar economic growth enabled drug companies to develop new drugs and governments to subsidize pharmaceutical benefits schemes. These developments permitted unrestrained growth in drug use, particularly the benzodiazepines, antipsychotics, and antidepressants. Psychiatrists and politicians promoted medical beneficence, and free-market operation of the drug companies. Ivan Illich, Michel Foucault, and anti-psychiatrists generally saw the resultant explosion of drug prescription as a form of social control (depicted dramatically in Ken Kesey's novel *One flew over the cuckoo's nest*).

From the 1970s, the development of more costly psychotropic drugs against a backdrop of slower economic growth, led to a cost blow-out, and accelerated the introduction of accountability. Other factors included an expanding community-based psychiatric population, particularly of the elderly and the chronically mentally ill. There was growing awareness in government and the health insurance industry of the need to balance care with cost.[127]

Unfortunately, the best drug may not always be the cheapest. More expensive new drugs include the SSRIs, and the new antipsychotics. In the case of SSRIs, their 'superior risk–benefit profile'[128] and greatly increased safety in overdose[19] clearly gives them a therapeutic advantage over the much more toxic tricyclics. The individual cost of the new drug over traditional standard medications is marginal. Rather, cost blow-outs relate to the increased volume of SSRIs prescribed, even extending to non-clinical groups. Secondary cost factors include those generated by the need to prescribe additional drugs to mitigate side-effects, e.g. hypnotics for insomnia.

Arguments for cost-containment equally extend to the new so-called 'budget busting' antipsychotic drugs, in particular, clozapine. Healey[129] reviewed the introduction of clozapine in comparison with other costly drugs; he acknowledged the inevitable role of psychiatrists as gatekeepers in societal drug-resource allocation, and the need to ration drug prescription. Healey examined cost–benefit in the context of patients' rights to expensive treatments, community budgetary constraints and, most problematic, pharmaceutical company pressures to prescribe. In his view therapeutic benefits are equivocal, and so increased costs are less than justified. Bosanquet and Zajdler[130] saw this view as short-term and static. Like McKenna and Bailey,[131] they regarded the introduction of clozapine as a positive development. They saw the true issue as fostering innovation, for example by ensuring competition from new compounds. These positive views were reinforced by the findings of Davies and Drummond[132] in their cost–benefit study of drug therapy in treatment-resistant schizophrenia. They demonstrated a net gain of nearly 6 years of life with either no or mild disability, and significantly reduced direct costs over standard psychotropic therapy, when the effect on all health-care resources was taken into account. They also demonstrated cost-saving or cost-neutrality under various conditions. Furthermore, several researchers in the US have demonstrated savings to society,[39] in terms of reduced hospital costs,[133] and improved economic generativity of otherwise chronically ill people.

Faced with the declining health dollar, governments in many countries have adopted authoritarian approaches to curb demand for prescribed drugs on the one hand, and perceived *laissez faire* medical attitudes on the other. There has been a trend to limit access to medication by reducing state subsidies, and by monitoring doctors' prescribing patterns. These actions threaten economically vulnerable psychiatric patient groups such as children, the elderly, migrants, indigenous populations, and the chronically and severely ill.

In the UK effective controls have been introduced on the total volume of prescribing, with doctors given written feedback about their own prescribing patterns, a process entitled 'Prescribing analysis and costs' (PACT).[134]

In Australia, with State Government cost-cutting, care of the public patient shifted from State-funded inpatient facilities to Federally-funded outpatient services, partly to private psychiatric practitioners and partly to GPs. At the same time, Federal government reduced prescription subsidies made through its Pharmaceutical Benefits Scheme. The overall result was less optimal supervision and greater drug cost to the patient. On a positive note,[135] the Australian Government agreed that a range of psychotropic medications should be available, and effectively allocated and monitored. They outlined a 'Quality use of medicines policy', with participation of governmental, pharmaceutical, and related bodies. This encourages research on comparing prescription practices of GPs and specialists and on the efficacy of providing information on adverse effects to patients. Its recommendations have been implemented as part of a National Mental Health Strategy instigated in 1993.[136] Guidelines for the use of long-term medication in readmission and chronic illness have been advocated by Bergen.[135]

Attempts to improve patient access to community-based psychiatric care have focused on cost-beneficial GP services. Governments regard these services as cheaper to fund and easier to regulate than specialist services. A number of GP incentive schemes are in place enlisting the support of psychiatric specialists. The latter will be expected to take on a supervisory rather than a direct treatment role. Upgrading the skills of GPs by their professional associations is also being encouraged, thereby extending their role in managing, for example treatment-resistant depression and patients with chronic schizophrenia. GPs have proved more sensitive and amenable to cost-containment. Thus, Beilby and Silagy[137] in reviewing the impact of providing information about costs to GPs, found that this modified their prescribing behaviour. However, there are limits to GPs' ability to diagnose and treat mental illness, and there are attendant ethical issues of access to the most appropriate providers of psychiatric care. Without specialist supervision of assessment, planning and implementing treatment, and without appropriate monitoring there could be increased risk to patients, such as suicide with failed treatment. If promoting non-specialists to contain costs is fraught with ethical dilemmas, creating psychiatric subspecialties (e.g. to treat depression) is no less ethically problematic in regard to cost-containment. Clearly a balance has to be struck between general and specialist practice of mental illness.

Prior to the 1960s, decisions about resource allocation were seen as beyond the purview of clinicians.[138] Since then psychiatrists have become managers of health care resources, with the dual role of caregiver and gatekeeper.[139] However, there are scant guidelines on how to allocate services on clinical or ethical grounds in the face of limited funds.[140] Psychiatrists must necessarily become more involved in managing health-care costs.[141]

Clinical services are increasingly faced with the ethical problem posed by the need to ration drugs.[142] Factors include: costly new drugs; ageing populations; patient expectations; psychiatrists' desire for effective preparations; and government restrictions on health-care costs. Solutions of equity and fairness must be equally acceptable to all protagonists. Calman[143] has similarly considered allocation of limited resources. Following his argument, drug prescription must balance patients' rights and benefits to the community. Allocation requires investment in research and development of new treatment strategies as much as evaluating the effectiveness and costs of existing treatments. He has advocated greater public involvement in the allocation process. Cost–benefit according to the Health Council of the Netherlands is considered as only one of four elements in resource allocation.[144] Factors also include necessary care as determined by the community, effectiveness, efficiency, patient's rights, and autonomy in decision-making. Chadwick and Levitt[144] explore two influential models of justice in resource allocation: distribution according to need and according to deserts. They noted that need is defined by economists as the capacity to benefit. Alternative quality-of-life (QOL) measures remain problematic.

Cost–benefit has become subsumed under managed care in the US and the Western World (see Chapter 19). This is a partnership between government, seeking to reduce their budgetary responsibilities, and third-party payers seeking to ensure profits on investment. In this system, prescribers have become answerable to the payers, with case managers and colleagues mediating and monitoring. Ostensibly this is to ensure fair access, but instead some feel that there has been a *de facto* devolution of power from the medical profession, and undermining of trust in the doctor–patient relationship through breaches of confidentiality and withholding of preferred or even essential treatments.

Limitations of physicians' choice of drugs as part of a project in an HMO unexpectedly led to increased use of services, and increased costs. Formulary restrictions resulted in more patient visits to physicians, more visits to the emergency room, more hospitalizations, and greater estimated costs of prescriptions.[145] Use of services also went up, and therefore costs, with greater use of generic drugs.

Psychiatrists face problems of double agency[146] when attempting to accommodate patients' right to effective treatment with economic constraints. Where are psychiatrists to turn for guidelines in their role as managers of the drug dollar for all those concerned: patients, governments, and insurers? Furthermore, doctors face legal challenges from patients and the community when they attempt to reduce access to treatment, either directly in the clinic or indirectly through restrictions in resource allocation. They have resorted to evidence-based medical guidelines, and defensive medicine, but cost-containment will require more creative solutions if patient care is not to be stifled.

In teaching the ethics of cost containment, Schneider-Braus[147] has emphasized heightening awareness of the dilemmas facing all parties (health-care managers, purchasers of health-care, public policy makers, and consumers of mental health care) and the development of practical ethical strategies.

Conclusion

Two psychotropic drug revolutions have occurred in the second half of the twentieth century. The first, the introduction of the principal drug classes in the 1950s, was followed by significant new antidepressant and antipsychotic preparations from the late 1980s. These drugs brought increased benefits, increased risks, and increased costs. The SSRIs, for example, were prescribed as panaceas by some, and promulgated as designer drugs by others. Although supported by brain studies linking structure and function and by meta-analyses demonstrating treatment efficacy, the new drugs manifested therapeutic and economic shortcomings.

At the same time, the locus of prescription control in the doctor–patient relationship began to shift from the doctor to the patient, and to third parties in society at large. Patients initially sought to ensure treatment access through the courts. This was followed by their demand for the right to refuse treatment and recently the right to effective treatment. Concomitant cost blow-outs occurred due to prescription of more expensive drugs, increased patient demand, and unrestrained drug company growth. Governments increasingly sought to regulate and contain drug usage and insurers introduced managed care.

Faced with these challenges psychiatrists have been forced to relinquish traditional treatment ethics. The 1990s have therefore witnessed the introduction of applied treatment ethics, in which the mediating role of the doctor has been widened to include not only the patient but also other significant parties in the professional, legal, business, and political realms.

References

1. Delay, J. and Deniker, P.: Le traitement des psychoses par une methode neuro-lytique derivee de l'hibernotherapie. *Congres des Medecins Alienistes et Neurologistes de France*, Luxemburg **50**:497, 1952.
2. Kuhn, R.: The treatment of depressive states with G22355 (imipramine hydrochloride). *American Journal of Psychiatry* **115**:459–64, 1958.
3. Sternbach, L. H.: Pharmacology of benzodiazepines, in *The discovery of CNS active 1,4-benzodiazepines (chemistry)*, ed. E. Usdin., T. J. R. Skolnick, Jr., *et al*. London, Macmillian, 1982, pp. 7–14.
4. Cade, J. F. J.: Lithium salts in the treatment of psychotic excitement. *Medical Journal of Australia* **36**:349–52, 1949.

5. Davis, J. M., Barter, J. T., and Kane, J. M.: Antipsychotic drugs, in *Comprehensive textbook of psychiatry*, ed. H. I. Kaplan. and B. J. Sadock. Baltimore, Williams and Wilkins, 1989.
6. Roth, L. H.: Four studies of mental health commitment. *American Journal of Psychiatry* **146**:135–7, 1989.
7. Goffman, E.: *Asylums: essays on the social situation of mental patients and other inmates.* Chicago, Aldine, 1962.
8. Scheff, T. J.: *Being mentally ill: a sociological theory.* Chicago, Aldine, 1966.
9. Thompson, I. E.: Fundamental ethical principles in health care. *British Medical Journal* **295**:1461–5, 1987.
10. Uhlenhuth, E. H., DeWitt, H., Balter, M. B., Johanson, C. E., and Mellinger, G. D.: Risks and benefits of long-term benzodiazepine use. *Journal of Clinical Psychopharmacology* **8**:161–7, 1988.
11. Hallstrom, C.: Use and abuse of benzodiazepines. *British Journal of Hospital Medicine* **41**:115, 1989.
12. Ballenger, J. C.: Benzodiazepines, in *Textbook of psychopharmacology*, ed. A. F. Schatzberg and C. B. Nemeroff. Washington DC, American Psychiatric Press, 1995, pp. 215–30.
13. Shader, R. I. and Greenblatt, D. J.: Use of benzodiazepines in anxiety disorders. *New England Journal of Medicine* **328**:1398–405, 1998.
14. Pantelis, C. and Barnes, T. R. E.: Drug strategies and treatment-resistant schizophrenia. *Australian and New Zealand Journal of Psychiatry* **30**:20–38, 1996.
15. Hirsch, S.R. and Barnes, T.R.E.: Clinical use of high-dose neuroleptics. *British Journal of Psychiatry* **164**:94–6, 1994.
16. Thompson, C.: The use of higher-dose antipsychotic medication: consensus statement. *British Journal of Psychiatry* **164**:448–58, 1994.
17. Kane, J. M. and McGlashan, T. H.: Treatment of schizophrenia. *Lancet* **346**:820–5, 1995.
18. Goldberg, D. and Huxley, P.: *Mental illness in the community.* London, Tavistock, 1980.
19. Cooper, G. L.: The safety of fluoxetine—an update. *British Journal of Psychiatry* **153**:77–86, 1988.
20. Pedersen, O. L., Kragh-Srensen, P., Bjerre, M., *et al.*: Citalopram, a selective serotonin reuptake inhibitor: clinical antidepressive and long-term effect—a phase II study. *Psychopharmacology (Berl)* **77**:199–204, 1982.
21. Leonard, B. E.: Pharmacological differences of serotonin reuptake inhibitors and possible clinical relevance. *Drugs* **43**(Suppl 2):3–10, 1992.
22. Tollefson, G. D.: Selective serotonin reuptake inhibitors, in *Textbook of psychopharmacology*, ed. A. F. Schatzberg and C. B. Nemeroff. Washington, DC, American Psychiatric Press, 1995, pp. 161–82.
23. Michelson, L. K. and Ray, W. J., ed.: *Handbook of dissociation. Theoretical, empirical, and clinical perspectives.* London, Plenum, 1996.
24. Oldham, J. M., Hollander, E., and Skodol, A. E., ed.: *Impulsivity and compulsivity.* Washington DC, American Psychiatric Press, 1996.
25. Aizenberg, D., Gur, S., Zemishlany, Z., *et al.*: Mianserin, a 5-ht2a/2c and alpha(2) antagonist, in the treatment of sexual dysfunction induced by serotonin reuptake inhibitors. *Clinical Neuropharmacology* **20**:210–14, 1997.
26. Potter, W. Z., Manji, H. K. and Rudorfer, M. V.: Tricyclics and tetracyclics, in *Textbook of psychopharmacology*, ed. A. F. Schatzberg. and C. B. Nemeroff. Washington DC, American Psychiatric Press, 1995, pp. 161–82.

27. Carpenter, W. T., Jr, Heinrichs, D. W., and Alphs, L. D.: Treatment of negative symptoms. *Schizophrenia Bulletin* **11**:440–52, 1985.
28. Barnes, T. R. and Liddle, P. F.: Evidence for the validity of negative symptoms, in *Schizophrenia: positive and negative symptoms and syndromes*, ed. N. C. Andreasen. Basel, Karger, 1990, pp. 43–72.
29. Breier, A., Buchanan, R. W., Kirkpatrick, B., *et al*.: Effects of clozapine on positive and negative symptoms in outpatients with schizophrenia. *American Journal of Psychiatry* **151**:20–6, 1994.
30. Barnes, T. R. E.: Tardive dyskinesia: can it be prevented? in *Dilemmas and controversies in the management of psychiatric patients*, ed. K. J. Hawton and P. Cowen, 1990. Oxford, Oxford University Press, pp. 157–69.
31. Marder, S. R. and Van Putten, T.: Antipsychotic medications, in *Textbook of psychopharmacology*, ed. A. F. Schatzberg. and C. B. Nemeroff. Washington DC, American Psychiatric Press, 1995, pp. 247–61.
32. Shalev, A., Hermesh, H., and Munitz, H.: Mortality from neuroleptic malignant syndrome. *Journal of Clinical Psychiatry* **51**:25, 1989
33. Baldessarini, R. J. and Frankenburg, F. R.: Clozapine: A novel antipsychotic agent. *New England Journal of Medicine* **324**:746–54, 1991.
34. Meltzer, H. Y.: The mechanism of action of novel antipsychotic drugs. *Schizophrenia Bulletin* **17**:263–87, 1991.
35. Gerlach, J.: New antipsychotics: classification, efficacy, and adverse effects. *Schizophrenia Bulletin* **17**:289–309,1991.
36. Hippius, H.: The history of clozapine. *Psychopharmacology (Berl)* **99**:53–5, 1989.
37. Lieberman, J. A., Saltz, B. L., Johns, C. A., Pollack, S., Borenstein, M., and Kane, J.: The effects of clozapine on tardive dyskinesia. *British Journal of Psychiatry* **158**:503–10, 1991.
38. King, D. J. and Green, J. F.: Medication and cognitive functioning in schizophrenia, in *Schizophrenia: a neuropsychological perspective*, ed. C. Pantelis., H. E. Nelson and T. R. E. Barnes. Chichester, Wiley, 1996, pp. 419–45.
39. Owens, M. J. and Craig Risch, S.: Atypical antipsychotics, in *Textbook of psychopharmacology*, ed. A. F. Schatzberg. and C. B. Nemeroff. Washington DC, American Psychiatric Press, 1995, pp. 263–80.
40. Alvir, J. M. J. and Lieberman, J. A.: A reevaluation of the clinical characteristics of clozapine-induced agranulocytosis in light of the United States experience. *Journal of Clinical Psychopharmacology* **14**:87–9, 1994.
41. Golden, R. N., Bebchuk, J. M., and Leatherman, M. A.: Trazodone and other antidepressants, in *Textbook of psychopharmacology*, ed. A. F. Schatzberg. and C. B. Nemeroff. Washington D.C., American Psychiatric Press, 1995, pp. 195–213.
42. Leo, R. J., Kreeger, J. L., and Kim, K. Y.: Cardiomyopathy associated with clozapine. *Annals of Pharmacotherapy* **30**:603–5, 1996.
43. Yung, A. R. and McGorry, P. D.: Is pre-psychotic intervention realistic in schizophrenia and related disorders? *Australian and New Zealand Journal of Psychiatry* **31**:799–805, 1997.
44. Morice, R.: Comment: should we walk before setting the PACE? *Australian and New Zealand Journal of Psychiatry* **31**:806–7, 1997.
45. Preskorn, S. H.: Clinically relevant pharmacology of selective serotonin reuptake inhibitors—an overview with emphasis on pharmacokinetics and effects on oxidative drug metabolism [Review]. *Clinical Pharmacokinetics* **32**(Suppl. 1):1–21, 1997.
46. Gullick, E. L. and King, L. J.: Appropriateness of drugs prescribed by primary care physicians for depressed outpatients. *Journal of Affective Disorders* **1**:55–8, 1979.

47. Catalan, J., Gath, D. H., Bond, G., Edmonds, P., Martin, J., and Ennis, J.: General practice patients on long-term psychotropic drugs. *British Journal of Psychiatry* **152**:399–405, 1988.
48. Yellowlees, P. M. and Kennedy, C.: Telemedicine: here to stay. *Medical Journal of Australia* **166**:262–5, 1997.
49. Crowe, G. R.: Telemedicine: solution of problem? *Medical Journal of Australia* **167**: 56, 1997.
50. Klerman, G. L., Dimascio, A., Weissman, M. M., Prusoff, B. A., and Paykel, E. S.: Treatment of depression by drugs and psychotherapy. *American Journal of Psychiatry* **131**:186–91, 1974.
51. Stockler, M. and Coates, A.: What have we learned from meta-analysis? *Medical Journal of Australia* **159**:291–3, 1993.
52. Adams, C., Anderson, J., Awad, G., *et al.*: Schizophrenia and the Cochrane Collaboration. *Schizophrenia Research* **13**:185–8, 1994.
53. Felson, D. T.: Bias in meta-analytic research. *Journal of Clinical Epidemiology* **45**: 885–92, 1992.
54. Stewart, L. A. and Parmer, M. K. B.: Meta-analysis of the literature or of individual patient data: is there a difference? *Lancet* **341**:418–22, 1993.
55. Eysenck, H. J.: An exercise in mega-silliness. *American Psychologist* **33**:517, 1978.
56. Sackett, D. L., Haynes, R. B., Guyatt, G. H., *et al.*: *Clinical epidemiology: a basic science for clinical medicine*. Boston, Little, Brown, 1991.
57. Sacks, H. S., Berrier, J., Reitman, D., *et al.*: Meta-analysis of randomized controlled trials. *New England Journal of Medicine* **316**:450–5, 1987, 13 March.
58. Normand, J-M.: France's unethical medics. *Le Monde*, 1993.
59. *Diagnostic and statistical manual of mental disorders, DSM-IV*, 4th edn. Washington DC, American Psychiatric Association, 1994.
60. Klerman, G. and Schechter, G.: Ethical aspects of drug treatment, in *Psychiatric ethics*, 1st edn, ed. S. Bloch. and P. Chodoff. Oxford, Oxford University Press, 1981, pp. 117–30.
61. Boon, S. and Draijer, N.: *Multiple personality disorder in the Netherlands: a study of reliability and validity of diagnosis*. Lisse, Swets and Zeitlinger, 1993.
62. Ball, J. R. B.: Massive sexual assault: a test of human resilience. *Journal of Law and Medicine* **1**:52–62, 1993.
63. Burges Watson, I. P.: 'Is violence a contagious disease?'—the social implications of post-traumatic stress disorder. *Irish Journal of Psychological Medicine* **7**:47–52, 1990.
64. Brown, P. and Van der Hart, O.: Memories of sexual abuse: Janet's critique of Freud, a balanced approach. *Psychological Reports* **82**, 1027–43, 1998.
65. *Diagnostic and statistical manual of mental disorders, DSM-III*, 3rd edn. Washington DC, American Psychiatric Association, 1980.
66. Kihlstrom, J. F.: The trauma memory argument. *Consciousness and Cognition: an International Journal* **4**:63–7, 1995.
67. Davidson, J. R. T. and van der Kolk, B. A.: The psychopharmacological treatment of post-traumatic stress disorder, in *Traumatic stress: the effects of overwhelming experience on mind, body and society*, ed. B. van der Kolk, A. C. McFarlane, and L. Weisaeth. New York, Guilford, 1996, pp. 510–24.
68. Krystal, J. H., Bennet, A., Bromner, J. D., *et al.*: Recent developments in the neurobiology of dissociation: implications for post-traumatic stress disorder, in *Handbook of dissociations: theoretical, empirical and clinical perspectives*, ed. L. K. Michelson. and W. J. Ray. New York, Plenum, 1996, pp. 163–90.

69. Trimble, M. R.: *Post-traumatic neurosis: from railway spine to the whiplash*. New York, Wiley, 1981.
70. Marin, D. B., Davis, K. L., and Speranza, A. J.: Cognitive enhancers, in *Textbook of psychopharmacology*, ed. A. F. Schatzberg, Jr. and C. B. Nemeroff. Washington DC, American Psychiatric Press, 1995, pp. 391–404.
71. Clark, W. H.: Ethics and LSD. *Journal of Psychoactive Drugs* 17:229–34, 1985.
72. Bosco, J. J. and Robbins, S. S., ed.: *The hyperactive child and stimulant drugs*. Chicago, Chicago University Press, 1976.
73. Wender, P.: *Minimal brain dysfunction in children*. New York, Wiley, 1971.
74. Main, T. F.: The ailment. *British Journal of Medical Psychology* 30:129–45, 1957.
75. Bloch, S.: Psychiatry: an impossible profession? *Australian and New Zealand Journal of Psychiatry* 31:172–83, 1997.
76. Dyer, A. R. and Bloch, S.: Informed consent and the psychiatric patient. *Journal of Medical Ethics* 13:12–16, 1987.
77. Winslade, W.J.: Informed consent in psychiatric practice: the primacy of ethics over law. *Behavioral Sciences and the Law* 1:47–56, 1983.
78. Mullen, P. D., Green, L. W. and Persinger, G. S.: Clinical trials of patient education for chronic conditions: a comparative meta-analysis of intervention-types. *Preventative Medicine* 14:753–81, 1985.
79. Sider, R. C. and Clements, C.: Psychiatry's contribution to medical ethics education. *American Journal of Psychiatry* 139:498–501, 1982.
80. Belmaker, R. H., Klein, E. and Dick, E.: Ethics and psychopharmacologic research, in *Pharmacology: impact on clinical psychiatry*, 2nd edn. ed. D. Morgan. St Louis, Ishiyaku Euro America, 1985, pp. 19–29.
81. Appelbaum, P. S. and Grisso, T.: The MacArthur treatment competence study. 1. Mental illness and competence to consent to treatment. *Law and Human Behavior* 19:105–126, 1995.
82. Clayton, E. W.: From Rogers to Rivers: the rights of the mentally ill to refuse medication. *American Journal of Law and Medicine* 13:7–52, 1987.
83. Kleinman, I., Schachter, D. and Koritar, E.: Informed consent and tardive dyskinesia. *American Journal of Psychiatry* 146:902–4, 1989.
84. Kleinman, I., Schachter, D., Jeffries, J., and Goldhamer, P.: Effectiveness of two methods for informing schizophrenic patients about neuroleptic medication. *Hospital and Community Psychiatry* 44:1189–91, 1993.
85. Kleinman, I., Schachter, D., Jeffries, J., and Goldhamer, P.: Informed consent and tardive dyskinesia: long-term follow-up. *Journal of Nervous and Mental Disease* 184:517–22, 1996.
86. *Rogers* v *Whitaker*: 175, C.L.R. 479, 1991.
87. Sexton. P.: *Rogers* v *Whitaker* revisited: Why do we have medical ethics? *Australian Medicine* 8:14, 1996.
88. Liddel, M.: Rational prescribing and professional standards. *Medical Journal of Australia* 160:564–7, 1994.
89. *SSRI antidepressants—information for patients*. Psychiatric Services Division, Victorian Government Department of Health and Community Services, Melbourne, 1994.
90. *Major tranquillisers—information for patients*. Psychiatric Services Division, Victorian Government Department of Health and Community Services, Melbourne, 1994.
91. *Psychotropic drug guidelines*, 3rd edn. Victorian Medical Postgraduate Foundation, Melbourne, 1995.

92. *The RANZCP guidelines for psychotropic drugs in psychiatric practice.* Royal Australian and New Zealand College of Psychiatrists, Melbourne, 1994.
93. Waddell, M., Doherty, P. J. and Schweitzer, A. P. I.: *The Australian psychotropic pharmacopoeia.* North Eastern Health Care Network, Melbourne, 1996.
94. Wood, J.: The challenge of individual rights. *British Journal of Psychiatry* **166**: 417–20, 1995.
95. *Wyatt* v. *Stickney*: 325 F. Supp.781 (M.D.Ala.), 1971.
96. *O'Connor* v. *Donaldson*: 422 US 563, 1975.
97. Applebaum, P. S. and Gutheil, T. G.: The right to refuse treatment: the real issue is quality of care. *Bulletin of the American Academy of Psychiatry and the Law* **9**:199–202, 1981.
98. Geiselmann, B.: Informed refusal: the patient's influence on long-term treatment. *Pharmacopsychiatry* **27**(Suppl.):58–62, 1994.
99. *Rennie* v. *Klein*: 720 F2d. 266 (3d Cir), 1983.
100. *Rogers* v. *Okin*: 478 F. Supp. 1342 (D.Mass.), 1979.
101. Gutheil, T. G.: In search of true freedom: drug refusal, involuntary medication and rotting with your rights on. *American Journal of Psychiatry* **137**:577–80, 1980.
102. Roth, L.: Mental health commitment: the state of the debate. *Hospital and Community Psychiatry* **31**:385–96, 1980.
103. *Mills* v. *Rogers*: 457 US 291.
104. *Rogers* v. *Okin*: 738 F2d. 1 (1st Cir.), 1984.
105. *Rogers* v. *Commissioner of Department of Mental Health*: 458 NE 2d. 308 (Mass.), 1983.
106. Beck, J. C.: Determining competency to assent to neuroleptic drug treatment. *Hospital and Community Psychiatry* **39**:1106–8, 1988.
107. Appelbaum, P. S.: The right to refuse treatment with antipsychotic medications: retrospect and prospect. *American Journal of Psychiatry* **145**:413–19, 1988.
108. Appelbaum, P. S. and Hoge, S.K.: The right to refuse treatment: what the research reveals. *Behavioral Sciences and the Law* **4**:279–92,1986.
109. Brooks, A. D.: Law and antipsychotic medications. *Behavioral Sciences and the Law* **4**:247–63, 1986.
110. Sidley, N. T.: The right of involuntary patients in mental institutions to refuse drug treatment. *Journal of Psychiatry and the Law* **12**:231–55, 1984.
111. Leong, G. B.: The expansion of psychiatric participation in social control. *Hospital and Community Psychiatry* **40**:240–2, 1989.
112. Rodenhauser, P. and Heller, A.: Management of forensic psychiatric patients who refuse medication—2 scenarios. *Journal of Forensic Sciences* **29**:237–44, 1984.
113. Schwartz, H. I., Vingiano, W. and Bezirganian Perez, C.: Autonomy and the right to refuse treatment: patient's attitudes after involuntary medication. *Hospital and Community Psychiatry* **39**:1049–54, 1988.
114. Hoge, S. K., Appelbaum, P. S., Lawlor, *et al.*: A prospective, multicenter study of a patient's refusal of antipsychotic medication. *Archives of General Psychiatry* **47**:949–56, 1990.
115. Marder, S. R., Mebane, A. and Chein, C.: A comparison of patients who refuse and consent to neuroleptic treatment. *American Journal of Psychiatry* **140**:470–2, 1983.
116. Marder, S. R., Swann, E. and Winslade, W. J.: A study of medication refusal by involuntary psychiatric patients. *Hospital and Community Psychiatry* **35**:724–6, 1984.
117. Kalman, T. P.: An overview of patient satisfaction with psychiatric treatment. *Hospital and Community Psychiatry* **34**:48–53, 1983.

118. Keisling, R.: Characteristics and outcome of patients who refuse medication. *Hospital and Community Psychiatry* **34**:847–8, 1983.
119. Ziegenfuss, J. T.: Conflict between patients' and patients' needs: an organisational systems problem. *Hospital and Community Psychiatry* **37**:1086–8, 1986.
120. Sider, R. C.: The ethics of therapeutic modality choice. *American Journal of Psychiatry* **141**:390–4, 1984.
121. Bloch, S. and Brown, P.: Can there be a right to effective treatment in psychiatry? *Changes—An International Journal of Psychology and Psychotherapy* **9**:101–12, 1991.
122. Klerman, G. L.: The psychiatric patient's right to effective treatment: implications of *Osheroff* v. *Chestnut Lodge. American Journal of Psychiatry* **147**:409–18, 1990.
123. Stone, A.: Law, science and psychiatric malpractice: a response to Klerman's indictment of psychoanalytic psychiatry. *American Journal of Psychiatry* **147**: 419–27, 1990.
124. Groenewoud, J. H., Vandermaas, P. J., Vanderwal, *et al.*: Physician-assisted death in psychiatric practice in the Netherlands. *New England Journal of Medicine* **336**:1795–80, 1997.
125. Block, S. and Billings, J. A.: Patient requests for euthanasia and assisted suicide in terminal illness: the role of the psychiatrist. *Psychosomatics* **36**:445–57, 1996.
126. Osinga, M.: But the patient has responsibilities as well. *Australasian Journal of the Medical Defence Union* 38–39, 1989.
127. Gennery, B.: The role of pharmacoeconomics. *British Journal of Medical Economics* **6**:3–4, 1993.
128. Boyer, W. F. and Feighner, J. P.: The efficacy of selective serotonin uptake inhibitors in depression, in *Selective serotonin uptake inhibitors*, ed. J. P. Feighner and W. F. Boyer. Chichester, Wiley, 1991, pp. 89–108.
129. Healey, D.: Psychopharmacology and the ethics of resource allocation. *British Journal of Psychiatry* **162**:23–9, 1993.
130. Bosanquet, N. and Zajdler, A.: Psychopharmacology and the ethics of resource allocation: comment. *British Journal of Psychiatry* **162**:29–32, 1994.
131. McKenna, P. J. and Bailey, P. E.: The strange story of clozapine. *British Journal of Psychiatry* **162**:32–7, 1988.
132. Davies, L. M. and Drummond, M. F.: Assessment of costs and benefits of drug therapy for treatment-resistant schizophrenia in the United Kingdom. *British Journal of Psychiatry* **162**:38–42, 1994.
133. Meltzer, H. Y., Cola, P., Way, L., *et al.*: Cost effectiveness of clozapine in neuroleptic-resistant schizophrenia. *American Journal of Psychiatry* **150**:1630–8,1993.
134. Bosanquet, N. and Zammitlucia, J.: The effect of competition on drug prices. *Pharmacoeconomics* **8**:473–8, 1995.
135. Bergen, J.: Report on 'Psychotherapeutic medication in Australia'. *Australasian Psychiatry* **5**:91–3,1997.
136. Whitford, H.: The National Mental Health Strategy: is it making any difference? *Australasian Psychiatry* **4**:313–15,1996.
137. Beilby, J. J. and Silagy, C. A.: Trials of providing costing information to general practitioners—a systematic review. *Medical Journal of Australia* **167**: 89–92, 1997.
138. Cassel, C. K.: Doctors and allocation decisions: a new role in the new Medicare. *Journal of Health Politics, Policy and Law* **10**:549–64, 1985.
139. Pellegrino, E. D.: Rationing healthcare: the ethics of medical gatekeeping. *Law Policy* **2**:23–45, 1986.

140. Daniels, N.: Why saying no to patients in the United States is so hard. *New England Journal of Medicine* **314**:1380–4, 1986.
141. Brody, H., ed.: *The healer's power*. New Haven, Yale University Press, 1992.
142. Bochner, F., Burgess, N. G. and Martin, E. D.: Approaches to rationing drugs in hospitals—an Australian perspective. *Pharmacoeconomics* **10**:467–74, 1996.
143. Calman, K. C.: Ethics, allocation of health care resources, education, outcome. The ethics of allocation of scarce health care resources—a view from the centre. *Journal of Medical Ethics* **20**:71–4,1994.
144. Chadwick, R. and Levitt, M.: When drug treatment in the elderly is not cost effective—an ethical dilemma in an environment of healthcare rationing. *Drugs and Ageing* **7**:416–19, 1995.
145. Horn, S.: Managed care cuts counterproductive. *Australian Medicine* Feb:10–11, 1997.
146. Dougherty, C. J.: Mind, money, and morality: ethical dimensions of economic change in American psychiatry. *American Journal of Psychiatry* **18**:15–20, 1998.
147. Schneider-Braus, K.: Exploring the ethics of cost containment in psychiatric training. *Academic Psychiatry* **20**:158–64, 1996.

13

Ethical aspects of the physical manipulation of the brain

Harold Merskey

In this chapter, I base my discussion of ethical issues in the physical manipulation of the brain on the following:

1. Physicians advise and do not impose their advice except in special circumstances. Thus treatment to save lives or relieve distress is usually ethical but it may not be so if imposed, even though legally allowed.
2. Children, and others in a condition which precludes them from deciding rationally, may have decisions taken for them by people (usually their next of kin) who have appropriate concern for their interests and welfare.
3. Physicians may ethically treat those who come under (2), but the treatment requires careful scrutiny as do the status and motives of the decision-maker.
4. Ethical actions may or may not be sanctioned by law. Physicians normally do not consider themselves bound to pursue ethical treatments for the patient's benefit if they are forbidden to do so by law, but a difficult situation arises, for example, if physicians wish to treat injured persons in secret when police or other security agencies are in pursuit.
5. Coercive treatment for the benefit of a third party is unethical. (To say, 'You must have this behaviour modification or drug or leucotomy which you do not want because otherwise we expect you to murder your mother' is not ethical).
6. The treatment of individuals against their wishes in order to change them for the sake of the needs of society or a political system is likewise ethically repugnant.
7. Patients may consent to treatment which benefits either themselves or others, but there are peculiar difficulties in confirming that consent is freely given in certain circumstances.

These rules partly reflect ethical considerations and partly reflect practical problems. The latter, as will shortly be seen, are capable of solution.

Clinical cost–benefit ratios

There are three major types of physical manipulation of the brain: electro-convulsive therapy (ECT); surgical ablation by scalpel or other technique which deliberately damages tissue; and the insertion of recording or stimulating electrodes, in essence an advanced form of surgery. All these have been attacked, often ignorantly. I wish here to sketch the reasonable basis for their use, if any, in terms of medical ethics. Much of the controversy turns on the usefulness of the procedures and the morbidity due to them. These are necessary aspects to consider in all treatment. They do not determine the ethical justification for the use of a treatment. Whether a treatment is justified or not must always pass the test that the likelihood of benefits outweighs the hazards. If the chance of benefit is held to outweigh the risk of suffering or loss from the morbidity and mortality of the treatment, the treatment is ordinarily given.

As every clinician knows these matters are often difficult to quantify. If radical mastectomy for breast cancer gives, say, an 80 per cent chance of five-year survival (with a 10 per cent chance otherwise), and less than a 1 per cent chance of operative death, the calculation is straightforward even though the operation also gives a near 100 per cent guarantee of transient pain and discomfort as well as certain other risks. It is harder to evaluate thalamotomy for chronic pain with perhaps a 70 per cent chance of significant relief at 12 months, a 20–30 per cent risk of exacerbation of the pain, and a 5 per cent risk of stroke or aphasia. Nevertheless, breast cancer continued to be treated by radical mastectomy so long as the above odds prevailed and no other treatment offered better prospects, whereas thalamotomy has been virtually discarded for pain (and not at all because it was an operation on the brain).

Procedures are assessed on the basis of informed knowledge of what they can offer patients. If ECT is attacked on the grounds of seeming barbaric because it incidentally causes convulsions this is an irrational view compared with the acceptance of surgery in which a breast may be mutilated or a larynx removed. Each procedure can be done for the benefit of the patient and in the light of information provided; he may ordinarily decide if the disadvantages are greater or less than the advantages.

Refusal of general surgery

If a competent adult chooses not to have a general surgical operation, despite knowing the risks, surgery is not pursued. One important practical reason is that patients undergoing operations without some degree of acceptance often fare poorly. Patients who fear their operations excessively are dreaded by the surgeon since clinical lore holds that they suffer serious complications and more often die. Patients' attitudes are therefore a factor in the cost–benefit equation. If it were not so, surgeons might be tempted to press necessary operations on patients more vigorously. Practical wisdom reinforces the ethical position of not doing things to patients who refuse to consent.

The wisdom of not operating on the strongly unwilling person applies equally to psychotic patients. If they refuse a general surgical operation there is no more chance of them doing well with it than if they were insightful. Children, however, are treated differently. Johnnie, aged 7, may protest that he does not want an appendectomy. He may be anaesthetized against his strongest expressed wishes and physical resistance. However, the operation is performed and he recovers nicely. It would take an unusual person, medical or lay, to maintain the child should have been allowed to refuse.

We can conclude that clinical wisdom limits the frequency with which non-cerebral operations are undertaken against patients' wishes. Nevertheless, in those who cannot decide for themselves (for example children), practice and feeling both hold that it is right to disregard their wishes when life or health is at risk. John Stuart Mill, often quoted by those who argue against compulsory treatment, says the following about the individual's right to take actions which might be harmful to his physical or moral health:

It is, perhaps, hardly necessary to say that this doctrine is meant to apply only to human beings in the full maturity of their faculties. We are not speaking of children, or of young persons below the age which the law may fix as that of manhood or womanhood. Those who are still in a state to require being taken care of by others must be protected against their own actions as well as against external injury.[1]

The unique status of the brain

When procedures are considered which affect the brain a fresh consideration arises. Even if the patient can consent we have to ask if it is right to alter, probably irreversibly, the structure of the organ on which the patient's volition and power to consider treatment is based. If he cannot consent or refuses to agree to treatment, is it justified to override his wishes so that one may physically abolish the elements of his brain which have enabled him to sustain his objection? In either case, with or without consent, would we be in the position of chopping off the hands not of a thief but of a man who has created a work of art which we do not like, or perhaps an idol of which we disapprove?

Many psychiatrists who practised in the 1950s have no difficulty with one aspect of the question. Although frontal leucotomy was overused, and sometimes crudely employed, there was a time when ECT was sometimes insufficient to treat effectively all cases of severe depression, and when antidepressant drugs were not available. From about 1945 a proportion of patients in continuing misery from depression were treated with leucotomy, and in well-selected cases the cost–benefit ratio was such that in the view of patient, family, and physician the operation was usually held to have been a substantial success. Formal studies reveal that the procedure, and especially some of its later modifications, was worthwhile in cost–benefit terms.[2–8]

Men and women who were ill had accepted that their structurally normal brains could be cut into, and had recovered, resuming happy and effective lives. Before surgery their mood was often appalling and their judgement of life and events was made irrational by that mood. They still had perhaps enough command of their thoughts to make a valid decision about whether to have an operation, and the consequences were beneficial for many. Yet the brain was both the organ of decision and the site of operation. In principle, and in practice, it is acceptable to operate on the brain to relieve emotional disorder provided that the patient can make a valid decision about the risks and benefits, and that these risks are small enough and advantages large enough.

A more specific argument could also be considered. The part of the brain subjected to treatment may not be involved in decision-making. Hence that part is open to operation on the same terms as a limb or abdominal organ. I find this argument unattractive, however, because profound disturbances of mood usually affect judgement; and it may be specious to claim that the site of operation does not have a function in the process of making decisions. It is better to rely on the presence of feelings and of reasoning which validate consent.

Similar considerations apply to the use of ECT in depression resistant to medication but which is of the type known to be likely to respond to ECT. If the patient is willing, there is no ethical problem in giving ECT. Hazards to life are minimal, any impairment of brain function is minimal or temporary, structural disturbance is highly unlikely from a well-conducted course of treatment, and therapeutic results are frequently dramatic.

This situation, however, represents the optimal circumstances for physical manipulation of the brain. The anticipated cost–benefit ratio is highly favourable: risk to life is low; substantial personality change is not an issue; the patients are suffering intensely; and they can reasonably expect good results and minimal disadvantage. More difficult problems arise with patients who refuse treatment, with patients whose treatment may be recommended for the sake of others because of their aggressive or other unacceptable behaviour, and in those constrained by circumstances like imprisonment so that obtaining consent to treatment may be felt to be forced upon them in some way by conditions which others impose. Some of these dilemmas require attention with respect to each type of physical manipulation of the brain.

Electroconvulsive therapy (ECT)

The status of ECT has been assessed in the valuable report of the American Psychiatric Association (APA) Task Force on the subject.[9] ECT is now mainly used for severe depression where suicide is a major risk.[10,11] Other unusual indications include some forms of schizophrenia[9] and mania.[9] The risk to life is very small,[12] as little as 1 in 28 000 treatments in one survey.[13] In five other reports the death rate ranged from nil to 0.8 per cent of patients treated.[9] The treatment's effects are both scientifically proven and highly regarded clinically. Compared with drugs ECT is the more effective treatment for severe depression, particularly psychotic depression.[9,14,15] ECT compared with 'mock' ECT is highly effective.[16] A double-blind, controlled trial which did not show a good result for ECT in depression[17] has been criticized as inadequate,[18] and also as permitting a possible favourable interpretation.[19] Other trials have favoured ECT moderately[20] or markedly.[21] Another trial[22] favoured ECT against placebo, although the treatment was complicated by the use of active medication in some subgroups. Costello,[23] who notes the failure of trials to be methodologically perfect, recognizes that ECT produces unique effects on memory which might not be mimicked by placebo so that a truly blind, controlled trial may be impossible to achieve.

Controlled trials are perhaps not necessary if the long-known work of Cronholm and Ottosson[24] is accepted. They showed a quantitative relationship between the amount of epileptic discharge produced and the remission of depression. This is probably the strongest evidence available for the significance and effectiveness of the actual convulsion. A consistent relationship has also been shown between the dose-response ratio with ECT and the overall results.[25] This has long been observed by practising psychiatrists gauging the response to treatments and looking for the typical stepwise improvement in the successful case.

The main complication of ECT is temporary impairment of memory. Objective tests indicate that after a conventional course (6–12) of bilateral or unilateral applications, ECT produces no detectable permanent loss of memory for prior years.[9] Memory is lost for events around the time of treatment but new learning is not detectably affected several months later.[26] Prospective research comparing patients having ECT and controls showed no relative impairment in the ECT group on an extensive battery of psychological tests.[27] However, two-thirds of patients who have had ECT, especially bilateral ECT, do complain of memory difficulty. Extended courses of 250 bilateral ECT have been shown to be associated with long-term memory impairment.[9] Three retrospective reports[9] found impairment on tests of memory and cognitive function, but, as the APA Task Force reports, there are alternative explanations in terms of the patients' diagnosis or treatment which might have been factors in causing the memory damage. It seems reasonable to assume that after six months, ECT rarely causes more than mild memory difficulty, but that the risk increases with successive treatments, particularly those given bilaterally. Brain damage is known to result from anoxia, which may cause gliosis. There are no convincing reports of these phenomena after ECT which can be dissociated from the occurrence of anoxia due to more primitive methods of treatment than are currently available. A thorough review of whether ECT alters brain structures concluded that there was no such evidence.[28]

Attempts have been made to ban or curtail the use of ECT, most notably in the state of Alabama, where in state hospitals no less than three specialists and five others have been required to approve the treatment for a patient.[29] In California, the law specifies that before ECT can be given to a voluntary patient, even in a private office, informed consent must be obtained from the patient according to a standard, written-consent form supplemented by the physician with appropriate information pertaining to the specific patient being treated. The information to be given includes 'significant risks ... especially noting the degree and duration of memory loss (including its irreversibility)' and that 'there exists a division of opinion as to the efficacy of the proposed treatment...'[30] Thus 'informed consent', as stipulated by law, includes a scientifically groundless criticism of the treatment and misleading allegation about its efficacy which disparages the available scientific information. ECT may not be given to minors (under 12 years of age) in California and only in an emergency, as a life-saving procedure and after three child psychiatrists have approved it, to those between 12 and 16 years. A court hearing is required as well as the consent of the appropriate relative or guardian to give ECT to a patient of any sort who is not competent to give consent. Winslade *et al.*[31] comment that interposing the law between physician and patient results in delay or denial of service while failing to resolve critical legal issues involving competence and consent.

Such political activity over a highly successful treatment owes little to knowledge of clinical practice and is also an interference with a patient's free choice of treatment. To some extent such measures are stimulated by claims that ECT is overused, for inappropriate conditions, and even to punish recalcitrant patients. Oddly, they seem to owe little if anything to the worst example of misuse of ECT, the practice of 'de-patterning' through frequent multiple treatments. That treatment, as advocated by Cameron,[32] produced memory changes and confusion, but was quickly ignored or rejected by almost all other psychiatrists.[33] These are matters for technical decision and competent clinical practice, and not arbitrary legislative interference. The currency which such wild law-making gains is to some extent due to irresponsible journalism. Psychiatry is a common subject for the news media and physical manipulation of the brain is a dramatic and appealing topic.

Whether ECT should be given to patients against their will is a more troublesome issue. The problem was common but is now infrequent; yet it occasionally still arises in patients with a severe (usually acute) depressive illness not responsive to medication or other measures. In a series of 315 patients examined retrospectively, 16 per cent were unable or unwilling to give informed consent.[34] A few such patients object strongly to ECT. Some have had it and developed a fear of it even though it is beneficial. Some of these may yield to sympathetic persuasion. Others remain adamant. There may be a serious risk of suicide or other self-harm, the patient's distress is often severe and his or her judgement disordered. This situation can be compared with forcible appendectomy in children. The patient stands to gain far more than he or she will lose but cannot decide rationally. The psychiatrist is ethically obliged to attempt to relieve suffering and to prevent suicide (see Chapter 21). Apart from the serious effects mentioned, other deleterious psychological, social, and financial results may occur. Yet there exists, nevertheless, a concept of a right to effective treatment.[35] On occasion I have seen ECT given against the patient's will. He or she has continued to accept both the treatment and the relationship with the psychiatrist long after the compulsory status has lapsed, the relatives were grateful, and no recrimination ensued. A legal system which does not provide such an effective measure to relieve suffering could be regarded as inhumane.

The APA Task Force[9] permits treatment where the patient is incompetent but refuses, and their report emphasizes correctly that the guiding principle should be good overall care with minimal delay and no restriction on the exercise of sound clinical judgement. In Victoria, Australia, ECT may be given despite a patient's refusal but subject to review procedures (Bloch, personal communication, 1997).

The practical qualifications in this context are important. The diagnosis and alternative treatments should be double-checked by independent psychiatrists (if the patient does not respond there may be underlying dementia or physical illness). The agreement of the principal carer is desirable on ethical grounds and also in some jurisdictions on legal grounds. If those who are likely to be most concerned for the patient do not approve the treatment, doubts should arise as to its justification. The psychiatrist should also be satisfied that the family support is given out of love and not out of antagonism and should be sure, also, that he is not himself responding out of irritation or frustration or other illegitimate motives. Granted that these conditions are met it is appropriate to insist on providing treatment. Not to give it could be regarded as negligence but, in my view, the decision to treat against a patient's wishes should always be validated by an independent professional colleague.

The position adopted in this discussion is paternalistic. However, the paternalism is shared with colleagues, and just as to have good parents is valuable for children so to have good fatherly (or motherly) physicians can be valuable to psychotic patients. It is not necessary to reject paternalism because it may be confused with authoritarianism. Although some readers may feel that a contractual relationship which relies on an ethic of partnership is a better option, and in my view, the patient has more to gain from a scrupulous fiduciary approach in which the professional does not take advantage of his inevitably greater knowledge of the illness and its treatment. Since physicians are expected anyhow to observe fiduciary self-restraint it seems mistaken to suppose that they are not influential in the outcome of the patient's decision.

Apart from its use in depressive illness ECT is rarely indicated today. Paradoxically, in view of the concern about memory, it has a role in some patients with organic brain disease. It can help those with depression and

Alzheimer's Disease[36] (or other dementia) where the use of drugs is limited; and it has long had a place in the treatment of Parkinson's disease with depression or delusional changes.[37] Rarely, manic or catatonic schizophrenic patients may require it briefly and the considerations that apply are essentially the same as those relating to severe depression. More often the issue of consent is a 'paper' issue. The patient will not sign a form or is not competent to do so but accepts preparation for treatment, fasts before the anaesthetic, knows that he or she will receive electricity to the brain, and receives the anaesthetic injection before treatment without complaint. As with depression, the doctor who fails to give ECT after all the above criteria are satisfied could be regarded as negligent morally, even if not legally.

Psychosurgery

The main neurosurgical procedures used in psychiatry are leucotomy and amygdalotomy, the former to control depression, the latter to control aggression, against the self or others. The former standard leucotomy is no longer used but stereotactic operations are now applied in carefully selected cases, at least in Australia, Britain, Canada, Sweden, and the United States.

Neurosurgical operations on putatively healthy brain tissue to relieve psychiatric symptoms are generally called psychosurgery. The definition requires care. A World Health Organization booklet[38] defines psychosurgery as 'the selective surgical removal or destruction ... of nerve pathways with a view to influencing behaviour'. Bridges and Bartlett[7] point out that this definition is incorrect because most modern psychosurgery is concerned with the treatment of severe, intractable affective illnesses without any intended effect on behaviour at all, although of course behaviour may alter where it is directly influenced by the illness. Unfortunately, the United States Department of Health Education and Welfare has taken the same view as the WHO booklet and has defined psychosurgery as: (1) surgery on diseased brain tissue of an individual not suffering from physical disease for the purpose of changing or controlling behaviour; or (2) surgery on diseased brain tissue of an individual if the sole object of the surgery is to control, change, or affect behavioural disturbances.[39] As Bridges and Bartlett state[7] 'a better definition of contemporary psychosurgery is: the surgical treatment of certain psychiatric illnesses by means of localized lesions placed in specific cerebral sites'. A formal change in the title of the treatment from psychosurgery to 'neurosurgery for mental disorder' is taking place. Freeman[40] points out that such a term, to be used in the UK, is in line with terms used in other countries such as Sweden and the US and is further justified for the following reasons: the term psychosurgery has become firmly linked with older, freehand operations which had little to do with modern psychosurgical techniques; the surgical technique is the same as that used for other conditions such as Parkinson's disease and pain; and the term further emphasizes that this is a treatment for specific conditions such as treatment-resistant, major depressive disorder and obsessive–compulsive disorder and is not a treatment for behaviour disturbance, aggression or anti-social traits. All this is correct, although it does still leave the need to use the term for occasional instances where help in controlling aggressive impulses is deliberately sought by individuals, as discussed below.

This matter is important, as will be seen, since the incorrect definition has served as a basis for unreasonable conclusions which are likely to affect the availability within the United States of certain valuable operations.

Operations for disturbed affect

Psychosurgery as we know it began with an operation on the frontal lobes. This was proposed by Egas Moniz, a neurologist, and undertaken by a surgeon, Almeida Lima, on 12 November, 1935.[41]

The earlier history of different forms of leucotomy was discussed in previous editions. In 1977 an enquiry in the United States[42] found that about 400 procedures, meeting the definition of psychosurgery which the Department of Health Education and Welfare has adopted, were being performed annually in the United States. No significant psychological deficits were attributable to the psychosurgery in the patients evaluated and the treatment was efficacious in more than half of the cases studied. The data presented did not indicate that the procedure had been used for social control (as had been alleged) or been applied disproportionately to minority or disadvantaged populations (as had been noisily claimed). Most psychosurgery patients were middle-class individuals referred to neurosurgeons by psychiatrists and were about equally divided between males and females. The National Commission for the Protection of Human Subjects of Biomedical and Behavioral Research in the United States found that psychosurgical treatment constituted a minuscule proportion (estimated to be less than 0.001 per cent) of psychiatric treatment in general.

Hussain *et al.*[43] have shown, in a follow-up of all cases from a defined urban population, that psychosurgery is of value particularly in those with depression, agoraphobia, obsessive–compulsive disorders, and certain forms of schizophrenia. Reports on stereotactic procedures continue to support this view,[44,45] particularly for intractable obsessive–compulsive disorders.[46,47]

The evidence reviewed indicates that some forms of psychosurgery are recognized procedures in that physicians refer patients for them, agree on indications, and can anticipate the outcome with considerable accuracy. It is therefore surprising that the US National Commission concluded that 'the procedure' did not constitute 'accepted practice', seeming to confound a range of different operations. The conclusion seems to have had more to do with political and social factors than with the merits of the case, even though the Commission was regarded as having produced a surprisingly favourable report on psychosurgery.

This is not to say that some psychosurgical procedures are not experimental but rather that certain operations are as well founded as many valid medical or surgical procedures. Stereotactic subcaudate tractotomy,[2,48] forms of limbic tractotomy,[4,44,49] and Crow's procedure[8] constitute such accepted forms, as probably do other modified leucotomy operations. Sachdev and Sachdev[50] after reviewing current practice conclude that psychosurgery is well established in a limited field.

Operations for pain

Although cerebral operations have been carried out to alleviate pain and have been briefly mentioned above they do not currently present an ethical issue. Those undertaken are always done with consent. Pain may be due either to physical lesions or to an emotional state.[51–53] It is accordingly defined as: 'an unpleasant sensory and emotional experience associated with actual or potential tissue damage, and described in terms of such damage'.[54] Whatever the cause the experience is subjectively the same, an unpleasant one in the body. Leucotomy for pain when done in the presence of an appropriate psychiatric illness such as depression was successful. However, in the last 30 years in regular work with patients with pain, I have only seen one who seemed to require an operation for pain and depression and he underwent a stereotactic subcaudate procedure. This modified version of leucotomy was used primarily because he was depressed. When depression was not the main cause, leucotomy for pain only worked if the lesion was so large as to damage the personality.[52,55]

Thalamic and mesencephalic operations have also been undertaken for pain but were largely unsatisfactory.[56] These were for patients presumed to have, usually, peripheral lesions causing pain. Hypophysectomy has been undertaken with benefit for pain from carcinoma,[57] but no one talks of this organ as sacrosanct. Thus operations for pain can either be assimilated to the argument concerning those for affective disorder or are not in significant use. Stereotactic cingulotomies are currently undertaken in a small number of centres for patients with cancer pain. It is hard to imagine anyone saying that they should not be done. This suggests that the wrong sort of distinction is made between psychiatric illness and physical illness, namely that it is all right to operate on the brain for a physical illness arising elsewhere in the body, but not for a psychological disturbance. This seems unfair not only to the patient who has pain for psychological reasons but also to all those patients who might benefit psychiatrically from brain surgery.

Operations for aggression

The human brain has highly developed anatomical and physiological systems which subserve self-protective and aggressive responses accompanied by emotional changes. Like some animal brains it may also provide for cool predatory aggression.[58] Most human aggression is affect-laden. When human aggression is not affect-laden it is probably unpredictable by anybody other than the aggressor. Much human aggression can also be linked to environmental triggers, cultural patterns, childhood experiences, and a variety of other social and psychological factors. Even so, predicting aggressive behaviour is extremely difficult, and for clinical purposes very unreliable, despite the fact that better prediction would be of enormous value for judges in passing sentence and in connection with offenders seeking parole. Nevertheless, there are a few people who engage in repeated aggression against themselves or others. As a result of animal work and from operations on patients who had temporal lobe lesions (often with epilepsy) it became evident that aggressive behaviour might be modified by means of surgical lesions, particularly in the region of the amygdala. Such stereotactic operations have been undertaken in retarded patients,[59] overactive and self-damaging children,[60] and violent offenders.[61–66] The number of operations in this last group is small in Britain and the United States, and other English-speaking countries. Several hundred operations in India[60] on children apparently required consent not only from the children's parents but from grandparents as well.

The outcome of such operations was reviewed by Smith and Kiloh[61] and Kiloh.[66] Some successes were obtained, although the results are not nearly as good overall as those for the modern stereotactic leucotomies. Nevertheless, Kiloh pointed out that these stereotactic procedures appear to be relatively safe and effective in 50–75 per cent at a 2-year or longer follow-up. Given time, the results might become as good as those for modern stereotactic leucotomies, but opportunities for development of the technique in suitable patients are circumscribed due to public concern.[42] Smith and Kiloh[61] point out with respect to operations for rage on non-epileptic patients with limbic lesions that: 'Whether such operations can benefit those individuals experiencing dangerous rage attacks with relatively minimal provocation whose behaviour is currently regarded as a socially defined deviation from the norm remains uncertain. But it seems unlikely in view of current State laws that in the foreseeable future this interesting and perhaps important problem can be solved.' The US National Commission for the Protection of Human Subjects of Biomedical and Behavioral Research was called into being after 'widespread expression of public and Congressional concern that these procedures were ... being used for "social control" of dissidents and violence-prone individuals and ... were performed disproportionately on members of minority populations'.[42] In the event, the results quoted indicate an enormous disproportion between the outcry and the facts. It is doubtful that, as already described, any operation was done for 'social control' and minorities were notably under-represented.

In Germany, surgery performed on the hypothalamus for sexually deviant behaviour has been abandoned.[67] The issues are whether the social considerations form an invalid part of the criteria to operate, and whether operations may be done without consent. The first question relates mainly to psycho-surgery for violence. The second relates both to surgery for mood states and to that for violence.

Brain surgery with consent

Whether we like it or not the attribution of the word 'disease' to a set of circumstances is still determined in many cases by social factors. Fabrega[68] has described how social behaviour is used as a criterion of disease in different societies. Disease patterns are determined, at least in part, by social expectations combined with biological features. More precise definitions of disease (or health) have long eluded agreement. Physicians see themselves as trained to recognize 'diseases' or 'conditions'. If they have something to offer in the treatment or care of a 'condition' they are willing to provide their professional services, whether by drug treatment, other physical treatment, psychological treatment, or modifying the environment. For example, patients with peptic ulcer or conversion hysteria alike might be recommended for discharge from the armed services, and so on.

This need not stop the physician from limiting his functions to those which are strictly 'medical'.[69] The physician who adheres to a traditional role will help a patient to achieve improved social conditions but will not, *qua* physician, seek automatically to change the conditions. In some cases (cholera due to contaminated water) his view of a social arrangement will be deservedly accepted. In others (the advisability of conscription for instance) he is wise if he is content only to exercise the role of an ordinary citizen.

Consider the situation of the physician with patients who are recommended for treatment of disorders of thought, mood, or behaviour. The disorder may be recognizable as a syndrome, with or without biological correlates. There is no reason not to treat if the patient asks for help. If it is not what the patient seeks, the doctor may then determine if this arises from disturbed reasoning. If so he might treat the patient who does not ask but does not oppose, provided that the proper representatives of the patient (family or guardian) request him to do so and they do not have a disproportionately selfish interest. (The wife of a depressed man once asked me if a leucotomy would help the impotence from which he had suffered even before depression supervened.)

If the patient clearly opposes treatment then the physician will only rarely, if ever, undertake it. Those circumstances where this might happen in relation to the brain will be discussed below. At this point it is sufficient to stress that our notion of illness is partly biological and partly social; treatment by physicians applies the 'medical model'; we may recognize and sometimes act in relation to social factors but only within the limits of our agreed function as physicians, which is to diagnose and promote cure where we can, and to advise on how individuals and society may take responsibility for prevention and control. I consider the ethics of psychosurgery from this standpoint.

Relevant considerations include, as always, the cost–benefit ratio. Another issue is more 'ethical' in nature: whether it is right to destroy putatively normal brain tissue in order to treat emotional distress. Edgar[70] points out that there is no objection to operating on the brain as such, e.g. to remove a tumour. He argues that in the face of evidence that a person's aberrant behaviour resulted from a tumour we would not reject surgery because it might be at a brain site related to personality or the 'will'. Thus, we are prepared to operate where there is evidence of structural brain change and accept possible effects upon personality. In individuals who can freely consent to accept a procedure which offers benefit in the absence of structural pathology there is no reason not to proceed; indeed their freedom is curtailed if we refuse permission.

General surgery also is not confined to abnormal tissue. Legs may be shortened, ears or noses reshaped (although healthy). Normal organs are removed; adrenalectomy for cancer or hypophysectomy for severe pain.[57] Operations have also been performed on putatively normal brain tissue in order to relieve pain attributed to organic disturbances elsewhere in the body.[56] Although it is sometimes technically difficult to do useful surgery on the brain there should be no objection to brain surgery for psychiatric disorder solely because the brain controls thought, feeling, judgement, and personality. Logically it is the most appropriate site of intervention in a consenting individual. But it is vital to consider in due course what constitutes valid consent.

The relevance of brain pathology is a practical issue. Mark and colleagues[64,65] rejected psychosurgery for aggression except in patients with brain lesions. They seemed to accept, in principle, that psychosurgery for aggression might be allowed without physical pathology but ruled it out in the short run. Physical pathology may be one source of evidence that intervention at a particular site is 'good medicine', especially if: (a) the patient's brain is damaged in a particular way; (b) most people who have such damage behave aberrantly as does the patient; and (c) this operation has changed that behaviour in others.[62] However, to limit operations to cases which only have physical pathology would make for several difficulties.

If a person is distressed and regrets his aggressive behaviour, why should he not have the opportunity to receive surgical help, assuming it is effective, just as much say, as, a man with phobias or a woman with chronic pain due to an emotional disorder or to a lesion outside the brain? There are also problems in defining pathology broadly and yet perhaps it should be so defined. While EEG abnormality is less easily related to disease than histological change it could have a valid association with pathophysiological disturbance in the temporal lobes. Relevant chemical abnormality or microanatomical differences will not be found before surgery.

Hostile community attitudes to psychosurgery have presumably contributed to a reduction in its provision. In Ontario a compulsorily hospitalized patient, even if competent, is not permitted the opportunity to consent to psychosurgery.[71]

In Britain, the control of medical decisions also covers modern procedures to the detriment of work at a highly respected specialist centre with exceptional experience. The Mental Health Act 1983, Section 57, empowers a Mental Health Act Commission, under a non-medical chairman, to supervise psycho-surgery. The patient, his general practitioner, his regular psychiatrist, and the specialist to whom he is referred may all concur that surgery is indicated. A separate medical commissioner and two lay persons are then required to confirm the validity of the patient's consent, but carry no responsibility for further care. The patient has to accept therefore an intrusion of a panel with no therapeutic role, which has the power to block the operation. Patients considering such treatment have to make difficult decisions in which discretion and careful evaluation of feelings are required from their advisors. A committee procedure and legal process are likely to help less than they hinder. Suicide followed one such refusal.[71-76] These arrangements, brought on by a combination of anti-psychiatry attitudes and bureaucratic officialdom, violate the patient's rights. The numbers affected may be few, but the breach of principle remains troublesome.

Brain surgery without consent

If it is humane and proper to undertake appropriate surgery to change the mood or behaviour in people who can make an appropriate judgement and provide valid consent, would it not also be humane and morally unobjectionable to operate for the same purposes on those who cannot give consent because they are too disordered? In principle, the answer appears to be 'yes' but special precautions are required. It should first be abundantly clear that the patient is unable to decide. Any hint of reluctance, expressed in behaviour like eating before an anaesthetic, or failing to cooperate with preliminary procedures, should be taken to indicate that consent is refused. The decision should also be made by more than one person, and should be subject to review and supervision. As usual, it should require the approval of the next of kin. Perhaps too it should be approved by independent, non-medical professionals. Although the participation of the latter in decisions about competent patients has just been rejected because it is an interference with their valid wishes, its disadvantages may need to be accepted in those who cannot themselves provide valid consent. Given that these conditions were satisfied it should be acceptable to treat patients who do not consent but who do not explicitly or implicitly refuse.

In my view it is unacceptable to perform brain surgery for psychiatric disorder on patients who decline explicitly or are implicitly unwilling. This differs from the case with ECT. The first reason is the minimal or absent risk of permanent brain changes with ECT compared to surgery. It is unacceptable to enforce even such infrequent hazards, as those of brain surgery, on unwilling patients. The second reason is still more fundamental. Even if there were no potential deleterious changes with surgery or if the manipulation were not physical, it is wrong to impose potentially permanent changes in a person's mental state against his or her wishes. In case this should seem to be at variance with my willingness to recommend ECT to patients who refuse it, I would point out that the effects of ECT are essentially temporary and ECT may be required as an emergency (even life-saving) treatment. Although neurosurgery for mental disorder may also be life-saving this is rarely an emergency issue and it is inconceivable that its effects could be classed only as temporary. Third, while compulsory ECT also violates a person's autonomy, he still has the opportunity to protest later. It does not carry the risk of permanently changing his original personality and basis of judgement or take away his opportunity later to seek redress himself for unfair treatment.

It is the case that social systems do sanction interventions on people's minds which may change them permanently. Reformatories, correctional institutions, and penal establishments usually have such aims but they are not founded on medical considerations. If we consider procedures dependent on medical expertise the refusal of consent is a fundamental objection to those which seek irreversible personality change. This position also safeguards against the appalling possibility of the use of psychosurgery on unwilling political prisoners.

There remains an important issue to do with consent, that of people detained in prison or similar institutions. Mark and Neville[65] argue that such detainees should receive psychosurgery. Against this view a hypothetical case may be raised of a prisoner who develops a depressive illness for which he would have a neurosurgical procedure if free. Provided that the conditions of his imprisonment and the length of his sentence have no bearing on the treatment recommended, which could, say, be a modified leucotomy, the question of an operation should be decided on the same basis as for a free person. However, psychosurgical operations suggested for prisoners do not always satisfy these requirements. They are in any case few in number. It is likely that there is a ratio of a score of articles on the topic to every operated prison case. But these operations are offered for aggressive behaviour and may change the overall personality as well as simply reduce the frequency of aggressive antisocial actions. Let us assume that such treatments work. The question arises whether it is right to suggest them to detainees, and if so under what conditions. Some patients engage in self-mutilation and other self-harm; they may be glad to undergo an operation which relieves them of this behaviour. Surgery in those cases may be as much justified as for depression.

Other patients deeply regret behaviour—say repeated assault—which they fail to control and which harms others. One such man sought treatment for his aggressive outbursts by attending a hospital out-patient department. An oral phenothiazine was included in his treatment and was partly helpful, but supposing surgery gave the best chance of success and that the risks were acceptable, would it be justified to operate? A conditional 'yes' seems the correct position. If so, the treatment should also be available to prisoners with the same motives and wishes. Again the right answer appears to be in the affirmative. However, prisoners present great difficulties.

At this point let us turn to established procedures with known benefits and hazards. The problem is whether the prisoner consents not because he wants to change his behaviour but to alter the terms of his sentence. A prisoner at the end of a sentence is unlikely to be influenced by the hope of early release. A prisoner with a longer sentence facing years of incarceration may well assent for just that reason. While his consent might not be called free it might be valid in his own interests. We are reluctant to accept that such an external constraint should influence the decision. In the one case the decision may be correct. But since constraints from the civil authority can be varied then a variety of new constraints might appear (perhaps with a new revolutionary government?) and psychiatrists would be asking surgeons to take on new cases because of new political changes. The thought is anathema. It is even not too far-fetched to imagine a society where imprisoned psychiatrists might be invited to accept some intracerebral lesion which would change their responses so that they would become more accepting of the tenets of the government of the day. Colleagues have been tortured in Argentina, or vanished without a trace. Doctors Semyon Gluzman and Anatoly Koryagin suffered in the Soviet prison system because of their adherence to medical ethics. Less resolute physicians (and who can say he would be a hero like one of these two?) might prefer the option of surgical treatment. It seems hard to assent voluntarily to any brain operations under conditions of constraint.

In the United States a court action was brought to prevent psychosurgery on a prisoner,[77] in prison for 18 years for murder (followed by necrophilia), who had satisfied an independent review committee consisting of a law professor, a priest, and an accountant that he wanted the operation. Ironically the attorney who brought the case, '*Kaimowitz* v. *Department of Mental Health*' (representing himself and members of the Medical Committee for Human Rights on behalf of John Doe), had never consulted the prisoner. The lawyer appointed to represent the prisoner thought that he desperately wanted the operation,[78] but proved to the court's satisfaction that the man was detained unconstitutionally. Despite the fact that the prisoner was therefore freed, the hearing continued on whether a prisoner could give free informed consent to psychosurgery and it was held that he could not. It has been argued[79] that the conclusion violates the right to treatment; it seems unlikely that the *Kaimowitz* case represents a definitive conclusion in United States law.

The issue may be hard for American lawyers or judges. It also presents a problem in practical ethics for doctors. It seems that physicians, lawyer, priest, and accountant all believed, probably correctly, that the prisoner wanted the operation. But after he was released, he changed his mind. Burt's account[78] gives clear reason to think that the circumstances of imprisonment and medical surveillance at least contributed to the prisoner's consent without any attempt being made by physicians to press the prisoner to agree.

Given this finding it can be argued that no prisoner's consent should be accepted for psychosurgery related to the type of behaviour which has led to his imprisonment. This however might be double jeopardy. It seems desirable to allow long-term, non-political prisoners (strictly defined) to obtain treatment for repetitive violence or enduring symptoms such as depression. One condition could be that the prisoner is aware that no early change is to be expected in his sentence. Only long-term evidence of change (say, a minimum of three years), would be acceptable thus leading to a reduction of the sentence. Such change should be equally helpful if it occurred in the absence of surgery. It would be up to him to decide whether he wanted the procedure to facilitate his own efforts. Second, a substantial independent review of the proposal would be required to assess if the consent was reasonable and consistently held and not linked to the hope of early release. With such safeguards few operations might be done, but it is likely they would be potentially beneficial. Prisoners should have a 'right to treatment'. (It is unthinkable that anyone who did not give consent should have psychosurgery under these conditions.)

On the basis that minors, prisoners, and committed mental patients should not be denied the benefits of treatment, the US National Commission concluded that psychosurgery should be available to them provided their rights were rigorously guarded.[42] The American Psychiatric Association (APA) supported the Commission's report but opposed psychosurgery on children because of insufficient data, and approved it only for prisoners if its indications were unrelated to criminal behaviour. The US Department of Health Education and Welfare decided however not to fund psychosurgery research or treatment in any of the institutions it supports for any of these groups.[42] This action, going against the recommendations of both the National Commission and the APA echoes the Commission's conclusion that psychosurgery is not 'an accepted procedure', and perhaps relates more to public noise than to the facts or merits of the matter.

In regard to children and the mentally incompetent I suggest that stringent procedures, similar to those outlined for prisoners, might be used to establish that the procedure offered potential benefit and was in the patient's interest, and consent was not implicitly refused.

To sum up this discussion I have argued that psychosurgery should never be forced but it might be done with non-competent individuals or prisoners subject to stringent safeguards, some of which have been considered.

Depth electrical stimulation

Electrical stimulation offers similar problems to the longer-established forms of surgery, and one additional problem. The similar problems arise because electrical stimulation is not without risk of permanent harm. Any electrode or sheaf of inserted electrodes might rupture a vessel. Indwelling electrodes, further, can give rise to a fibrotic reaction—particularly when used for repeated electrical stimulation. These risks require assessment in relation to any electrical stimulation procedures; those of a haemorrhage are minimal but those of fibrotic reactions may be greater than is currently anticipated and implanted electrodes for dorsal column stimulation in the treatment of chronic pain have given rise to fibrotic reactions. Intracerebral electrodes, no matter how sophisticated, might do something similar, or promote other forms of continuing damage to cells. Nevertheless, both Heath *et al.*[80] and Crow[8] appear satisfied that this technology is minimally harmful; in any event it is not intended for permanent implantation. Only occasional operations with indwelling brain electrodes have been performed for the alleviation of pain[81] and they do not appear to be very successful.[82] They have been used for chronic pain from peripheral lesions. As with the unsuccessful thalamic operations it is hard to imagine moral objections being raised to these treatments in the event of their being successful.

The additional problem of indwelling electrodes is that they may lead to pleasurable self-stimulation. This is not common, but if it were someone would be sure to want to stop it. Patients may be given batteries which they can switch on and off and which deliver stimulation via the implanted electrodes. When this is done with animals taught to perform certain acts, such as lever-pressing, to initiate self-stimulation they may work assiduously to stimulate themselves, and do little else,[83] even neglecting food, water, and natural functions. For a further account see Valenstein,[84] who indicate that these phenomena are rare and difficult to reproduce consistently in either animals or man.

Apart from these practical considerations there is a theoretical issue. Medicine has so far aimed mostly at correcting abnormalities, not at obtaining a subjective Elysium. Self-stimulation which achieves the latter would be socially objectionable. Should we pay heed to such a consideration? Perhaps not if we accept the principle of self-determination. Again, in practice, the operation would probably not get far since it would be biologically disadvantageous, leading to failure of reproduction as well as death. These reasons appear to be sufficient for physicians to avoid supporting the achievement of 'super-normality' through self-stimulation.

There are hypothetical situations in which surgery and especially self-stimulation could make people function more effectively. Perhaps intelligence could be improved. Mark and Neville[65] point out that this makes the medical profession an authority on what constitutes the good life. A case could be argued for that conclusion without suggesting that we are the sole authorities, but we are probably neither ready nor willing to assume such a role.

The dangerous attraction of electrical brain stimulation is that it offers possibilities for investigation of the brain in patients with psychoses and perhaps some other conditions. We would clearly like to know more about patterns of activity in different parts of the brain in various psychiatric conditions—and even non-medical circumstances. This motive is not a legitimate guide to the ethical management of patients. The advantages of electrical stimulation are greater precision in placing lesions, and graded ablation of tissue. After stimulation in a given part, tissue may be destroyed by increasing the current used, with only small amounts needing to be destroyed at any one time. Painstaking steps can be taken to secure relief without personality change. Despite the problems outlined, this is presumably the optimal way to conduct psychosurgical ablation.

Surgical innovation

We have so far covered operations where established knowledge is extensive and sound, and hypothetical situations. Most controversy attaches to innovations in treatment. This is a difficult subject in any branch of medicine. Is the first patient to have a particular procedure being treated ethically? If not, how can new operations be developed? It is clear that procedures should not ordinarily be introduced on those who cannot provide consent. This might be qualified to the extent that the new procedure is likely to be less risky than established treatments. A coronary patient may be able to give valid consent for a new type of graft if it is carefully explained. But can psychiatric patients needing treatment for mood, thought, or behaviour respond similarly to unproved treatments? The answer is uncertain, but it is equally uncertain whether a patient with say advanced cancer can make a free, valid judgement on a last-chance new procedure. Commentators like Mark and Neville,[65] recommend the criterion of physical pathology. In the development of techniques this is plainly sound. If we start from a base where verification of the facts is relatively easy, we have more chance of finding beneficial new procedures with the least risk.

However, neither psychiatric nor cancer patients should be excluded from the possibility of being helped by an unproven treatment which has scientific merit. Innovations which carry hazards should therefore be allowed with due precaution for both of these groups. Innovative treatments are now subject to increasing control through special review mechanisms. It seems best to argue that they may occur in consenting free patients without physical disease, that the review procedures will be maintained and that they will not be done on prisoners or incompetent patients. But if an innovation were suggested which could only help prisoners or the incompetent this conclusion might need to be revised.

Some practical issues

In all the procedures discussed the outstanding precondition is that they should be capable of yielding benefit, at minimal risk, and the benefit should be significantly greater than that from alternative less traumatic procedures. By this criterion ECT is distinctly attractive. Its morbidity rate is much less than that of antidepressants. It causes transient memory disturbance, very few fatalities, and little other trouble. First-generation, antidepressant drugs which are still much used, frequently cause discomfort (dry mouth, constipation, blurred vision), and quite often cause hypotensive faint feelings, and can provoke a variety of significant illnesses such as prolapsed haemorrhoids from constipation, epileptic fits, retention of urine, and, theoretically, glaucoma. The cardiotoxic effects of the antidepressants probably also cause fatalities several times more frequently than does ECT. Even the more recent SSRIs and other second-generation, antidepressants have a quota of such effects.

Although leucotomy-like procedures are rarely performed the modified versions have high standing, as described above, because their morbidity is low and their therapeutic effects are recognized.[2,5,8] They have a proper place in psychiatric treatment.

Among the psychosurgical procedures, amygdalotomy, amygdalectomy, and hypothalamic operations[85,86] are less well established. This is not only due to opposition to treating behaviour rather than emotional distress, but also because knowledge of their benefit and risk has been available for a much shorter time and research methodology (criteria for selection of patients and for assessment of results, etc.) is still embryonic. There is also an inherent difficulty in assessing aggression compared with depression, obsessive–compulsive disorders, or schizophrenia because its manifestations are usually intermittent. Although some patients assault themselves or others continuously, major violence tends to be committed by those with 'over-controlled hostility'.[87,88] The prediction of dangerousness is handicapped by the infrequency with which it occurs. Cocozza and Steadman[89] for instance, developed a measure which correctly predicted dangerous behaviour in 11 of 14 patients who did behave dangerously. A further 25 patients were predicted as dangerous but did not prove to be so. Thus, although the measure produced highly significant results statistically they were clinically insufficient. The best conclusion we can draw is that operations for aggression should be developed first for those who frequently make assaults, so that a time-span of one or two years will permit a more valid assessment of outcome.

The difficulty in prediction provides a further reason to avoid surgery in prisoners where outcome is a condition for release. Psychiatrists function on the principle that the patient who is interested in cure will be frank with them. This does not necessarily hold for some aggressive prisoners. Psychiatric skill is reasonably good in treating psychotic and neurotic patients but less so with those who intend to deceive, and we need not be ashamed of this since we do not or should not purport to be detectives. We are another type of investigator. Assessing patients who might say they are cured by operation so as to promote their release is fraught with difficulty. On the other hand, it seems wrong to deny them the benefits of potentially effective surgery. Sufficient safeguards are therefore required to allow psychosurgery on consenting prisoners. A novel instance, derived from the Detroit case,[77,78] would be to conduct a legal review of a prisoner's sentence, such that the opportunity for him to challenge his incarceration could be pursued before psychosurgery.

References

1. Mill, J. S. *On liberty* (1859). London, Watts, 1929.
2. Knight, G. C.: Further observations from an experience of 660 cases of stereotactic tractotomy. *Postgraduate Medical Journal* 49:845–54, 1973.
3. Tooth, G. C. and Newton, M. P.: *Leucotomy in England and Wales 1942–1954*. Reports on Medical Subjects, No. 104. London, HMSO, 1961.
4. Dax, E. C.: The history of prefrontal leucotomy, in *Psychosurgery and society*, ed. J. S. Smith and L. G. Kiloh. Oxford, Pergamon, 1977, pp. 19–24.
5. Mitchell-Heggs, N., Kelly, D., and Richardson, A.: Stereotactic limbic leucotomy —a follow-up at sixteen months. *British Journal of Psychiatry* 128:226–40, 1976.
6. Goktepe, E. O., Young, L. B., and Bridges, P. K.: A further review of the results of stereotactic subcaudate tractotomy. *British Journal of Psychiatry* 126:270–80, 1975.
7. Bridges, P. K. and Bartlett, J. R.: Psychosurgery: yesterday and today. *British Journal of Psychiatry* 131:249–60, 1977.
8. Crow, H.: The treatment of anxiety and obsessionality with chronically implanted electrodes, in *Psychosurgery and Society*, ed. J. S. Smith and L. G. Kiloh. Oxford, Pergamon, 1977, pp. 71–3.
9. American Psychiatric Association: *Electroconvulsive therapy*. Task Force Report No. 14, Washington DC, 1978.
10. Guze, S. and Robins, E.: Suicide and primary affective disorders. *British Journal of Psychiatry* 117:437–8, 1970.
11. Huston, P. E. and Locher, L. M.: Involutional psychosis: course when untreated and when treated with ECT. *Archives of Neurology and Psychiatry* 59:385–94, 1948.
12. Beresford, H. R.: Legal issues relating to electroconvulsive therapy. *Archives of General Psychiatry* 25:100–2, 1971.
13. Barker, J. C. and Baker, A. A.: Deaths associated with electroplexy. *Journal of Mental Science* 105: 339–48, 1959.
14. Bruce, E. M., Crone, N., Fitzpatrick, G., *et al.*: A comparative trial of ECT and Tofranil. *American Journal of Psychiatry* 117:76, 1960.
15. Medical Research Council: Clinical trial of the treatment of depressive illness. *British Medical Journal* 5439:881–6, 1965.
16. Sainz, A.: Clarification of the action of successful treatments in the depressions. *Diseases of the Nervous System* 20:53–7, 1959.
17. Lambourn, J. and Gill, D.: A controlled comparison of simulated and real ECT. *British Journal of Psychiatry* 133:514–19, 1978.
18. Ottosson, J. O.: Simulated and real ECT. *British Journal of Psychiatry* 134:314, 1979.
19. Watt, J. A. G.: Simulated and real ECT. *British Journal of Psychiatry* 134:314, 1979.
20. Johnstone, E. C., Deakin, J. F. W., Lawler, P., *et al.*: The Northwick Park ECT trial. *Lancet* ii:1317–20, 1980.
21. Brandon, S., Cowley, P., McDonald, C., Neville, P., Palmer, R., and Wellstood-Eason, S.: Electroconvulsive therapy: results in depressive illness from the Leicestershire trial. *British Medical Journal* 288:22–5, 1984.

22. Wilson, I. C., Vernon, J. T., Guin, T., *et al.*: A controlled study of treatments of depression. *Journal of Neuropsychiatry* **4**:331–7, 1963.
23. Costello, C. G.: Electroconvulsive therapy: is further investigation necessary? *Canadian Psychiatric Association Journal* **21**:761–7, 1976.
24. Cronholm, B. and Ottosson, J. O.: Experimental studies of the therapeutic action of electroconvulsive therapy in endogenous depression. *Acta Psychiatrica Scandinavica* **35**:(Suppl. 145)69–97, 1960.
25. Price, T. R. P., MacKenzie, T. B., Tucker, G. J., and Culver, C.: The dose response ratio in electroconvulsive therapy. *Archives of General Psychiatry* **35**:1131–6, 1978.
26. Squire, L. R. and Chace, P. M.: Memory functions six to nine months after electroconvulsive therapy. *Archives of General Psychiatry* **32**:1557–64, 1975.
27. Weeks, D., Freeman, C. P. L., and Kendell, R. D.: ECT III. Enduring cognitive deficits? *British Journal of Psychiatry* **137**:26–37, 1980.
28. Devanand, D. P., Dwork, A. J., Hutchinson, E. R., Bolwig, T. G., and Sackeim, H. A.: Does ECT alter brain structure? *American Journal of Psychiatry* **151**:957–70, 1994.
29. *Wyatt v. Hardin*, No.3195-N (M.D. Ala. 28 Feb. 1975, modified 1 July 1975): I. *Mental Disability Law Reporter* **55**, 1976.
30. California Welfare and Institutions Code, 1979. SS.5325.1, 5434.2, 5326.7, 5326.8.
31. Winslade, W. J., Liston, E. H., Ross, J. W., and Weber, K. D.: Medical, judicial and statutory regulation of ECT in United States. *American Journal of Psychiatry* **141**:1349–55, 1984.
32. Cameron, D. E.: Production of differential amnesia as a factor in the treatment of schizophrenia. *Comprehensive Psychiatry* **1**:26–34, 1960.
33. Gillmor, D.: *I swear by Apollo*. Montreal, Eden Press, 1960.
34. Galletly, C. A., Field, C. D., and Ormond, L.: Changing patterns of electro-convulsive therapy use: results of a five-year survey. *Australian and New Zealand Journal of Psychiatry* **25**:535–40, 1991.
35. Leong, G. B. and Eth, S.: Legal and ethical issues in electroconvulsive therapy. *Psychiatric Clinics of North America* **14**: 1007–20, 1991.
36. Duffy, J. D. and Coffey, C. E.: Depression in Alzheimer's disease. *Psychiatric Annals* **26**:269 –73, 1996.
37. Höflich, G., Kasper, S., Burghof, K. W., *et al.*: Maintenance ECT for treatment of therapy resistant paranoid schizophrenia and Parkinson's disease. *Biological Psychiatry* **37**:892–4, 1995.
38. World Health Organization: *Health aspects of human rights.* Geneva, WHO, 1976.
39. *Determination of Secretary regarding recommendation on psychosurgery of the National Commission for the Protection of Human Subjects of Biomedical and Behavioural Research.* Federal Register, 15 Nov. 1978. Part VI, pp. 53241–4.
40. Freeman, C.: Neurosurgery for mental disorder in the U.K. *Psychiatric Bulletin* **21**:67–9, 1997.
41. Moniz, E.: Les Premieres tentatives operatoires dans le traitement de certains psychoses. *Encephale* **31**:1, 1936.
42. US National Commission for the Protection of Subjects of Biomedical and Behavioral Research involving Psychosurgery: *Report and Recommendations with Appendix.* Bethesda, MD: US Department of Health, Education and Welfare, Publication No. (OS)77-0001 and (OS)77-0002, 14 March 1977.
43. Hussain, E. S., Freeman, H., and Jones, R. A. C.: A cohort study of psychosurgery cases from a defined population. *Journal of Neurology, Neurosurgery, and Psychiatry* **51**:345–52, 1988.

44. Snaith, R. P., Dove, E., Marlowe, J., *et al.*: Psychosurgery: description and outcome study of a regional service. *Psychiatric Bulletin* **21**:105–9, 1997.
45. Mindus, P. and Nyman, H.: Normalization of personality characteristics in patients with incapacitating anxiety disorders after capsulotomy. *Acta Psychiatrica Scandinavica* **83**:283–91, 1991.
46. Mindus, P. and Jenike, M. A.: Neurosurgical treatment of malignant obsessive compulsive disorder. *Psychiatric Clinics of North America* **15**:921–38, 1992.
47. Hay, P., Sachdev, P., Cumming, S., *et al.*: Treatment of obsessive–compulsive disorder by psychosurgery. *Acta Psychiatrica Scandinavica* **87**:197–207, 1993.
48. Bridges, P. K., Bartlett, J. R., Hale, A. S., Poynton, A. M., Malizia, A. L., and Hodgkiss, A. D.: Psychosurgery: stereotactic subcaudate tractotomy an indispensable treatment. *British Journal of Psychiatry* **165**:599–611, 1994.
49. Baer, L., Rauch, S. L., Ballantine, H. T., *et al.*: Cingulotomy for intractable obsessive–compulsive disorder. Prospective long-term follow-up of 18 patients. *Archives of General Psychiatry* **52**:384–92, 1995.
50. Sachdev, P. and Sachdev, J.: Sixty years of psychosurgery: its present status and its future. *Australian and New Zealand Journal of Psychiatry* **31**:457–64, 1997.
51. Beecher, H. K.: *Measurement of subjective responses.* New York, Oxford University Press, 1959.
52. Merskey, H. and Spear, F. G.: *Pain: psychological and psychiatric aspects.* London, Baillière-Tindall and Cassell, 1967.
53. Sternbach, R. A.: *Pain: a psychophysiological analysis.* New York, Academic Press, 1968.
54. Task Force on Taxonomy of the International Association for the Study of Pain. *Classification of chronic pain: descriptions of chronic pain syndromes and definitions of pain terms.* Seattle, ISAP Press, 1994.
55. Elithorn, A., Glithero, E., and Slater, E.: Leucotomy for pain. *Journal of Neurology, Neurosurgery, and Psychiatry* **21**:249–61, 1958.
56. Cassinari, V. and Pagni, C. A.: *Central pain: a neurosurgical survey.* Cambridge, Mass., Harvard University Press, 1979.
57. Moricca, G.: Pituitary neuroadenolysis in the treatment of intractable pain, in *Persistent pain: modern methods of treatment*, ed. S. Lipton. London, Academic Press, 1977, pp. 149–73.
58. Sheard, M. H.: Neurobiology of aggressive behaviour, in *Aggression, mental illness and mental retardation: psychobiological approaches*, ed. D. Zarfas and B. Goldberg. University of Western Ontario, London, Ontario, pp. 76–93, 1978.
59. Kiloh, L. G., Gye, R. S., Rushworth, R. G., Bell, D. S., and White, R. T.: Stereotactic amygdalotomy for aggressive behaviour. *Journal of Neurology, Neurosurgery, and Psychiatry* **37**:437, 1974.
60. Balasubramaniam, V. and Kanaka, T. S.: Amygdalotomy and hypothalamotomy in a comparative study. *Confinia Neurologica* **37**: 195, 1975.
61. Smith, J. S. and Kiloh, L. G.: Psychosurgery and deviance, in *Contemporary themes in psychiatry: a tribute to Sir Martin Roth*, vol. 48, ed. K. Davison and A. Kerr. London, Gaskell, pp. 492–500, 1989.
62. Narabayashi, H., Nagao, T., Saito, Y., *et al.*: Stereotaxic amygdalotomy for behaviour disorders. *Archives of Neurology* **9**:1, 1963.
63. Heimburger, R. F., Whitlock, C. C., and Kalsbeck, J. E.: Stereotaxic amygdalotomy for epilepsy and aggressive behaviour. *Journal of the American Medical Association* **198**:741–5, 1966.

64. Mark, V. H. and Ervin, F. R.: *Violence and the brain*. New York, Harper and Row, 1970.
65. Mark, V. H. and Neville, R.: Brain surgery in aggressive epileptics: social and ethical implications. *Journal of the American Medical Association* **227**:765–72, 1973.
66. Kiloh, L. G.: The treatment of anger and aggression, in *Symposium on psychosurgery and society*, ed. J. S. Smith and I. G. Kiloh. Oxford, Pergamon, 1977, pp. 37–53.
67. Schmidt, G. and Schorsch, E.: Psychosurgery of sexually
68. Fabrega, H., Jr: *Disease and social behaviour: an interdisciplinary perspective*. Cambridge, Mass, MIT Press, 1974.
69. Merskey, H.: A variable meaning for the concept of disease. *Journal of Medicine and Philosophy* **11**:215–32, 1986.
70. Edgar, H.: Regulating psychosurgery: issues of public policy and law, in *Operating on the mind: the psychosurgery conflict*, ed. W. M. Gaylin, J. S. Meister, and R. D. Neville. New York, Basic Books, 1975.
71. *Mental health Act*; Section 35 Toronto, 1980, revised, 1987.
72. Bridges, P. K.: Psychosurgery and the Mental Health Act Commission. *Bulletin of the Royal College of Psychiatrists* **8**:146–8, 1984.
73. Bridges, P. K.: Addendum to 'Psychosurgery and the Mental Health Act Commission. *Bulletin of the Royal College of Psychiatrists* **8**:172, 1984.
74. Lord Colville: The Mental Health Act and second opinions. *Bulletin of the Royal College of Psychiatrists* **9**:2–3, 1985.
75. Thompson, C.: An open letter to Lord Colville. *Bulletin of the Royal College of Psychiatrists* **9**:100, 1985.
76. Bridges, P. K.: The Mental Health Act Commission and second opinions. *Bulletin of the Royal College of Psychiatrists* **9**:120, 1985.
77. *Kaimowitz v. Department of Mental Health*. Cir. Ct. Wayne City, Mich., Civil, No. 73-19434 AW, 10 July 1973.
78. Burt, R. A.: Why we should keep prisoners from the doctors. *Hastings Center Report* **5**:25–34, 1975.
79. Greenblatt, S. J.: *New York Law School Law Review* **22**:961–80, 1976–7.
80. Heath, R. G., John, S. B., and Fontana, C. J.: Stereotaxic implantation of electrodes in the human brain: a method for long-term study and treatment. *IEE Transactions on Biomedical Engineering* **23**296–304, 1976.
81. Hosobuchi, Y., Adams, J. E., and Linchitz, R.: Pain relief by electrical stimulation of the central gray matter in humans and its reversal by Naloxone. *Science* (New York) **197**:183–6, 1977.
82. Gybels, J.: *Electrical stimulation of the central gray for pain relief in humans*. Pain Abstract 1:170, 2nd World Congress on Pain. Montreal, International Association for the Study of Pain, 1978.
83. Delgado, J. M. R.:*Physical control of the mind: toward a psychocivilized society*. New York, Harper and Row, 1969.
84. Valenstein, E. S.: *Brain control*. New York, Wiley, 1973.
85. Sano, K.: Sedative neurosurgery, with special reference to posteromedial hypothalamotomy. *Neurological Medico-Chirurgica* **4**:112, 1962.
86. Sano, K.: Sedative stereoencephalotomy: fornicotomy, upper mesencephalic reticulotomy. *Progress in Brain Research* **21**:350, 1966.
87. Megargee, E. I.: A critical review of theories of violence, in *Crimes of violence*, ed. D. J. Mulvihill, M. M. Tumin, and L. A. Curtis. Washington DC, US Government Printing Office, 1969.

88. Quinsey, V. L., Pruesse, M., and Fernley, R.: A follow-up of patients found 'unfit to stand trial' or 'not guilty' because of insanity. *Canadian Psychiatric Association Journal* **20**:461–7, 1975.
89. Cocozza, J. J. and Steadman, H. J.: Some refinements in the prediction of dangerous behaviour. *American Journal of Psychiatry* **131**:1012–14, 1975.

14

Ethics and child psychiatry

Philip Graham

Ethical dilemmas usually result from conflicting principles; those involving child psychiatry are no exception. Consider a few illustrations. Parents have a right to bring up their children in privacy, but the state has a duty to protect children from cruelty and neglect. So long as children are competent to make decisions, they have a right to choose how they will spend their time, but the state has a duty to ensure all children receive education in school. The needs of a mother with incapacitating mental illness may best be met by keeping her children with her, but her children may thrive better in an adoptive or foster family. In this chapter I aim to clarify the ethical dilemmas facing mental health professionals who work with parents and children. As will already be apparent, there are no easy solutions; however several principles are available to assist professionals. While the thoughtful professional reflects carefully on ethical quandaries, a considerable body of case law, professional guidelines and relevant articles and chapters provide a helpful steer. The United Nations Convention on the Rights of the Child also offers a useful framework of principles that should govern policies affecting children.[1]

Child protection

A historical perspective.

Until well into the twentieth century children were regarded as their parents' property, and, in particular, that of their father's. This changed in 1925 when the Guardianship of Infants Act named the 'first and paramount consideration' in matters of custody and upbringing to be the child's welfare. This was the first time this principle had been articulated in English law. (I shall confine myself, for convenience, to English law when dealing with legislative provisions.) The legal position is similar in other Westernized countries, although English law has lagged behind other countries in child welfare. For example, in 1987 England became the last European country to make it illegal for teachers to beat children. In the 1990s England has the lowest age (10 years of age) of criminal responsibility in Europe.

Only in 1970 did it become firmly established in England that a court's determination of the child's best interests should override parental claims and other considerations. The Children Act of 1989 went further, making local authorities responsible for identifying children in need, providing services for their families, and preventing abuse and neglect. Children in need were defined as those unlikely to achieve or maintain a reasonable standard of health or development without provision of services by the local authority, or where health or development was likely to be significantly impaired without such provision, or where the child was disabled. The health authority's duties also involved the identification of children in need, and cooperation with relevant social services. Since the 1990s these authorities are duty bound to deal with cases that come to their attention, and to seek out those in need because of inadequate care in their families.

Conflicts of principle

The need to meet legislative requirements may result in ethical dilemmas for mental health professionals working with children and their families. For instance, an adult psychiatrist sees a patient with schizophrenia whose eight-year-old son suffers neglect because his single mother is hounded by hallucinations. This situation has arisen in the past, the patient always responding rapidly to appropriate medication. Should social services be informed even though this might antagonize the mother and jeopardize the therapeutic relationship?

A child psychologist treats a three-year-old girl with anxiety. During a session the therapist learns that her five-year-old brother, far from being over-protected like his sister, is neglected by his depressed mother. She has been preoccupied with the loss of her own mother for several weeks. Should the psychologist inform social services when again this might antagonize the mother?

In the two examples, both of which are commonly encountered in clinical practice, several principles clash. The duty to maintain confidential information conflicts with the duty to do what is best for the child. The duty to do what is best for the parent conflicts with what is best for the child. The duty to obey the law may collide with the duty to do what is best for the child. The duty to do one's best for a patient clashes with the duty to what is best for a non-identified but impaired sibling. In considering how to act ethically in these situations, the professional should bear the following in mind.

1. The welfare of a child is paramount when what is best for the child and what is best for the adult conflict. However, the welfare of the child is not the sole consideration; a minor benefit to the child may be outweighed by a major benefit to the adult.

2. The degree of chronicity in the situation is pertinent. For example, in the first example the fact that the mother has a chronic mental illness, lives alone with her child and has had long-standing psychotic symptoms

indicates that social services should have been actively involved for some time.

3. The likely benefit of contacting social services is noteworthy. The clinician familiar with resources available to other agencies in the district in which he or she works will be able to anticipate their capacity to respond appropriately. In the second example above, it is unlikely that any social services can do more than the psychologist. Indeed, with any hint of suicidal ideas in the mother, the psychologist is likely to consider referral to a child or general psychiatrist for a detailed assessment. There are however circumstances in which referral to social services is indicated even when its resources are stretched. These include situations when the child is at serious risk. How serious is serious? If in doubt, the professional should consult with a colleague. Discussion does not axiomatically mean referral.

4. The attitude to a referral of the parent, *and*, where appropriate, the child needs to be considered. In the two case examples above, I have suggested that both mothers would resist a referral to social services. However, this cannot be taken for granted. The attitudes of doctors to referrals to social services differ. Such attitudes may colour their perceptions as to the likely attitudes of parents. They should be aware of this possibility. Where possible, the consent of parents and, where appropriate the child, should be obtained prior to a referral. In the first case, it is ethically doubtful to refer without consent. In the second, it is ethically doubtful *not* to refer regardless of consent.

Ethical issues in relation to interagency working

A referral to another agency may accentuate ethical problems revolving around issues of confidentiality and interagency differences of opinion. Agencies may have contrasting policies concerning confidentiality. There is, however, no substitute for a trusting relationship between all involved agencies and family members. Legislation requiring open communication has facilitated the development of trust. However, it has also led to professionals taking greater care in the information they record in writing. This issue is also dealt with in Chapter 7.

Differences of opinion between agencies and their repercussions generate specific matters when children are involved. It is not infrequent for those working in mental health agencies to wish that social services would remove a child from the care of his parents more rapidly when he is at risk. The reverse may also be the case. Mental health professionals need to recognize that it is the legal responsibility of social services to decide on a child's optimal placement. They may wish to make clear in writing that they disagree with decisions taken by social workers, but they must recognize basic matters of legal responsibility. The more closely mental health professionals and social workers can work together, the more the service will work effectively for the benefit of the child. It is salutary for psychiatrists to remember, in particular, that many social workers regard the use of psychotropic medication in children as unethical, but are powerless to intervene.

Ethical issues relating to consent

Involvement of children and adolescents in decision-making in psychiatric and psychological interventions raises ethical issues often ignored by both parent and professional. The legal position is complicated in most countries since two sets of legislation, one for child protection (e.g. in England and Wales, the Children Act 1989) and one for the care of people with mental illness (e.g. in England and Wales, the Mental Health Act 1983), may be invoked in situations when compulsory intervention is desirable. Most dilemmas arise where compulsion is not in question; I consider these first.

When a child or adolescent is referred to a psychiatric clinic parents are expected to give implicit or explicit consent at various points. Shall they accept a referral to such a facility in the first place? At the first appointment shall they agree to observers or a video-recording? Shall they consent to physical or psychological investigations? If there is an offer to treat shall this be taken up? Shall treatment be discontinued if it appears ineffective or harmful? At all these various points to what degree has the child or adolescent been part of the decision-making process? Are his views freely given? Are they taken seriously?

There are at least five reasons why children *should* participate in decision-making.[3]

1. The principle of self-determination holds for children to the degree they are competent to exercise judgement.
2. Children's involvement improves communication between professionals and family members.
3. Children involved will cooperate more fully in treatment.
4. Such children will enjoy a greater sense of self-control.
5. These children will sense the professional's respect for their capacities, so providing opportunities for social development.

Naturally, there may be concern that children and young people are undesirably burdened with decision-making beyond their competence. Further, many children may well be able to contribute, but prefer that parents or others take the responsibility. While these are appropriate concerns, it is more common for decisions to be taken over children's heads (often literally so!), even though they are able and willing to contribute to decisions affecting their treatment.[4]

A useful basis to consider the desirability or necessity of obtaining consent of children and young people was provided by two English judges in 1985.[5]

Victoria Gillick, the mother of five daughters, sought to prevent her health authority from issuing guidance to family doctors allowing them, in some circumstances, to provide contraceptive advice to girls under the age of 16 years without informing their parents. The High Court dismissed her case, but an appeal court unanimously found in her favour. The case was finally taken to the House of Lords, but here Mrs Gillick lost by a majority verdict. Lord Fraser concluded that a girl under the age of 16 had the legal capacity to consent to contraceptive advice, examination, and treatment provided she had sufficient understanding and intelligence to know what they entailed. For Lord Scarman the legal principle was that:

parental rights were derived from parental duty and existed only so long as they were needed for the protection of the person and property of the child. Parental right yielded to the child's right to make his own decisions when he reached sufficient understanding and intelligence to be capable of making up his own mind.

This case provides a basis for others in which there is disagreement about whether a child's consent is desirable or necessary (not only those when contraception is involved). It follows that mental health professionals caring for children should regard it as a duty to determine a child's competence to consent to proposed interventions and involve the child to the maximum of his capacity. In most cases, this means checking informally that the child knows what is proposed and agrees to it.

Many parents and professionals underestimate how much children and young people do understand. Weithorn and Campbell[6] gave four groups aged 9, 14, 18, and 21 complex tasks to assess their competence to consent as judged by evidence of choice, capacity to evaluate a reasonable outcome, to produce a rational basis for their choice, and to show inferential understanding. While 9-year-olds were less competent than the young adults, they were nevertheless able to contribute significantly to decision-making. The 14-year-olds were as competent as the two adult groups.

If a child disagrees with a proposed action, then, assuming he is 'Gillick competent', i.e. can reasonably understand what is proposed, the professional should not proceed. However, the action may be necessary for the child's health or safety. Even life may be endangered. In these circumstances, in Britain and in most Western countries, one can invoke mental health or child protection legislation. The older the child and the more clear-cut it is that he is mentally ill, the more appropriate to invoke mental health law. With younger children, child protection legislation is more apt.

Practical and ethical difficulties have arisen over compulsory treatment for children under the age of 16 who suffer from anorexia nervosa but refuse treatment. Psychiatrists and parents may appeal to the courts for permission to pass a nasogastric tube to feed the child against her will. Contradictory judgments have resulted. While child protection law usually allows the child more opportunities to present her case, mental health law is appropriate if the young person suffers from a mental illness and her behaviour is a danger to herself. In England, the Mental Health Act Commission published guidelines in 1997 clarifying the use of the 1983 Mental Health Act in these circumstances.

Diagnostic labelling

Ethical aspects of diagnosis are discussed in Chapter 10. Certain matters arising in children require specific consideration. In particular, the act of attaching a diagnostic label has been questioned ethically.

The position of the child psychiatrist involved in diagnosing behavioural problems which revolve around deviance and troublesome behaviour is ethically fraught. It is easier for the psychiatrist to limit attention to severe disorders which result in maladaptation to a better than average (if not to an optimal) domestic or school environment. Many argue that the psychiatrist's task when faced with non-conformity and deviance involves not only adequate assessment, but also a full appraisal of the environment in which the child is apparently, and perhaps only apparently, creating difficulties. Assessment of a child who shows disruptive school behaviour should therefore incorporate a consideration of teaching methods and the means applied to achieve classroom control.

Referring to the 'medicalisation of maladjustment and distress', Goodman[7] has sought to distinguish between social and educational problems that have no identifiable health component, and 'other disorders that need the sort of input that only health service professionals are likely to provide'. Examples of social and educational problems include conduct disorders, whereas health service problems include the hyperkinetic syndrome and anorexia nervosa. While sometimes clothed in ethical garb, the controversy over Goodman's views relates to the efficient use of resources (which is only indirectly an ethical matter). These issues are discussed further in relation to treatment.

The negative effects of labelling are discussed by Hobbs,[8] who points out forcefully that a diagnosis like 'mental retardation' can stick for life inappropriately, adversely affecting opportunities. However labels can also exert positive effects. A child pressured inappropriately may be given a learning programme more suited to his needs and abilities after a label of 'brain damage' has been applied. Excellent facilities for children with autism may only open their doors once a label has been assigned. Furthermore, the use of labels is a pragmatic as well as an ethical issue. Do labels act to the detriment of children? Findings are not clear-cut. In a much quoted study by Rosenthal and Jacobson,[9] children were given randomly assigned intelligence scores which were then passed to their teachers. At the end of the academic year, children allocated low scores achieved significantly less well than those allocated high scores. However, attempts to replicate have not obtained such clear-cut findings, and, even in the original the results held for younger but not older children. Research has also been done on the effects of labelling by comparing the outcome of boys charged and found guilty of certain offences with that of boys who had shown equivalent antisocial behaviour, but had not been involved in legal proceedings.[10] Here evidence supports negative effects of labelling.

Most psychiatrists are aware of the dangers of the use of labels when communicating with a person whose attitude to them is uncertain or unknown. They should regard it as an essential part of their job to explain the terms they use and so ensure these are understood, at least at the time of an interview. This is a counsel of perfection as, once a report has been despatched, psychiatrists often have little control over the way their words are interpreted. The issue of confidentiality, discussed elsewhere, is of considerable relevance in this context.

Treatment

Ethical aspects of psychotherapy and drug therapy are dealt with in Chapters 11 and 12. However, special issues pertain to children.

Psychotherapy with children

Various types of psychotherapy bring different ethical issues.

Psychodynamic therapies

Broadly speaking, these derive from the theories of Sigmund Freud, though much psychodynamic practice has a tenuous connection with Freud's original ideas. Usually dynamic therapy is concerned with bringing unconscious thoughts and feelings into consciousness and the way past events, often forgotten and traumatic, impinge on current behaviour. Various ethical issues arise when this approach is used in children. Orthodox analysts such as Diatkine[11] regard social adaptation and symptomatic criteria of change irrelevant. This can lead to difficult situations when parents want their child's behaviour to change. (This is not a problem for those psychodynamic therapists for whom behavioural change is a focus.) The privacy of the therapy sessions may become problematic. In contrast to past practice, most therapists do discuss aspects of the therapy with parents. But the therapist may undermine parental authority by retaining as secret some material that emerges during the child's treatment. Finally, as Diatkine makes clear, the therapist may be overly bound to ideas derived from theory which influence his interpretations, even if the theory is not relevant to the particular child in question.

Cognitive and behavioural therapies

These therapies also pose special ethical issues when applied to children.[12] The emphasis is either on behavioural change or on altering cognitions regarded as exerting a deleterious effect on the child's emotional health. Especially with younger children, treatment is done in collaboration with parents, who may be responsible for carrying out procedures under the therapist's supervision. Ethical problems may arise given the focus on social conformity, perhaps at the expense of the child's individuality. This issue is pertinent in treating conduct or oppositional disorders when a child's behaviour might be a legitimate response to an intolerable situation. Achieving classroom tranquillity through behavioural methods can hardly be regarded as justified unless, as a result, improved opportunities are created for learning, which enable targeted children to benefit as well as their peers. Gender identity disorders raise similar issues. How appropriate is it for parents and therapists to collude in treating tomboyish behaviour in girls or effeminate behaviour in boys, or even gender identity disorders in either sex, when the children themselves are satisfied with their own identities.[13]

As Marcus and Schopler[4] note when discussing ethical issues in relation to behavioural therapy, 'a further problem arises because the behavioural experimental models and paradigms are reductionistic and do not reflect the wide range of factors that influence and enrich human behaviour'. Finally, although this problem may not arise anywhere nearly as frequently as opponents of behaviour therapy suggest, focus on symptoms alone may result in ignoring salient, covert psychological problems. Depression, for example, may underlie antisocial behaviour; a depressed child may also be suffering from covert sexual abuse.

Family therapy

Family therapy with its emphasis on treating individuals as members of a family, risks jeopardizing family structures that do not fit preconceived notions of 'good' family functioning. For example, family therapists commonly insist that the father attends sessions. His participation may lead to altered family functioning, whereby his role and authority are threatened; this is likely to apply to working-class families, in which responsibilities of parents tend to be rigidly defined. Most family therapists appreciate this danger but a danger it remains.

Many parents are reluctant to 'criticize' their children to the therapist in front of them, and hesitate to do so. Family therapists, however, encourage expression of negative feelings, in the reasonable belief that the child knows what the parent feels anyway, and that unless honest acknowledgement of these aspects of communication prevails, improved family relating is unlikely. It remains a concern that parents will develop a pattern of negative thinking about their children which they would otherwise not have adopted. Another question is the therapist's use of potent procedures, such as family sculpting and paradoxical injunction; they may be applied without the therapist being aware of the degree to which he engages in paternalistic manipulation.[15]

Common problems

Some problems are common to all forms of child psychotherapy. One is the issue of the child's consent. For young people over 16 years of age in the UK, the young have an overriding right to accept or refuse treatment. For those under 16 the earlier discussion about consent is relevant in initiating or continuing treatment. Another issue is offering treatment, especially psycho-dynamic forms (although this is also true of much cognitive and behaviour therapy), that has not been adequately evaluated, or has been found to be relatively ineffective.[7] All therapists should avoid exaggerating the likelihood of success, especially if the family is going to invest their time, and possibly their money, into the therapy.

Medication

Different ethical issues arise with various forms of medication.

Stimulants

The delineation of the hyperkinetic or attention-deficit hyperactivity syndrome is well established; a genetic component in their aetiology is likely.[16] Methyl-phenidate and dextroamphetamine sulphate improve learning task perform-ance in laboratory research; they also reduce distractability, impersistence, and disruptive behaviour in the classroom. This effectiveness is not only limited to children diagnosed as hyperactive, but also, at least in the experimental situation, the drugs enhance performance in normal children.

Notwithstanding the research, the use of stimulants has been criticized on the grounds that unusually active children through inappropriate expectations in the classroom, but otherwise normal, are given drugs instead of better teaching and more individualized attention. In fact, in children who have been fully assessed and diagnosed as showing the hyperkinetic syndrome, improved teaching and other forms of management at home are relatively ineffective compared to stimulants.

The diagnostic validity of attention-deficit hyperactivity disorder, used more commonly in North America, is less securely based than that of hyperkinetic disorder. Medication is used much more frequently to treat it, raising grounds for ethical concern. North American paediatricians apparently accede fre-quently to the wishes of parents and teachers and medicate difficult and disruptive children. Child psychiatrists in the US and physicians elsewhere are more conservative, taking the view that it is not their task to smooth out ordinary variations in learning ability. This is especially the case when improved levels of concentration are only achieved with the loss of vivacity, curiosity, and exploration, all of which may be lost with exposure to medication. On the other hand, many children outside North America who suffer from a severe hyperkinetic syndrome are denied this treatment either because of their doctors' inexperience in the use of medication or their ideological objections to its use, or due to a governmental policy which impedes or even bars the prescribing of stimulants.

Antidepressants

Interesting ethical issues emerge with the use of antidepressants in children. Although numerous, sound meta-analyses confirm that tricyclic antidepressants are ineffective in children and younger adolescents, clinicians continue to prescribe them.[17] This is not the only example of widespread use of a form of medication demonstrated to be ineffective, but, given the far from negligible mortality among children and adolescents from accidental and non-accidental poisoning with tricyclics, their continued use is a matter of particular ethical concern.

The selective serotonin-uptake inhibitors seem effective in children, but have not been adequately evaluated in this age group because of legislation restricting the conduct of trials in minors. Clinicians commonly prescribe this medication for children and adolescents notwithstanding the pharmaceutical companies' recommendations against this practice. This inconsistency obviously needs resolution, but clinicians occupy a tricky ethical position in the meantime. Legislation enacted in the US in 1997 requires testing of drugs in children prior to their general clinical use in this age group.

Finally, use of antidepressants in young people may lead to insufficient attention being paid to basic factors underlying their sadness. Medication becomes a poor substitute for potentially effective and clearly indicated social and personal interventions. The dilemma is further compounded by parents concealing pertinent aetiological factors for which they are responsible or which they find difficult to face. A clinician acts unethically if he or she only prescribes antidepressants and has not attempted to identify and deal with personal and social stresses that obviously contribute to the clinical picture.

Psychosurgery and electroconvulsive therapy (ECT)

Trenchant criticism of both procedures has been made on ethical grounds when used in children under the age of 16 years. Temporal lobectomy is indicated in some cases of uncontrolled seizures arising from a unilateral lesion. Temporal lobe epilepsy is often accompanied by psychiatric features, of which aggression may be prominent. Although such behaviour often improves following surgery which leads to reduced seizure frequency, behavioural criteria alone should not determine the decision to operate or not.

While ECT is rarely used in prepubertal children[18] and infrequently in adolescents,[19] it has a role in catatonic and severe depressive states that have not responded to psychotherapy and adequate medication. Providing ECT is administered competently and after alternative treatments have failed, and a check is made on memory and other cognitive functions, ethical objections are not justifiable. Indeed, withholding an effective treatment like ECT might well, in certain clinical circumstances, be unethical.

Alternative treatments

Mental health professionals working with children and families may be asked to offer their views and refer to alternative therapies, including dietary manipulation in hyperkinetic disorders, holding treatment and facilitated communication in autism, and cranial osteopathy in a variety of disorders. They may be told that their patient is to see an expert (even in another country) at great expense, whose methods are questionable. It is ethically problematic how to respond. Having worked in the National Health Service in the UK (free at the point of delivery), I have felt inclined to protect parents planning to spend considerable time and money on unevaluated treatments by reducing parental expectations of the outcome to realistic levels, and expressing appropriate scepticism. It also helps to reassure the family that they should feel free to return if the alternative therapy turns out to be ineffective. The therapist may need to act more decisively, for example in the case of facilitated communication with autistic children, since the treatment may involve serious exploitation. Finally, it is salutary to remember that today's alternative therapy may be conventional therapy tomorrow. This has, to a degree, been the case with dietary therapy, which is validated, at least for some patients, in the hyperkinetic syndrome.[20]

Special inpatient hospital and residential educational provision

While separate educational provision for disturbed and slow-learning children has been traditionally seen as advantageous, and indeed as a form of positive discrimination, attitudes have swung noticeably since the 1970s. It is thought preferable to educate children with exceptional needs wherever possible alongside ordinary children, in order to reduce stigmatization and ensure as normal a school experience as possible. In the US, this is reflected in state and federal law. For example, the Individuals with Disabilities Act, PL102-109 rules that children with disabilities be educated in the least restrictive environment possible; similar legislation has been enacted in many other countries. Notwithstanding the basic change in attitude, most experts agree that *some* special provision is necessary and desirable, at least for severely disabled children. In so far as psychiatrists advise on special educational needs, their decisions have a distinctly ethical dimension. Consider, for example, the question of special provision for a child who is benefiting from his current education, but is disruptive and disturbing others; or placing a child in a special residential school, since, while a special school is necessary, limited resources mean the unavailability of day placement.

Teachers often press psychiatrists and educational psychologists, quite understandably, to use their influence to remove extremely difficult children and adolescents and place them in special educational, or even hospital institutions. Conflict between education, health, and social services as to who bears responsibility in these circumstances often results in an ethical dilemma for child psychiatrists. They are faced with a series of questions which challenge their sense of integrity. Has all been done in order to maintain the child in ordinary school; for example, has individualized attention in the form of a teaching assistant been given a fair trial? If such a step has been considered and rejected, has the authority compared the costs of the alternatives, including special school placement? Will the latter actually help? If not, has this been stated openly to parents and teachers, so that no one is in doubt for whose benefit removal from the regular school is planned? How aware is the child of the real reasons for the proposed placement? Allocating limited resources is, of course, always problematic, and is especially so when mental health professionals are responsible for recommending expenditure of funds from a range of public sources.

Research

Scanty knowledge about the cause, prevention, and effective treatment of psychiatric disorders in children and adolescents highlights the need for vigorous research. Indeed, conducting research may be ethically more justified than unevaluated clinical practice. The non-researching clinician may be surprised to hear that those who participate in both clinical psychiatry and research are more ethically comfortable in research pursuits than in applying treatment of dubious validity in a possibly spurious effort to alleviate suffering. Non-therapeutic research into behavioural and emotional disorders has already brought considerable benefit to children. For example, many children with enuresis have been spared unnecessary physical and psychological investigations by knowledge gained from community surveys about its benign natural history. Lack of published trials on the effectiveness of various forms of medication commonly used with children poses greater ethical problems for the clinician than would the conduct of such trials for the researcher.

Most ethical matters affecting research in children are similar to those encountered in adults, and are dealt with in Chapter 22). (See Munir and Earls[21] for a helpful review.) Issues especially relevant in child psychiatric research include consent, confidentiality, assessment of risks and benefits, ethics review committees, and the advantages of participation in research for the socialization of children.

Many aspects of consent to participation in research resemble those covered above in relation to treatment. They have been usefully discussed in the context of biological research and physical disorders by the British Paediatric Association[22] and the Institute of Medical Ethics.[23] In most countries, parents consent on behalf of their children under the age of 16. However, children should be approached as well. Any dissent (regardless of the proxy's decision) should be taken seriously and should usually preclude participation. Children of normal intelligence over seven years of age are likely to understand sufficiently for their judgement to be significant. Indeed the ability of children to comprehend quite complex matters is widely underestimated.[6] Information provided to parents should be stated as clearly as possible to their children.[24] Parents should be keenly encouraged to discuss with their children what will transpire, and parents and researchers should not resort to coercion.

The risk–benefit ratio is a crucial concept in research with children. Although a universally agreed classification of risk is unavailable, the following four-category schema is useful:

(1) minimal risk, (risk is no greater than that faced in everyday activities such as crossing the road);

(2) greater than minimal risk with prospect of direct benefit to the subject (such as might arise in the trial of a new antidepressant);

(3) greater than minimal risk without such direct benefit, but likely to yield knowledge about the subject's condition; and

(4) not otherwise approvable, but provides an opportunity to understand, prevent, or alleviate a serious health problem.

In general, non-therapeutic research involving more than minimal risk is unethical. However, the risk rating of a procedure may vary. The British Paediatric Association guidelines, for example, regard venepuncture as carrying more than minimal risk. But a one-year follow-up of seven-year-olds after this procedure found only trivial distress.[25] Venepuncture is more reasonably regarded as a minimal risk, providing the child consents. Do psychiatric interviews pose more than minimal risk? Clearly, if a child is asked questions which provoke anxiety and where no opportunity for discussion is available, the risk is potentially more than minimal. But it is impossible to predict which children might feel distressed.[26] All children interviewed in community studies should probably be given an opportunity for debriefing. This is not obligatory, but should be incorporated as an option for those who seek it; parents suspecting a distressing response in their children should be positively encouraged to request debriefing for themselves and their children.

Information about children is subject to special considerations that apply less markedly to adults. A videotaped research interview may, for example, portray a child in a way that he is unhappy to have shown to researchers at a later point. Information about a child's detected or undetected delinquencies fall into a similar category. Records that could provide identifiable information should therefore be destroyed after a specified period.

It is important that research ethics committees should include members expert with younger age groups. If they do not, significant issues may be ignored. These include the way in which children's consent may be obtained, the role of parents during experimental procedures, developmental considerations in assessing anxiety in research subjects, and whether comparable information could be obtained by studying adults.

Participation in research is so common a part of adult experience that it might be regarded as desirable for it to form part of a child's socialization experience. Children need to know about the research process, consent, and confidentiality. Furthermore, while children's altruism might be 'played upon', a greater danger lurks of children being debarred from altruistic activity because of overprotective adults. Research involving children can be virtually obstructed because of an overriding concern for their rights. Advances in knowledge for the benefit of the afflicted necessitate inconvenience in people who do not themselves suffer; the privilege of participating in such activity should not be denied to children.

Conclusion

Clinical practice and research in child psychiatry raises special ethical problems given the special status of children and adolescents. The special position of parents as trustees for their children's welfare, or the role of the state in providing clinical services for parents who have difficulty fulfilling their responsibilities are also noteworthy. Mental health professionals who are constantly aware of their ethical responsibilities towards children and their families will find their work more time-consuming, but are likely to offer a more thoughtful, child-orientated service.

References

1. *United Nations Convention on the Rights of the Child.* New York, United Nations, 1991.
2. Bainham, A.: *Children, parents and the state.* London, Sweet and Maxwell, 1988.
3. McCabe, M. A.: Involving children and adolescents in medical decision making: developmental and clinical considerations. *Journal of Pediatric Psychology* **21**: 505–16, 1996.
4. Shield J. and Baum, D.: Children's consent to treatment. *British Medical Journal* **308**:1182–3, 1994.
5. Dyer, C.: Contraceptives and the under 16s: House of Lords ruling. *British Medical Journal* **291**:1208–9, 1985.
6. Weithorn, L. and Campbell, S.: The competency of children and adolescents to make informed treatment decisions. *Child Development* **53**:1589–98, 1982.
7. Goodman, R.: Child mental health: who is responsible? *British Medical Journal* **314**:813–14, 1997.
8. Hobbs, N.: *Issues in the classification of children.* San Francisco, Jossey-Bass, 1975.
9. Rosenthal, R. and Jacobson, J.: *Pygmalion in the classroom: teacher expectation and pupils' intellectual development.* New York, Holt, Rhinehart, and Winston, 1968.

10. West, D. J.: *Delinquency: its roots, careers and prospects*. London, Heinemann, 1982.
11. Diatkine, R.: The ethics of child psychoanalysts, in *Ethics and child mental health*, ed. J. Hattab. Jerusalem, Gefen, 1994.
12. Guidelines to good practice in the use of behavioural and cognitive treatments. *Bulletin of the Royal College of Psychiatrists* (In press).
13. Rosen, A. C., Rekers, G. A., and Bentler, P. M.: Ethical issues in the treatment of children. *Journal of Social Issues* **34**:122–36, 1978.
14. Marcus, L. M. and Schopler, E.: Ethics and behaviour therapy with children, in *Ethics and child mental health*, ed. J. Hattab, Jerusalem, Gefen, 1994.
15. Lindley, R.: Family therapy and respect for people, in *Ethical issues in family therapy*, ed. S. Walrond-Skinner and D. Watson. London, Routledge and Kegan Paul, 1987.
16. Goodman, R. and Stevenson, J.: A twin study of hyperactivity: II The aetiological role of genes, family relationships, and perinatal adversity. *Journal of Child Psychology and Psychiatry* **30**:691–710, 1989.
17. Fisher, R. L. and Fisher, S.: Antidepressants for children. Is scientific support necessary? *Journal of Nervous and Mental Diseases* **184**:99–102, 1996.
18. Cizadlo, B. and Wheaton, A.: Case Study: ECT treatment of a young girl with catatonia. *Journal of the American Academy of Child and Adolescent Psychiatry* **184**:332–35, 1995.
19. Walter, G. and Rey, J.: An epidemiological study of the use of ECT in adolescents. *Journal of the American Academy of Child and Adolescent Psychiatry* **36**:809–15, 1997.
20. Schmidt, M. Mocks, P. Lay, B. H-G., *et al.*: Does oligoantigenic diet influence hyperactive/conduct-disordered children—a controlled trial. *European Child and Adolescent Psychiatry* **6**:88–95, 1997.
21. Munir, K. and Earls, F.: Ethical principles governing research in child and adolescent psychiatry. *Journal of the American Academy of Child and Adolescent Psychiatry* **31**:408–14, 1992.
22. British Paediatric Association: *Guidelines for the ethical conduct of medical research involving children*. London, Royal College of Paediatrics and Child Health, 1992.
23. Nicholson, R. (ed.): *Ethics and medical research in children*. Oxford, Oxford University Press, 1987.
24. Alderson, P.: 'Will you help us with our research?' *Archives of Disease in Childhood* **72**:541–2, 1995.
25. Smith, M.: Taking blood from children causes no more than minimal harm. *Journal of Medical Ethics* **11**:127–31, 1985.
26. Herjanic, B. Hudson, R., and Kotloff, K.: Does interviewing harm children? *Research, Community, Psychology, Psychiatry Behavior* **1**:523–531, 1976.

15

Ethics in old age psychiatry

Catherine Oppenheimer

Even a little knowledge of ethical theory will suffice to convince you that all important questions are so complicated, and the results of any course of action are so difficult to foresee, that certainty, or even probability, is seldom, if ever, attainable. It follows at once that the only justifiable attitude of mind is suspense of judgement ... At this point the arguments for doing nothing come in; for it is a mere theorists's paradox that doing nothing has just as many consequences as doing something. It is obvious that inaction can have no consequences at all.[1]

Ethical issues crop up with remarkable frequency in the practice of old age psychiatry, and in a variety of forms. Arguments about real-life problems often turn out to rest on a handful of general themes and assumptions, so we should consider these first. We then discuss some common situations in which ethical difficulties arise, particularly those where specific remedies exist or are proposed. Lastly, we shall tease out some of the ambiguities in our approach to patients in this branch of psychiatry.

Not all issues could be covered in the space available. The most important omissions are the principles of palliative care at the end of life; research in dementia and the problem of ensuring that the interests of non-competent patients are protected (without denying them opportunities they might have valued); and the tension between confidentiality and essential sharing of information when colleagues in different professions or employed by different agencies work cooperatively in the care of a mentally ill person.

General issues

Who are the elderly?

Why is there a separate chapter on older people in this book? Old age *in itself* does not mark off a person as ethically different in any way from someone in middle age or youth. But many circumstances that do give rise to specific ethical problems—circumstances such as physical illness, mental incapacity, dependence on help from others, and vulnerability to cruelty or exploitation—become statistically commoner in people as they grow old. Discussion of 'the elderly' frequently focuses on people in such circumstances. Hence the proper image of an old person as healthy, independent, and fully able to protect himself, is constantly subject to erosion. This is an example of the halo effect—the halo of disability conferred on all older people.

The halo effect operates also in another direction. 'Old age' refers to an ill-defined age-group that can span the years from 65 to 95 or more. The use of a single category to encompass the whole range obscures the vast differences between people in different parts of the age-band, let alone the differences between individuals irrespective of age. The real problems faced by many 90-year-olds may falsely be attributed also to 65-year-olds, simply because of the 'elderly' label that they bear.

The tendency to view 'the elderly' as a homogeneous mass is related to another tendency, also hard to avoid—viewing old age too much from the perspective of youth. Mostly it is younger (or middle-aged) people who write about the problems of old age. Pehaps this does not matter where the material is strictly factual; but where feelings, beliefs, or rights are at issue, there is much room for subjectivity and unexamined assumptions to infiltrate the arguments. The likely sources of untested assumptions are the professionals' second-hand experience of old age, through their observation of the people they have cared for, and possibly also of relatives and friends. In addition, their opinions may well be coloured by their beliefs and wishes about their own future old age. We should question how accurately one can look into one's future in this way: would we accept a view of middle age that emerged from a discussion among teenagers? The imaginative leap of empathetic understanding is a technique widely used in psychiatry and psychotherapy, but it is safe only when tempered by corrective information from the person being empathized with. The problem with old age—our own or others'—is that such corrective information may be difficult or impossible to get.

So there are potential injustices contained in our assumptions when we consider people as *old* rather than *individual*. But even the attempt to 'accord respect to the individual', in order to escape from these damaging stereotypes, has its difficulties. Do you respect me as a human being with universal human attributes, or as a person of advanced age and therefore worthy of respect, or as myself—unique me? You cannot respect me (uniquely) without knowing who I am.

When a person holds all the information that needs to be known about her, and can communicate it to others, there is no problem in respecting her individually. (No ethical problem, anyway—though in practice the time needed to allow such communication is often not accorded.) But there *is* a problem when a person cannot speak for herself, and the information that would allow her uniqueness to be respected has to be found from other sources. The usual sources in such circumstances will be the patient's relatives, and any people currently looking after her, such as nurses or care staff in a home. Probably the relatives will draw on their knowledge of how she was in earlier times, and they may infer her current preferences and attitudes from what they remember of her previous feelings and way of life. On the other hand, care staff are likely to try and understand her through their observations of the way she is now, coloured also by their experiences with other old people who have passed through their care.

These two frameworks of perception may or may not agree, because the sources of their assumptions are different. So the attempt to 'respect the individual' may founder on the problem of *who* the individual is. Is she the person we meet now, expressing herself (obscurely perhaps) in her current behaviour, or is she the person who was quite different before, and who, for 60 years or more, would not have wanted to be what she is now?

Two further points should be mentioned here. Each involves a problem of labelling, and the clutch of attitudes that goes with each label. These labels are 'ill' and 'helpless'.

Psychiatric illness is common in old age, and the diagnosis can be more difficult to make than in younger people. Experienced psychiatrists may there-fore set the threshold lower for identifying such illness in older people than they do for the young. Non-medical people who are anxious about an old person may give impetus to this process, if their anxieties can be relieved by attaching a medical label to the problem they are grappling with: the responsibility for solving the problem then passes to medical powers (for example, through admission to hospital). So problems can acquire a medical label that may not belong to them. But there is also the opposite risk that, out of a laudable wish to preserve a person's freedom, signs of illness are missed and the ill old person is denied necessary and effective treatment. Affective disorder is an example of a condition whose ambiguous boundaries and multiple causes makes it particularly subject to these conflicting pressures, and where the act of making a diagnosis entails far more than a simple medical calculation.

The other label concerns helplessness or 'dependency'. Older people are frequently limited in one aspect or other of their lives, and they are thereby obliged to accept help from someone. The more they accept outside help, the more their lives become public to others. At the extreme comes institutional life (residential care or a hospital ward), but many people experience lesser breaches of their privacy, with the entry of helpers into their lives at home. The painful process of subjecting oneself to public scrutiny may happen at any age, but for younger people it is more likely to be a transient experience. In old age, it is often feared in advance, and once begun it is likely to continue. The surrender of privacy in accepting outside help brings with it other surrenders. The person must share with other clients in the help that is being offered, and fit in with a system that is shaped by the requirements of the caregivers as well as the needs of the cared-for. Other people's perceptions of her life will guide her future, and she risks being treated as helpless in areas where help is not needed.

In this, older people have common cause with young disabled people. The young woman in the wheelchair is assumed not to be able to speak for herself, just as older people are expected to need the protection of society. The very existence of special categories of people (geriatricians, social workers in elderly care, members of Age Concern) sets apart the group whose rights they wish to affirm. It is a process that tends to reduce all people under the label to the lowest common denominator. Mrs Amanda Smith, aged 75, who delivers meals on wheels and campaigns for a day-centre for her local pensioners' group, has a clear sense of her own identity. It is very different from the view of those who would recognize her only as one of 'the rising tide of the elderly' who burden society today.

The first general theme—autonomy versus paternalism

In the 1970s and 1980s the major preoccupation in the literature on ethics in old age care was the issue of life versus death. Arguments about the appropriateness of life-saving interventions in very sick older patients, about the scope allowed (whether by public or professional opinion) for withdrawal of life-support measures, and the polarization of views between 'death with dignity' and 'life at all costs', provoked wide interest and strong feelings, and were reflected in important legal decisions in test cases in various countries.

A principle often invoked in those 'life-versus-death' arguments was that of autonomy, or self-determination: the right of individuals to choose how to live their lives, even if (in this context) the choice they make is to die. 'Autonomy' then was pitted against 'paternalism'—the propensity of carers and professionals to make decisions on behalf of a patient, rather than allowing him to decide.

The pejorative implication contained in the term 'paternalism' is this: however well intentioned the professional, she cannot possibly be as well informed as the patient is about his own preferences and goals in life, so that any decision she makes on his behalf will stray further from the fulfilment of these goals than his own decision would do. Furthermore, it is argued, there is an intrinsic value in being able to make one's own decisions, however ill-judged they may turn out to be: we none of us like to be bossed or interfered with; the sense of self-determination is something that we enjoy for its own sake.

Yet the autonomy/paternalism debate would not exist if there were never any justification for deciding on behalf of patients. When a person is ill, he may willingly give up his right to decide, and ask a professional to make a decision for him; he may be physically incapable of making and communicating a decision (for example, if he is unconscious); or he may be judged by others to be incapable of making a decision that is valid.

The last of these three possibilities is the one where tension between self-determination and determination by others is most apparent. It acknowledges that there are situations in which a person's clearly spoken intentions and wishes concerning his or her own life can be invalidated or discounted by others.

During the 1990s the focus of ethical discussion in the care of older people has accordingly moved on somewhat, to considering the meaning and scope of autonomy—particularly where older people with mental illness are concerned —and to working out the conditions under which infringements of autonomy can be justified. Competence, decision-making capacity, risk-taking, advance directives, all form part of this discussion. They will be considered in the second part of the chapter, while here we stay with the general issues.

The second general theme—autonomy is not enough

Underneath the shift in interest from end-of-life issues to self-determination, there has at a deeper level been a unifying theme: that of power. It concerns the power of professionals over the lives of those in need of medical care, set against the power of individuals to resist their efforts (whether benignly intended or malign). This is a theme that makes for invigorating argument, and its importance—including the seriousness of the risk that power might be abused—cannot be dismissed. Nevertheless in practice, in the field, there is something about it that is one-dimensional and incomplete.

No working psychiatrist can ignore the fact that people do not live as isolated individuals but as participants in relationships—as members of friendships, enmities, families, neighbourhoods, and institutions. The view of professionals as 'doers' and patients as 'done-to' is a thin, monochromatic view: it presents the people concerned through only one of their attributes. A different dimension, that cuts across this, might perhaps be called 'relatedness', as a way of expressing the following idea.

The essential significance of people, their impact on the world, depends at least as much on their connections with other people as on the degree of independence that they exercise. In the practice of old age psychiatry this is a matter of common experience, but it is rarely elevated to the status of an ethical principle. Old age psychiatrists daily see patients who experience some threat to their autonomy, and a minority of our patients, at some point in their lives, can scarcely be said to make autonomous decisions at all. Yet we see that these patients, for all their impaired autonomy, play an immensely significant part in the lives of the people who are connected to them. They are participants in relationships that can be joyful and rewarding; or troublesome, full of pain and guilt; relationships deeply rooted in the past, or fresh encounters between a new carer and the person needing care. It is the emotional context of these relationships (or their absence) that determine how much the person flourishes or withers, how much his potential for affection, enjoyment, humour, and the vivid communication of feeling, are stifled or expressed. Autonomy, or lack of it, plays only a secondary role here.

In this field, therefore, there are two important questions. Not only: 'Can we regard this person as autonomous?', but also: 'We recognize that this person has impaired autonomy: nevertheless, how can we help him to exert as much power and independence as possible; how can we help to preserve his relationships?' Of course, the wording of both these questions reveals that the power still lies with us: *we* make the judgement about a person's capacity for autonomous decision-making (though we can be challenged); *we* proffer help (or fail to do so) designed to support the choices of the patient who has lost the right of independent choice. This is a kind of modified paternalism: a paternalism bent on reducing its own scope as much as possible.

In practice, it is often the 'relatedness' of people, their connections to others and to their past, that forces decisions into a broader field than that marked out by the autonomy/paternalism dimension. Loving children cannot bear to see their elegant, fastidious mother become dishevelled and abusive, however much she protests against their interference; neighbours cannot tolerate for long their anxiety for an elderly man who wanders the streets at night, whether they feel they have any responsibility towards him or not.

The interaction between the 'autonomy dimension' and the 'relatedness dimension', and their effect on decisions when illness brings about the involvement of professionals, is depicted in Fig. 15.1.

The third general theme—the worth of older people with mental illness

The capacity for autonomous decision-making, as we shall see later when we discuss competence, is assessed very much on cognitive criteria. For example, memory, the ability to weigh disparate evidence together, and to predict out-comes, are likely to be taken into consideration when judgements are made about a person's ability to decide matters for himself.

But we should question the effect on our thinking that is created by the habit of measuring people by their cognitive ability. Might it lead us into the careless assumption that those with less cognitive ability are also of less *value*?

This question is most eloquently put by Post[2] in his book *The moral challenge of Alzheimer's disease*. He writes:

A new ethics of dementia care will not accept the postulate of some ethicists that rationality and memory are the features of the person that give rise to moral standing and protection. Too great a value emphasis on rationality and memory, arguably the cardinal values of modern technological societies, wrongly excludes people with dementia from the sphere of human dignity and respect ... Instead of mirroring the inequalities of a hypercognitive culture, the ethics of dementia attaches no moral relevance to mental acuity or decline. The value of a human being is not diminished by even profound forgetfulness...

The richness and sweep of Post's discussion as he develops this approach —outwards to philosophical and religious principles, inwards to personal experiences of dementia and the practical details of caring—cannot be properly conveyed here. His chief philosophical target is the contemporary attempt to define (or at least describe) 'personhood', in a way that makes the

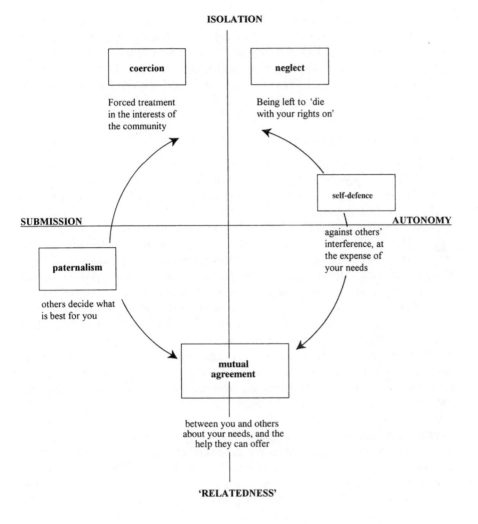

Fig. 15.1 The interaction between autonomy and 'relatedness' in mental illness in old age.

philosophical category of 'persons' smaller than the biological category of 'human beings'. In other words, some human beings—among whom are people with dementia—are excluded from 'personhood' by these definitions. Post argues convincingly that such exclusion from the status of 'person' will put these human beings at risk of devaluation, neglect, and abuse by their societies. We know from historical example that this is no imaginary risk: most notoriously in the case of Nazi Germany.[3]

Post's view is that 'a task of ethics is to include rather than exclude the vulnerable' and to preserve in our morality the significance of virtues like dedication, solicitude, and self-denying love. The virtues spring from the qualities of the giver—they are not entitlements due to the qualities of the receiver—and on them we should build our ethical understanding of people with dementia.

The fourth general theme—the claim on resources

Not very distant from this argument about the moral (or existential) 'value' of vulnerable older people lies the question of their value in economic terms.

It is perfectly legitimate for societies to practice good housekeeping—to count up their responsibilities and commitments, to calculate the resources that can be drawn on, and to juggle the one against the other. It is also legitimate—in fact essential—to use money as the language of measurement in making these calculations. But a simple-minded use of this approach would put older people into a disastrous position. No longer economically productive (as measured by a wage), insatiable consumers of resources (as measured by the costs of medical and social care), they are takers from society, not generators of wealth; in fact it would be better for society (on this view) if everybody died instantly on retirement.

Of course this is a ludicrous picture, and there are broadly two lines of approach to correcting it. The first is to look more comprehensively at the contributions which older people make to society and (if the argument requires it) to find measures which can show that contribution in financial terms—even if they do so only indirectly.

The second line of approach looks at the life history of people rather than at their status at any given moment. We have no difficulty in recognising that we work during one part of the day in order to be at leisure later on: we do not regard our working self and our leisure self as two different people. Likewise the person who works and the person who is retired are the same person—the time-scale is a little different, that is all. So the rational member of society will want to see his society making good provision for retired people out of simple self-interest, expecting to benefit from that provision himself in due course. (See Daniels[4] for a full treatment of the latter argument).

The obvious absurdity and inhumanity of the proposition (when it is starkly put) that 'older people are nothing more than a drain on society' doesn't unfortunately prevent it creeping in, half-believed and mostly unspoken, to the political and administrative decisions which affect the allocation of resources to illness in old age—and especially to the dementing illnesses.

This is partly because the risk of becoming mentally ill in old age is relatively small compared to the high probability of reaching retirement age, so it is easy for each of us, when debating what 'society' should provide, to retreat into imagining provision for 'them' rather than for 'me'. As with illness in any age group, the question here needs to focus not on what the person contributes to society but on what he ought to receive to treat his illness. And with a comprehensive health service, funded from taxation and free at the point of use, the arguments about allocation of resources to different categories of illness are necessarily political and emerge at national level—even though innumerable implicit rationing decisions are taken, often without discussion, at a local level every day.

There has been no serious suggestion that a treatable mental illness like depression, occurring in old age, should be regarded as less deserving of resources than depression in younger people. With the dementing illnesses however, other issues complicate the picture. The question of *entitlement* becomes entangled in debates about effectiveness of treatments—in this case, treatments for dementia, the rationale of interventions (active or palliative) in terminal illness, and the legitimacy of bringing long-stay care under the umbrella of social (rather than medical) budgets. We shall return to some of these specific issues later.

The general question of *justice in the distribution of resources*—between the old and the young, between the healthy and the ill, between mental illness and other diseases, between curative treatment and humane supportive care—cannot be taken further here. It is worth just stopping to note, however, that the less favoured category in all four of these pairs—old, ill, mentally ill, and incurable—applies to people with dementia. Alertness to ethical issues in old age psychiatry brings a constant realization that, where generalized, thought-less and poorly informed perceptions of society hold sway, our patients are unwanted and unloved.

(See Dilnot and Taylor[5] for a more detailed discussion of economic principles in this field, and Hope and Oppenheimer[6] for a brief account of rationing theories.)

Specific issues

Competence and consent

We referred earlier to circumstances where a patient's freedom to act autonomously is not respected, and his decisions are not regarded as valid. What entitles health professionals to do this? When is it reasonable for us to move into this paternalistic position, making decisions ourselves on behalf of our patients?

The notion of autonomy belongs to ethical theory, but the practical consequences of respecting, or invalidating, a patient's decisions are so important that the law has to play a part here. The meaning of 'capacity to make decisions' has been argued out in legal settings, and it is the law that gives authority to health professionals to make the necessary judgements in individual cases.

The words 'competence' and 'decision-making capacity' tend to be used almost interchangeably in this area, except that 'competence' is favoured in the ethical literature, and 'mental capacity' has been used, and defined, in the legal sphere—in English law at any rate. In this chapter, the examples described will reflect English law and the British health services, but the principles that they illustrate do not respect national boundaries.

The compulsory admission of mentally ill patients to hospital is a special case of the general issue, and it hinges on impaired capacity in one particular respect. Here, the decision that the patient is asked to make is the decision whether to accept treatment for a mental illness. If it is judged (by the people authorized in law to do so) that his illness prevents him from making a rational decision on this, and the risks of not deciding are sufficiently grave, then compulsory admission to hospital is lawful. The further implications of this special case are discussed by other authors in this book (e.g. Peele and Chodoff).[7]

However, we shall stay with a broader notion of mental capacity, and consider what enables us, as competent beings, to take any decision—whether on questions of health, finances, living arrangements, or anything else.

In law, and in everyday life as well, there is a presumption that everyone is capable of making the decisions which concern his own life, and that his right to do so cannot be taken away without very good reason. Other people may regard his decisions as foolish, hasty, or unfair to others. If so, they can only try to argue with him, to persuade him, or to sue him. But if it can be shown that he lacks the abilities needed for the *process* of making this decision, then—and only then—is it proper to discount his decision.

To discount a person's thinking on the grounds of lack of capacity has to be an all-or-nothing act. Either he is sovereign at this moment and in this decision, or he is subject to someone else's judgement.

However, for the psychiatrist the assessment of the different abilities that make up mental capacity is often quantitative rather than absolute: abilities are more commonly lost gradually than wholesale. Furthermore, we recognize that complicated decisions demand more of a person's mental abilities than do simple decisions. These considerations lead us to see capacity (or competence) as a graded and variable attribute of the person, rather than as something either present or absent.

Fortunately, the legal necessity for making an absolute decision (yes or no) can be reconciled with the clinical recognition of competence as a relative concept, in the following way: The clinician is expected to judge capacity *in relation to the specific decision that has to be made,* and she will decide whether the abilities that she is assessing have crossed a threshold appropriate to that decision. In principle this is no different from many other clinical decisions we make, where judgements on continually varying characteristics lead to binary (yes or no) decisions.

So much for the principles. What about the method of assessing competence? Buchanan and Brock[8] discuss the 'capacities needed for competence': and here they mean the mental abilities needed in decision-making. They identify two: 'the capacity for understanding and communication' and 'the capacity for reasoning and deliberation'. Of course the four words they use are themselves very complex, and could be broken down into more refined subdivisions. Within these terms are included memory and language ability, and also the crucial ability to *envisage future outcomes*.

Understanding the consequences of a decision is a complicated task. It seems to require a cognitive process of calculating probabilities and the risks attached to them, as well as a more emotional process of imagining what the different outcomes will *feel* like, specifically and uniquely for the person concerned. Not only cognitive but also emotional obstacles (such as anxiety or depression, denial, or external pressures) can therefore hinder this process of weighing up future outcomes.

Case 1

A 75 year old woman was admitted to hospital for the fourth episode of depression in three years. Her depression tended to respond well to medication in hospital, but as soon as plans for her return home were made her mood declined, though she always said how anxious she was to be at home to look after her husband. The psychiatric team knew that her husband drank heavily and they suspected that she was very unhappy in her marriage, but she would never admit this. She had difficulty in concentrating and her thinking became vague and indecisive whenever the staff attempted to discuss her situation with her. There was a serious question as to her competence to decide on whether she should return home, where the likelihood of a relapse and a readmission was very high, and where staff feared she was at risk of abuse, or whether plans should be made for her to live apart from her husband. *He* was very sure that she ought to return home, and there were no other relatives to share in the decision.

One possibility here would have been to bring her under guardianship and to make the decision for her. She was certainly unable to marshall all the information relevant to the decision, or to foresee the consequences of a decision either way in a realistic manner. This was probably because she was frightened of her husband and also fearful for her safety, she was denying the risks at home, she didn't like the idea of any alternative place to live, and her misery about her dilemma was impairing her concentration. However, rather than determining her incompetence, the staff tried to improve her competence. They decided that she would need a prolonged stay on the ward if she was to arrive at her own decision; and they were able to give her the security of knowing she would not be hurried. They felt that she needed to experience life in a residential setting—neither in hospital nor with her husband—and they negotiated with a neighbouring home to provide her with several successive stays there. Domiciliary care was provided for her husband (when he would accept it), so that her anxiety about him was partly relieved. Six months later she made an informed and settled decision that she would like to become a permanent resident in the home, and her husband accepted her decision. (Two years later still, she happily moved into an independent flat; her husband visits her regularly and their relationship has improved.)

It is seldom easy for a clinician to determine whether a person is competent to make a decision. Impairments of attention, memory, language, and logical reasoning can be assessed fairly objectively. But where the patient's difficulty lies in the more subtle process of predicting and 'imaginatively sampling' alternative futures for himself, the clinician has to fall back on more subjective criteria.

The most recent guidance available in English law (the Court of Appeal in 're MB'[9]) uses concepts similar to those discussed by Buchanan and Brock. The legal judgment in this case concerned capacity to agree to medical treatment.

A person lacks capacity if some impairment or disturbance of mental function renders the person unable to make a decision whether to consent or to refuse treatment. That inability to make a decision will occur when:

a) the patient is unable to comprehend and retain the information which is material to the decision, especially as to the likely consequences of having or not having the treatment in question

b) the patient is unable to use the information and weigh it in the balance as part of the process of arriving at the decision.

It seems fitting that this statement uses metaphor ('to weigh in the balance') in its analysis of decision-making. It is an acknowledgement that objective, scientific descriptions of such processes do not yet exist (and may never do so). So, in summary, we accept that judgements about a patient's competence should be made in relation to a specific decision; and must also accept that these judgements, however much they can draw on general guidelines and particular tests, are ultimately subjective in each individual case.

Two further general points must be considered before we leave the topic of competence: whether the *threshold of competence* should be set differently for decisions that have different risks attached to them; and the duty to *optimize the conditions* for competent decision-making, before judging that competence has been lost.

Setting the threshold

Buchanan and Brock[8] argue that, in evaluating a person's competence, it is not enough just to examine the person's mental capacity for making the decision in question. They suggest that 'the standard of competence ought to vary in part with the expected harms or benefits to the patient of acting in accordance with the patient's choice'. From this would follow that: 'just because a patient is competent to consent to a treatment, it does not follow that the patient is competent to refuse it, and vice versa. For example, consent to a low-risk life-saving procedure ... should require only a minimal level of competence, but refusal of that same procedure ... should require the highest level of competence.'

Such an asymmetry seems troubling and illogical. If competent decision-making involves looking at all the outcomes of a decision, both risky and safe, then surely the process of looking is the same, whichever choice is afterwards arrived at. Making the safer choice cannot be an easier *process* (unless it was spuriously made easier by not really considering the alternatives).

Yet there is a genuine issue here. In real life, a patient making a decision that seems to fly in the face of his own interests, and in defiance of professional advice, is bound to make others wonder if he is capable of deciding at all. The cynical view might be that this is an issue of power once more: if professionals cannot prevail over a patient through the advice they give, they will be tempted to prevail instead by declaring him incompetent. There is indeed some danger of this occurring—which is one reason why the competence of a patient should be judged not by the outcome of his decision but by the process through which he takes it. And although Buchanan and Brock, in the passage quoted, are talking not about how to evaluate competence, but about the level of competence that should be required (the threshold that should be set), they do come dangerously close to confirming the cynics.

Is there any other way of understanding competence in the light of risky and ill-advised decisions by patients? There are three possibilities. First, the 'risky' decision by the patient might *prompt* the professionals to consider the patient's competence. The evaluation would rest on other evidence, but the patient's decision would have started the process. Second, the professionals might decide that a very stringent standard of *care in evaluating* competence should be set, where a patient has made a risky decision. The standard of competence itself would not be set differently, but a high degree of certainty would be required before agreeing that the patient met that standard.

Third, it may be that we are talking about *two different decisions* here. One is the patient's decision with respect to the professional advice he is given—to accept or to reject it. The other is his own decision on the merits of the case—on the facts concerning the advantages and disadvantages of the proposed treatment and any possible alternatives. Everyday life is full of people deciding to accept professional advice in matters which are too complicated or technical for them to assess properly themselves; and it seems reasonable to argue here that deciding to trust and accept advice, or to reject it, might require a lesser degree of competence than evaluating and deciding a complex matter on one's own.

The patient who chooses to ignore medical advice on treatment might be competent to decide whether he feels able to trust his doctor or not, but, having decided to reject advice, he will need to take his own independent view on the question of treatment. His competence in carrying out that deliberation must be separately evaluated, against a standard that reflects the complexity of the treatment decision.

This view of competence in treatment decisions resembles the position of the Enduring Power of Attorney (in English law) where financial decisions are concerned. It is recognized that a person can be competent to grant this Power of Attorney and at the same time lack competence to manage his financial affairs himself. The standard of competence involved in granting the power is less than that required to manage financial transactions: it involves only the ability to understand what the power is and what its implications are, and the ability to choose a person to undertake the duty. (See Jacoby[10] for a discussion of the case law which established this principle.)

We should note here, incidentally, that both cases—the medical and the financial—raise the issue of trust in others: trust in the doctor in one case, and in the chosen 'attorney' in the other. The patient may trust, and may competently describe his trustful state of mind; but whether the person on whom he relies is indeed trustworthy, and whether the patient is competent to make *that* judgement, is a separate question. We shall return to it later.

Optimizing the conditions—general principles

Assessing competence is a subjective matter, not only because there is no reliable way of measuring the mental faculties involved, but also because the values of the assessor are inevitably brought into play in setting the threshold. As Buchanan and Brock show, all judgements on competence require one to balance the risk that the patient may be making decisions contrary to his own enduring interests, against the risk of unreasonably depriving a person of the power of independent choice. 'More or less stringent standards of competence in effect strike different balances between the values of patient well-being and self-determination'.[8]

However, the day-to-day practice of old age psychiatry addresses the conflict between these two principles rather differently from the pure laboratory method envisaged by ethicists. The occasions when one has to make the clear-thinking balancing act between opposing principles are relatively rare. Mostly we move in muddier waters. So many of our patients have difficulty in thinking through decisions—whether for cognitive, emotional, or delusional reasons—that our working practices accommodate the possibility that *everyone* will have some such difficulty. Our transactions with patients are built on a pragmatic mixture of informing, discussing, and persuading; allowing events to happen as a way of testing out beliefs; building relationships and fostering trust; creating safe settings in which people can think in new ways, relieved from the distorting effects of anxiety or external pressure.

The unifying spirit within this mixture of activity seems to be the desire by professionals to enlarge the scope of decision-making by patients in all the directions that seem (to the professionals) to be beneficial to the patients. The formal evaluation of patients' competence, testing their irrational decisions and establishing an entitlement to override them, is not really the essence of old age psychiatry. Instead, the approach is implicit, diplomatic, and protective: tending to work round conflict rather than confronting it, seeking to foster trustfulness as well as to shore up independence.

The difference between everyday practice and the pared-down ethical dilemma is illustrated by a common situation: the problem of a cognitively impaired woman who will not accept a little help in her own home.

Her judgement that she needs no help is seen as *mistaken,* by professionals and family alike, who base their opinion more on the consequences of her decision (they see her weight loss, her unhappiness) than on explicit evaluation of her competence in this regard. The *method* by which these others try to alter the situation is not by reasoning and argument, nor yet by overruling her in face-to-face conflict, but by persuading her to accept the friendly overtures of a home carer. This carer may then spend weeks carefully building up the woman's trust so that in the end her agreement to receive the carer's help is willingly given. And the *aim* of the family and the professionals, by which they decide their actions, is of course to give help—the help that they judge necessary for the woman's happiness and welfare—but to do so in a way that allows her to exercise as much choice as is feasible, and to feel as autonomous as possible in the march of events.

This is the 'modified paternalism' we mentioned earlier. It is paternalism, because the professionals (and families) are making decisions about the need for intervention, the overall aims of the treatment plan, and the methods to be used, often without full discussion with the patient concerned. It is 'modified', because one of the paternalistic aims embodied in the plan is the aim of opening up autonomous choices for the patient.

Another variant illustrates the ambivalent mixture of paternalism and auto-nomy more clearly still. Imagine an elderly man, moderately cognitively im-paired, who is insisting on remaining at home, although he is barely able to look after himself there, and whose willingness to accept help with feeding or hygiene is erratic at best. Yet he can argue fluently and forcefully about his attachment to his home and his determination never to go into any kind of institutional care. It may be hard to judge whether he is expressing a competent choice in this matter, because personal preference and values play such an important part in it. Suppose he develops a chest infection which causes him to become significantly more confused and at greater risk to his life, so that he is brought (without much protest, because he is so ill) into hospital. In that environment, he accepts the help and care of the nursing staff, and enjoys the company of other patients; and when he is offered a period of convalescence in a residential home, he is equally happy there. He is now able to make a choice between residential care and a return home on the basis of real experience rather than—as before—on the basis of a merely theoretical idea. But what enabled him to make this important and autonomous choice was the semi-coercive (though beneficent) action of bringing him into hospital without his consent.

Of course other cases occur in which a patient refuses any intervention with such determination that all persuasion is fruitless. Here it is usually necessary to wait until the risks to the patient are so evident, and his failure to under-stand them or give them due weight so clearly demonstrates his impaired competence, that action in direct conflict with his expressed wishes can be justified. Then he may be admitted compulsorily to hospital. Yet even in those conditions the staff who care for him will be trying to maximize his opportunities for free choice where that can be allowed, and trying to help him understand why some of his choices are disallowed.

This last category comprises the rarer cases. For much of the time, the competence of patients who do not actively refuse help is not questioned. Even when a patient is reluctant to accept help, persuasion is seen as the right way of proceeding where that is possible. Tacitly it is justified as acting in the patient's best interests; rarely is it critically examined as a potential infringement of the patient's autonomy.

Let us look again at the contrast we have drawn. On the one hand is the philosophically pure weighing up of opposing principles, the clean decision as to whether a person is competent or not. On the other, is a picture of messy pragmatism: doctors and nurses making paternalistic decisions which they hope will promote their patient's sense of making his decisions himself.

We should ask ourselves which approach is more respectful of the patient's autonomy. Perhaps his sense of self-determination is better safeguarded by accepting his compliance (having coaxed him towards it) without explicitly questioning his competence. Or is it better safeguarded by opening up the issue, exposing his inability to make a valid decision, and formally taking on the right to decide for him? Which should we value more on behalf of our patients—the kindness implicit in the first approach or the honesty expressed through the second?

This dilemma echoes the dilemma built in to the Mental Health Act 1983 in English Law, where the duty to follow proper procedure if the patient's liberty is to be infringed is set alongside the duty to use the least coercive alternative in securing the patient's treatment. At the time that the Act was passed, the view was that a person not actively refusing to come into hospital for treatment should be regarded as agreeing to do so. If a new law, superseding the 1983 Act, is enacted in the next few years (as is proposed), then the theoretical question we ask ourselves here may be debated in Parliament and answered in legislation.

Optimizing the conditions—practical measures

It is worth reminding ourselves of the measures that professionals can take to maximize a patient's competence in tackling a crucial decision: how they can create circumstances that enable the patient to mobilize his abilities at their optimum level, so that the decision is as far as possible his own rather than a decision by others.

These measures are:

1. Improve the patient's health by all reasonable means. If his condition fluctuates, take advantage of his best times to bring the decision to him for discussion.

2. Reduce the emotional pressure associated with the decision. This pressure may be intrinsic to the decision—the alternatives in prospect may all seem

frightening, for example. Or it may come from external sources—such as conflicting views among different family members. (Sometimes an admission to hospital is justifiable for this reason—to provide safety and containment while the patient undertakes a difficult decision.)

3. Find the clearest and most comprehensible methods for presenting the information relevant to the decision, and help the patient to understand and retain the information. This can include simplifying the language of discussion; creating opportunities for actual experience—as in the examples above; using written materials or lists of points; breaking discussion into small sub-items, presented step by step over time; and so on.

4. Lastly, clinical experience suggests that, where efforts are made to assist cognitively impaired patients in making choices in areas where they readily feel competent, then their confidence in their ability to make larger autonomous choices can be enhanced.

Decision-making for non-competent patients

When patients cannot make decisions for themselves, two questions arise: who can make the decision for them; and what information should guide that person?

Treatment decisions in common law

In 1989 the legal position in England and Wales was clarified by a case (*Re F*) which, because of the importance of the principles it embodied, was taken to the House of Lords (the highest court in the country). The principles established were these:[11]

- No-one can give consent on behalf of another adult (including a non-competent adult).
- In the absence of consent, it is lawful for a doctor or a dentist to give treatment, provided that it is in the patient's *best interests*.
- 'Best interests' means that treatment 'which is necessary to preserve the life, health, or well-being of the patient'.
- Treatment lawfully given without consent may include 'even simple care such as dressing and undressing and putting to bed'.
- The clinician providing treatment must act in accordance with practice accepted at that time by a responsible body of opinion skilled in the relevant field.
- It is good practice, in making the decision, to consult with relatives and others concerned with the care of the patient (but they cannot give or withhold consent).

- Certain difficult decisions will require a declaration from the court that the treatment is indeed in the patient's best interests.

(It is worth clarifying here that treatment for mental illness in detained patients is governed by different arrangements, under the Mental Health Act 1983.)

For treatment decisions under these principles, there is little scope for the non-competent patient to influence the decision-maker. It is the doctor who decides, relying primarily on medical information, although some attempt at assessing the patient's values might contribute to judging what his *best interests* are.

Proxy decisions

The Enduring Power of Attorney (in England) is a good example of a mechanism for establishing a legally recognized proxy decision-maker. By this, a person when competent nominates another person (or more than one) to make decisions on his behalf when he becomes non-competent. In this instance the choice of decision-maker is left entirely to the (presently competent) person; and it is he who decides in advance how much scope in the decision-making he wishes his proxy to have. At present the Power applies only to financial matters, but there are proposals currently under consideration[12] for a Continuing Power of Attorney that would encompass medical and other matters as well.

Substituted judgement

People who have to make a decision for a non-competent person will try to respect his individuality as far as possible by making the decision in line with his own values and interests. Two issues arise: how to discover what those values and interests are, and how much weight to give to information derived from the past, as against what can be observed in the present.

The purpose of consulting relatives (for example in treatment decisions) is to gain a better understanding of the patient's values through the eyes of people who have known him longer and more intimately than the doctor does. Unfortunately, there is evidence[13,14] that relatives are not a very accurate guide to the patient's views, especially on matters that were never explicitly discussed between them.

Advance directives

A better way of ensuring that the values and interests of the non-competent person influence decisions which others take for him is through the mechanism of an advance directive. This is a statement made by a competent person about treatments that he does or does not wish to receive if the time comes when he cannot contribute actively to the decision.[15]

Again there are practical issues here: the difficulty for the person in foreseeing future situations accurately and comprehensively enough to give clear guidance about his wishes; and the fact that treatment decisions, even with competent patients, take into account the patient's wishes but are not wholly determined by them. For example, a patient cannot legitimately demand that his doctor give him treatment that will be ineffective or harmful.

It seems likely that in practice, even where an advance directive exists, doctors will still be the decision-makers in most cases, and will be taking decisions on grounds of 'best interests'; but the advance directive will ensure that the doctor is better informed about the interests which the patient values most. This is particularly important in circumstances where the patient's interest lies in *not* having life prolonged: otherwise, as we saw earlier, the legal formulation of 'best interests' is predisposed towards saving life. In English common law, advance *refusals* of a particular form of treatment are already regarded as binding; the status of advance statements more generally is currently under discussion.[12]

There is also an interesting theoretical difficulty about advance directives: is it right that a decision made by a person at one time should be binding on him at another time? Normally we allow people to 'change their minds'—to reverse a decision that they have made, perhaps in the light of new information, or as a consequence of a change in themselves. But the non-competent person is deprived of this chance: he cannot 'change his mind' in this sense (precisely because it is irretrievably changed in another sense).

This may be only a theoretical worry, if the non-competence is so severe that the person is incapable of understanding or communicating any kind of decision at all. Who then could be in a better position than his former self to decide for him? But if the impairment is only moderate, the person may communicate his preferences and interests in non-verbal ways, even when he cannot make complex cognitive decisions. Suppose such non-verbal communications seem to run counter to his wishes as expressed in an advance directive: suppose he had previously said that, if he was demented and struck by a life-threatening illness, he was not to have any life-saving treatment; yet now he appears to be happy and enjoying life. What decision would best reflect *his* interests if he were now to fall ill with a treatable, life-threatening illness? Is *he* the person who wrote the directive, or the person who is enjoying life now?[6]

Nobody can seriously believe that a demented person has become someone entirely different from his former self. If we did believe that, then, as Buchanan and Brock[8] point out, we would have to read wills, and pursue all the other measures that signal the legal end of a person's life, in order to make way for the new person in their place. On the contrary, there is a sense in which a dementing person's established identity and characteristics are kept alive—in defiance of the changes in him that are taking place—by the people who knew him best during his life. This is part of the 'relatedness' discussed earlier. Friends wish to see the person with dementia being helped to act in ways consistent with his former disposition, and to receive care which acknowledges his former identity. They feel that they act on his behalf when they do so; and such devices as advance statements, which capture the views of the person more directly, give expression to the same feeling.

Conflicts of interest between families and patients

Conflicts are liable to arise over the participation of a family member in the care of a patient, or over financial issues; and often both together. The role of the authorities—mainly doctors or social services—in these situations can be complicated and ambiguous. The following case serves to illustrate some of the issues.

Case 2

Mrs Adams, a widow on a modest pension, offered her teenage grandson a home with her when his parents' marriage broke up. She cared for him and supported him through school and periods of unemployment. Twelve years have passed (making the grandson an adult and therefore freeing both his parents from any obligation to support him). Mrs Adams has developed a dementing illness, and now depends on care from others (though she does not realize the extent of her dependence). A home carer visits twice daily to attend to her personal needs; the rest of the day she is on her own, but her grandson is there at night. He is now attending a college course, and still financially dependent on his grandmother and on the home she provides for him. She still thinks of him as a teenager, and the demands she makes on him for company and attention cause ugly conflicts between them.

At this point her social worker and her general practitioner must make two crucial decisions. Is she at risk (of neglect or actual harm from her grandson) and is she competent to take part in the necessary discussions around this question? Up till now, the social worker has done her best to introduce appropriate care, working round Mrs Adams' reluctance to receive it, aware that the grandmother is denying herself so as to give money to her grandson, but feeling that the authorities have no right to intervene in Mrs Adams' free choice as to how she spends her money.

Now, if the grandmother is not competent to judge the risks in this situation, others must act for her, trying to decide in her *best interests* how to provide for her care. In terms of her health and physical comfort, there is no doubt that a move to a residential home would be preferable to staying in her current circumstances. If she moves, her pension will have to go towards paying for her stay in the residential home. The authorities who take over from her the right to decide on her health and safety thereby also take on the right to decide how her money will be spent. (The legal means for doing so might be, in English law, through the Social Services taking powers of guardianship for her under the Mental Health Act 1983.) Yet Mrs Adams herself has always preferred, and still vigorously asserts that she prefers, to spend her money on her grandson rather than herself, and she would rather live with him than move elsewhere.

In making judgements about her competence, the doctors must consider how well she is able to assess her own needs and the risks associated with them; *and also* how well she is able to weigh up the choice between generosity to her grandson and care for herself, considering what kind of return she may expect for her generosity, and how much her grandson can be trusted to respond to this expectation (whether by studying hard, or giving her his time, for example).

If she is not competent to do these things, and others have to decide in her best interests, do those interests include enabling her to continue acting altruistically rather than 'selfishly'? There is a similarity here with the question of 'best interests' in treatment decisions. There, the law makes an assumption that 'best interests' entail the preservation of life, but an advance directive forbidding life-prolonging treatments can override that assumption. Here, legal arrangements for managing another person's finances make the assumption that his best interests are served by spending his money on himself. There is as yet no form of directive that allows a person to say in advance that he would prefer, for example, his money to go to his heirs rather than being spent on expensive care for himself when he becomes non-competent.

The matter is further complicated by the interests of the state: if a person's own money can pay towards his care, then the state pays less: if the money is diverted elsewhere, then the state has to pay for the person's care—he cannot be left to die uncared for, even if when competent he stated a preference not to live at all if his independence had gone.

One further aspect of this case needs to be mentioned: the role of authority (doctors or social workers) in safeguarding the interests of carers and other family members. People who become dependent but who have only partial insight into their needs can make demands on family carers that are intolerable to the carer. In the case described, the grandmother called to her grandson throughout the night, every night, presumably because she didn't see him in the day and slept then herself.

Attention to the needs of family members and other carers is justifiable on grounds of the patient's own interests: his care depends on the health and well-being of the carers. And if a carer (or the needs of the patient) have reached a point where it is impossible for the carer to do any more, then professional intervention is undoubtedly warranted, not least to prevent neglect or abuse. In practice of course, wherever possible the intervention is made earlier, out of justice to the carers and to prevent foreseeable distress.

Truth-telling and deceit

How much of the truth to tell a patient is a question often asked, in many different contexts. Should I explain to this patient that I think he has Alzheimer's disease? Will it help this person with a paranoid illness if I try to persuade her that the tax inspector is not interested in her misdeclaration in

1952? When I go to visit a new patient, should I introduce myself as 'a psychiatrist' or 'a specialist in the care of older people'? When the old gentleman in the nursing home insists on going home to his mother, is it cruel to tell him that she died many years ago? Is it right to hang a curtain over the exit door so that the confused resident cannot see that it is a door? If a non-competent patient is used to taking medication for a physical condition, should we explain to her that we have added a drug to calm her agitation, or let her accept the additional pills without question?

In many instances these are partly practical or clinical questions as well as ethical ones, and in many (the question of communicating a diagnosis, for example) the issues arise equally in other branches of medicine. But an interesting general question is brought out especially clearly (though not uniquely) by patients with dementia. This is, what does telling 'the truth' mean, when someone is already deceived by their illness?

We cannot know exactly what is in the mind of the man who feels the need to return to his mother. Yet it seems reasonable to deduce that psychologically he is existing in a time when he lived with her and needed her to care for him. If we try to enter his world imaginatively, it is cruel to confront him with the absence of his mother's support, and it is true only in 'our' time and in our world, that she is dead now. What is true, both in 'our' world and in his as far as we understand it, is that there are people now who can take the place of his mother in caring for him, who wish to comfort him and enable him to feel safe. Communicating emotional truths of this kind, in preference to barely factual truths, is one of the key messages in validation therapy,[16] and in other nursing approaches in dementia that have developed from Feil's work and others.

Similar arguments perhaps apply to the various practical methods—architecture and furnishings—that are used to divert people from persistent attempts to leave a place where they are safely cared for. Knowing that in dementia, people's ability to reason about their environment is decreased, and that 'stimulus bound' behaviour increases, we can understand that a door with an obviously recognisable handle is giving a message to the person with dementia. The door says 'open me'. The carers (knowing that he is at risk and they are empowered to keep him indoors) say, 'don't go out, Fred, it's raining and you'll get wet'. Is it deceitful then to ensure that the door no longer conveys a message to him, which he will in any case not be allowed to obey?

Questions about truth-telling at the beginning of a dementing illness rather than near the end raise different dilemmas, but at least they are ones where the person affected may have a view of his own, and can therefore participate in the decisions about how much he wants to pursue investigations, to be told their results, and so on; people with early dementia can also act as informed participants in empirical studies on these questions, in a way that people with advanced dementia cannot. The advance of understanding about the genetics of dementing illnesses raises further questions still, which are only now beginning to be discussed. The most difficult issue is that of predictive testing for the relatives of a person with dementia. In early-onset Alzheimer's disease the situation resembles that of Huntington's disease, where extensive research has underpinned the development of workable guidelines concerning the ethics and practical organization of genetic counselling for families. In late-onset Alzheimer's disease there are no causative genes identified as yet: the different phenotypes of the *APOE* gene act as risk factors for the development of Alzheimer's disease (and probably other types of dementia also), but even the most risky of the phenotypes is 'neither necessary nor sufficient' for the development of the disease.[17] Whether, in the light of this, it will be of any advantage for people to know their own APOE status is questionable, and a question to be answered rather empirically than ethically. However, genetic studies in dementia are advancing rapidly and the ethical complications are likely also to multiply in the future (see Chapter 23).

Resources again—public policy and decisions about individuals

Younger people (below the age of 65) with dementia are disadvantaged by being few in number—their group is too small yet to have stimulated the growth of services adapted to their particular needs. On the other hand, older people with dementia are disadvantaged by being members of a very large group—so large that they have frightened the policy-makers. The high prevalence of dementia among people of 75 and older, and the rapid growth in this portion of the population, mean that any policy decision concerning them may have substantial repercussions on the financing of the National Health Service (NHS) and other institutions.

This is the context in which national policy decisions on the provision of long-stay care in the later stages of dementia, and on the use of medical treatments in the early stages of Alzheimer's disease, have been taken.

In the first case, there has been a shift (initially in practice, then cemented in legislation) in the provision of long-stay care away from the NHS and into the independent sector and social services. Long-stay provision within the NHS (and therefore at no cost to the patient) is reserved for the most severely disabled who meet formal eligibility criteria for this provision. Other people needing care pay for it with their own money, unless their income and assets fall below a threshold which qualifies them for financial support through social services.

The ethical difficulties encountered by doctors who take part in managing these arrangements arise partly through their role as gatekeepers to different elements of service provision, and affect their decisions over individual patients. But the difficulties are more acutely felt at a different level, by clinicians who regard themselves as advocates for their patients collectively, and who want to influence policies that have such a serious effect on them. In their eyes it is wrong for the resources of some patients (who are not poor but who have dementia) to be tapped in order to safeguard resources for other patients who are both demented and poor—instead of calling on additional resources from those who are not ill at all—that is, from society at large.

Short of civil disobedience, however, these clinicians must acquiesce in arrangements they think unjust, and use them as fairly as they can in the interests of all the patients they are concerned for. Doctors (and other professionals) are here being made to carry ethical dilemmas which properly fall on the politicians, who for their part would rather make unsustainable promises of high standards of care in chronic illness than take the decisions needed to supply the resources for that care.

The situation concerning medication for symptomatic treatment in early Alzheimer's disease is different but equally uncomfortable. Donepezil, the only medication so far licensed in the UK for this purpose, is relatively expensive and the evidence for its efficacy is disputed. Local health authorities in different parts of the country, who hold substantial responsibility for funding health care for their populations, have relied on expert advice which mostly recommends that the benefit offered by the drug does not justify the expense of widespread use in patients with early and middle-stage dementia, and they have therefore decided not to finance it for their populations. On the other hand, those who support its use point out that group outcome measurements obscure the finding that some individuals—unpredictably—benefit substantially and for a sustained period from use of the drug. For any individual patient, therefore, it may be worth taking a gamble and trying the drug to see if it works for them. In a health district that has decided not to fund it, however, they must pay for it for themselves (though a doctor must prescribe it, and the health authority decision on funding does not prevent the doctor from prescribing). The ethical difficulties here include problems of equity (patients with the same needs will be treated differently, depending on their means and on where they live) and a perception that a rationing decision has been unfairly dressed up as an efficacy decision. The same strict view on efficacy does not seem to be applied retrospectively to treatments already in common use, with other illnesses and other age groups, and where the number of potential patients (and therefore the cost of the decision) is not so large.

Professional roles

At many different points in this chapter we considered the actions of professional people—usually doctors but also others who hold authority—in situations of ethical uncertainty or conflict. I shall conclude with some general reflections on this topic.

It will be clear by now that when we act, we do so under different *domains of regulation* of ethical behaviour. For guidance we may look to our individual consciences, to agreed practice among immediate colleagues, to codes of conduct in our profession, to common (judge-made) law or statute law, or to political and administrative arrangements agreed at national level. It depends on the exact situation in question; and a specific problem that begins in one domain may well shift to another—for example, when a patient at risk in his own home is made subject to the Mental Health Act.

Likewise historically. A class of problematic situations can be dealt with at one time under the umbrella of individual or professional conscience, until disquiet about the informality and inconsistency entailed leads to more formal arrangements being set up. The move from individual ('conscience-led') treatment decisions on non-competent patients, to legal guidance on this process, to statutory mechanisms for advance directives, would be an example of this process.

The variety of regulatory systems is reflected in the great variety of roles that professionals play in the ethical arena. Someone working with older mentally ill people may act at a political level as a voter, an activist in organisations promoting the cause of older people, or even as a source of advice to national or local government bodies. As a professional she may take part in associations of colleagues, and through them may contribute towards improving arrangements for the care of older patients with mental illness.

Besides influencing policies at these levels, however, she must also implement them—even those with which she personally disagrees. Her professional responsibilities require her to subordinate her decisions about an individual patient to rules set up politically or administratively that determine the distribution of resources to different types of need. For example, as we discussed, in deciding whether a patient's condition makes him eligible for a certain level of (free) health care, she may feel that she has compromised his welfare in order to safeguard resources for other patients who are marginally more in need than he is.

Even at a local and personal level, decisions *for* one patient may mean a decision *against* another where resources (such as hospital beds, or professional time) have to be shared. She will also find herself, willingly or not, acting to adjudicate between the different members of a family in conflict: the act of diagnosing a person as mentally ill and, even more so, of determining that he is not competent in some respect, can drastically influence the distribution of power and the nature of the transactions between relatives. Often the doctor is the herald, and sometimes also the agent, of irreversible changes in the life of a couple or an entire family.

It is not only the content of decisions made by clinicians that is important. Their style of practice, the manner in which they implement their decisions, can have a critical effect on the happiness or distress of the people they care for. And the way in which a professional functions will also have important educational and moral consequences for her immediate colleagues: all the members of a clinical team play their part in creating the ethical climate in which the whole team operates.

These many different guises in which an ethically minded professional works—as advocate for patients, agent of government, adjudicator, maker of diagnoses, prescriber, communicator, and teacher—can prove bewildering in practice, especially when the role confusion is only half-recognized by its victim.

The best defences against this confusion are to work out, in any specific instance, just what the overlapping expectations are and where they come from. It is essential to discuss the problem with colleagues—especially with those who see the situation from a different standpoint—before deciding how to act.

Finally, the irony in our opening quotation is not misplaced. Ethical dilemmas never allow us simply to suspend judgement and do nothing.

References

1. Cornford, F.M.: *Microcosmographia academica.* Bowes and Bowes, Cambridge, 1908.
2. Post, S.J.: *The moral challenge of Alzheimer's disease.* London, Johns Hopkins University Press, 1995.
3. Mueller-Hill, B.: Psychiatry in the Nazi era, in *Psychiatric ethics*, 2nd edn, ed. S. Bloch and P. Chodoff, Chapter 22. Oxford, Oxford University Press, 1991.
4. Daniels, N.: *Am I my parents' keeper: an essay on justice between the young and the old.* Oxford, Oxford University Press, 1988.
5. Dilnot, A. and Taylor, J.: The economics of long-term care provision, in *Psychiatry in the elderly*, 2nd edn, ed. R. Jacoby and C. Oppenheimer, Chapter 23. Oxford, Oxford University Press, 1997.
6. Hope, T. and Oppenheimer, C.: Ethics and the psychiatry of old age, in *Psychiatry in the elderly*, 2nd edn, ed. R. Jacoby and C. Oppenheimer, Chapter 38. Oxford, Oxford University Press, 1997.
7. Miller, R.: The ethics of involuntary commitment to mental health treatment, in *Psychiatric ethics*, 2nd edn, ed. S. Bloch and P. Chodoff. Oxford, Oxford University Press, 1991.
8. Buchanan, A. E. and Brock, D. W.: *Deciding for others: the ethics of surrogate decision-making.* Cambridge, Cambridge University Press, 1990.
9. Times Law Reports 18th April 1997 *re MB,* cited by Luttrell, S.: Assessing mental capacity for decisions about medical treatment. *CME Bulletin Geriatric Medicine* **1**:19, 1997.
10. Jacoby, R.: Manging the financial affairs of mentally disordered persons in the UK, in *Psychiatry in the elderly*, 2nd edn, ed. R. Jacoby and C. Oppenheimer, Chapter 41B. Oxford, Oxford University Press, 1997.
11. Department of Health. Health Circular HC(90)22: a guide to consent for examination or treatment. Department of Health, NHS Management Executive, 1990.
12. Lord Chancellor's Department by Command of Her Majesty: *Who decides? Making decisions on behalf of mentally incapacitated adults*, Green Paper Cm 3803, 1977.
13. Seckler, A. B., Meier, D. E., Mulvihill, M., and Paris, B. E. C.: Substituted judgement: how accurate are proxy predictions? *Annals of Internal Medicine* **115**:92–98, 1991.
14. Volicer, L., Rheaume, Y., Brown, J., Fabiszewski, K., and Brady, R. Hospice approach to the treatment of patients with advanced dementia of the Alzheimer type. *Journal of the American Medical Association* **256**:2210–13, 1986.

15. BMA (British Medical Association).: *Advance statements about medical treatment.* British Medical Journal, London, 1995.
16. Feil, N.: *The validation breakthrough: simple techniques for communicating with people with Alzheimer's type dementia.* Health Professions Press, Baltimore. 1993.
17. Lovestone, S.: Molecular biology and molecular genetics of dementia, in *Psychiatry in the elderly*, 2nd edn, ed. R. Jacoby and C. Oppenheimer, Chapter 7. Oxford University Press, Oxford, 1997.

16

Ethics and forensic psychiatry

Thomas G. Gutheil

Definition

Historically, debate and the resolution of disputes took place in an open, public space called, in Latin, *forum*, and in English, courtyard, or court. From *forum* comes forensic, an adjective applied to legally relevant activities that range from forensic dentistry (e.g. identifying corpses by dentition) to forensic entomology (e.g. determining the age of corpses by the associated insect life) to forensic pathology (e.g. the whole panoply of postmortem examinations and laboratory studies).

Unlike the foregoing specialties, forensic psychiatry deals with the living *and* the dead. *Like* them, forensic psychiatry employs a scientific specialty (psychiatry) to assist the legal system. More formally, we might cite the definition of forensic psychiatry employed by a national organization of forensic psychiatry, the American Academy of Psychiatry and Law (AAPL), in its code of ethics:

Forensic psychiatry is a subspecialty of psychiatry in which scientific and clinical expertise is applied to legal issues in legal contexts embracing civil, criminal, correctional or legislative matters; forensic psychiatry should be practiced in accordance with guidelines and ethical principles enunciated by the profession of psychiatry.[1]

The second sentence raises some complexities that are addressed in the next section.

Note for clarity that, in the days of the 'alienists', the term forensic psychiatry was limited to the field of narrow determinations directly connected with criminal law, such as competence to stand trial and insanity (or criminal responsibility). In current usage, however, forensic psychiatry has expanded to include a host of new areas of interest and function, including civil and other matters such as civil competencies, psychiatric malpractice, workman's compensation, psychiatric disabilities, and child custody; primarily regulatory issues, such as informed consent requirements and the right of patients to refuse treatment; clinical topics with legal implications, such as assessment of dangerousness and risk management; and decision-making that requires testimony, such as hearings before licensing boards or ethics committees of professional organizations.

A different relationship

A critical distinction with profound ethical implications between forensic and general psychiatry is the altered relationship between the psychiatrist and the object of psychiatric attention. For the general psychiatrist, that relationship is the traditional one of doctor and patient, wherein the customary duties, obligations, and standards apply, as in general medicine. In most forms of forensic psychiatry, however, the doctor–patient relationship does not apply; rather, the relevant relationship is 'examiner–examinee' or 'evaluator–evaluee' (there are some exceptions, such as when a forensic psychiatrist renders treatment to an inmate or offender, where the more traditional relationship may well apply).[2,3]

There are several reasons for this alteration. First, the general psychiatrist is 'employed' by the patient, even when third parties pay the bill. The patient's interests, needs, and goals predominate in the work. Even more fundamentally, the bedrock obligation of the physician is captured by the Latin axiom, '*primum non nocere*', which may be translated: 'as a first priority, do no harm'.

In contrast, the forensic psychiatrist is 'employed' by the court or an officer thereof, such as an attorney or judge. The final result of the forensic psychiatric examination may be testimony that ultimately harms the examinee. For example, the forensic witness's testimony may be that a defendant is criminally responsible; if accepted and ratified by the court, this testimony may lead to punishment of the defendant—an obvious harm. Yet the adversarial system of justice commonly requires psychiatric input in just this form to educate the decision-maker about issues, disorders, and psychiatric principles involved.

The adversarial setting: serving two masters

A thorny problem in forensic psychiatry is the question of agency: for whom does the forensic psychiatrist work? Does the fact that the 'employer' is the legal system mean that all obligations to the patient are erased? And how does the forensic psychiatrist's position compare with other established dual-agency contexts such as military psychiatry, school psychiatry, and industrial psychiatry, as well as psychiatry in employee assistance plans?

The ethical tension in dual agency is best resolved by the understanding that —while one's employment 'contract' is usually with a part of the legal system— the forensic psychiatrist owes certain duties to the examinee, particularly one of disclosure. That is, in order to prevent deceiving one's examinee—even inadvertently—it is of paramount importance that the examinee be fully informed—indeed, warned—about the implications of the *different relationship* that applies with the forensic examiner compared to the treating doctor. There are several reasons for the ethical importance of this warning.

First, persons seeing a doctor tend to have certain expectations, be they unexamined assumptions or transferences, as to what the rules are. People expect confidentiality of their disclosures and expect medical efforts to be directed solely to their benefit, excluding other considerations. Those forensic examiners who are also gifted clinicians and interviewers compound these tendencies by establishing good rapport and an atmosphere that promotes sharing confidences.[4]

Fundamental fairness requires that examinees be informed *from the outset* that the usual rules do not apply. This goal is accomplished by non-traditional *warnings* as to the altered situation. A typical warning might include several points:

1. That the content and results of the examination are not confidential and may be transmitted to attorneys and judges, and may be revealed in open court under some circumstances.
2. That the examination does not involve treatment, in that the examiner, though *a* doctor, is not the *examinee's* doctor in the treatment sense.
3. That the examinee need not answer questions, though that refusal may be noted.

Other ethical concerns dictate informing the examinee about which side of the case (prosecution or defense) retained the examiner and about the right to take reasonable breaks from the examination.

For completeness, let us consider the other side of the coin: actual treatment in a forensic psychiatric context, such as treatment of prisoners, pre-trial detainees, parolees, inmates on probation or conditional release. In those and other situations the doctor–patient relationship is present in the classic sense, with patients' interests predominating. However, the earlier comments about dual agency apply here.

In the present context the forensic treater is ethically bound to inform the *patient* of any limitations on confidentiality and reporting requirements to which the forensic psychiatrist may be subject. The latter requirement may be dictated by institutional policies and procedures, which the forensic treater may help develop. Ambiguous situations should be resolved by ethical analysis of goods and harms.[5]

Case 1
An inmate being treated for depression told his psychiatrist that he had overheard plans for a riot to cover an escape attempt the next day. The psychiatrist, acting in accord with his previous warning to the patient, alerted prison authorities without naming the source. A lock-down averted the riot. Though worried about retaliation, the patient accepted the necessity of the treater's action to prevent widespread injury.

The present chapter

The present discussion of the ethics—the tensions between goods and harms—of forensic psychiatry could be organized in several ways. A useful approach might be to follow the Code of Ethics of the American Academy of Psychiatry and Law to unpack the decision-making in each principle and to provide illustrative examples of ethical dilemmas that a forensic psychiatrist might confront.

For completeness, note that the ethical guidelines of the AAPL do not govern ethical complaints to the Academy about its members; such complaints are referred to the American Psychiatric Association (APA) Ethics Committee and to district branches. Recently, the incorporation of some aspects of the AAPL ethics code into the APA code has been considered. The purpose of this step would be to guide and protect psychiatrists working in the different setting of the forensic context with the altered relationship noted above. In brief, these additions deal with the absence of the typical doctor–patient relationship; honesty, striving for objectivity and respect for examination subjects; the fact that contingency fees should not be accepted; the need to interview all parties in a custody dispute; the need to place claims of expertise on a basis of actual experience; and the need to maintain confidentiality within legal limits.

The AAPL guidelines may further inform and perhaps influence decision-making in other settings as well. The actual standards of the AAPL are presented as displayed paragraphs below.[1]

The confidentiality standard

Respect for the individual's right of privacy and the maintenance of confidentiality are major concerns of the psychiatrist performing forensic evaluations. The psychiatrist maintains confidentiality to the extent possible given the legal context. Special attention is paid to any limitations on the usual precepts of medical confidentiality. An evaluation of forensic purposes begins with notice to the evaluee of any limitations on confidentiality. Information or reports derived from the forensic evaluation are subject to the rules of confidentiality as applies to the evaluation, and any disclosure is restricted accordingly.

Many of the implications of this standard have already been addressed in the earlier discussion of dual agency (see also ref. 6). An important additional issue stressed in the commentary to this standard is the need for the examiner's alertness *during* the examination for the examinee's possible lapse into a 'clinical mind-set' incompatible with the self-preserving guardedness appropriate to forensic evaluation, which is not predicated on therapeutic beneficence. Indeed, Appelbaum *et al.*[7] and others have noted that even research subjects, exposed to the extensive disclosure consistent with human studies regulations, may still slip into the idea that they are getting treatment.

Case materials may also be subject to certain confidentiality requirements, which may affect not only the various established documents connected with a case (records, reports, depositions, etc.), but also the results of the expert's own evaluations. To complicate the issue, differing jurisdictions have different discovery rules. Thus, in one jurisdiction, disclosure may be total: nothing that one side obtains or generates is hidden from the other. In a different jurisdiction, 'work product' protections may be so extensive that even the *name* of the opposing expert, much less the opinion, is kept from the attorneys until trial—a veritable 'trial by ambush'.

Ethical conduct by the forensic psychiatrist includes adherence to these relevant rules and efforts to keep case material confidential.

Case 2
Amid a hotly-contested high-profile custody battle, a psychiatrist without forensic training was serving as an expert witness. Just after testifying, she held an impromptu press conference on the steps of the courthouse, emphasizing her position, opinion and beliefs which had, of course, been challenged in the courtroom. She was subsequently sanctioned for, *inter alia*, breach of confidentiality during an ongoing case.

Consent

The informed consent of the subject of a forensic evaluation is obtained when possible. Where consent is not required, notice is given to the evaluee of the nature of the evaluation. If the evaluee is not competent to give consent, substituted consent is obtained in accordance with the laws of the jurisdiction.

Despite the alteration in the clinical relationship, informed consent of the examinee is obtained whenever possible for reasons which flow from the ethical principle of respect for persons. In forensic work, certain exceptions may apply, for example in court-ordered evaluation or treatment, legally authorized involuntary commitment, and the like.

The AAPL Guidelines make clear the ethical distinction between consent for *evaluation* (which may be overridden by court mandates) and consent for *treatment* which may be governed by jurisdiction-specific statute, regulation or case law. A number of cases (e.g. *Washington* v. *Harper*,[8] *Riggins* v. *Nevada*[9]) have identified the right to refuse treatment of individuals at various stages of the defendant's course through the legal system. Forensic psychiatrists are expected to be familiar with local rules bearing on their practice.

A complex consent issue

It is common for defendants to be sent to forensic institutions for a combined evaluation for competence to stand trial and criminal responsibility (insanity). Both of these evaluations are ultimately made by the court, with input from the forensic psychiatric opinion. A problem arises when the competence examination suggests the patient is *not* competent to stand trial. If true, this finding implies that the defendant may not understand the warnings against self-incrimination that are so essential a part of evaluation for criminal responsibility; hence, the latter examination may be ethically compromised.

Even though the forensic examiner's opinion about incompetence is not a judicial finding, the ethical examiner should suspend the evaluation, seek guidance from the court, or refer the defendant to his/her attorney before proceeding. The rationale for this step is the likely impairment of the defendant's consent to proceed.

Honesty and striving for objectivity

This—the most complex, most nearly central and most provocative standard—reads as follows:

Forensic psychiatrists function as experts within the legal process. Although they may be retained by one party to a dispute in a civil matter or the prosecution or defense in a criminal matter, they adhere to the principle of honesty and they strive for objectivity. Their clinical evaluation and the application of the data obtained to the legal criteria are performed in the spirit of such honesty and efforts to attain objectivity. Their opinion reflects this honesty and efforts to attain objectivity.

Since honesty is an accepted virtue, one might ask why it is necessary to assert it as a standard. The answer lies in the unique pressures on the forensic practitioner in an adversarial situation.

First, there are the pressures from the attorney who retains the forensic psychiatrist as an expert witness. The attorney is always partisan in the adversary system because his or her own ethical code requires zealous and aggressive representation of the client. The attorney's task is the very opposite of the balanced, non-judgmental therapeutic position. In attempting to win the best outcome for the client, the attorney may exert pressure on the expert witness to slant or tilt an opinion in the most favorable direction. Complementary to these external pressures are forces internal to the forensic psychiatrist, such as identification with the retaining attorney, wishing to please or cooperate with that attorney, and the wish to present a strong, consistent, or coherent case (even if the facts of the case do not permit these qualities to emerge).

Finally, simple financial motivations may constitute powerful pressures against the honesty of the expert's opinion, as discussed at greater length below as the 'hired gun' problem.

These pressures generally constitute temptations that the ethical practitioner resists. As the AAPL guidelines commentary puts it:

Being retained by one side in a civil or criminal matter exposes the forensic psychiatrist to the potential for unintended bias and the danger of distortion of his opinion. (ref. 1, p. 3)

Honesty and striving for objectivity can thus be understood as the counterforce to bias and distortion.

How are honesty and striving for objectivity to be achieved? The relevant information (records, interviews, etc.) should be reviewed as thoroughly and extensively as possible, or as permitted by rules of discovery or admissibility; and an objective and dispassionate opinion drawn therefrom. This opinion, 'warts and all', should be communicated to the retaining attorney; the attorney then decides if the opinion is useful for the case or usable at hearing or trial. If the opinion does not help the attorney's case, the attorney can make litigation decisions (e.g. to settle) or attempt to find another expert—both legitimate legal strategies.

A specific example of this issue commonly occurs in psychiatric malpractice questions about the standard of care, typically defined as the care of the 'average reasonable practitioner'. The objectivity of the forensic expert is often challenged by the hindsight bias and the expert's *own* standard practice which—even if lower or higher than the average—is not the proper yardstick.

Another relevant forensic area is child-custody litigation.[10] A comprehensive examination of all parties and observers prevents the forensic psychiatrist from being influenced by the sometimes energetic demands for custody and criticism of opposing parties that are common features of this 'ugliest form of litigation'.

An additional ethical dimension here is that most scholars in this area agree that an evaluator should examine *all* parties—parents, children, observers, other members of the household, etc.—in order to obtain a comprehensive view of the family situation. Examination of, say, one parent would constitute a potential source of bias and an impairment of objectivity in assessing parenting capacity.

Forensic opinions in the absence of examination

The AAPL standards note:

Impartiality and the adequacy of the clinical evaluation may be called into question when an expert opinion is offered without a personal examination. While there are authorities who would bar an expert opinion in regard to an individual who has not been personally examined, it is the position of the Academy that if, after earnest effort, it is not possible to conduct a personal examination, an opinion may be rendered on the basis of other information. However, under such circumstances, it is the responsibility of the forensic psychiatrist to assure that the statement of his opinion and any reports or testimony based on this opinion expressed is thereby limited.

The issue of opinion without examination commonly arises in the following contexts:

1. *Psychological autopsy*: in these cases the decedent's mental state may be at issue. Some life-insurance policies, for example, are void for 'rational suicide', but valid for suicide under conditions of mental aberration, variously defined. A psychological autopsy may be relevant also to the next category.

2. *Malpractice alleged in suicide*: as part of a malpractice case, misdiagnosis and mistreatment of the deceased may be alleged. To discuss the case intelligently, the examiner needs to grasp the patient's mental condition; however, this is available only through records and observers.

3. *Postmortem will contest*: the testamentary capacity (competence to make a will) may be challenged by heirs after the testator's death. Such claimants, moreover, may not be the most impartial of witnesses. Nevertheless, the forensic psychiatrist may ethically proffer opinions as to whether the testator did or did not meet criteria for testamentary capacity based on data from observers, medical and mental health personnel, writings of the deceased, and similar data. The limits of such data must be acknowledged; moreover, a fully acceptable conclusion may be: 'I don't know'.

In all three cases above the potential examinee is already dead. The situation may also arise that the attorneys on the other side of the case refuse to *allow* examination of a plaintiff (or defendant). The ethical expert factors this into the opinion as missing data which, if later supplied, might change the opinion given, which must perforce be based on all the data then available.

A specific ethical pitfall that sometimes arises when a potential examinee is already dead is the temptation for the expert to claim to have a more accurate diagnosis by hindsight that those of the contemporary clinical observers. In the absence of grotesque misdiagnosis by contemporary treaters, the ethical expert yields the benefit of the doubt to direct observers, who had access to a wealth of data (body language, facial expression, tone of voice, observer's emotional response and empathy) that rarely makes it to the cool written record.[11,12] Though unwritten, such subjective data may have a decisive impact on decision-making.

A closely related ethical pitfall is the temptation for the expert to apply his or her *own* standard of practice as the yardstick for the standard of care in a malpractice case. This violates the standard of 'striving for objectivity', since the requisite standard is that of the *average* reasonable practitioner (or similar language). The requirement of objectivity mandates that the forensic examiner put aside personal approaches and use the average standard.[3] Of course, experts should explain the basis for their knowledge of the 'average'.

If, after the above efforts, the opinion *is* helpful to the attorney, the ethical tension is not yet resolved. The final threshold of ethical practice is honesty on cross-examination.[3] The reason is straightforward. On direct examination the opinion is brought out in an organized way reflecting careful preparation and planning with the attorney. It is on cross-examination that the unexpected query is posed and any limits, inconsistencies, and 'holes' in the opinion are demonstrated and probed. The ethical practitioner must frankly acknowledge the contradictions, unknown areas, and limitations of the available data on cross-examination. This is the true test of expert integrity.

Treater vs. expert

For a host of reasons, treating-clinicians are sometimes called on to serve as expert witnesses on their own patients. These reasons include: attorneys wishing to economize by having a treater do 'double duty' without expert fees; attorneys ignorant of any conflict between the roles; and treaters swept away by a passion for advocacy in the service of helping their patients. The ethical irreconcilability of the treater and expert roles are extensively described elsewhere[13,14] but the crux of the matter is a twofold conflict, in which each role vitiates important elements of the other.

The noxious effect of the treatment role on the expert role flows from the inescapable—perhaps even therapeutically desirable—bias introduced by the treater's therapeutic alliance[15,16] with the patient. Though essential for treatment, the alliance is a likely distorting force exerted on the expert's needed objectivity.

Conversely, the mandates of the expert role leave impacts on treatment. For example, as noted in an earlier section of this chapter, the patient enters treatment with broad expectations about confidentiality—expectations which often cannot be honored in the legal setting of expert-witness work. Moreover, the patient in customary treatment is usually not warned about future courtroom disclosure since such disclosure is not expected; indeed, to do so would contaminate the clinical work. Thus, the absence of an initial understanding about the ultimate non-confidentiality of the interviews—in effect, an absence of 'informed consent' as well—renders ethically doubtful the treater's participation as an expert.

A special problem in this area merges issues of informed consent with confidentiality. In a situation that is growing increasingly common in this litigious society, a patient in traditional therapy becomes involved in litigation totally unconnected to the therapeutic endeavor (e.g., an automobile accident). The patient may elect to proffer a claim for 'emotional injuries' stemming from the accident. What the patient may fail to realize is the fact that such a claim effectively waives privilege for the entire mental health history, including present therapy. To make matters worse, consultative experience reveals that many attorneys fail to inform their clients, for a variety of reasons, about this exposure of clinical data.

The treating psychiatrist is ethically constrained to alert the patient to this problem and encourage attorney/client discussion of the issue. Such dialogue may result in withdrawal of the claim, psychological preparation of the patient-litigant for the exposure, or other useful outcome.

The 'hired gun' problem

Tension, confusion, and rancor about the 'hired gun' question comprise much of the controversy swirling around forensic psychiatric testimony even today.

Indeed, every high profile insanity trial, since and including the fabled *M'Naghten* case in England in 1843[17] (pronounced Mc-Naw-ten) has been followed by outcry from public, press, and politicians for various changed laws, altered rules, and sweeping reforms, as well as expressions of professional embarrassment from general psychiatry and even medicine; these affective responses are commonly coupled with cries for de-adversarialized approaches such as expert panels appointed by the court. The hurly-burly around such public cases appears to stem from the perception that a newspaper reader can form an accurate picture of a suspect's mental state at the time of a remote crime and thus can just *tell* whether a psychiatrist is trying to get a felon 'off;' such perceptions also ignore the far more determinative role function of judge and jury. Underlying these curious views is the notion that—while the average layperson would not think of considering him or herself a DNA expert—many people view themselves as sound psychologists and thus able to detect malingering from the televized image of a defendant in court.

But behind all this noise and smoke is a serious matter: the perception and reality that venal forensic psychiatrists corruptly vend opinions based, not on 'honesty and striving for objectivity', but on whatever the attorney wants them to say. The distinction between corrupt and ethical experts is sometimes further aphorized as: 'The ethical expert sells time, the hired gun sells testimony'.[3] Note that this reasoning also justifies the statement in the AAPL's Code commentary that forensic psychiatrists should reject contingency fees (fees tied to the *outcome* of a case) as a potentially biasing factor. The expert's testimony then should be 'outcome-neutral.[18]

Alas, for simplicity, the matter is not always so cut and dried. Experts within all realms of psychiatry do frequently disagree, at times acrimoniously. Such disagreement, seen whenever psychiatrists gather, does not imply venality. My disagreement with some aspect of your testimony, as reported in the papers, may tempt me to paint you with the hired-gun brush, but this is inappropriate; media reportage of trial testimony is often erroneously selective or highly distorted. Thus, accurate assessment of the validity of testimony can be challenging.

Note in this context that opinions in court, because of the complexity of forensic issues, are not proffered as 'certainty', only as 'reasonable medical certainty'. This more modest standard suits the inherent uncertainty of forensic assessment.

Additional ethical conflicts may arise from issues intrinsic to the case itself. Examples might include cases which touch on personal aspects of the expert's own life or cases which place the expert on the defense side of perpetrators of heinous crimes, evil corporations, and the like; or on the plaintiff's side of frivolous or wrongheaded litigation. The ethical expert's path must lie between two poles: (1) everyone is entitled to a day in court or to a defense; and (2) experts need not take on any case which they find incompatible with personal values. While some stress and discomfort is expected in dealing with the sometimes horrific content of forensic cases, at a certain level of extreme personal discomfort the expert is fully entitled to withdraw.

Ethical experts, then, validate their opinion by thorough assessment, adherence to honesty and striving for objectivity, and resistance to the various pressures from retaining attorneys or other sources.

Qualifications

Expertise in the practice of forensic psychiatry is claimed only in areas of actual knowledge and skills, training and experience.

Arguably, this standard extends the 'honesty' standard from before to apply to frank acknowledgment by the expert of 'real' experience. If you have only treated three alcoholic patients, say so; if this is your first post-traumatic stress disorder (PTSD) assessment, admit that fact. Ideally, such experiential strengths and weaknesses are discussed with the retaining attorney from the outset. The goal of this standard is clearly to attempt to avoid misrepresentation of the level of expertise actually possessed by the testifying witness.

The tension between forensic questions and essentially moral or social ones constitutes an area of ambiguity that may enter into the issue of qualifications. As the guidelines state, psychiatric principles are applied by the forensic psychiatrist to legal matters. Question of moral blameworthiness, ultimate responsibility for behavior, conscious versus unconscious motivation, predictions of the future, may all be posed in different forms to the forensic expert in the course of civil and criminal litigation:

'Don't you think Doctor, that what happened to this poor woman was a crying shame?'

'Doctor—can you truthfully say you blame this man for what he did?'

The 'ultimate question' issue

An area of some controversy is the question of whether forensic psychiatrists should express on the witness stand their conclusions as to the ultimate (legal) issue in the case. The ultimate issue may be, say, the criminal responsibility or non-responsibility of a defendant—findings which are the province of the fact-finder (judge or jury).

Some scholars have suggested[2] that for the forensic witness to state the ultimate issue as an opinion—'This defendant is (or should be found) not guilty by reason of insanity'—would be to invade the province of the fact-finder. Such scholars recommend that the forensic witness testify to opinions just short of the ultimate issue, as in: 'The defendant lacks substantial capacity to appreciate the wrongfulness of the act'. By addressing the *criteria*, the witness leaves the ultimate *finding* to the fact-finder.

Others have suggested that *all* forensic evidence is opinion anyway, and that opining only about criteria without coming to the obvious implied conclusion is an unnecessary nicety; moreover, judges' instructions usually inform juries about the weight to be given to the expert's opinion. Some judges even insist that the expert go on to the ultimate opinion to make it clear to the jury that the expert's opinion has obvious implications. The ethical expert should be guided by local custom and the attorney's advice.

Areas of ethical controversy

The above standards alone do not represent the universe of possible ethical issues in forensic work. A number of other areas have raised concern among both practitioners and the general psychiatric public.

Pre-arraignment examination

The controversy in this area relates to the question of whether a forensic psychiatrist should examine a suspect during the period immediately after they have has been arrested and detained, and possibly before they have been assigned legal counsel.[19] The general argument is as follows. Traditionally— except for *emergency* treatment—forensic psychiatrists are expected to wait for and insist upon legal counsel's assignment to a suspect so that the examinee can be advised of all relevant rights and privileges that may apply to their situation. The AAPL guidelines commentary (ref. 1, p. 2) notes: '... ethical considerations preclude forensic evaluation prior to access to, or availability of legal counsel. The only exception is an examination for the purpose of rendering emergency medical care and treatment.' The purpose of this restriction is to prevent the suspect's disclosure of potentially self-incriminating statements to the psychiatrist, whose presumed skill at obtaining information may place the suspect at a disadvantage. Thus, the examiner avoids the possibility of exploiting an examinee through the latter's ignorance of areas they may not be required to answer, restrictions on confidentiality and the like.

The other side of the argument is that many patients can be informed, by appropriate warnings, of the most important relevant rights and privileges, and that the data that emerge from an examination, immediately after an alleged crime has occurred, are extremely valuable and relevant to later determinations of criminal responsibility; if the search for truth is primary, such a timely evaluation, the argument goes, would provide the best access to the best data: the earliest data are the best data. At present, the ethical position of the American Academy of Psychiatry and Law is to delay or refrain from examination until legal counsel has been assigned and has had an opportunity to consult with the potential examinee. Here, certain competing ethical goals may be easily identified.

Obviously, a Solomon-like solution here would be to separate treatment and examination functions by dividing them between two clinicians, thus preventing contamination of roles—a solution still problematic in settings with limited resources.

The insanity defense

Participation in the insanity defense by forensic psychiatrists (or 'alienists' in an earlier era) must be considered one of the wellsprings of the field. As earlier noted, the issue is also the wellspring of much acrimony, calamity and calls for reform whenever high-profile cases appear.

A reality often lost in the media storm around such cases is the fact that—while at least two psychiatrists present opinions about a defendant's mental state—only the judge or jury, in a finding, actually decides who is insane and hence exculpated.[2]

The core of the insanity issue—application of legal (usually statutory) criteria to a mental condition in a defendant at the time of the act in question to determine whether he or she should be held responsible—requires the most careful, precise, and subtle bridging of the gap between clinical and legal realms; indeed, perhaps no other forensic question requires such attention to this conceptual bridging.

Beside these rigorous professional demands, the subject terrain presents certain ethical pitfalls. The honesty and objectivity earlier noted may be tested by such factors as: the examiner's identification with criminal defendants, especially palpably mentally ill ones, (tending perhaps to lower the threshold for an opinion of insanity); identification with victims (tending perhaps to raise the threshold for an opinion of insanity); and countertransference reactions to the heinousness or bizarreness of a particular crime (tending perhaps to promote confusion of the apparent 'craziness' of the act with the criteria-driven test for legal insanity). Those specific criteria dictate the apparent paradox: a defendant may be 'crazy' (that is, mentally ill), but not insane (that is, with the illness meeting the criteria).

Personal injury cases

Cases alleging psychological injury are common subjects of forensic psychiatric involvement. The ethical challenges commonly include: the delicate question of malingering or exaggeration of symptoms; the often challenging determination of the causal linkage between the alleged injurious act and the present emotional condition, especially when the history contains much previous trauma and abuse; and the challenge of remaining objective when confronting a person who may be suffering as intensely as one of our patients in treatment, thus challenging us to remain clear that we here face an examinee.

Consultative experience reveals that perhaps the most confounding examination in this area requires peeling apart the disparate impacts of serial traumata that may have been inflicted by different perpetrators/defendants.

The psychiatrist in the forensic hospital and in the prison system

While both these institutions involve incarceration, the ethical issues in each show both similarities and differences. Both settings may involve dual agency as noted before. Both settings may involve treatment, hence may return the treater from the role of examiner to the role of physician. As before, separation of the examination and treatment functions between separate clinicians is extremely desirable but may be prevented by limitation of resources.

An ethical dilemma unique to the forensic hospital may be posed when a defendant has been found not guilty by reason of insanity, and duly committed, but has been found on examination not to have the underlying illness! Glib psychopaths who persuade a jury of their insanity might be such cases.

A baroque example occurred years ago when a policeman shot a young man because the latter was allegedly planning to shoot; however, no gun was found. Charged with the killing, the policemen pleaded insanity based on alleged temporal lobe epilepsy. Forensic hospital staff, examining him after his commitment, found no evidence of this condition; however, the court refused to permit his release and insisted on continued 'treatment'. The policeman then sued the police for failure to pick up and treat his 'disability'! Though unusual, the case captures the conflicting forces and agendas that may combine in the forensic hospital.

The prison psychiatrist faces a 'captive audience' but is challenged to offer appropriate assessment and treatment within the walls. Ethical challenges may include prisoners who spontaneously confess to other crimes; who use drugs prescribed for themselves as contraband traded on the prison 'underground market'; and those who disclose, within a treatment setting, rape, murder, escape or riot plans. While these examples offer no clear general solutions, a fundamental issue again is the importance of disclosure to the prisoner of the dual agency and confidentiality restrictions that may appear.

Issues relating to the death penalty

Almost a dozen years ago, the US Supreme Court found in the case of *Ford* v. *Wainwright*[20] that prisoners have a right to be competent to be executed and that an incompetent prisoner may not be executed when sentenced to the death penalty. One of the most intense controversies in this area rages about the question of whether psychiatrists can perform such competence examinations. The intensity of the conflict is clearly influenced by a number of factors including personal, clinical, and official attitudes toward the death penalty; the difference between the psychiatrist as physician and as forensic examiner (in which latter context, a doctor–patient relationship arguably does not occur); and the question of 'how close to the execution one should stand', in order to be enmeshed in the prohibition against physicians participating in actual execution—a standard common to both the American Psychiatric Association and the American Medical Association. Each of these ethical dilemmas requires some examination.

First, since the court has established the need for competence to be executed as a right of prisoners, the need for some sort of examination has been defined; and one may legitimately take the position that only by such examination can some incompetent prisoners be spared death by the commutation of their sentence to life imprisonment. Indeed, some advocates have suggested that a resolution to the ethical dilemma in this regard is for psychiatrists only to perform competency evaluations on those persons whose sentence has already been commuted, whereby the sentence to life imprisonment would be a pre-condition for the examination itself. Of course, the possibility that certain individuals may be saved from death by a finding of incompetence must be balanced against the finding of competence as eliminating a potential last obstacle to an execution. Here, personal attitudes toward the death penalty are certainly relevant and influential.

Another point made in this area by scholars of the issue is that once one has accepted the idea that the forensic psychiatrist is not a doctor in a doctor–patient relationship, but is an examiner of an examinee, the ethical principles are no longer those of the healing treater, but are those of honesty and respect for persons, an argument that was extensively discussed at a 1997 American Psychiatric Association annual meeting debate on this issue.[21] The affirmative view, that death-row competence examination was ethical, was put forth by Drs Paul S. Appelbaum and Steven K. Hoge. The points stressed, among others, were: failure to perform such examinations deprived prisoners of the possibility of uncovering a mental disorder that might save them from execu-tion; other potentially harmful examinations were considered ethical and dis-tinguishing them from other exams was 'artificial and logically indefensible' (ref. 21, p. 18).

The negative view, presented by Drs Alfred Freedman and Lawrence Hartmann, proposed, among other points: the Nuremberg principles' position that it is unethical for physicians to take part in proceedings that can lead to executions; the affirmative view (above) is 'immoral' (ref. 21, p. 18); partici-pation in the capital punishment pushes the issue 'beyond the ethical breaking point' (p. 18).

The debate will probably not reach consensus soon. One might argue that although the possibility of harm is in this case extreme (i.e. death), the expert is in no different an ethical position from other potentially harmful opinions that may emerge from civil, criminal, workman's compensation, emotional injury, custody, or other forms of litigation. An argument extending the reasoning in the debate above is the idea that the psychiatrist who refuses to perform such examinations, on the one hand, withholds needed services from a needy population and, on the other, leaves the field open to less trained or qualified individuals to perform a service that the Supreme Court has defined as necessary.

Finally, the question of how close one stands to the fire, as it were, is another area of debate. A psychiatrist who testifies honestly and objectively for the prosecution, in a case in which the death penalty is one of the possible sentencing outcomes, may be seen as sufficiently remote from the ultimate death of the defendant to be ethically untarnished. From another viewpoint, however, the psychiatrist could be seen as pushing the first domino in a chain which ultimately leads to the defendant's death. The degree to which functioning at various points along the way from trial to execution represents 'too close to the execution' to be ethically pure is an area of hot controversy in the field, and, again, one which will not soon be resolved.

Conclusion

Jonas Rappeport said it well in the second edition of this text:

Forensic psychiatry is not a field into which a psychiatrist should step without a good deal of forethought. It contains many ethical pitfalls. The contract of the forensic psychiatrist is essentially not with the patient, but with the latter's lawyer or the court. In fact, the 'patient' is not really a patient in the usual doctor–patient sense. This needs to be made clear to the *examinee* at the outset. Another house is being entered, not the house of medicine but that of law—with its different motives, goals, and rules of conduct. In medicine we communicate openly, in the law we may not. In medicine we listen to everything, and may discuss it with colleagues. In the law, the attorney by whom we are employed may not want us to do this. He may even wish us to omit information which he believes will harm his client; we may want to omit material which we feel is irrelevant. We may be tempted to say too much or too little, or, in our zeal, advance ideas and theories which have no foundation, or allow our personal bias to appear as professional opinion. These are only some of the ethical problems which arise in the forensic arena.[22]

Acknowledgment

The author acknowledges his indebtedness to Jonas Rappeport for providing inspiration and guidance.

References

1. *American Academy of Psychiatry and the Law ethics guidelines for the practice of forensic psychiatry.* Adopted 1987, revised 1989, 1991, 1995. Baltimore, MD.
2. Appelbaum, P. S. and Gutheil, T.G.: *Clinical handbook of psychiatry and the law,* 2nd edn. Baltimore, Williams and Wilkins, 1991.
3. Gutheil, T.G.: *The psychiatrist as expert witness.* Washington DC, American Psychiatric Press, 1998.
4. Stone, A. A.: The ethics of forensic psychiatry: a view from the ivory tower, in Rosner, R. and Weinstock, R. (ed.), *Ethical practice in forensic psychiatry and the law.* New York, Plenum, 1990, pp. 3–17.

5. Reiser, S., Bursztajn, H., Gutheil, T. G., and Brodsky, A.: *Divided staffs, divided selves: a case book of mental health ethics.* Cambridge, Cambridge University Press, 1987.
6. In the service of the state: the psychiatrist as double agent. *Hastings Center Report* **8**(Suppl.):1–23, 1978.
7. Appelbaum, P. S., Roth, L. H., Lidz, C. W., Benson, P., and Winslade, W.: False hopes and best data: consent to research and the therapeutic misperception. *Hastings Center Reports* **17**:20–24, 1987.
8. *Washington* v. *Harper* 100 S.Ct. 1028 (1990).
9. *Riggins* v. *Nevada* 60 U.S.L.W. 3302 (1991).
10. Goldzband, M. G.: *Custody cases and expert witnesses: a manual for attorneys,* 2nd edn. Clifton, NJ, Prentice-Hall, 1988.
11. Gutheil, T. G., Bursztajn, H., and Brodsky, A.: Subjective data in suicide assessment in the light of recent legal developments. Part I: Malpractice prevention and the use of subjective data. *International Journal of Psychiatry and Law* **6**:317–329, 1983.
12. Gutheil, T. G., Bursztajn, H., and Brodsky, A.: Subjective data and suicide assessment in the light of recent legal developments. Part II: Clinical uses of legal standards in the interpretation of subjective data. *International Journal of Psychiatry and Law* **6**:331–350, 1983.
13. Strasburger, L. H., Gutheil, T. G., and Brodsky, A.: On wearing two hats: role conflict in serving as both psychotherapist and expert witness. *American Journal of Psychiatry* **154**:448–456, 1997.
14. Schouten, R.: Pitfalls of clinical practice: the treating clinician as expert witness. *Harvard Review of Psychiatry* **1**:64–65, 1993.
15. Gutheil, T. G. and Havens, L. H.: The therapeutic alliance: contemporary meanings and confusions. *International Review of Psycho-Analysis* **6**:467–481, 1979.
16. Gutheil, T. G., Bursztajn, H., and Brodsky, A.: Malpractice prevention by the sharing of uncertainty: informed consent and the therapeutic alliance. *New England Journal of Medicine* **311**:49–51, 1984.
17. *M'Naghten* case: 8 Eng. Rep. 718, * Eng. Rep. 722 (1843).
18. Schultz-Ross, R. A.: Ethics and the expert witness. *Hospital and Community Psychiatry* **44**:388–389, 1993.
19. Goldzband, M. G.: Pre arraignment psychiatric examinations and criminal responsibility: a personal Odyssey through the law and psychiatry west of the Pecos. *Journal of Psychiatry and the Law* **4**:447–466, 1976.
20. *Ford* v. *Wainwright* 477 U.S. 399, 106 S.Ct. 2595 (1986).
21. *Psychiatric News*, June 20, 1997, pp. 6, 18.
22. Rappeport, J.: Ethics and forensic psychiatry. in Bloch, S. and Chodoff, P. (ed.) *Psychiatric ethics*, 2nd edn. Oxford, Oxford University Press, 1991, pp. 391–413.

17

Ethics in community psychiatry

George Szmukler

Community psychiatry, as adopted in many developed countries, involves radical changes in practice. It differs distinctively from previous hospital-based or office-based practice, and some treatment approaches depart dramatically from what we have previously known. Developments have occurred rapidly; in the first two editions of this volume on psychiatric ethics no need was perceived for a separate review of the ethics of community psychiatry.

Just how far-reaching the changes might prove is attested by a 1993 editorial by Bell:[1]

By 2000, mental health laws will have swung back in the direction of permitting involuntary treatment of severely and persistently mentally ill patients based on psychiatric need: stringent commitment criteria will no longer allow patients who seriously need help to go untreated. Further, the restrictive confidentiality laws that inhibit mental health professionals' communication with family members about patients' conditions and treatment plans will be long gone ... Problems with continuity of care will be lessened by a unified computer network that provides authorised access to medical records and permits knowledgeable treatment of patients regardless of where they seek care ... More CMHCs (Community Mental Health Clinics) will be involved with residential alternatives and vocational training ... [There will be] linkages with correctional facilities that will make after care available to incarcerated mentally ill persons after their release ... The increase in partnership between family members and CMHCs will form a strong lobby that will bring a common sense approach to the care of patients most in need.

Ethical implications of the new kinds of practice in community psychiatry have been neglected. It is not clear why this is so; perhaps the forces, ideological and fiscal, driving change are too powerful to be questioned. The ethical basis for deinstitutionalization is discussed in another chapter of this book.

My aims in this chapter are:

(1) to outline the new model of care and the climate in which it has developed;
(2) to identify the ethical challenges resulting from this new model of care and the need for an appropriate ethical framework;
(3) to look at practical approaches to these challenges.

There will be a British bias in this chapter, but the examples presented will almost certainly be paralleled by similar ones in most other countries and services.

Philosophy and practice of community psychiatry

I here present a fairly detailed account of community psychiatry since many are still not aware of its philosophy, objectives, and organization.

Community psychiatry involves a change in the locus of care (from hospital to community), funding arrangements, and treatment techniques (many derived from theories of social psychiatry). It aims to establish a network of services offering crisis intervention, continuing treatment, accommodation, occupation, and social support which together help people with mental health problems to retain or recover social roles, as close to normal as possible for them.[2] In most countries, the focus of the services is on those with serious mental illness, especially the psychoses. A useful perspective is to see community services as attempting to provide outside the old mental hospitals, the complex range of care once provided within. These covered not only health needs but also social, accommodation, occupational, and leisure facilities, as well as the provision of asylum.

The scale of deinstitutionalization has been astonishing. In England, the number of psychiatric beds decreased from a peak of 152 000 in 1954 to 39 500 in 1993, a reduction of 74 per cent. This has been associated with a large increase in admissions but also a greatly decreased number of patients with a protracted stay in hospital. In the US, occupied psychiatric beds in state hospitals have fallen from 339 per 100 000 population in 1955 to 29 per 100 000 in 1994 (cited in Lamb).[3]

Case management and assertive community treatment

To ensure that patients in the community receive the benefits of the range of services which they may require, the widespread practice of 'case management' has been adopted. The aims of case management are to ensure continuity of care, accessibility to often fragmented and independently managed services, accountability, and efficiency. The core functions usually include: assessing patient needs; developing a comprehensive care plan; arranging service delivery; monitoring and assessing services; evaluating progress and follow-up.[4,5]

Although the practice of case management varies, two general approaches can be identified. Service 'brokerage' case management sees the 'case manager' as an enabler, systems coordinator, or broker of services. In 'clinical' case management on the other hand, the professional has a direct treatment relationship with the patient, often being personally involved with aspects of the patient's psychological, physical and social care.[6] In the public sector, case management is seen as ensuring access to care for those too disabled to seek it themselves. Within the private sector, as sometimes in the US, case management may be used as a mechanism of utilization review, limiting access to some services in order to contain costs.[7]

Research on simple implementations of case management tends to show relatively poor effectiveness.[8,9] As a result a more intensive model of case management is being increasingly adopted in community mental health services, usually known as Assertive Community Treatment (ACT). ACT aims to provide a comprehensive care package including treatment and support services via a multidisciplinary team within the community. It includes frequent contacts with patients in the community (often at home), 24-hour availability, direct responsibility of staff for a broad range of interventions, and low staff:patient ratios.

The ACT model was first evaluated in the early 1970s in Madison, Wisconsin,[10] and has been followed by a number of replication studies in Australia, Michigan, California, and London.[11] Most ACT programmes result in a reduction in the use of psychiatric inpatient care partially offset by additional use of other community-based services. Positive effects on symptoms, social functioning, and disability are less evident. They do have a positive impact on residential stability and result in better retention in treatment.[9] Cost savings result where there has been a reduction in the use of inpatient care. Costs are shifted to community-based services but there is often a net saving despite this.[12,13]

A major focus of ACT is to prevent the severely mentally ill patient from dropping out of treatment, since loss of contact is likely to lead to relapse and the need for admission to hospital. Admission tends to be seen as a last resort, and as often representing a failure of continuity of care. An assertive approach, bringing treatment *to* the patient aims at preventing the patient falling through gaps in the net of services. Lapsing from treatment may be an early sign of relapse. The community team may then actively seek out the patient to re-establish contact. Uninvited visits to the patient's home and sharing concerns about the patient's risk with other agencies may follow. Interventions may occur in public places so that patients, their treatment, and the role of mental health teams become more visible to the public.

In contrast to the hospital, the community is a complex environment in which to provide care. Patients with severe mental illness have a complex range of needs that can only be met by a range of separate services and agencies. For the patient to have access to these, there needs to be a substantial flow of information between them concerning the patient. Furthermore, the key-worker or other members of the multidisciplinary team tend to develop a special kind of relationship with the patient. They provide a broad treatment approach. As well as medication and conventional psychological interventions, they work with the patient in their ordinary community settings to rehabilitate basic living skills. They may help with budgeting, shopping, cooking, attend appointments with the patient to see other professionals, advocate for services, and work closely with carers, housing offices, and other figures in the patient's social network. This special relationship may be used to encourage the patient to comply with treatment, especially prophylactic medication.

In the background may loom important issues of another kind. The shift from hospital to community may exert pressure to discharge patients as quickly as possible. Still symptomatic and disabled patients then require intense and controlling management in the community. Lack of responsiveness from other agencies (for example, one responsible for finding suitable accommodation) may provide a temptation to withdraw some responsibilities in an effort to stimulate a response.

The community's response to community psychiatry

Public fears are common that care in the community for mentally ill persons will be a failure. At times this fear may amount to a 'demonization' of the mentally ill who are seen as posing a serious risk to innocent members of the public. Responses to these fears by government and others may significantly affect the practice of community mental health teams.

In England, for example, such fears have been fuelled by highly publicized incidents involving people with mental illnesses. In December 1992 Christopher Clunis, a man with schizophrenia, stabbed to death a complete stranger on an underground station platform. This led to a prominent public inquiry, the Ritchie inquiry, which described Clunis' care as 'a catalogue of failures'.[14] Amongst the report's many recommendations were the need for improvement in care planning and interagency working, for highly intensive care for difficult patients, for training of 'key-workers' (case managers), and for better assessments of risk. Subsequently, almost every homicide by a person with a history of contact with mental health services has been publicized, often sensationally, and has been the subject of an independent public inquiry. These have all reached more or less the same conclusions: that contributing to the tragic outcome have been poor communication between agencies, poor assessment of the risk of violence, poor liaison with police and probation services, and barriers posed by 'confidentiality and professional ethics'.[15]

In England, the government's response to the public's fear has been to issue 'guidance' and new legislation. The former has taken the form of the 'Care Programme Approach' (CPA) and the 'Supervision Register'. The CPA essentially institutionalizes the core principles of case management—assessment of the health and social needs of people accepted by specialist psychiatric services; formulation of a care plan which addresses these needs; appointment of a key-worker to keep in close touch with the patient and monitor care; and, regular review, and if need be, agreed changes to the care plan. Health purchasing authorities monitor the implementation of this approach including the requirement that registers of patients on the CPA be maintained. In 1994 the government introduced guidance for 'Supervision Registers' for patients identified, during a Care Programme review meeting, as being at 'significant risk of committing serious violence or suicide, or of severe self-neglect in some foreseeable circumstances which it is felt might well arise in this particular case (eg. ceasing to take medication, misusing drugs or alcohol, loss of a supportive relationship, or of accommodation)'.[16,17] In practice, their focus has usually been on the risk of harm to others. Services are required to identify and give priority, of an only vaguely suggested nature, to these patients within the CPA framework. Health authorities (the purchasers) must ensure, through their contracts for mental health services that providers draw up, maintain, and use Supervision Registers of those patients who are at risk. Supervision Registers will be discussed again later when we examine questions of privacy.

In 1995 legislation was passed establishing 'supervised discharge'—'after care under supervision' for vulnerable former inpatients previously detained compulsorily under the Mental Health Act. This provides powers 'to convey' a patient to a place of treatment, occupation, education, or residence by a community supervisor (e.g. case manager) but does *not* permit compulsory treatment itself. Indeed, the guidance accompanying the legislation requires that before enforced conveyance, the supervisor should have reason to believe that such conveyance is likely to change the patient's mind about accepting treatment. Guidelines also suggest that the power may be used to take home urgently a patient putting themselves or others at risk. Essentially the legislation amounts to a power of arrest, but to no apparent purpose. The effects of such powers on relationships between patients and staff can be anti-therapeutic. The legislation has been rarely used to date. It is intended to be used when it is 'likely to help to secure' that the patient receives the aftercare services to be provided; as it does not compel treatment, it could presumably only work for a patient who accepts the care plan—but such a patient would not require an order. Most clinicians view supervised discharge as ill-considered and unworkable.[18]

These measures are a 'half-way house', between—on the one hand—the recommendations of the Ritchie inquiry for a supervised discharge order with the power to recall a patient defaulting on treatment, together with a national register of patients 'at risk' to allow tracking across services, and—on the other hand—obstacles to such an order raised by professionals' resistance to such an approach as being anti-therapeutic, and its likely contravention of Article 5 of the European Convention on Human Rights.

Most commentators see the CPA and the Supervision Register as having two implicit functions—firstly, identifying individuals (key-workers) who can be held responsible for the dangerous behaviour of their patients, while deflecting attention from resource deficiencies.[19] (The recommendation by the Ritchie inquiry that special teams be set up for difficult-to-engage patients, comprising community nurses with low caseloads, has been ignored.) Second, a political purpose, to reassure the community that they are being protected from dangerous patients. The term adopted, '*supervision*' register rather than say, '*at-risk*' or '*priority*' register, supports this contention.

As a result of such fears and reactions to them clinical practice has changed in ways which have ethical import. Between 1989 and 1993 the number of compulsory admissions to hospital increased by 27 per cent. Mental health professionals recognize that a public inquiry following a homicide by one of their patients (or ex-patients) threatens their professional reputation and badly damages the morale of their service. Under such circumstances it would not be surprising to find their practice moving in the direction of greater control over their patients at the expense of autonomy.[19]

Responses also occur at an institutional level. Increasing attention is being given to 'clinical risk management' in psychiatry. Lipsedge[20] has summarized the factors contributing to the clinical risk in psychiatry. These include: 'professional arrogance combined with a reckless tolerance of deviance leading to a failure by mental health professionals to heed reports by carers and members of the public about disturbed behaviour'; 'undue emphasis on the civil liberties of psychiatric patients at the expense of tolerating grave suicidal risk and the danger of violent behaviour'; 'failure to pass on information about potential dangers to other professionals, such as hostel staff, for reasons ranging from inertia, inefficiency, or over work to a misguided overprotective view of the patient at the expense of the safety of potential victims'. Ethical implications abound, as we shall see in the next section.

Harrison[21] has summarized the current position in England as follows: 'The danger is that given the low predictability of risk factors in relation to individual patients, large numbers may be drawn into supervision programmes having a custodial and coercive therapeutic focus.... Many patients require intensive care, perhaps over long periods of time. But there is a significant risk that mental health professionals will resort to inpatient care, or to over-restrictive styles of therapeutic care, because of risks not to their patient but to *themselves* should something go wrong.'

While especially prominent in England, similar pressures inflate anxieties of psychiatrists elsewhere. Appelbaum[22] from an American perspective, has noted the tendency to err on the side of involuntary commitment because of societal pressure. In some states in the US there is a '*Tarasoff*-type' duty to protect, and if necessary to warn, potential victims when a patient poses a serious threat of physical harm. At least one state, Vermont, has extended the duty to protect to include property.[23] The potential for litigation by third parties harmed by patients has probably changed clinicians' behaviour significantly, but the negative effects of *Tarasoff*-like court decisions have in the main been less damaging than feared. Subsequent judicial, legislative, and clinical responses have muted the more unrealistic expectations.[24]

In relation to community psychiatry it is noteworthy that the original Californian *Tarasoff* decision occurred at a time when mental hospitals were being viewed increasingly negatively and commitment laws were becoming more restrictive;[25] there nevertheless remains a persistent demand—if not met by walls then by duties to protect imposed on professionals charged with the care of the mentally ill—for the public to be kept safe from the 'insane'. Well-publicized local incidents may result in a temporary increase in admissions; in England, where nearly all are publicized, the effect becomes persistent.

Ethical dilemmas

In this section I attempt to characterize the core ethical issues arising in community clinical practice. They can be grouped under four headings: privacy, confidentiality, coercion, and conflicts of duty.

Privacy

Assertive treatment programmes bring treatment to the patient, often in the patient's residence whether it be home, hostel, or boarding house. If the patient is regarded as being at risk of relapse, visits may be made by members of the community mental health team even when uninvited. Indeed, visits may continue even when the patient's explicit desire is that they cease. Since much treatment occurs in the community, there is also an increased risk that it becomes public. The curiosity of neighbours may be aroused, particularly with repeated visits, and especially if attempts to gain entry are rebuffed by the patient. Neighbours and other members of the public may deduce that a mental health team is involved and that the person being visited is a patient.

Furthermore, as treatment becomes more visible to the public, new expectations may be generated that a community mental health team can be called to deal with a disturbed or difficult person suspected to be a patient. Even if a public assessment is not carried out, an acknowledgement by the mental health team that they may have a role may reveal to bystanders that the difficult person is a mental patient (if already so) or label them as one (if not).

The 'Supervision Register' in England, discussed earlier, illustrates most of my points concerning privacy. An aim is for the key-worker to maintain contact with the patient. The Register is meant to act as a 'flagging device' to staff that there is a significant risk. It is also meant to ensure that identified patients receive the care they need, and that resources are targeted on this group, even though the introduction of Supervision Registers was not accompanied by any increase in resources. It may be difficult for some patients ever to be discharged from the Register as many of the factors suggesting a risk of violence—a past history of violence, for example—will persist. If the patient defaults from treatment, the key-worker and other members of the team are enjoined to make every effort to re-establish contact. This includes contacting the carer or family, consulting the general practitioner, checking with local accident and emergency departments for any contacts, and checking with neighbouring mental health units. Immediate consideration is also to be given 'to the need to inform the police service if contact is lost with a patient who could pose a significant risk to him/herself or others'.[17] The nature of the relationship between clinician and patient may shift from care to supervision, akin to that between a probation officer and client. Is the Supervision Register more likely to ensure that patients receive the care they need, or to stigmatize them with the label of 'dangerous', leading to exclusion from community services or amenities, including housing?

The patient has a right to know that he or she is on the Register, unless it would cause 'serious harm to his or her physical or mental health'. The patient may request removal, but it is up to the psychiatrist in discussion with the multidisciplinary team to decide. If the patient remains dissatisfied, the normal channels for complaint and the right to a clinical second opinion apply.

The status of 'guidance', such as that issued concerning Supervision Registers,[16] is not law but, if challenged, the clinician is liable to criticism, for example by an independent inquiry, and possibly to a charge of negligence, if he or she cannot show that account was taken of the guidance. The impact on practice is thus major.

Confidentiality

Confidentiality may be considered an aspect of privacy in which information obtained from a patient on the assumption that it will not be disclosed to others, is disclosed. As the patient is commonly treated by a multidisciplinary team, sharing of information among its members is common. Patients may not know that this is to be expected. More complex is the sharing of information between agencies—health, social, voluntary, housing, and so on. Very needy patients' access to benefits and other goods may depend on information about them being revealed to those in a position to supply them. Since information may flow frequently, confidentiality may receive less emphasis. There may be what might be called the 'cat already out of the bag' phenomenon, and an attitude that 'the patient has less to lose by certain breaches of confidentiality than other kinds of patients do'.[26]

Confidentiality may be breached ostensibly in the interests of the patient as above, or for the protection of others. The latter is considered below, including the interests of family and carers.

Coercion

'Coercion' is a complex notion. A range of pressures may be exerted by community mental health teams to gain the patient's cooperation with treatment. The least problematic is 'persuasion', an appeal to reason. Since the key-worker may have established a relationship with the patient, broader in scope and more intimate than the conventional patient–clinician relationship, opportunities for other kinds of pressure arise. 'Leverage' or 'interpersonal pressure' may be exercised through the patient's emotional dependency on the key-worker.[27] A vague threat may be implied of something being removed, or the patient may simply want to please someone who has proved helpful. More obvious threats, veiled or direct, may be employed. For example, the patient may be threatened with the loss of a valued aspect of their treatment or of a social benefit if they fail to comply with treatment, especially medication.

When does 'leverage' become 'coercion'? A helpful account by Wertheimer[28] suggests that no simple definition can be offered for the term 'coercion'. The issue for us in mental health care is whether there are morally relevant distinctions between different kinds of pressure or force on patients to comply with treatment. A helpful view of coercive proposals may be that 'threats' coerce, but 'offers' do not. The former threatens to make the recipient worse off than they are at present, while declining an offer does not. Whether the subject is worse off depends on what has been termed the 'moral base line'. Threatening to remove something to which the subject is 'entitled' (e.g. a housing benefit determined by statute) makes the subject worse off if he or she does not accede. An offer of something which is not an entitlement but is in the nature of special assistance (e.g. a mental health worker having a connection with a second-hand furniture dealer who gives special discounts) made on condition that the patient complies with the treatment would, if rejected, not make the patient worse off compared with the relevant moral baseline—what his or her position would have been if the offer had never been made. One imposes a penalty, the other offers a reward.

On this account, 'coercion' can be distinguished from other kinds of pressure —for example, persuasion or inducement (by making offers). It refers to propositions which, under normal circumstances, ought not to be made and which are aimed at motivating a person to act in a way desired by the coercing agent. Thus, conditional access to monetary benefits (statutory entitlements), as occurs when some patients in the US have a 'representative payee' under Supplemental Security Income/Social Security Disability Insurance (SSI/SSDI) who only gives the patients their benefits when they comply with treatment is coercive.[27] Other features of coercion may include a feeling of constraint in the subject, a restriction on autonomy, a reduction of choice, and the mitigation of moral or legal responsibility (including freely given consent).

Deception, less equivocally seen as morally wrong, may be another way of inducing patient compliance. It is possible that some outpatient commitment orders depend for their effectiveness on a patient's misconception concerning the consequences of not complying. The patient may falsely believe that transgression of the order will result in re-hospitalization or enforced treatment, but it may in fact only permit the conveying of the patient to a treatment facility (as in 'supervised discharge' in England, discussed earlier).

The most direct form of force is a compulsory treatment order. With a change of treatment to the community, a number of jurisdictions have introduced outpatient commitment orders carrying varying powers. They may allow commitment to outpatient treatment instead of inpatient treatment as a less restrictive alternative; permit earlier conditional release from inpatient commitment; or allow preventative commitment.[27] The third category is the most controversial since it may allow the compulsory treatment of a patient who is not currently at risk. Based on a proven record of relapse when treatment is discontinued, and of dangers previously demonstrated when relapse has occurred, compulsion is used to avert future risk. Outpatient commitment orders are dealt with in another chapter in this book.

Increasing financial constraints set limits on what is possible in a mental health service. It has been suggested that some calls for increased coercion on patients to comply with treatment are an inappropriate attempt to compensate for money-starved, poor quality services. Clinicians may find themselves having to discharge patients before they are really ready because of insufficient beds and to consider controlling treatments in the community as a consequence. A patient may prefer to forgo medication after discharge from hospital despite a high risk of relapse and readmission. If admissions are expensive or beds are scarce, clinicians may sometimes be inclined not to consider such a patient's wishes adequately.

Conflict of duty to patient versus others

Risk of harm to others

As previously discussed, the current climate in which community psychiatry is practised often raises the question of the degree to which the psychiatrist has a duty to protect others. If a specific risk to an identified person is established, the clinician's duty to protect that person is clearer. When the risk to others is general, judgements are harder.

An important statistical fact is germane to the risk of serious violence to others. Despite the public's fears, acts of serious violence are rare. The prediction of a rare event inherently lacks precision. A predictive instrument, even with high sensitivity and specificity, will seriously err in the direction of false-positives. This can be demonstrated by a study involving patients treated by my own community mental health team in Camberwell, South London. Of 320 patients seen in one month, 73 were assessed by clinicians as posing a moderate or severe risk of violence to others over the next six months. Using the best available predictive statistics from large-scale predictive studies we determined that 7 of the 73 patients were likely to be violent to person in the next six months. But so also were 10 of the 247 low-risk patients. Indeed, more violent incidents would thus occur in the low-risk group than the high-risk group! This limitation in prediction must be borne in mind. What is the social and moral cost of unnecessarily restricting a large number of patients in order to prevent (probably inefficiently) harm by a few? Prediction is better the higher the base rate of violence in the population of patients who might pose a risk, for example in forensic patients. Not able to be easily assessed is the possibility that clinicians are better able to predict danger in the very short term (that is, in the next few hours or days).

The often visible nature of community treatment may change expectations of members of the public. For example, the mental health team may be asked to intervene by members of the public (for example, neighbours or shopkeepers) when they are disturbed by a patient's behaviour. They may be frightened or simply wish that a nuisance be removed. A further aspect of such situations may be the possibility that if the team does not act, prejudice against the patient will increase and his or her community tenure be threatened. The balance between the clinician's duty of care to the patient and to the local community may be difficult to determine. An intervention by a worker in a public place to allay anxiety may have serious implications for the patient's privacy and confidentiality.

Community psychiatrists are expected to be competent in assessing risk to others as well as to patients themselves. This often requires information from a range of informants, particularly concerning previous incidents of violence and risk factors such as substance abuse. Sometimes, the mere seeking of information from others concerning the patient's past behaviour may reveal that the person is being treated by a psychiatric team. It may even raise unwarranted anxieties in their minds.

Informal carers

Informal carers, usually family, are central to a successful policy of community care. However, the extent to which their own needs should be met is cloaked with uncertainty. Where there is a danger of serious physical harm to the carer, the clinician's responsibility is usually straightforward. Far more common are less serious threats to their well-being which none the less cause substantial suffering. They may experience difficulty in coping with burdensome behaviours, lack important knowledge about their relative's illness, and may not know to whom to turn for support.[29,30] The patient may prohibit the clinician any contact with the family. In these circumstances it is unclear to what extent the community mental health team owes a duty of care to the family. This question has been largely ignored in the literature.

Approaches to ethical problems in community psychiatry

In this last section I shall suggest ways of helping clinicians resolve the ethical dilemmas discussed above.

Increasing patient involvement in their care

Patients are likely to feel less coerced the more they play an active role in their treatment. The current trend for increased service users' consultation and involvement in determining the shape and nature of local mental health services may be helpful in this regard. There are also initiatives at the individual patient level worth exploring. In Britain, 'Crisis cards' originated as a voluntary sector initiative to facilitate access to an advocate and to state a patient's preferences for treatment in an emergency when he or she might be too unwell to express their wishes coherently.[31] They are designed to be carried by the patient and have the potential to record a range of useful information about the patient's treatment plan as well as advance statements. Crisis cards have usually been drawn up by the patient alone, without discussion with the treatment team. There is scope for this idea to be developed in to what we have termed 'joint crisis plans'. Here the content of the card, while still ultimately determined by the patient, is negotiated with the treatment team. The aim is to reach agreement on the care plan. This occurs when the patient is well enough to make competent judgements about what is in his or her best interests.

We have studied the utility of crisis cards and joint crisis plans in Camberwell. Participation was offered to all patients with a psychotic illness who had had at least two previous admissions to hospital: 40 per cent wished to develop a card. They chose to include a wide range of information including diagnosis, current treatment, contact information for carers and professionals, first signs of relapse and the preferred treatment for these, treatment preferences and refusals for an established relapse, indications for admission, and practical requests (e.g. who should ensure that domestic arrangements are not neglected in the case of admission). Independent assessment of the process showed that it was experienced by the patient as non-coercive and that they felt their voice was heard. Follow-up 6 to 12 months later showed that for patients who had experienced a crisis, the card was consulted in most cases. The information was considered helpful by patients and mental health professionals. Over 50 per cent of the patients reported feeling more involved in their care, more positive about their situation and more in control of their mental health problem. In addition, 40 per cent of patients reported feeling more likely to continue with their treatment as a result of developing the card. We concluded that a joint crisis plan could serve both a manifest, practical function in a crisis—to provide important information when the patient is too ill to do so, as well as a latent, psychological one—positive effects on patients' attitudes to themselves, their illness and treatment, and their relationship with the clinical team.

Cards such as these also have the potential for further transformation into 'psychiatric advance directives' which would be legally binding. Such a directive, anticipating relapse of a psychosis develops the concept of the 'living will'. It could reconcile two apparently contradictory themes in the current practice of psychiatry—on the one hand, the call to provide non-consensual treatment in the community, and on the other, the promotion of patient autonomy.[32] They could for some be an alternative to community treatment or outpatient commitment orders. Challenges to their implementation are discussed by Halpern and Szmukler[32] and include the problem of evaluating the patient's competence—when is it adequate to make a directive, sufficiently inadequate to trigger its application, and adequate to revoke a directive;

ensuring the absence of coercion in drawing up the directive; mechanisms for appeal in cases of dispute; resource implications; and, clarifying relationships between advance directives and existing mental health legislation. Psychiatric advance directives are possible now in some jurisdictions in the US,[33,34] but they have been little taken up presumably because of such difficulties. Despite this, advance directives might still find a place for some groups of seriously mentally ill patients.

Crisis cards and their variants could significantly reduce the number of situations in which clinicians find themselves needing to act against the patient's wishes expressed when he or she is unwell rather than well. Many of the ethical dilemmas discussed above occur at precisely such times of crisis.

Grounds for paternalism

Most invasions of privacy, breaches of confidentiality and uses of coercion rest on a paternalistic justification—'intentional non-acquiescence or intervention in another person's preferences, desires or actions with the intention of avoiding harm to or benefiting the person'.[35] There is debate whether overriding the wishes of a person who is unable to exercise substantial autonomy is paternalistic. For the clearly non-autonomous person acting beneficently may be termed 'paternal'.[36]

Despite the differences in views concerning the exact nature of paternalism, given the instances in which clinicians in the community may act without the patient's agreement, staff in community mental health teams must develop a working knowledge of acceptable grounds for paternalistic interventions. This may be difficult to achieve: 'developing a position on issues of paternalism is a matter of appreciating the limits of principles and the need to give them additional content, while attempting to render one's consequent rules and judgements as coherent with other commitments as possible. The problem of medical paternalism is the problem of putting just the right specification and balance of physician beneficence and patient autonomy in the patient– physician relationship. It is a messy complicated problem, and coherence is difficult to achieve. Paternalistic intervention requires persons of good judgement as well as persons with well-developed principles able to confront contingent conflicts'.[35] We should aim to train such persons.

The approach to paternalism by Culver and Gert[36] is helpful. A person is acting paternalistically to another if his action benefits the other; his action involves violating a moral rule with regard to the other; his action does not have the other's past, present, or immediately forthcoming consent; and the other is competent to give consent. Culver and Gert regard the subject as able to give consent if he is able to understand the information and to appreciate it (i.e. to understand why it is being asked for). Consent here is taken to include simple and possibly 'valid' consent. In attempting to justify a paternalistic act, at least five questions can be asked:

1. What are the moral rules which are violated when the clinician acts against the patient's wishes (e.g. deceit, limiting freedom of choice, causing psychological pain)? What are the evils thus to be perpetrated on the patient and for how long will they last?

2. What is the seriousness of the evils to be avoided through the paternalistic intervention (e.g. death, disability, worsening of the psychiatric disorder), and what is their likelihood?

3. How does the clinician rank the sets of evils above compared to the patient?

4. Is the patient's preference when comparing the evils to be avoided with the evils to be incurred, irrational?—that is, the patient has no rational reason to prefer an outcome with apparently greater evils.

5. Can the clinician advocate *publicly* for his ranking of the evils to be perpetrated compared to those to be avoided? In other words, would all or most rational people agree that this kind of moral violation should in such circumstances be universally allowed?

Conflicts of duty

Risk of harm to others

There is a distinction to be drawn between the danger to self (leading to paternalistic interventions) and a danger to others. As Culver and Gert[36] point out, in the latter, the question of the patient's 'rationality' is barely relevant, only being so in relation to the longer term harms it could be anticipated will be suffered by the patient as a result of his or her violent actions to another. The key question is whether the potentially dangerous person has volitional ability to refrain from acting dangerously, that is, the degree to which 'unvoluntariness' is present. The ethical basis for the Supervision Register in England seems to confuse these issues. Dickenson[37] points out that if the purpose of the register is to ensure that a key-worker is held responsible, or to protect the community against risk, there is no justifying argument from 'benevolence' or paternalism. On what basis then is it proper for a patient to be fit to be discharged from hospital, yet to not be well enough to enjoy the civil rights of those never mentally ill? What level of risk to others justifies such an infringement of autonomy; is a non-specific risk to the community sufficient?

Risk assessment is now at the crux of managing potentially dangerous behaviour. It thus becomes essential that clinicians adopt risk assessment approaches which represent best practice and are based on the best available research evidence. A process of self-interrogation regarding whether a particular assessment is defensible scientifically as well as clinically is desirable. Discussion with colleagues, both in and outside the multidisciplinary team, helps. The high proportion of false-positives must also be remembered. Factors such as a history of previous violence (and its details), potential disinhibiting factors (especially substance misuse, provocative social settings), treatment compliance, stresses and available social supports, and particular features of the mental state (threat/control override symptoms, emotions related to violence, specific threats) need special consideration.[38] Collateral information from informants is essential. It is important to establish the relationship between dangerousness and the patient's mental illness; psychiatric interventions are only justified when the mental illness significantly increases risk. On the basis of the risk assessment a clinical management plan can be devised which offers the least restrictive approach to the patient.

Elements of the 'crisis card' can also be brought in if possible. Discussion with the recovered patient, previously violent, may lead to agreement between patient and clinician at precisely what point (e.g. recurrence of a specific delusion; an unprovoked outburst of anger to a specified person) it would be appropriate to intervene against the patient's wishes if a relapse were to occur.

At the same time, community psychiatrists should engage in a dialogue with those representing the community about the balance to be struck between risk to others and restrictions on the liberty of mentally ill people. The public must be helped to recognize that risk-taking is fundamental to community care and that inevitably there will be tragedies. It should also be pointed out that despite media perceptions, there is no good evidence of an increase in homicides by the mentally ill as a result of the implementation of community care policies.

Duties to carers

As mentioned above, carers raise important questions in relationship to community psychiatry. Szmukler and Bloch[39] have argued for clarification of the ethical basis for working with families of psychotic patients. Much can be achieved in avoiding later dilemmas by an ethically sensitive approach to family engagement at the outset. This essentially involves spelling, out through the process of obtaining informed consent from patient and family, the basis on which care will proceed. The clinician's position in respecting the relative interests of family members and on confidentiality within the family is made explicit although subject to re-negotiation with the family as treatment proceeds.

Szmukler and Bloch[39] also consider justifications for involving a psychotic patient's family without the patient's consent out of *concern for the family's wellbeing* (short of serious, physical danger). Legislation in England as well as Victoria (Australia) suggests that carers' interests are beginning to be formally recognised. This is likely to grow in parallel with the expanding role of informal carers as members of the 'care team' in the community. For example, the Victorian Mental Health Act, amended in 1995 (Section 120A) allows the giving of information relating to a patient by a member of staff to a guardian, family member or primary carer of the person to whom the information relates if:

i) The information is reasonably required for the ongoing care of the person, and
ii) The guardian, family member or primary carer will be involved in providing that care.

At least three arguments can be adduced for involving relatives primarily for their own benefit, but against the patient's wishes. The first is to view the family as the 'unit of treatment', given that the family has much to contribute to the patient's care and the impact of the illness on them is usually so profound. This would represent a radical departure from conventional notions of medical confidentiality. The second invokes the principle of justice or 'fairness'—the needs of the family would merit distinctive attention if resources required to meet these needs reside in major part within the treatment team, but not outside it. The third, and probably most compelling argument is to reframe relatives' relationship to the patient as not only familial but also as 'carer'. As such they should enjoy rights intrinsically attached to all carers, whether relatives or not. These would cover, for instance, an account of the illness and guidance about how to deal with the patient's problems in so far as they impinge on the carer's life. This might include details about other agencies that offer help. This would bring the family's position into alignment, for example, with that of a hostel support worker. This argument is consistent with the trend in legislation which views 'carers' as having special status *vis-a-vis* the patient.

Whether any of these arguments will be adopted remains to be seen. However, what seems clear is that in this era of community care we expect much from informal carers but this has not been balanced yet by mapping out our duties towards them.

Conclusions

The ethical dilemmas discussed in this chapter are not new. However, they present in sufficiently different guises to warrant reconsideration in their new context. Diamond and Wikler[26] note that staff working in ACT-like services do not ordinarily view their work as raising significant ethical problems. Their diagnosis of why this is so is in accord with my own observations. They ascribe it to the pragmatism of community mental health team workers:

It is obvious that their work has beneficial effects. Patients who once bounced in and out of hospitals and jails come to live reasonable lives, with apartments and friends and enjoyable activities. It seems reasonable that any clinical intervention that produces such positive effects must be ethically justified. Moreover, these are very difficult patients, and community treatment is very difficult work. Staff are busy trying to prevent mayhem and develop creative treatment plans, develop their clinical skills, give each other needed support, soothe the concerns of the community, and deal with many other social agencies. The constraints of confidentiality, voluntariness, and other moral requirements whose application to the community treatment context is unclear often seem to be issues of bureaucratic nicety, important to rule makers but remote from the real concerns of patients and staff

This describes the context and sense of beleaguerment often encountered in the community. However, for community psychiatric practice to survive and to develop it must rest on an acceptable ethical base. If traditional modes of analysis are wanting, then new ways of tackling the problems must be found which do justice to changing circumstances.

Fear of the mentally ill is omnipresent. Care in the community treads a fine line. If it is not managed successfully 'there is a danger that progress over recent decades in emphasising the individuality of patients and affirming their rights (and responsibilities) within a therapeutic relationship could be compromised by early resort to unnecessary inpatient supervision and coercive models of care'.[21]

References

1. Bell, C. C.: The new community psychiatry in 2000 A.D. *Hospital and Community Psychiatry* **44**:815, 1993.
2. Strathdee, G. and Thornicroft, G.: Community psychiatry and service evaluation. In *The essentials of postgraduate psychiatry* ed. Murray, R., Hill, P., and McGuffin, P., 3rd edn. Cambridge, Cambridge University Press, 1997, pp. 513–33.
3. Lamb, H. R.: The new state mental hospitals in the community. *Psychiatric Services* **48**:1307–10, 1997.
4. Intagliata, J.: Improving the quality of community care for the chronically mentally disabled. The role of case management. *Schizophrenia Bulletin* **8**:655–74, 1982.
5. Holloway, F., Oliver, N., Collins, E., and Carson, J.: Case management: a critical review of the outcome literature. *European Psychiatry* **10**:113–28, 1995.
6. Holloway, F.: Case management for the mentally ill: looking at the evidence. *International Journal of Social Psychiatry* **37**:2–13, 1991.
7. Sledge, S. H., Astrachan, B., Thompson, K., *et al.*: Case management in psychiatry: an analysis of tasks. *American Journal of Psychiatry* **152**:1259–65, 1995.
8. Chamberlain, R. and Rapp, C. A.: A decade of case management: a methodological review of outcome research. *Community Mental Health Journal* **27**:171–88, 1991.
9. Marshall, M., Gray, A., Lockwood, A., and Green, R. Case management for severe mental disorders. *The Cochrane Library*: 1997, Issue 3.
10. Stein, L. I. and Test, M. A.: Alternative to mental hospital treatment: I. Conceptual model, treatment program, and clinical evaluation. *Archives of General Psychiatry* **37**:392–7, 1980.
11. Burns, B. J. and Santos, A. B.: Assertive community treatment: an update of randomised controlled trials. *Psychiatric Services* **46**:669–75, 1995.
12. Weisbrod, B., Test, M. A., and Stein, L.: Alternative to mental hospital treatment II: economic benefit cost analysis. *Archives of General Psychiatry* **37**:400–5, 1980.
13. Knapp, M., Beecham, J., Koutsogeorgopoulou, V., *et al.*: Service use and costs of home based versus hospital based care for people with serious mental illness. *British Journal of Psychiatry* **165**:195–203, 1994.
14. Ritchie, J. H.: *The Report of the inquiry into the care and treatment of Christopher Clunis*. London, HMSO, 1994.

15. Lelliott, P., Audini, B., Johnson, S., and Guite, H.: London in the context of mental health policy. In *London's mental health: the report for the King's Fund London Commission*, ed. Johnson, S., Ramsay, R., Thornicroft, G., *et al.* London, King's Fund, 1997, pp. 33–44.
16. Department of Health. Introduction of supervision registers for mentally ill people from 1 April 1994. HMSO, London, 1994.
17. Department of Health (England and Wales): *Building bridges: a guide to arrangements for interagency working for the care and protection of severely mentally ill people*. London, HMSO, 1996.
18. Eastman N.: The Mental Health (Patients in the Community) Act 1995. A clinical analysis. *British Journal of Psychiatry* **170**:492–6, 1997.
19. Holloway, F.: Community psychiatric care: from libertarianism to coercion: moral panic and mental health policy in Britian. *Health Care Analysis* **4**:235–44, 1996.
20. Lipsedge, M.: Clinical risk management in psychiatry. In *Clinical risk management*, ed. Vincent, C. London, BMJ, 1995, pp. 276–93.
21. Harrison, G.: Risk assessment in a climate of litigation. *British Journal of Psychiatry* **170**(Suppl. 32):37–9, 1997.
22. Appelbaum, P. S.: The new preventive detention: psychiatry's problematic responsibility for the control of violence. *American Journal of Psychiatry* **145**: 779–85, 1988.
23. Stone, A. A.: Vermont adopts *Tarasoff*: a real barn-burner. *American Journal of Psychiatry* **143**:352–55, 1986.
24. Appelbaum, P. S.: *Almost a revolution: mental health law and the limits of change*. New York, Oxford University Press, 1994.
25. Stone, A. A.: *Law psychiatry and morality*. Washington, DC, American Psychiatric Press, 1984.
26. Diamond, R. J. and Wikler, D. I.: Ethical problems in community treatment of the chronically mentally ill. In *Training in community living model: a decade of experience*. New Directions for Mental Health Services, No. 26, ed. Stein, L. I. and Test, M. A. San Franscisco, Jossey-Bass, 1985, pp. 85–93.
27. Berg, J. W. and Bonnie, R. J.: When push comes to shove: aggressive community treatment and the law. In *Coercive and aggressive community treatment: a new frontier in mental health law*, ed. Dennis, D. L. and Monahan, J. New York, Plenum, 1996, pp. 169–96.
28. Wertheimer, A.: A philosophical examination of coercion for mental health issues. *Behavoural Sciences and the Law* **11**:239–58, 1993.
29. Szmukler, G. I., Burgess, P., Herrman, H., Benson, A., Colusa, S., and Bloch, S.: Caring for relatives with serious mental illness: the development of the 'Experience of Caregiving Inventory'. *Social Psychiatry and Psychiatric Epidemiology* **31**: 137–48, 1996.
30. Bloch, S., Szmukler, G. I., Herrman, H., Benson, A., and Colusa, S.: Counselling caregivers of relatives with schizophrenia: themes, interventions and caveats. *Family Process* **34**: 413-425, 1995.
31. Sutherby, K. and Szmukler, G.: Crisis cards and self-help crisis initiatives. *Psychiatric Bulletin* **22**:3–7, 1998.
32. Halpern, A. and Szmukler, G.: Psychiatric advance directives: reconciling automony and non-consensual treatment. *Psychiatric Bulletin* **21**:323–7, 1997.
33. Appelbaum, P. S.: Advance directives for psychiatric treatment. *Hospital and Community Psychiatry* **42**:983–4, 1991.

34. Perling, L. J.: Health care advance directives: Implications for Florida mental health patients. *University of Miami Law Review* **48**:193–228, 1993.
35. Beauchamp, T. L. and Childress, J. F.: *Principles of Biomedical Ethics*. 4th Edition. New York, Oxford University Press, 1994.
36. Culver, C. N. and Gert, B.: *Philosophy in medicine: conceptual and ethical issues in medicine and psychiatry*. Oxford, Oxford University Press, 1982.
37. Dickenson, D.: Ethical issues in long term psychiatric management. *Journal of Medical Ethics* **23**:300–4, 1997.
38. *Assessment and clinical management of risk of harm to other people*. Council Report 53. London, Royal College of Psychiatrists, 1996.
39. Szmukler, G. I. and Bloch, S.: Family involvement in the care of people with psychoses: an ethical argument. *British Journal of Psychiatry* **171**:401–5, 1997.

18

Ethical issues in mental health resource allocation

James E. Sabin and Norman Daniels

On a world-wide basis, a large proportion of psychiatric treatment—most likely the majority—is financed by tax revenues or insurance premiums, rather than being paid for by the individuals receiving the treatment. When individuals pay for their own treatment they allocate their own resources according to their own values and priorities. When public or third-party funds pay for treatment, however, important ethical questions about resource allocation inevitably and unavoidably arise.

In this chapter we will address the ethics of resource allocation in psychiatry at a series of levels, each of which raises distinctive theoretical and practical questions.

- Within the total allocation that a population, insurance pool, or society makes to health care, how much should be allocated to mental health? This is a 'macro level' question concerned with resource allocation to the different sectors of health care.
- Within the mental health sector, how should resources be allocated among the multiple potential patients, conditions, and types of intervention? These are questions of psychiatric priority setting.
- Within a particular area, such as schizophrenia, how much resource should be allocated to the different potentially useful treatment elements that could be offered, ranging from prevention and early intervention to rehabilitation and support? These can be viewed as questions about treatment guidelines and disease management strategies.
- Finally, as to the care of an individual patient, how much treatment is 'enough?' This is a 'micro level' question about resource allocation, or, in current US terminology, a question of 'utilization management' and 'medical necessity'.

In the first four sections we discuss the major ethical issues that arise for each of these levels of resource allocation and review some of the approaches to these issues in real-world situations. Next we consider the question of legitimacy and fairness in resource allocation policy—that is when does a patient, a clinician, and the public have sufficient reason to accept the outcome of a resource allocation process as legitimate and fair? In the concluding section we suggest some ways in which societies can move along a learning curve with regard to health-care resource allocation, limit-setting, and possible rationing.

While we believe that for purposes of analytic clarity it is useful to distinguish these four levels of resource allocation, policy determinations actually entail complex, sometimes messy interactions between levels. Resource allocation decisions are not made by a sequential deductive process that moves in logical steps from 'macro level' to 'micro level', but by interactions that sometimes clarify, enrich and deepen the deliberative process, and at other times involve raw assertions of interest by different stakeholder groups and political forces that may have little to do with mental health issues. In the first four sections we consider each level in isolation. In the next two sections we shift to a more process-oriented view of resource allocation and focus on the applied ethics of making allocational policy.

Resource allocation to mental health within a total health-care budget

Although the question, 'How much of the health-care budget should be devoted to psychiatry?' is commonly posed in real-world resource allocation situations, it is important to challenge the question itself. Why should resources be allocated to psychiatry as a sector, rather than among all medical conditions, levels of impairment, or in some other way?

The answer is bureaucracy as opposed to principle. Systems and budgets are typically organized in terms of sectors, so it is natural for managers and policy makers to ask how much to allocate to psychiatry, pediatrics, surgery and the like. The reason we ask how much to allocate to psychiatry as a sector is primarily due to managerial convenience.

Posing the question of resource allocation in terms of psychiatry as a sector influences the way the question is answered. For example, from the inception of health insurance in the United States more than 60 years ago, psychiatric services have been treated much more restrictively, limiting the amount of hospital or outpatient care in ways not applied to other sectors of medicine.[1] Sometimes insurance programs completely omit mental health and substance abuse care. This categorical distinction between psychiatric and other sectors of health care must be regarded as unethical for both theoretical and practical reasons.

The theoretical rationale for arguing that mental health services should compete on equal footing with other sectors of health care for priority in the resource allocation process turns on our view of the moral importance of health care itself, and the moral grounding for the widely recognized societal obligation to ensure a basic level of health care for all. In this chapter we presuppose that the distinctive importance of health care comes from its role in protecting and promoting fair equality of opportunity for members of a society. Disease impairs the species-typical capacity to pursue our life plans. Effective health care prevents, restores, corrects or limits the degree to which disease impedes the ability to form and pursue our conceptions of the good life.[2] Because it contributes in a significant manner to fair equality of opportunity, basic health care is not simply a commodity to be distributed according to ability to pay, but must be regarded as a societal obligation.

If there were reasons for considering mental health care *per se* as fundamentally less important to fair equality of opportunity than general medical care, there would be justification for placing mental health services on a lower footing as different in kind from other health services. In fact, mental health conditions cause substantial impairments of species-typical capacity, equal to or greater than many chronic medical diseases about which there is no controversy regarding insurance coverage.[3] Similarly, if there were reasons for regarding mental health treatment as uniquely ineffective to a degree that it did not help ameliorate the impairments created by mental disorders, justification would again exist for omitting mental health services from basic health care. In fact, mental health treatment is comparable in effectiveness to most other areas of medical treatment.[4]

Consequently, it is possible to make a strong moral argument on behalf of the proposition that 'mental and physical health should be fully integrated in any priority-setting plan; mental health research and services should not be discriminated against in favor of physical health'.[5] A particular health system may reasonably decide to give the mental health sector more or less priority relative to other sectors. There is no single 'right' answer to the question of how much of a total health-care budget should be allocated to mental health. However, it is not ethically defensible to keep the mental health sector from competing for resources on a level playing field.

The practical reason for regarding the common practice of imposing distinctive limitations on mental health services in the macro resource allocation process as unethical comes from the Oregon priority-setting process. Oregon is arguably the best example of open and explicit priority setting and rationing that has occurred to date. Oregon provides the clearest test of what happens in a democratic process when mental health conditions 'compete' not as a sector, but as individual disorders, comparable to diabetes, pneumonia and appendicitis.

If the Oregon priority-setting process had systematically ranked psychiatric disorders below all other medical and surgical conditions, it would have provided evidence that the widespread practice of allocating resources for mental health services by coverage rules that uniquely disadvantage the mental health sector at least reflected true public opinion. What happened was actually quite different.[6] Schizophrenia ranked just behind asthma and respiratory failure in the priority listings. Chemical dependencies ranked just behind treatment of closed hip fracture. Attention-deficit disorder ranked just ahead of hypertension. The relatively small number of mental health conditions that fell below the cut-off point for coverage created by the legislatively determined budget included only hypochondriasis, transsexualism, and personality disorders other than borderline or schizotypal.

The Oregon experience provides important practical lessons for resource allocation and efforts to set politically acceptable limits on health-care expenditures.[7] Before the state passed the 1989 legislation that began its priority-setting process, it had conducted a multi-year program of grassroots education and reflection about the goals and objectives for health care and the need to control costs in order to expand access. In Dr John Kitzhaber, first as senate president and later as governor, it had a political leader unusually courageous and skilful in shaping public reflection and debate.

The final ranking of conditions depended on assessment of the severity of impact of the condition and the effectiveness of treatment.[8] Most mental health conditions fell into the groups for which treatment (a) prevents death with full recovery (top priority), (b) prevents death with less than full recovery (third), and (c) improves lifespan and quality of life. The few conditions that were not covered were judged to be less responsive to currently available methods and therefore fell into lower priority groups, for which (d) repetitive (meaning extensive) treatment improves quality of life (thirteenth) or (e) treatment causes minimal or no improvement in quality of life (seventeenth and last). Thus even the conditions that fell below the cut-off point for funding were seen as significant in terms of the impairment they produce.

The fact that the citizens of Oregon gave psychiatric disorders comparable priority with all other medical and surgical disorders supports the theoretical argument that there is no principled basis for selectively disadvantaging mental health services at the macro level of resource allocation. A just resource allocation process will put the mental health sector on the same footing as other sectors and will subject it to the same forms of priority setting and management. Oregon shows that this kind of process can actually be done in practice.[9]

Resource allocation within the mental health sector

Given the fact that in actual health-care systems and insurance programs mental health usually has its own budget, resource allocation within the psychiatric sector is an extremely important practical issue. Thus, for instance, state commissioners of mental health and psychiatric medical directors for insurance programs in the United States and district authority leaders in the United Kingdom must decide how much of their budget will go to patients with severe and persistent disorders (e.g. schizophrenia and bipolar disorder) and how much to devote to the larger group with less severe forms of mental illness (e.g. anxiety, depression, and adjustment disorder). In similar fashion, they must also decide what proportion of funds will go to hospitals and to community-based services.

Unfortunately, what has been called the indeterminacy of distributive principles[10] precludes an elegant theoretical answer to the resource allocation decisions state commisioners, insurance program medical directors, and district managers regularly face. We expect the state commissioner, medical director, and district manager to give priority to those who suffer the greatest pain and impairment, but aside from the practical problem of comparing degrees of pain and impairment, we cannot give them a principled basis for deciding how much priority—and resource—to give. Further, we expect them to seek maximum value for the money in their budgets, but we do not want them to deprive patients less likely to benefit from treatment of all chances of achieving their potential. Finally, we expect mental health program leaders to recognize and attend to common conditions highly prevalent in the population, but we can offer them no principles for deciding how to aggregate small benefits for the many and weigh them against larger benefits for the few.

By what appears to have been an entirely serendipitous process, the British National Health Service (NHS) appears to have developed a unique form of structured advocacy to address the absence of a principled basis for allocating mental health resources within a fixed budget.[11] Although the health districts within which front line resource allocation occurs create their individual priorities, district managers are subject to a national policy set by the Department of Health which clearly states that 'people who are most disabled by mental illness should be afforded the highest priority'.[12] Under this policy the NHS has established three targets for mental health resource allocation, which focus on the severely impaired: 'to improve significantly the health and social functioning of mentally ill people'; 'to reduce the overall suicide rate by at least 15 per cent by the year 2000'; and, 'to reduce the suicide rate of severely mentally ill people by at least 33 per cent by the year 2000'.[13]

At the same time, but through another mechanism, the NHS gives considerable resource allocation authority to general practitioners, who predictably give priority to the more common but less severe conditions they regularly encounter in practice. In other words, rather than seeking to set ordered priorities as Oregon did, the NHS has created a system of balanced advocacy that pits district managers and the national policy of giving priority to the sicker few against general practitioners who give priority to the healthier many. The outcome for resource allocation is not driven by a principle-based selection of priorities or an effort to quantify need and benefit, but rather by political give and take between advocates for different segments of the mentally disordered population.

If widely accepted principles of distributive justice could provide principle-based resource allocation priorities that were specific enough to be useful in practice, the NHS system of balanced advocacy would have to be rejected as an unprincipled power-based process. In the absence of such principles, a strong case can be made for doing what the British call 'muddling through elegantly'.[14] As we will argue in pp. 393–96, if the NHS process of balanced advocacy involves a publicly accessible form of debate and deliberation based on clinical information and explicit reasoning about how the proposed choices provide the best 'value for money' for the population being served, then it should be regarded as a legitimate way of allocating resources. However, if it plays out in practice as a hidden process of bargaining between competing interest groups, it cannot be defended in this way. Although some general practitioners[15] and district health authorities[16] are trying to explicate the reasoning behind the process of 'muddling through', there is simply not enough information available to assess the NHS system of balanced advocacy for psychiatric resource allocation.

In an effort to overcome stigmatizing views of mental illness as fundamentally different from and less 'worthy' than 'physical' illness, advocacy groups in the United States have argued that 'biologically-based brain disorders' (generally defined in legislation as schizophrenia, schizoaffective disorder, bipolar disorder, major depression, obsessive–compulsive disorder, and panic disorder) should be funded on the same terms as 'physical' disorders. This is frequently an effective political strategy, but it is hard to see why presumed etiology should give priority to one disorder over another. The fact that these conditions cause severe and enduring impairment of opportunity to form and pursue life plans would appear to be a more important basis on which to argue for their priority. Further, as research reveals—as it surely will —that some less serious disorders are also 'biologically based', and that some extremely serious disorders, such as post-traumatic syndromes, are 'experience-based', arguments for priority based on etiology will lose their coherence.

Many of the most heated struggles about resource allocation within the mental health sector must be understood as reflecting politics more than principle.[17] From a sociological perspective it is not surprising that different components of the chronically stigmatized mental health sector end up competing with each other rather than forming broad coalitions that allow a more comprehensive approach to resource allocation policy. Thus, while in terms of best clinical practice hospital and community services should be part of an integrated spectrum, in many societies they compete fiercely for their share of the limited mental health budget, as much (or more) out of concern for jobs and other economic benefits as out of a set of beliefs about service priorities. Different mental health professions compete in a similar guild-like manner. Advocates for specific populations, such as the developmentally disabled or elderly, tend to fight for their own target rather than allying with other mental health advocates to advance a principle-based argument for equity for the entire mental health sector *vis-a-vis* other health sectors.

Resource allocation within mental health conditions (treatment guidelines)

Once a health-care system decides to give a certain level of priority to a particular mental health condition decisions must be made about which of the many alternative treatment approaches to use. Currently, this level of the resource allocation process is frequently addressed via efforts to develop organized, evidence-based approaches in the form of treatment guidelines, algorithms, and disease management strategies. The central ethical issues regarding resource allocation that arise in developing treatment guidelines involve the selection of the treatment outcome objectives and the forms of treatment selected to achieve these outcomes.

From the perspective this chapter takes on the goals of health care, it follows that third-party insurance funds should be devoted to treatments aimed at restoring normal function (equal opportunity) by decreasing the impact of disease or disability, and should not be used to enhance well-being or general capability, however desirable those goals may be in themselves.[18] The language of health insurance in the US, however, obscures the fundamentally ethical question about the appropriate goals of health care by making insurance coverage contingent on what could appear to be a question about the medical facts—whether the proposed course of treatment is 'medically necessary' or 'optional'. In the context of insurance 'medically necessary' correlates with 'eligible for coverage by insurance funds' and 'optional' correlates with 'ordinarily to be paid for by the individual'. Properly understood, a 'medically necessary' treatment is a means for attaining a specified end (health outcome).

In mental health it is especially important to be clear about the goals of the treatment process because a number of psychiatric treatments can be helpful even in the absence of a mental disorder. Psychotherapy is the most widely recognized example. Well-conducted psychotherapy can provide substantial benefit for people struggling with normal developmental or existential issues. And, more recently, it has been recognized that medications, notably the selective serotonin reuptake inhibitors (SSRIs), may provide benefit for what we have heretofore thought of as ordinary human variation in such traits as shyness or charm.[19] Diminished shyness, increased charm, and heightened effectiveness in coping with life's typical challenges may well be regarded as desirable outcomes, but unless the clinical target is alleviation of the impact of a recognized mental disorder, the process is better described as 'enhancement' than 'treatment'. Third-party health-care resources are not ordinarily allocated for 'enhancement'.

Once the outcome objectives have been specified individual patients and their clinicians typically have preferences—often held quite strongly—between alternative ways of achieving the objectives. Certainly patient preferences carry significant moral weight for treatment planning, as does respect for the considered clinical judgment of health professionals. However, if patient and clinician preferences would consume more of the available resources than comparably effective alternatives, stewardship of collective resources unavoidably comes into conflict with respect for patient preference and professional judgment.

Although few health systems have applied considerations of cost-effectiveness across disease categories, primarily because of the great difficulty of publicly deliberating about the relative value of relieving arthritis versus schizophrenia, or even schizophrenia versus post-traumatic stress disorder or panic disorder, within a single disease category considerations of cost become paramount. A particular treatment (e.g. intensive psychotherapy or a costly new medication), may be known to be effective, but the practical demands of resource allocation within a limited overall budget require asking whether the treatment is more effective than less costly alternatives and, if so, whether an increment in effectiveness is worth the cost.

If the treatment proposed in the guideline as the most cost effective way of achieving the outcome objectives is close in kind to the patient or clinician's preference—such as cognitive therapy for depression as opposed to psychoanalytic psychotherapy—the conflict between individual preference and stewardship of collective resources is relatively small. But if the modalities proposed by the guideline and preferred by the patient are significantly different, such as pharmacotherapy versus psychotherapy, or, more starkly, electroconvulsive therapy versus psychotherapy, the conflict becomes more serious. Perhaps the commonest clinical situation in which patient preferences come into serious conflict with resource allocation is when patients with episodic conditions like bipolar disorder or schizophrenia refuse to take medication. The ethical commitment to respecting a patient's right to refuse treatment, supported by precedents established in case law, give strong protection to the right to refuse medication. That refusal, however, has the potential to generate substantial costs via otherwise avoidable hospitalization. Within a limited pool of funds the patient who refuses to accept recommended treatment may thereby diminish the resources available to provide beneficial care desired by others. Another common situation arises when the guideline proposes a treatment approach that makes substantial demands on a family, such as keeping a highly symptomatic patient at home rather than using the hospital. When a family refuses to support a treatment approach that may be as effective, or possibly more effective, than a more costly approach, that refusal creates a claim on collective resources.

One resolution for the dilemmas created by competition between individual and collective claims on mental health resources would be to allow patients to exercise choice, but to require them to take responsibility for the difference in cost between what treatment guidelines recommend and their preferred approach. The theory behind the concept of 'managed competition' in the US is that patients choose insurance alternatives in the light of their own values and preferences. If the American health-care system actually offered patients a range of insurance choices, including providing the poor with more than a single 'Medicaid' level of basic coverage, it would be reasonable to expect individuals to accept the treatment guideline that their chosen system offered. However, many patients have only the one choice their employer provides, creating the moral problem of how best to handle strongly held but more costly patient preferences.

Moreover, the question of what constitutes 'treatment' is surprisingly complicated. Many interventions that will help patients with mental disorders—like better housing, employment opportunities, or educational remediation—fall outside the sphere we conventionally think of as health care. This leads to a paradox: treatment guidelines for a mental disorder may include clinical interventions that produce less benefit than 'non-health' interventions might produce. If individuals were spending their own resources they might purchase better housing or job support, not psychotherapy or medication. How should mental health resource allocation respond to this paradox?

The divisions societies make between sectors—health, housing, education and the like—represent an effort to divide social responsibility in a useful way. The divisions are philosophically arbitrary, though socially useful if well defined and well managed. The relative hypertrophy of health expenditures and deficiency of support for other sectors that would improve the status of patients with mental disorders cannot be rectified at the level of treatment guidelines. Using 'health' allocations to pay for 'non-health' interventions undermines the social division of labor, but ignoring the importance of the 'non-health' factors to patient well-being is clinically irresponsible.[20]

One practical solution has been to include coordination of services and advocacy as part of the treatment guideline, either by educating patients and their families in advocacy skills or by providing coordination and advocacy as part of treatment itself. With this approach 'health' allocations are used to maximize the availability of 'health-relevant non-health' resources. Another solution has been the effort to unify separate funding streams so that collective monies are not divided into spheres like health, housing and education, but focused on improving the well-being of a particular population. These efforts are extremely complex and politically difficult to implement when they are targeted at large and diverse populations, but show some promise when smaller, highly impaired and costly populations, like those with severe and persisting mental illness, are involved.[21]

Resource allocation within the care of the individual patient

When individuals pay for their own treatment they commonly specify their own view of 'good enough treatment'. When their resources are limited they may choose to forgo objectives that both they and their clinician regard as desirable. When collective funds pay for the treatment the question of deciding what constitutes 'good enough treatment' implicitly involves third parties along with the dyad of patient and clinician. The question will be answered differently depending on the amount of resource available to the system within which the treatment is occurring. With more total resource available more extensive goals can be pursued. With less resource, treatment goals will have to be less ambitious. To date, societies have not done much explicit deliberation about how to set treatment limits with and for individuals in the light of overall resource limitations.[22]

Largely in reaction to the fear that mental health treatment may be prolonged and costly, many insurance programs limit objectives to relief of symptoms and return to baseline functioning. For conditions such as adjustment disorder in a previously healthy, well-functioning person, relief of symptoms and return to baseline functioning is an entirely reasonable outcome objective. But given the recurrent nature of many psychiatric conditions, and the frequency with which the disorder that brings the person to treatment is preceded by a chronic condition of milder but significant impairment, a rigid policy of limiting treatment goals to relief of acute symptoms and return to baseline appears to be a highly questionable resource allocation policy.

Similarly, it is common for insurance programs to set limits and seek objectivity and ease of administration by restricting treatment goals to alleviation of measurable dysfunction, such as poor work performance or impaired self-care. Here too it would seem that as long as treatment is directed to alleviating the negative impact of a mental disorder, has a reasonable chance of attaining the desired outcome, and is planned in a cost-effective manner, it is reasonable to expect that even in the absence of any externally measurable dysfunction, relief of subjective suffering should be a valid treatment goal. These questions arise most sharply in treating depression, where some patients are able to function well by most criteria but suffer significant inner misery, sometimes to the point of suicidality.

Because hospital costs form such a substantial percentage of total mental health expenditures, reducing hospital length of stay is a common cost-containment strategy. When the resources that would have been allocated to hospital care can be withheld without causing harm to any of the important stakeholders, the strategy is clearly ethically admirable. However, the need for hospital containment is often a function of how much is expected of alternative caregivers. Even significantly suicidal or psychotic individuals can be treated in the home environment if family and friends are prepared to take responsibility for safety. There has been little explicit ethical consideration of how to weigh allocating collective resources in the form of paying for hospital care as opposed to expecting the patient's family and friends to allocate their own resources by providing a high level of supervision at home.[23]

The question of whether it is ethical for mental health clinicians to consider wider societal concerns about resource allocation in the context of their work with patients has been hotly contested, especially in the US. The preamble to the American Psychiatric Association's *Principles of medical ethics* (see Appendix) would appear to provide the potential basis for a moral vision that would include some form of balance between patient-centered (beneficence/fidelity) and communitarian (stewardship) ethics. It states:

As a member of this profession, a physician must recognize responsibility not only to patients, *but also to society* [emphasis added], to other health professionals, and to self.[24]

However, none of the mental health professions have yet explicated in any detail the nature of this responsibility to society, and how it could best be harmonized with the clinician's primary responsibility, which is of course to his/her patients. It is likely that most mental health clinicians, at least in the US, would embrace the moral ideal that Norman Levinsky captures in his passionately argued, influential essay on *The doctor's master*. He states:

physicians are required to do everything that they believe may benefit each patient without regard to costs or other societal considerations. In caring for an individual patient, the doctor must act solely as that patient's advocate, against the apparent interests of society as a whole, if necessary.[25]

Since all health care, including mental health care, occurs within the context of limited resources, there is every reason to believe that even in the most well-financed, efficiently run, health-care system, some potentially beneficial treatments will have to be withheld. Clinicians who truly hold to Levinsky's view believe they must advocate for any treatment that may benefit their patient, no matter how small the benefit or how large the cost. This view, and the behavior it entails, have profound implications for the allocation of resources in day-to-day practice. In so far as pressures from patients and clinicians ensure that the mental health sector gets fair treatment in relation to other sectors (pp. 384–6), that patients at risk of relative neglect (e.g. those with severe mental illness or developmental disabilities) get fair treatment within the mental health sector (pp. 386–8), or that individual patients who could receive substantial benefit, but have not been properly diagnosed and treated, receive care (pp. 391–3), the pressure the Levinsky position generates is all to the good. But in so far as it interferes with the recognition by clinicians, patients, and the general public that limit-setting is inevitable and that attempting to do it fairly is a moral imperative, it impedes engagement with the crucial social task of defining equitable and socially acceptable ways of setting priorities and limits. The latter issue is addressed in the next section.

Legitimacy and fairness in resource allocation

Virtually all societies are currently struggling with tensions generated by growing public expectations for health care and the increasing costs of health-care budgets. The bland phrase 'resource allocation' denotes policies and decisions that inevitably create disappointment for those who fare poorly in the allocation process, and suffer harm when that process deprives them of services that would enhance their ability to pursue life's opportunities.

Because health-care is not the only important social good, health care resources will inevitably be limited. And given that there are more potentially beneficial health-care services that could be provided to patients than the public is prepared to pay for, making basic health care available to all citizens entails hard resource allocation choices. Justice requires that we promote fair equality of opportunity by ensuring basic health care. Providing basic health care requires hard choices. Hard choices cause pain.

The question of when and why patients, clinicians and the public should see painful resource allocation decisions as legitimate and fair has tremendous clinical and political importance. Clinically, health care—and above all, mental health care—requires trust and collaboration. Patients and families who are left bitter and distrustful by the results of the resource allocation process will be more difficult to treat, and practitioners who are bitter and disappointed will be less effective clinically. Although the public balks at paying higher taxes or higher insurance premiums, a government perceived as unfairly depriving individuals of health care that is important to basic life functions is in danger of political attack and ouster, and an insurer perceived as doing the same is likely to be the target of litigation.

If individuals purchased health care in a well-functioning market, choosing their insurer with the kinds of information and choice available when they purchase a car, there would be no broad issue of legitimacy and fairness; if they did not like the policies of one insurance program they would be free to choose another. However, though market-based organization and distribution of health care is currently the official policy for the United States, any effort to claim legitimacy and fairness on the basis of the market analogy fails, as most of the insured actually have little relevant information and few (or only one) insurance choices available to them—and more than 40 million uninsured have no access whatsoever to this deeply flawed market.

Similarly, if we had clear, compelling, and widely accepted principles from which we could derive answers to our resource allocation questions it would be possible to respond to challenges about legitimacy and fairness within the framework of these shared principles. In pluralistic societies, however, there is little likelihood that publicly acceptable principled solutions will emerge in the foreseeable future to answer questions concerning how to distribute resources across a population of patients suffering a variety of disorders that range from severe and persistent illness to less severe, but clinically meaningful conditions, or how to allocate services among the subgroups of child, adolescent, adult and elderly patients.

We have argued in detail elsewhere[26] that the most promising avenue for achieving patient, clinician, and public acceptance of resource allocation policies and limit-setting decisions as fair and legitimate is through processes that meet the following four conditions:

1. The resource allocation policies and limit-setting decisions must be publicly accessible. This condition is especially important in the US, where the competing insurers and managed-care organizations created by the strategy of market competition have sometimes treated their 'medical necessity' criteria as confidential proprietary information.

2. These policies and decisions should be based on a comprehensible and plausible interpretation of how they meet the mental health needs of a population under reasonable resource constraints. The rationale for policies must refer to clinical needs and show how the particular resource allocation choices can be construed as providing the best 'value for money' for the population in the light of the available resources. If a drug formulary restricts the agents that can be used, clear explanations of the rationale, supported by clinical data and acknowledging relevant trade-offs, should be presented. If a category of treatment, like intensive individual psychotherapy, is given less priority than group psychotherapy, a similar explanation should be provided.

Experience and common sense support this second condition. When people recognize that the basis of their disappointment arises from legitimate considerations, they—and others looking at the situation—are better prepared to see it as painful but not unfair. Thus when a US health maintenance organization (HMO)—after extensive consultation with members and clinicians—reallocated its mental health budget in order to provide unlimited outpatient care to the sickest patients, but at the same time introduced a co-payment for the less sick patients after the eighth outpatient session to stay within the total budget, virtually no patients and families who had to pay the new co-payment saw the policy as unfair, even though they were not happy about having to pay more under the new policy.[27]

3. There must be a mechanism for dealing with challenges and disputes regarding policies and limit-setting decisions, as well as a process that ensures learning from these challenges so that policies can be altered in accord with experience. More than establishing a bureaucratic requirement for an appeals process, this guarantees that questions, challenges and appeals are treated as an opportunity for change when warranted, and that patients, clinicians and the public are educated about the soundness and shortcomings of allocational policy.

4. There must be voluntary or public regulation of the process that allocates mental health resources to ensure that the first three conditions are met.

The process we envision is analogous to clinical methods familiar to most mental health clinicians: explicit presentation of the reasoning upon which decisions are based; readiness to enter into reflective give-and-take about what one has said; and a commitment to learning from experience. This form of deliberative dialogue must occur for each of the four levels of resource allocation, so it inevitably involves societal consideration of the total allocation to health care, consideration by the involved population regarding allocation to and within the mental health sector, and consideration between clinician and patient at the level of treatment planning for the individual patient.

It is important to note that many astute observers do not share our commitment to an open process and recommend using an *implicit* rather than *explicit* process for resource allocation and limit-setting. Mechanic,[28] who makes the strongest case for implicit rationing in health care, is concerned that explicit priorities and allocation policies will give preference to some who care less about treatment than others who care much more, but who fall lower on the priority list. He fears that openly acknowledging that we are choosing not to provide treatment to particular individuals will undermine trust between clinician and patient, and argues that a more implicit, less rule-bound approach gives the most flexibility for responding to individual needs and preferences.

Mental health resource allocation in the future—where do we go from here?

On the assumption that there will be future editions of the current version of this text, we predict that from their perspective it will be clear in retrospect that as of the late 1990s, societies internationally were in the early phases of a learning curve concerning health-care resource allocation. We further predict that the current debates as to whether it is ethical to set resource allocation priorities and ration health care will have been replaced by intensive international efforts to fathom how to conduct these necessary activities in a way that the public, patients, and clinicians can support as legitimate and fair.

The combination of continued rapid development of the scientific basis of psychiatric practice, treatment effectiveness research, and increased skill at managing the provision of psychiatric care within resource constraints make it highly likely that the lamentable tradition of stigma towards mental disorders and discrimination against the psychiatric sector within general health-care resource allocation will continue to wane. In whatever ways future societies decide to govern overall health-care resource allocation, the psychiatric sector will almost certainly compete on equal footing with other sectors for resources much more commonly than occurs at present. For all of the controversy that the managed behavioral health-care movement has elicited in the US, one undeniably useful outcome is diminished fear among policy makers and health-care leaders that removing all distinctive limits from the mental health sector and treating it no worse (or better) than other sectors will create a 'Pandora's Box' or 'bottomless pit' effect.

Putting the mental sector on a par with other health-care sectors will make it imperative that clinicians, patients, policy makers, and society develop a clear understanding of the goals of mental health treatment. While the promotion of positive mental health and well-being is a valid and important societal goal, it is unlikely that societies will opt to use their limited health-care resources for these purposes. We have argued that a proper understanding of the goals of health care in terms of its contribution to equal opportunity through alleviating the impairment of species-typical function created by mental disorders provides a principled basis for setting limits of this kind.[18] While there will clearly always be a gray zone of debate about the boundaries between treatment directed to diminishing the impacts of mental disorders and treatment directed at enhancement of well-being, the distinction itself is a meaningful one for purposes of policy. If we recognize that although counseling and psychotherapy directed at coping with life's vicissitudes may be extremely beneficial to individuals and families, there are ethically sound grounds for not paying for these services with collective health insurance funds, we may find it less tempting to stigmatize these services as directed to the 'worried well' as a justification for not covering them.

Callahan has provided a very useful general map and set of recommendations for future mental health resource allocation activities.[29] He argues that effective allocational policy can only emerge from a middle way between extremes he terms 'pure numbers' (efforts to deduce resource allocation priorities from clinical and economic facts or from first principles, which we described in pp. 386–8 as an illusory hope) and 'raw politics' (the clash of interests and power, decided solely through political strength). We believe that the four conditions for defining fair resource allocation procedures presented on p. 395 provide an initial practical characterization of just such a middle path.

Developing ethical, effective, and publicly acceptable approaches to resource allocation, limit-setting, and rationing in health care is a crucial learning challenge for all societies. Because different national approaches to health care create different configurations of challenge and opportunity, we believe that the requisite learning process can best be accomplished by looking at the issues in an international context. With regard to mental health resource allocation, the profusion of managed behavioral health-care programs in the United States makes the country the potential prime contributor to international learning about algorithms, disease management strategies, and micro-management of resource allocation at the level of the individual patient.[30] However, the decentralized, competitive health-care strategy that currently governs the American health-care system makes the US—with the exception of the Oregon process—ideally unsuited for learning about systematic approaches to more macro-level resource allocation. To learn about these broader levels of mental health resource allocation we will need to look to examples like the British National Health Service or countries like Holland, New Zealand and Australia which govern provision of health care on a more centralized basis.

Two to three decades ago clinicians believed it was cruel and harmful to tell the truth to patients about terminal diagnoses, especially cancer. Since then patients, clinicians, and the public have become much more skilful about collaborating with regard to treatment planning in the face of the ultimate limit set by mortality. We anticipate that through a similar learning process, during the next two to three decades we will witness a comparable increase in our capacity to collaborate with regard to the limits created by the finitude of economic resources.

References

1. Grob, G.: *From asylum to community: mental health policy in modern America.* Princeton, NJ, Princeton University Press, 1991.
2. Daniels, N.: *Just health care.* Cambridge, Cambridge University Press, 1985.
3. Hays, R. D., Wells, K. B., Sherbourne, C. D., *et al.*: Functioning and well-being outcomes of patients with depression compared with chronic medical diseases. *Archives of General Psychiatry* 52:11–19, 1995.
4. National Advisory Mental Health Council: Health care reform for Americans with severe mental illnesses. *American Journal of Psychiatry* 150:1447–65, 1993.
5. Boyle, P. J. and Callahan, D.: *What price mental health: the ethics and politics of setting priorities.* Washington, DC, Georgetown University Press, 1995.
6. Sabin, J. E. and Daniels, N.: Setting behavioral health priorities: good news and crucial lessons from the Oregon Health Plan. *Psychiatric Services* 48:883–9, 1997.
7. Garland, M.: Justice, politics, and community: expanding access and rationing health services in Oregon. *Law, Medicine and Health Care* 20:67–81, 1992.
8. Pollack, D. A., McFarland, B. H., George, R. A., *et al.*: Ethics and value strategies used in prioritizing mental health services in Oregon. *Healthcare Ethics Committee Forum* 5:322–39, 1993.
9. Pollack, D. A., McFarland, B. H., George, R. A. *et al.*: Prioritization of mental health services in Oregon. *Milbank Quarterly* 72:515–50, 1994.
10. Daniels, N.: Rationing fairly: programmatic considerations. *Bioethics* 7:224–33, 1993.
11. Sabin, J. E. and Daniels, N.: Lessons for U.S. managed care from the British National Health Service, II: setting priorities. *Psychiatric Services* 48:469–70, 482, 1997.
12. Jenkins, R.: The health of the nation: recent government policy and legislation. *Psychiatric Bulletin* 18:324–7, 1994.
13. Department of Health: *Mental illness key area handbook.* London, HMSO, 1993.
14. Klein, R., Day, P., and Redmayne, S.: *Managing scarcity: priority setting and rationing in the National Health Service.* Buckingham, Open University Press, 1996.
15. Crisp, R., Hope, T., and Ebbs, D.: The Asbury draft policy on ethical use of resources. *British Medical Journal* 312:1528–31, 1996.
16. Ham, C.: Priority setting in the NHS: reports from six districts. In *Rationing in action.* London, BMJ, 1993.
17. Mechanic, D.: Establishing mental health priorities. *Milbank Quarterly* 72:501–14, 1994.
18. Sabin, J. E. and Daniels, N.: Determining 'medical necessity' in mental health practice. *Hastings Center Report* 24:5–13, 1994.
19. Kramer, P.: *Listening to Prozac.* New York, Viking, 1993.

20. Forrow, L., Daniels, N., and Sabin, J. E.: When is home care medically necessary? *Hastings Center Report* **21**:36–8, 1991.
21. Babigian, H. M. and Reed, S. K.: Capitation and management of mental health in the public sector. In *Managed mental health care: administrative and clinical issues,* ed. J. Feldman and R. J. Fitzpatrick. Washington, DC, American Psychiatric Association Press, 1992, pp. 111–24.
22. Sabin, J. E. and Neu, C.: Real world resource allocation: the concept of 'good enough' psychotherapy. *Bioethics Forum* **12**:3–9, 1996.
23. Sabin, J. E.: General hospital psychiatry and the ethics of managed care. *General Hospital Psychiatry* **17**:193–8, 1995.
24. *The principles of medical ethics: with annotations especially applicable to psychiatry.* Washington, DC, American Psychiatric Association, 1995.
25. Levinsky, N. D.: The doctor's master. *New England Journal of Medicine* **314**: 1573–5, 1984.
26. Daniels N. and Sabin, J. E.: Limits to health care: fair procedures, democratic deliberation, and the legitimacy problem for insurers. *Philosophy and Public Affairs:* **26**:303–50, 1997.
27. Sabin, J. E.: Organized psychiatry and managed care: quality improvement or holy war? *Health Affairs* **14**:32–3, 1995.
28. Mechanic, D.: Dilemmas in rationing health care services: the case for implicit rationing. *British Medical Journal* **310**:1655–9, 1995.
29. Callahan, D.: Setting mental health priorities: problems and possibilities. *Milbank Quarterly* **72**:451–70, 1994.
30. Moffic, H. S.:*The ethical way: challenges and solutions for managed behavioral healthcare.* San Francisco, Jossey-Bass, 1997.

19

The ethics of managed mental health care

Stephen A. Green

Escalating medical costs over the past three decades have highlighted the growing pressure on health-care resources universally, and perhaps most dramatically in the United States. Annual health-care costs in America, which were approximately $1 billion in 1965, increased to $750 billion by the 1990s, accounting for more than 14 per cent of the GDP. Many believe these data reflect a fundamental systemic flaw, namely fee-for-service (FFS) medical care driven by patients' demands for services, guided by practice standards primarily defined by medical professionals, and supported by retrospective indemnity insurance. This system lacks incentives for cost-efficiencies, is financially burdened by administrative expenses and an oppressive litigious atmosphere, and invites provision of unnecessary care with a potential for clinicians to act irresponsibly or with intentional avarice. Governmental oversight is primarily concerned with protecting the public from the harm of unqualified or substandard care, as well as distribution and regulation of monies for publicly funded care.

This chapter will focus on the shift to managed care in the United States, which has become increasingly prevalent in an attempt to mitigate the detrimental impact the above issues impose on medical treatment. Some details of the discussion are distinctive to America; however, consideration of the ethical dilemmas inherent in managed care is relevant to all health systems which must balance individual needs against the welfare of society.

A significant factor contributing to the rise in health care expenditures in the United States has been the cost of mental health care.[1] In the 1960s monies became increasingly available for the treatment of mental and substance abuse disorders, with passage of the Community Mental Health Center Act of 1963, the implementation of broad public subsidies (e.g. Medicare and Medicaid), and the expansion of mental health benefits in private insurance programs. During the 1980s psychiatry increasingly fell under the control of market forces, particularly in regard to inpatient treatment, with a dramatic increase in the number of psychiatric beds and admission rate for children, adolescents, and people suffering from substance abuse disorders. The average length of hospitalization increased nationally, the per diem rates of private psychiatric hospitals rose more than that of general hospitals, and profit margins were higher in private hospitals than in non-profit hospitals.[2,3] By 1988 almost two-thirds of all inpatient facilities were privately owned, most by corporate chains. The increasing commercialization of mental health care was not necessarily in conflict with quality of care, though there was clear concern about the ethical implications of some prevailing practices, such as utilizing inpatient care when other levels of treatment could have sufficed, subjecting patients to inappropriately lengthy hospitalizations which depleted their insurance benefits at a faster rate than necessary, and rationing the availability and intensity of psychiatric treatment largely on the basis of insurance coverage. Moreover, legal settlements suggested that some treatment was unnecessary and/or fraudulent.[4] Despite the percentage of GDP devoted to health care (the highest percentage in the industrialized world), tens of millions of Americans remained uninsured or underinsured,[5] and a demonstrated need for mental health care persists;[6] this is particularly disturbing in light of the Epidemiologic Catchment Area Study[7] which found that mental and substance abuse disorders afflict 52 million Americans, representing 25 per cent of the population. In sum, the growing influence of market forces on psychiatric care during the 1980s failed to contain costs or improve access to treatment, and had a questionable impact on quality of care. These aggregate results prompted a shift in the financing and delivery of mental health care to a managed-care model grounded in a fundamental philosophy of increased efficiency.

Managed care and efficiency

Managed care, a generic term, applies to varied principles, practices, and structures for providing health care to groups of patients. Efforts to infuse more efficiency into health care began with the inception of health maintenance organizations (HMOs), corporate configurations of health providers which share the following features: contracts with selected physicians and hospitals to furnish a comprehensive set of services to enrolled members, usually for a predetermined monthly premium; utilization and quality controls that contracting clinicians agree to accept; financial incentives for patients to use the clinicians and facilities associated with the plan; and the assumption of financial risk by doctors, thus fundamentally altering their role from serving as agents who protect a patient's welfare to balancing his/her health needs against the goal of cost control.[8] HMOs initially employed administrative barriers to manage access to mental health benefits, thereby reducing costs of care. This progressed to a period of managed benefits, which relied heavily on utilization review to distribute patients' benefits, and ultimately evolved into the current system of managed-care.[9] Each phase progressively diminished the practitioner's autonomy, and increasingly brought clinical decision-making under the authority of managed-care organizations (MCOs).[10,11]

Proponents of managed care argue that it promotes a fundamental moral goal; namely, conserving scarce health-care resources by insuring their efficient distribution. Opponents of managed care criticize the efficiency principle because, in an effort to balance individual needs against welfarist concerns of society, it undermines the fundamental moral commitment of medical practice—advocacy for the individual patient. The debate regarding the ethics of managed care is formed along this central focus. Hume's moral theory,[12] which is concerned with the competing moral claims of fairness to the individual and promoting the well-being of society, provides an excellent perspective for this debate. As Hume discussed, the condition of scarce resources fosters activities requiring social rules, conventions emanating from a community's standards and historical tradition; these, in turn, define social justice, as they are grounded in principles of utility and beneficence. To Hume, both cooperation and conflict are required for justice because they compel members of society to establish guiding moral judgments that advance individual needs, as well as societal needs which convey benefit to individual citizens (e.g. social stability). In order to achieve just distribution of resources, Hume argues that humankind must resolve the tension between providing for the individual and advancing the public good. Managed care must realize that same goal if it is to claim moral legitimacy, which requires the preservation of fairness in an environment driven by efficiency.

Efficiency and fairness

Efficiency is based in consequentialist theory which holds that the right in any given situation, judged from an impersonal standpoint, produces the best outcome that affords equal weight to every person's interests.[13] Utilitarianism, the most familiar version of consequentialism, argues that the best state of affairs from among many contains the greatest net balance of aggregate human pleasure or happiness or satisfaction. Regarding health care, an accepted method of ranking from an impersonal standpoint involves examining the impact of treatment on quality of life as measured in quality-of-life years (QALYs).[14] Efficient health care generates low cost per QALY and, according to the principles of managed care, should receive priority over non-efficient treatments. Proponents of efficiency argue that in addition to the economic advantages that derive from QALY maximization, clinical decision-making driven by medical effectiveness is blinded to arbitrary discriminatory factors (e.g. age), therefore allowing for a convergence of economic efficiency and fairness.[15] However, others argue that the QALY approach can systematically disadvantage particular groups, and therefore violate the principle of fairness, by denying certain people an equal claim to health resources. Harris,[16,17] for example, believes that health policy based on efficiency suffers from 'economism', a bias favoring treatments and illnesses that require the least amount of resources. As a result, he believes that QALY determinations profess a *prima facie* impartiality while imposing *de facto* discrimination and, as such, are morally indefensible. Harris's concerns reflect a criticism of consequentialism; namely, its potential to disadvantage the individual because it is not directly weighted to consider justice or fairness in the distribution of goods.[18]

These challenges to efficiency as a principle to allocate resources do not necessarily suggest fairness as an alternative guiding principle. Given the conflicting goals of medical services (e.g. research, preventive care, treatment of acute and chronic illness), it is difficult to determine who has the greatest moral claim to finite resources. It is also difficult to justify a system which, in an attempt to meet these diverse needs, depletes resources in situations where care is futile or has little probability for success. For example, some consider expending resources on patients in a permanent vegetative state an immoral aspect of the FFS system when those considerable costs could fund guaranteed benefit to large numbers of patients (e.g. immunization against infectious disease). These types of arguments suggest that although the efficiency principle is not impartial in its distribution of resources, it is not necessarily immoral. More specifically, allocational criteria are only unjust when they convey immoral systematic disadvantage, since justice does not always require that 'we do not allow certain sections of the community to become the victims of systematic disadvantage' (see ref. 19, p. 48). Indeed, this is the justification for a health-care system which provides quality universal care in the context of centralized budgets that necessarily deny certain benefits to some members of society, but can be defended on the grounds of fairness because of considerations of justice in allocating resources.[20]

The legitimacy of claims to limited resources depends on circumstances which tug at our reason and emotions, particularly when we attempt to resolve difficult choices with rigid application of normative moral principles. Efficiency may be intuitively disturbing, but it can be discriminatory in ways that are both morally acceptable and unacceptable. As Broome argues, QALYs should not 'be condemned as worthless because they take no account of fairness', as there are circumstances when 'it will almost certainly be right to sacrifice some good in total for the sake of fairness ... [and] to tolerate some unfairness for the sake of the greater good' (see ref. 21, p. 64). Allocating health resources on the basis of efficiency or fairness has the potential to convey moral harm, and the need to effect a balance between the two principles is central to the debate concerning the ethics of managed mental health care. A consequentialist approach may discriminate against individual patients; however, recognized shortcomings of psychiatric treatment cause many to believe a degree of efficiency-driven health policy is ethically necessary.[22—24]

Given this background I now explore the ethical dilemmas associated with the treatment of mental and substance abuse disorders in a managed-care setting, by focusing on the therapeutic relationship, confidentiality, informed consent, quality of care, access to care, and implications for training. The discussion considers whether or not these dilemmas undermine the moral legitimacy of managed mental health care.

The therapeutic relationship

A fundamental dimension of the Hippocratic tradition is the trusting relationship that enables people to consign their well-being to a physician who, in turn, serves as the central figure in the health-care system with responsibility to advocate 'for the benefit of the sick'. This obligation of fidelity is reflected in diverse ethical justifications: it is grounded in consequentialism, which holds that promoting patients' interests maximizes the good; in deontological theory's commitment to moral duty based in rules of reason, specifically, the respect for autonomy; and in the Aristotelian tradition of virtue ethics, which holds that physicians should be individuals of good character who act justly and in a morally correct manner towards patients (see ref. 25, pp. 62—69).

The growing commercialization of medical care has steadily shifted the locus of clinical decision-making away from the physician–patient relationship due to the increasing influence of negotiations between clinicians and payers, with a significant impact on the obligation of fidelity. As the American Medical Association's Council of Ethical and Judicial Affairs notes,[26] a managed-care environment encroaches on advocacy for the individual patient by promoting conflicting loyalties in physicians in two ways. First, it places patients' interests in conflict, potentially preventing clinicians from acting as effective agents for an individual patient. Distributing resources across groups of patients in order to respond to welfarist needs does not necessarily convey moral harm; however, the potential for moral harm is ever-present if efforts to control costs lead to a rigid policy based on 'uninformed' clinical decisions predominantly sensitive to economic priorities (see ref. 27, p. 24). Empirical evidence suggests that managed mental health care has infringed on clinicians' obligation to fidelity in this manner. For example, it is difficult to imagine that the dramatically reduced duration of hospitalizations has resulted from the more efficient treatment of major mental illness. More likely, decisions regarding inpatient care are driven by managed-care protocols that are less sensitive to the clinical needs of the individual patient and more 'about who can provide care for the least number of dollars and get away with it'.[28]

The second way managed care can interfere with the principle of fidelity is by placing financial interests of physicians in conflict with patients' needs. Clinicians' income varies considerably in the context of managed care based on the type of treatment they provide. This raises the danger that care will be motivated more by economic than clinical concerns, which may cause physicians to withhold care, or knowledge about various treatment, or financial information that influences clinical decision-making (see ref. 27, p. 21). Moreover, recognition of potential conflict over finances can erode the trust necessary for an effective therapeutic relationship, and it is public knowledge that managed-care plans have attempted to induce physicians to reduce their use of services (e.g. by providing incentives to order fewer tests or medications, or basing a proportion of their salaries on the volume of work).[29,30] Unquestionably physicians' financial interests conflict with clinical care in the FFS system, when marginal or unwarranted treatment is prescribed primarily to generate income; the practice has resulted in lawsuits against particular psychiatric hospitals.[4,31] However, managed care provides financial incentives to *limit* treatment, perhaps more ethically problematic as it can more readily predispose to inadequate care.

Given these potential conflicts around advocacy, there is a need to define the ethical limits of fidelity in the context of managed care. Morreim (see ref. 27, p. 24) suggests that the therapeutic relationship requires clinicians to provide 'ordinary and reasonable care, with the provision that in times of scarcity, what is reasonable will depend in part on what is available', and to assist the patient 'through the growing maze of regulations and guidelines' in order to help them oppose rules which distribute resources unjustly. Physicians can pursue these goals at the micro- and macro-levels. Regarding the former, they should educate patients about available treatment alternatives, including potentially beneficial treatments not offered in a particular plan, and participate actively in appeals procedures when they believe such actions are clinically indicated.[32] There is clear precedent for clinicians to advocate for patients when the principle of fidelity conflicts with third-party interests, (e.g. opposing a Jehovah's Witness family's wish not to transfuse a child) (see ref. 25, pp. 130—131); similar moral reasoning applies when the third party is an MCO. Physicians should also disclose to patients any financial incentives they may realize from working in a particular health plan. At a macro-level, physicians are obliged to advocate for changes in policy that minimizes the negative impact of standard criteria on individual patients. Physicians should also be integrally involved in establishing clinical guidelines, both by contributing their expertise and advocating for justice within their profession and managed-care organizations.[33]

Confidentiality

Since medical confidentiality can be construed narrowly or broadly[34] clinicians define it along an axis, reflecting the fact that it is more a subjective judgment than an objective norm. For example, practitioners have varied opinions as to when a patient's threat to suicide is serious enough to warrant notifying a third party against the patient's wishes. The moral justification for confidentiality is grounded in a consequentialist argument which posits that breaches of confidentiality hamper treatment by causing patients to withhold relevant information, and in the extreme, forego care. This line of argument was specifically discussed in the *Tarasoff*[35] dissent and subsequently endorsed in a US Supreme Court decision which emphasizes that effective counseling depends on an 'imperative need' for confidentiality and trust.[36] Justifying confidentiality also rests on the deontological principles of fidelity and respect for autonomy, which are concerned with intrinsic values, as opposed to the consequences of actions. Fidelity, as previously discussed, entails implicit and explicit promises including a pledge of confidentiality. Respect for autonomy refers to the Kantian notion of a self-legislating will that endorses self-direction over control by others. The principle of respect for autonomy 'carries over the idea of having a domain or territory of sovereignty for the self and a right to protect it', which is closely linked to the right of privacy; granting access to oneself in the medical environment (e.g. by relating intimate thoughts to a therapist) is an exercise of that privacy right (see ref. 25, p. 410).

On the basis of either consequentialist or deontological principles, confidentiality is recognized as a prima facie obligation, as opposed to an absolute condition of medical practice. An obligation to violate confidentiality increases when there is substantial probability that harm may befall the patient or others. This is highly relevant in the context of managed mental health care which intrudes on the confidential patient–therapist relationship by design for the explicit purpose of promoting public interest through conservation of resources. Third parties have established claims to confidential information (for example, when the public interest is at risk, or to justify insurance reimbursement) which suggests that procedures (e.g. utilization review) seeking to evaluate the need for, or progress in, treatment are ethically justifiable. Valid social and medical reasons for reviewers to access privileged information concerning an individual's mental health care include an obligation to protect him/her from treatment that might have adverse effects, insure that treatment is guided by the clinical condition rather than by arbitrary benefit entitlements, and conserve society's limited resources.[22] However, prospective utilization review has the potential to affect the entire basis of confidentiality in the therapeutic relationship because reviewers can request increasingly detailed data in order to determine if a patient's problem warrants treatment, and, if so, its form and level of intensity. This shift of control from professional care to entrepreneurial pursuits[37] has moral relevance depending on how MCOs use and protect clinical data.

The ethical limits of confidentiality remain intact if those working in a system of managed care only use information necessary to accomplish their work and, additionally, appropriately protect its dissemination. There is, unfortunately, evidence that MCOs depart from this guideline in ways that convey moral harm to patients. To begin, an MCO often requires patients to sign disclosure forms so general in scope that people are unaware of all the parties to whom they grant access to confidential medical information.[38] The argument that patients authorize such disclosure is questionable, especially when the potential consequences of blanket authorization are considered, such as the refusal of disability or health insurance, and informing other medical specialists of a patient's history of a mental or substance abuse disorder (and even the details of their treatment). MCOs often insist clinicians provide full access to their files, another invasion of privacy about which patients may be inadequately informed. Apart from these practices which threaten confidentiality, a widespread perception prevails that privacy is always at risk in a system of managed mental health care.[39] This is reflected in individuals' decision to leave therapy after a records' audit by an MCO or not to use insurance to pay for treatment, and in the observation by some therapists that patients withhold certain information because they fear the consequences if it appears in treatment notes or records. Some clinicians have even provided written material to patients informing them of the potential dangers of storing private medical data in electronic databanks, a legitimate concern given some inexcusable failures of MCOs, such as allowing detailed notes of psychotherapy sessions to become available to patients' co-workers.[39]

If managed care is to protect patients' privacy it must fulfill reasonable expectations of confidentiality by providing the same degree of confidentiality found in the therapeutic relationship.[40] Without that guarantee people may forego treatment in order to protect their privacy, which can not only harm the individual patient, but also compromise the common good (e.g. by contributing to public and domestic violence).[41] The challenge to policy makers is 'to balance the need for confidentiality essential to the therapeutic process with the need for access to otherwise confidential information when necessary to protect legitimate public interests' (see ref. 42, p. 183).

Steps towards this end have already been incorporated into law; a 1996 statute in the State of Massachusetts limits the amount of information that can be revealed to third-party payers, requires genuine confidential review of appealed cases, requires informed consent from patients before their medical information can be entered into a computerized network, and prevents release of any clinical data until patients use up to $500 in medical benefits. Gostin et al.[43] have recommended comprehensive measures to replace the patchwork of federal and state law in the United States regarding confidentiality. In general, confidentiality should be expanded to cover the therapist–patient–MCO relationship, in order to reassure patients that disclosure of medical information by an MCO occurs as a good faith discharge to other parties with a corresponding interest and duty to secure that information, and that legal recourse is available when these conditions are not met. Given these circumstances managed-care personnel can retain proper ethical standards of medical confidentiality.[42]

Informed consent

Informed consent, the degree to which patients understand and agree to a proposed treatment, is concerned with the protection and facilitation of autonomous choice. As Beauchamp and Childress comment, informed consent is a complex process consisting of several distinct elements (see ref. 25, pp. 142—170). First, a *threshold element* is concerned with competence to consent, the capacity for decision-making as it relates to a specific task.[44] Second, there are *information elements* concerned with disclosure and understanding of pertinent information. This is possibly 'the most important element in the process of obtaining informed consent' (see ref. 25, p. 147) as patients require a core set of data (e.g. facts, descriptions, professional opinions) in order to exercise autonomous decision-making about proposed treatments. Adequate understanding of the information provided rests on an adequate opportunity for patients to discuss and reflect on medical data so that they have justified beliefs about the nature and consequences of their actions. Finally, informed consent involves *consent elements*, the voluntariness of decision-making and the degree to which patients' actions represent active authorization as opposed to passive acceptance. People must be free of coercive influences (e.g. presenting information in a way that alters the understanding of a situation) that may undermine independence of their actions.

Managed mental health care employs overt and covert practices which interfere with patients obtaining relevant information thus limiting autonomous choice. Research on HMOs shows that the quality of the communication between clinician and patient is lower in prepaid settings for general medical care compared to fee-for-service arrangements;[45] the evidence similarly applies to mental health care.[46] In particular, the organizational structure of managed care (e.g. imposing time constraints on the clinical interaction or failing to provide patients with the same caregivers over time) disrupts the communication necessary for patients to obtain information to reach an informed decision. Some MCOs impose 'gag rules' on the clinician, prohibitions which prevent discussion of treatments which are not included in services provided by their plan. Though these rules have been prohibited with certain groups of patients,[47] they remain legal in the United States pending legislative action.[48] Additionally, when patients join a health plan they evaluate the services available, but may be unaware of the criteria of 'medical necessity' which must be met to obtain those services. Because many MCOs consider these parameters proprietary, patients cannot know, when entering a health plan, the circumstances under which they will be eligible for specific treatments. Moreover, they are denied a forum to discuss eligibility since they do not communicate with the clinical reviewers who make those determinations. At best, patients can initiate an appeal after they have already joined an MCO in order to insist they receive information necessary to give informed consent. Finally, as noted earlier, limits imposed on informed consent by MCOs have significant implications for confidentiality, which patients would be likely to object to if properly informed of the scope of their authorization for release of clinical data. Appelbaum[49] offers suggestions for limiting the harms that may result from this practice.

In sum, managed mental health care can deny patients an adequate understanding of the treatments available to them both at the time of entry into a health plan and at the point of clinical service. Because these practices impede informed consent, they may undermine autonomous decision-making, causing moral harm to patients whose judgment may already be impaired by mental illness.

Quality of care

Criticisms of managed mental health care regarding the quality of treatment include: the use of less costly providers (e.g. non-physician therapists) and treatments; lower intensity of care or amount of services;[22] reliance on 'gate-keepers' (physicians who triage patients to specialist care) who may be insufficiently trained about the diagnosis and treatment of mental and substance abuse disorders;[50,51] using clinical guidelines based on outcome data whose accuracy is questionable;[52] determining quality of treatment solely by measuring its length and cost;[53] containing cost simply by shortening the duration of treatment;[1,54] and implementing efficiencies that may well reduce efficacy of treatment.[55] Professed concerns by managed-care organizations for quality of care is not supported by clinical reality[56,57] and fuel the criticism that they are good at keeping healthy people healthy, but do not respond adequately to the seriously ill. MCOs reply to their critics that they apply management procedures that insure the availability of necessary care whose quality is more defined than that provided in a FFS system. This argument rests entirely on the definition of 'medical necessity', which becomes a subjective standard given diverse treatment approaches and positions about the intensity of interventions required for particular mental and substance abuse disorders.

One method to determine the criteria of necessary care is to establish a morally acceptable level of quality;[22] this, in turn, requires consideration of the basis for a moral claim to health care. As I have suggested elsewhere,[41] this is best explicated by Daniels,[58] who argues that health-care needs are special since illness imposes a burden on individual opportunity. Social justice therefore requires maintenance of health to protect what the philosopher John Rawls calls a 'fair equality of opportunity', namely that 'those with similar abilities and skills should have similar life chances ... the same prospects of success regardless of their initial place in the social system' (see ref. 18, p. 73). Daniels defines disease as 'deviations from the natural functional organization of a typical member of a species' whose impact is to reduce 'the range of opportunity open to the individual' (see ref. 58, p. 28). In this manner he uses the impairment of normal opportunities as a gauge to meet different health-care needs, thereby extending Rawls' concept to cover provision of health care to society's members. Daniels' argument is grounded in rational autonomy as a condition to achieve fair equality of opportunity; those lacking resources to respond to the disadvantages imposed by ill health have a reduced opportunity range because of compromised autonomy, thereby impairing their ability to construct a 'plan of life' or 'conception of the good'. For example, people lacking health care needed to treat schizophrenia have fewer options in their lives than those who consistently receive appropriate care.

According to Daniels' theory, mental health care should be included in services necessary to maintain a normal opportunity range because of the effect of mental illness on autonomous functioning. However, there is much debate about what constitutes illness as opposed to psychopathological difficulties of living and, consequently, a parallel debate occurs about the degree to which society is morally obliged to insure treatment of mental dysfunction through public or private financial arrangements.[59] Sabin and Daniels address this issue by describing three conceptions of 'medical necessity',[60] reflecting increasing degrees of inclusiveness along a treatment spectrum. They conclude that the normal functioning model—essentially the clinical equivalent of Rawls' notion of fair equality of opportunity—is the most ethically acceptable since it satisfies criteria of fairness, practicality, and affordability to society. Whether or not their formulation is the most reasonable, it highlights the degree to which value judgments affect the medical criteria used for the design of insurance plans and the determination of quality of care, decisions which translate into clinical policies about the scope of services needed to provide medically necessary care.

Consensus about these issues usually (though not always) apply to the extremes; for example, sharp limits on inpatient treatment for severely psychotic patients will undoubtedly raise questions about quality of care. Widely accepted standards are more debatable in less extreme instances, a task complicated by conflicting empirical data concerning quality of care. Despite some proven shortcomings of prepaid mental health coverage,[61] the data yield contradictory conclusions. For example, the Medical Outcomes Study demonstrated that patients with depression treated in HMOs fared worse than patients treated under other insurance arrangements;[46] while limits placed on psychotherapy, common to many managed-care arrangements, correlated with more severe symptoms, reflected in increased duration and frequency of hospitalizations.[62] On the other hand, a study conducted by the US government suggests that States that utilize managed care for their indigent (Medicaid) populations provide the same quality as FFS treatment;[63] this is consistent with Lurie *et al.*'s observation that—at least in the short run—no harmful effects result from a prepaid care system for chronically mentally ill Medicaid patients as compared to FFS treatment of similar patients.[64] Other findings resist ready interpretation regarding quality of care.[65]

An alternate means to assess quality of care in a managed-care setting, which avoids the difficulty of resolving conflicting empirical data, is to investigate ways the system affects clinical care. This approach suggests that central aspects of managed mental health care detract from the quality of care. First, communication between caregiver and patient is diminished in managed-care settings,[45,66] particularly when implementation of practice efficiencies leads to more patients being seen in the same amount of time. Since a basic task in medical treatment, especially mental health care, is to appreciate the patient as a person with particular fears, wishes, and needs, any impediment to such appreciation threatens quality of care. Second, managed care often encroaches on the continuity of the relationship between patients and caregivers,[66–68] potentially disrupting the relationship in several ways. A patient may be compelled to end long-standing associations with physicians when employers contract with an MCO that does not include them in their clinical network. This situation becomes more common when employers offer a single health plan, thereby restricting employees to a preselected group of physicians or requiring them to assume a co-pay if they wish to see other doctors. Moreover, employers often contract with the least expensive health plan which may induce them to change plans frequently, thereby interrupting the relationship between patient and physician.[69] Beyond these tangible effects, a system that relies on incentives 'to switch plans to reward low prices' erodes patients' expectations that consistent, appropriate care is desirable or will be made available (see ref. 70, p. 1195). Third, MCOs rely increasingly on non-psychiatric clinicians whose inability to diagnose and treat mental disorders appropriately has been demonstrated.[46,51] Almost half the patients who present to general practitioners with depressive disorders remain undiagnosed,[71] despite research showing the high prevalence of recurrent depression in this group.[72,73] Moreover, recognition of mental illness is not a sufficient condition to guarantee delivery of appropriate treatment;[61] in fact, correct diagnosis does not necessarily correlate with better outcome.[74] Many clinicians prescribe psychoactive medications incorrectly; others fail to use appropriate psychotherapeutic interventions because they 'receive virtually no training in office counseling or psychotherapy'. Furthermore, general practice is not conducive to the time-intensive clinical interview 'essential to the detection and evaluative understanding of mental illness, its course, and its determinants'.[61]

No standard indicators are available with which to evaluate the quality of mental health care, and criteria which are employed are faulted for applying overly subjective measures (e.g. patient satisfaction) or are too broad to distinguish between different levels of quality of care. Until sophisticated, universal quality assurance indicators are adopted routinely, assessing the quality of care must be derivative. In the interim, the burden rests on MCOs to demonstrate that health care based on the efficiency model does, indeed, achieve an acceptable quality.

Access to mental health care

Proponents of managed care contend that integration of treatment with case management promotes efficiencies that improve increased access to care. Utilizing a continuum of services that provides patients with care in the most relevant setting throughout the course of their illness, managed care has reduced reliance on expensive hospitalization, and purportedly reduced treatment costs by 30–40 per cent, making 'possible the delivery of more care to a greater number of patients'. Optimizing efficiency may 'yield the greatest value for each health-care dollar spent' (see ref. 75, pp. 215–216), but it does not necessarily translate into better access. Indeed, as observations about the delivery of medical care in the United States suggest, managed care can compromise individuals' opportunity to obtain treatment by limiting access to health plans, as well as to specific services in those plans.

Although managed mental health care has steadily expanded in America—unmanaged indemnity insurance supports only 10 per cent of mental health services[75]—so has the proportion of Americans with unmet mental health needs. The ranks of the uninsured and the underinsured continue to grow; people with mental disorders among the uninsured population are estimated to be as high as 50 per cent.[6] Moreover, those insured and suffering from mental and substance abuse disorders are still undertreated due to lack of parity benefits compared to general medical care. In light of these data, the argument that efficient provision of mental health care necessarily increases access is questionable. An alternate explanation is that insurers and MCOs have achieved efficiency by limiting access to mental health care; by selectively marketing to healthier patient groups, or offering plans that exclude certain treatments, they are able 'to select enrollees who are likely to use fewer and cheaper services' (see ref. 66, p. 237). There is precedent for these types of limitation. In the 1970s and 1980s insurance carriers restricted mental health benefits of large patient groups, such as government employees, while HMO contracts excluded coverage for specific patient groups (e.g. the mentally retarded, the chronically mentally ill).[76] Further restrictions were imposed on mental health benefits through cost-sharing (e.g. co-payments and deductibles), mandatory time periods between hospitalizations, and lifetime reimbursement ceilings that were substantially lower than those for general medical care. Applying these practices insurance companies and managed-care organizations have sought to select enrollees likely to use fewer and cheaper services, though unmet mental health need in the United States continues.

Even if access to mental health care is not affected by the above factors, it may still be limited to people who are enrolled in a health plan by some managed-care practices. For example, many plans utilize gatekeepers, usually general practitioners, to authorize mental health care. Their demonstrated limited clinical experience to diagnose and treat mental and substance abuse disorders[46,50,51,72,73] can be a serious impediment to accessing needed care. MCOs also invoke cost to justify using physicians with minimal psychiatric training, as well as increasing numbers of non-medically trained mental health personnel (e.g. social workers) to 'manage conditions that are best handled by specialists;'[66] patients' access to needed treatment may be curtailed because of the limited clinical experience of these caretakers. The issue of how necessary care is defined, as discussed above, also affects patients' access to treatment. When enrolling in a health plan people may believe they are entitled to certain benefits, but learn that those services are available only when deemed 'medically necessary' by administrators of the plan. Patients may theoretically have access to an excellent range of services (e.g. long-term, psychodynamic psychotherapy), whereas in reality they are confined to highly circumscribed treatment due to strict guidelines which endorse less intensive interventions (e.g. time-limited cognitive therapy). MCOs may also limit access to certain medications since pharmaceutical formularies are largely determined on the basis of cost. As a result, new enrollees to a health plan who were previously treated with a selective serotonin reuptake inhibitor may be prescribed a tricyclic antidepressant despite the clear effectiveness of the current medication or the possibility that a different medication will cause previously unexperienced side effects. Similarly, some HMOs authorize a monthly drug budget to groups of physicians, penalizing them if they exceed it and allowing them to share savings if they remain below it. When a medical practice is allocated $8 per month per patient (half of what many physicians consider to be reasonable),[77] access to proper treatment is at clear risk of being compromised. Finally, gag rules can prevent enrollees from learning about treatments which may not be available in their plan, a circumstance which can deny them access to appropriate care.

According to Geraty and Fox, achieving greater efficiency in the delivery of mental health care imposes administrative costs equaling 20–25 per cent of total cost reduction, a price they consider 'well worthwhile' since cost-effectiveness enhances access to high-quality care (see ref. 75, p. 222). Their judgment is questionable. It is unclear whether the expansion of managed care in the United States has increased the number of people covered by health insurance, and whether those whose care is administered by MCOs are effectively denied treatment due to obvious or covert benefit restrictions. If, as some suggest,[28] financial gain is the basic motivation for MCOs to employ direct and indirect limits on access to mental health resources, then they are acting unethically.

Training and research

A key responsibility of psychiatrists is to promote their professional competence; this requires that they be trained in diverse treatment modalities in order to address patients' varied needs.[78] A significant issue is whether managed mental health care impedes that effort, given that its basic goal of cost-effectiveness inevitably conflicts with teaching and research activities of academic medical centers. Meyer and Sotsky[79] note how the culture, administrative organization, and goals of teaching institutions have traditionally not concerned themselves with the impact of market forces, by offering a broad range of clinical services, regardless of profitability, in order to support a rich learning environment. Academic medical centers attract a greater proportion of seriously ill patients who typically undergo expensive diagnostic testing, extensive specialist consultation, continuing detailed monitoring, and lengthy periods of hospitalization. Such activities promote and maintain medical education; however, financial restraint imposed by MCOs have profoundly affected these endeavors, with a notable impact on psychiatric training. The shift from indemnity insurance has limited inpatient treatment, which historically generated the bulk of income for psychiatry departments. As the length of hospitalization has declined training programs have been unable to secure revenue that covers unfunded or underfunded costs of education and research. Furthermore, requirements imposed by insurers and MCOs curtail (and may even eliminate) the interaction between psychiatric trainees and patients. These include time limits on doctor–patient sessions, the requirement that treatment is provided by a physician, not a trainee, and denying reimbursement unless care is directly supervised by a faculty member. The ethos of managed mental health care is also incompatible with the training goals of certain clinical settings; for example, the rapid discharge of patients from full or partial hospital programs diminishes the opportunity to observe their psychodynamic interactions with members of a treatment milieu.

The implications for mental health care resulting from the above issues is very disquieting. Trainees may learn how to provide efficient care, but not about core transferential aspects of the therapeutic relationship. They may become expert in pharmacologic treatment, but not gain adequate experience in supportive and insight-oriented psychotherapies.[80] Moreover, a growing proportion of the psychotherapies is being delivered by non-physician mental health professionals, and research indicates that allocating professional tasks in this manner means that less than a half of the current number of psychiatrists in the United States will be needed to meet mental health needs in the future.[81] Each of these factors may, in turn, contribute to the declining number of American medical students choosing to specialize in psychiatry.

As a profession we must consider whether these changes are ethically acceptable. Can we allow tomorrow's psychiatrists to complete training with such a circumscribed exposure to the psychotherapies? What are the ethical implications of endorsing a system of health care that will lead to a radical reduction in the number of psychiatrists, physicians who have a unique understanding of human development, normal and abnormal responses to illness, and the doctor–patient relationship? In light of these issues, efficiency arguments that posit an 'excess' of psychiatrists become less convincing.

An effort by all concerned parties is required to mitigate the danger which managed care poses to training. First, academic centers themselves must improve prevailing inefficiencies, and prevent external groups from dictating terms of that process. Teaching programs should be developed which support cost-effective care by including less traditional activities (e.g. crisis intervention), or preserving fundamental educational goals (e.g. studying the therapeutic relationship) by requiring trainees to maintain their involvement

with patients throughout the clinical course, even if they move to other treatment settings.[79] Second, government has a responsibility to support training.
In America, several states have decreased funding of medical education in
both public and private institutions, while federal monies (Medicare indirect
medical education (IME) adjustments) for hospitals are being reduced, unacceptable policies if society wishes to train health professionals to advance the
public good. Given the detrimental effect of MCO-derived financial constraints
on training there is a consequentialist-based argument for them to contribute
to psychiatric education. That claim is further supported by circumstances
stemming from contractual arrangements between some MCOs and academic
centers receiving IME adjustments for teaching costs. Hospitals that establish
risk-contracts with an HMO do so on negotiated reimbursement levels (most
commonly per diem payments) that generally do not reflect teaching costs. As a
result, even though Medicare teaching adjustments are included in monies
Medicare pays MCOs, those funds may not be included in the capitation rates
subsequently established between the MCOs and teaching hospitals. (see ref.
82, pp. 86–87). That training suffers in order that corporate profits increase
imposes an obligation on MCOs to subsidize at least some educational costs.
If this cannot be achieved by voluntary efforts (and representatives of the
managed-care industry have disclaimed responsibility (personal communication, 1996)) then legislation may be needed to designate a percentage of the
profits of MCOs for training and research.

Conclusion

A health-care system is ethically acceptable if it effects a just balance between
an individual's needs and those of society, in an effort to provide equality of
opportunity to all. In principle, an efficiency-based model can achieve that
goal; however, in an attempt to realize cost-effectiveness, managed mental
health care tends to undermine interests of the individual patient to a degree
that causes moral harm. Moreover, managed care cannot claim that its quest
for distributing health resources efficiently has advanced societal good by
improving quality of care or enhancing access to it—though its commitment
to efficiency has resulted in considerable profits[83] and generous executive
salaries.[84] I do not mean to suggest that an ethical system of managed mental
health care is unobtainable, although I do agree with Stone's observation that
'physicians alone cannot hope to counter the for-profit sale of health care
with ethical arguments'.[28] Insuring that a system of managed care is morally
acceptable depends on public debate and political activity, similar to that
which culminated in the Oregon Plan.[85,86] (See Chapter 18 for a more detailed
discussion of this issue.) This calls for increased responsibility on the part of
patients, who must become informed about policies affecting their health care,
and physicians, who have a duty to educate and advocate for patients. The net
outcome is heightened public awareness about aspects of health policy which

advance or detract from the welfare of individuals and/or society. A growing backlash against managed care in the United States[87,88] has already been translated into legislation which increases portability of health insurance, as well as administrative decisions by MCOs, such as ending the practice of performing a mastectomy as an outpatient procedure. Goals to be pursued in the area of managed mental health care include defining a package of mandatory benefits, insurance reform, protection of confidentiality, and guaranteed support for education and research. The ethical legitimacy of managed mental health care increases as these ends are realized.

References and notes

1. Jellinek, M. and Nurcombe, B.: Two wrongs don't make a right: managed care, mental health, and the marketplace. *Journal of the American Medical Association* **14**:1737–9, 1993.
2. Oss, M. and Krizsy, J.: Industry statistics: psychiatric room rates continue to increase faster than average hospital rates. *Open Minds* **2**:1, Newsletter, 1991.
3. McCue, M. and Clement, J.: Relative performance for for-profit psychiatric hospitals in investor-owned systems and nonprofit psychiatric hospitals. *American Journal of Psychiatry* **150**:77–82, 1992.
4. Kerr, P.: Charter and Texas settle a case. *New York Times* January 1, 1993, D3.
5. Powers, M.: Justice and the market for health insurance. *Kennedy Institute of Ethics Journal* **14**:307–23, 1991.
6. Berk, M., Schur, C., and Cantor, J.: Ability to obtain health care: recent estimates from the Robert Wood Johnson Foundation National Access to Care Study. *Health Affairs* **14**:138-46, 1995.
7. Robins, L. and Regier, D. (eds.): *Psychiatric disorders in America: the epidemiologic catchment area study*. New York, Free Press, 1991.
8. Iglehart, J.: The American health care system: managed care. *New England Journal of Medicine* **327**:742–7, 1992.
9. Geraty, R.: General hospital psychiatry and the new behavioral health care delivery system. *General Hospital Psychiatry* **17**:245–50, 1995.
10. Schlesinger, M., Dorwart, R., and Epstein, S.: Managed care constraints on psychiatrists' hospital practices: bargaining power and professional autonomy. *American Journal of Psychiatry* **153**:256–60, 1996.
11. Tischler, G.: Utilization management and the quality of care. *Hospital and Community Psychiatry* **41**:1099–102, 1990.
12. Hume, D.: *An enquiry concerning the principles of morals,* ed. J. Schneewind. Indianapolis, Hackett, 1983, pp. 13–106.
13. See Scheffler, S. (ed.): *Consequentialism and its critics.* Oxford, Oxford University Press, 1988, pp. 1–13.
14. QALY reasoning rests on defining a year of healthy life expectancy to be worth a value of one, and any less healthy life expectancy to be worth a lesser value. According to this schema health policy that maximizes medical benefits on the basis of a QALY calculus is ultimately founded on three factors: the length of one's life, the quality of one's life, and the comparative costs of medical treatments expressed in monetary units. See Williams, A.: Ethics and efficiency in the provision of health

care, in *Philosophy and medical welfare*, ed. J. Bell and S. Mendus. Cambridge, Cambridge University Press, 1988, pp. 111–26.

15. Eddy illustrates the clinical application of this approach across a population of patients. See Eddy, D.: Principles for making difficult decisions in difficult times. *Journal of the American Medical Association* **271**:1792–7, 1994; Eddy D.: Cost-effectiveness analysis: will it be accepted? *Journal of the American Medical Association* **268**:132–6, 1992; Eddy, D.: Cost-effectiveness analysis: a conversation with my father. *Journal of the American Medical Association* **267**:1669–75, 1992.

16. Harris, J.: QALYfying the value of life. *Journal of Medical Ethics* **13**:117–23, 1987.

17. Harris, J.: More and better justice, in *Philosophy and Medical Welfare*, ed. J. Bell and S. Mendus. Cambridge, Cambridge University Press, 1988, pp. 75–96

18. See Rawls, J.: *A theory of justice*. Cambridge, MA, Harvard University Press, 1971. One of Rawls' fundamental goals in this classic work is to articulate a theory of social justice superior to that of utilitarianism.

19. Lockwood, M.: Quality of life and resource allocation, in *Philosophy and Medical Welfare*, ed. J. Bell and S. Mendus. Cambridge, Cambridge University Press, 1988, pp. 33–55.

20. Daniels, N.: Why saying no to patients in the United States is so hard: cost-containment, justice and provider autonomy. *New England Journal of Medicine* **314**:1380–3, 1986.

21. Broome, J.: Good, fairness, and QALYs, in *Philosophy and medical welfare*, ed. J. Bell and S. Mendus. Cambridge, Cambridge University Press, 1988, pp. 57-73.

22. Boyle, P. and Callahan, D.: Managed care and mental health: the ethical issues. *Health Affairs* **14**:7–22, 1995.

23. Sabin, J.: Caring about patients and caring about money: the American Psychiatric Association Code of Ethics meets managed care. *Behavioral Sciences and the Law* **12**:317–30, 1994.

24. Schlesinger, M.: Ethical issues in policy advocacy. *Health Affairs* **14**:23–9, 1995.

25. Beauchamp, T. and Childress, J.: *Principles of Biomedical Ethics,* 4th edn. New York, Oxford University Press, 1994.

26. American Medical Association, Council on Ethical and Judicial Affairs: ethical issues in managed care. *Journal of the American Medical Association* **273**:330–5, 1995.

27. Morreim, E.: Cost containment: challenging fidelity and justice. *Hastings Center Reports* **18**:20–5, 1988.

28. We're not winning managed care battle. *Psychiatric News* **32**:1. American Psychiatric Association, Washington, DC, 4 July, 1997.

29. Hillman, A., Pauly, M., and Kerstein, J.: How do financial incentives affect physicians' clinical decisions and the financial performance of health maintenance organization? *New England Journal Medicine* **321**:86–92, 1989.

30. Insufficient patient care. *Wall Street Journal* 3 October, 1994, A1.

31. Florida psychiatric clinics sued in alleged health insurance scam. *Washington Post* 14 December, 1996, A6.

32. Wickizer, T., Lessler, D., and Travis, K.: Controlling inpatient psychiatric utilization through managed care. *American Journal of Psychiatry* **153**:339–45, 1996.

33. Sabin, J.: General hospital psychiatry and the ethics of managed care. *General Hospital Psychiatry* **17**:293–8, 1995.

34. Winslade, W.: Confidentiality, in *Encyclopedia of bioethics*, ed. W. Reich. New York, Free Press, 1978, pp. 194–8.

35. *Tarasoff* v *Regents of the University of California.* 529 P.2d 553 (Cal 1974); *551 p. 2d 533 (Cal 1976).*
36. *Jaffe* v *Redmond.* US U20012 (1996).
37. Hall, R.: Social and legal implications of managed care in psychiatry. *Psychosomatics* **35**:150–8, 1994.
38. Lazarus, J. and Sharfstein, S.: Changes in the economic and ethics of health and mental health, in *Review of Psychiatry,* vol. 13, ed. J. Oldham and M. Riba. Washington, DC, American Psychiatric Press, 1994, pp. 389–413.
39. Questions of privacy roil arena of psychotherapy. *New York Times,* 22 May, 1996, A1.
40. Corcoran, K. and Winslade, W.: Eavesdropping on the 50-minute hour: managed mental health care and confidentiality. *Behavioral Sciences and the Law* **12**:351–65, 1994.
41. Green, S.: An argument for a right to mental health care. Masters Thesis, Department of Philosophy, Georgetown University, Washington, DC, December, 1995.
42. Smity-Bell, M. and Winslade, W.: The impact of law on privacy, confidentiality, and privilege in psychotherapeutic relationships. *American Journal of Orthopsychiatry* **64**:180–93, 1994.
43. Gostin, L., Turek-Brezina, J., Powers, M., *et al.*: Privacy and security of personal information in a new health care system. *Journal of the American Medical Association* **270**:2487–93, 1993.
44. Buchanan, A. and Brock, D.: *Deciding for others: the ethics of surrogate decision making.* Cambridge, Cambridge University Press, 1989.
45. Luft, H.: *Health maintenance organizations: dimensions of performance.* New York, John Wiley, 1981.
46. Rogers, W., Wells, K., Meredith, L., *et al.*: Outcomes for adult outpatients with depression under prepaid or fee-for-service financing. *Archives of General Psychiatry* **50**:517–25, 1993.
47. Medicare prohibits gag orders. *Psychiatric News* **32**:1. American Psychiatric Association, Washington, DC, 17 January, 1997.
48. Congress to consider anti-gag legislation. *Psychiatric News* **32**:1. American Psychiatric Association, Washington, DC, 21 March, 1997.
49. Applebaum, P.: Legal liability and managed care. *American Psychologist* **48**:251–7, 1993.
50. Wells K., Hays, R., Burnam, M., *et al.*: Detection of depressive disorder for patients receiving prepaid or fee-for-service care: results from the Medical Outcomes Study. *Journal of the American Medical Association* **262**:3298–302, 1989.
51. Eisenberg, L.: Treating depression and anxiety in the primary care setting. *Health Affairs* **11**:149–56, 1992.
52. McCarthy, P., Gelber, S., and Dugger, D.: Outcome measurement to outcome management: the critical step. *Administration and Policy in Mental Health* **21**:59–68, 1993.
53. Sharfstein, S., Dunn, L., and Kent, J.: The clinical consequences of payment limitations: the experience of a private psychiatric hospital. *Psychiatric Hospital* **19**:63–6, 1988.
54. Van Gelder, D.: Surviving in an era of managed care: lessons from Colorado. *Hospital and Community Psychiatry* **43**:1145–7, 1992.
55. Thompson, J., Burns, B., Goldman, H., and Smith, J.: Initial level of care and clinical status in a managed mental health care program. *Hospital and Community Psychiatry* **43**: 599–607, 1992.

56. Shore, M.: Reinventing the wheel. *Hospital and Community Psychiatry* **43**:205, 1992.
57. Bornstein, D.: Managed care: a means of rationing psychiatric treatment. *Hospital and Community Psychiatry* **41**:1095–8, 1990.
58. Daniels, N.: *Just health care*. Cambridge, Cambridge University Press, 1985.
59. Chodoff, P.: Ethical dimensions of psychotherapy: a personal perspective. *American Journal of Psychotherapy* **50**:298–310, 1996.
60. Sabin, J. and Daniels, N.: Determining 'medical necessity' in mental health practice. *Hastiness Center Report* **24**:5–13, 1994.
61. Wells, K. and Sturm, R.: Care for depression in a changing environment. *Health Affairs* **14**:78–89, 1995.
62. Gabbard, G., Lazar, S., Hornberger, J., and Spiegel, D.: The economic impact of psychotherapy: a review. *American Journal of Psychiatry* **154**:147–55, 1997.
63. Medicaid: states turn to managed care to improve access and control costs. *GAO report to the chairman, subcommittee on oversight and investigations, committee on energy and commerce*, House of Representatives. Washington, DC, General Accounting Office, March, 1993.
64. Lurie, N., Moscovice, I., Finch, M., *et al.*: Does capitation affect the chronic mentally ill? Results from a randomized trial. *Journal of the American Medical Association* **24**:3300–4, 1992.
65. Cole, R., Reed, S., Babigian, H., *et al.*: A mental health capitation program: I. patient outcomes. *Hospital and Community Psychiatry* **45**:1090–6, 1994.
66. Emanuel, E. and Dubler, N.: Preserving the physician-patient relationship in the era of managed care. *Journal of the American Medical Association* **283**:323–9, 1995.
67. Macklin, R.: *Enemies of Patients*. New York, Oxford University Press, 1993.
68. Brock, D.: The ideal of shared decision-making between physicians and patients. *Kennedy Institute Journal of Ethics* **1**:28–47, 1991.
69. Emanuel, E. and Brett, A.: Managed competition and the patient–physician relationship. *New England Journal of Medicine* **320**:1489–91, 1989.
70. Brock, D. and Daniels, N.: Ethical foundations of the Clinton administration's proposed health care system. *Journal of the American Medical Association* **271**:1189–96, 1994.
71. Regier, D., Hirschfeld, R., Goodwin, F., *et al.*: The NIMH depression awareness, recognition and treatment program: structure, aims, and scientific basis. *American Journal of Psychiatry* **145**:1351–7, 1988.
72. Katon, W., Von Korff, M., Lin, E., *et al.*: Distressed high utilizers of medical care: DSM-III-R diagnosis and treatment needs. *General Hospital Psychiatry* **12**:355–62, 1990.
73. Katon, W.: The epidemiolgy of depression in medical care. *International Journal of Psychiatry and Medicine* **17**:93–112, 1987.
74. Tiemans, B., Ormel, J., and Simon, G.: Occurrence, recognition, and outcome of psychological disorders in primary care. *American Journal of Psychiatry* **153**:636–44, 1996.
75. Geraty, R. and Fox, R.: The economic case for the continuum of care, in *Managing care not dollars: the continuum of mental health services*, ed. R. Schreter, S. Sharfstein, and C. Schreter. Washington, DC, American Psychiatric Press, 1997.
76. Schlesinger, M.: On the limits of expanding health care reform: chronic care in prepaid settings. *Milbank Quarterly* **64**:189–215, 1986.
77. Some HMOs now put doctors on a budget for prescription drugs. *Wall Street Journal* 22 May 1997, A1.

78. Chodoff, P.: The responsibility of the psychiatrist to his society, in *Psychiatric ethics*, 2nd edn, ed. S. Bloch and P. Chodoff. Oxford, Oxford University Press, 1991.
79. Meyer, R. and Sotsky, S.: Managed care and the role and training of psychiatrists. *Health Affairs* **14**:65–77, 1995.
80. How large a part should psychotherapy get in training? *Psychiatric News* **32**:4. American Psychiatric Association, Washington, DC 18 July 1997.
81. Melek, S. and Pyenson, B.: *Actuarially determined capitation rates for mental health benefits.* Washington, DC, American Psychiatric Press, 1995.
82. Fox, P. and Wasserman, J.: Academic medical centers and managed care: uneasy partners. *Health Affairs* **12**:85–93, 1993.
83. The Business Week 1000. *Business Week* 27 March 1995, pp. 89–165.
84. Penny-pinching HMOs showed their generosity in executive paychecks. *New York Times* 11 April 1995, D1.
85. Pollack, D., McFarland, B., George, R., *et al.*: Prioritization of mental health services in Oregon. *Milbank Quarterly* **72**: 515–50, 1994.
86. Boyle, P. and Callahan, D.: Minds and hearts: priorities in mental health services. *Hastings Center Report* (Special Supplement) **23**:1–23, 1993.
87. Pioneering state for managed care considers change. *New York Times* 14 July 1997, A1.
88. Shortchanging the psyche. *Newsweek* 25 August 1997, p. 78.

20

The ethics of involuntary treatment and deinstitutionalization

Roger Peele and Paul Chodoff

Are there ever circumstances under which people should be deprived of their liberty and subjected, without their consent, to psychiatric treatment? Subjected to treatment in a regimented setting of strangers? Subjected to treatment that may change their thoughts, moods, behaviors, and attitudes? Subjected to treatment, which, although very beneficial for some, will not be of any help for a few, only partially effective for many, and may even harm some of them permanently?

The manner in which this question, which has philosophical roots in debates about liberty,[1] has been addressed over the past three decades has had a substantial impact on psychiatric practices in the United States and, to a lesser degree, other countries.[2] Until the 1960s, the questions were largely answered by physicians, operating within an ethical context that valued the reduction of human suffering through the provision of treatment, even when treatment was delivered under conditions of allegedly benign paternalism that suspended patient self-determination and autonomy.[3] The 1960s saw the ascendency of individual liberty interests and a degree of tethering of the state's police powers in a variety of social and legal contexts.[1–3] In the United States, this resulted in legislation and court decisions that narrowed the power of medicine, including its role in mandating involuntary treatment, and contributed to a massive deinstitutionalization.[4] These developments led to further questions.

Are there circumstances under which the public bears no responsibility for the welfare of its most vulnerable citizens, the psychiatrically ill? When protecting afflicted individuals or the public from the dangerous consequences of mental illness, is mere physical segregation or containment sufficient, or should the public insist upon treatment that has the power to liberate people from painful and disabling psychiatric illnesses?

These issues, each of which generates protean ethical, legal, and moral questions, have been widely debated over the past several decades. The positions taken have reflected the core values underlying the historical roles, responsibilities, and missions of the several discussants: the health and legal professions, the judiciary, legislatures, the executive branches, law enforcement, accrediting bodies, managed-care organizations, and advocacy organizations. These players were responsible for a multiplicity of values and ethical contexts, sometimes concordant and compatible, but more often not. Even within bodies or groups—health-care providers included—there has not been unanimity regarding priorities, methods, and values—the substrata of ethics.

Thus the debate over involuntary treatment and deinstitutionalization has taken place at the interface of competing values and ethical contexts. Unfortunately, debate and drift threaten to supplant initiative. Now, conditions exist that amount to abandonment of tens of thousands of severely afflicted persons, not because any single player is behaving unethically—each player, it can be argued, is behaving ethically within the context of his unique priorities, methods, and values—but because there has been a diffusion of focus and accountability regarding the treatment needs of the severely psychiatrically ill. The result is the fundamentally ethical question that serves as the primary focus on this chapter. Who should be responsible for the psychiatrically ill and how should psychiatrists maintain their ethical probity as they deal with these complicated questions?

We begin by presenting the values and ethical contexts of the various players involved in the debate, contrasting those from outside with those from within health professions. This done, we will address the major ethical issues of involuntary treatment and deinstitutionalization.

The values of the players

The law

The methods and ethical values of the law and medicine are inherently in conflict:

1. Whereas the goal of the law is to achieve justice through conflict resolution (adversarial process), the goal of medicine is to restore health through consensus[5,6] between patient and doctor. The law assumes that there is a conflict inherent in the pursuit of justice, whereas medicine assumes a consensus inherent in the desire to attain health. For the law, involuntary treatment is primarily a restriction of individual liberty that carries due process burdens (e.g. proper execution of petition for emergency hospitalization, representation by counsel, probable cause, adversarial hearings, burdens of proof, etc.) whereas for most of medicine, involuntary treatment is primarily an effort to bring about restoration of health. Since the 1960s the former view has gained ascendency in the United States.

2. Whereas the law pursues its factual determinations formally, adversarially, and in accordance with rules of evidence, medicine operates informally, cooperatively, and scientifically. For the involuntary treatment process, the procedural values of the law have been superimposed on the way medicine

would prefer to deal with these matters—and discouraged some clinicians from pursuing involuntary treatment because of a distaste for the legal culture and its emphasis on conflict.[5,6]

3. Whereas the law's concern about error is expressed in the sentiment that it is better that ten guilty people go free than that one innocent person be punished, medicine adheres to the position that saving a patient from death is worth an occasional unnecessary hospitalization. Here we have vastly different ethics and principles, illustrating the difficulty in making unequivocal moral judgments in these complex matters. The law perceives hospitalization, or even the giving of medications over a patient's objections, as inherently harmful and undesirable, depriving the patient of liberty/privacy, while medicine perceives these as acts of caregiving likely to benefit the recipient on the road to health.

4. Whereas the law, to preserve the premise of moral agency that underlies determination of culpability (*mens rea*), assumes there is a free will, medicine assumes sufficient determinism to allow predictability. Every therapeutic act involves a prediction as to what the act will produce. A medication, an interpretation of a dream, or placement in an Alcoholics Anonymous (AA) group involves a prediction based upon empirical evidence or upon a concept of illness. A treatment's underlying rationale cannot allow free will at any of its syllogistic junctions, because that would remove predictability and deprive the treatment of its justification. This basic difference in values can color many a conflict about involuntary treatment.

The law has introduced the concept of 'least restrictive setting' as an underlying value.[7,8] This is a negative goal that does not require any positive results for the patient, even tolerates neglect, and is in conflict with the more positive goal of medicine: to reduce suffering and improve functioning. For example, patients disabled by permanent and severe mental illnesses may, from a medical view, be best served in a highly protective setting to attain their greatest day-to-day freedom from the symptoms and consequences of their illness. Given legal values, it is difficult for the courts to endorse this concept of protective asylum, especially for the involuntary patient.

The legislation

While many public representatives desire to pass legislation that will achieve a social good or abolish a social evil, the need to choose among many options often leads to shortchanging the psychiatrically ill because (1) there are few voters among them, and (2) the stigma of mental illness has resulted in social and political disenfranchisement. These are considerable obstacles. The values of the political marketplace contribute to the undervaluing of the needs and interests of the psychiatrically ill, and influence the debates on involuntary treatment.

This limited legislative support brings up its own separate ethical question: Is it justified to take someone's liberty away under the promise he will be helped and then place him in a marginal institution? This is not to say that all public facilities are marginal. Despite inadequate financing, they even attract voluntary patients and do compare favorably with some private hospitals. Even their large size can be an advantage since it can mean more programs and more options for patients. Still, proponents of involuntary hospitalization can be embarrassed by many of the public hospitals to which involuntary patients are sent. To address this issue, the American Psychiatric Association has taken the position that any involuntary patient should only be hospitalized in an accredited hospital.

Considering the low political priority of the mentally ill, it is surprising that legislatures in the United States authorized as much support as they have over the years. Until the 1960s, it was not unusual for a state's largest budget item to be its psychiatric hospitals. When, however, the opportunity to be less responsive arose in the 1960s, legislatures did allocate proportionally less money,[4] particularly in response to the criticism of state hospitals by the civil rights movement. Also in the 1960s, three huge federal programs—SSI, Medicare, and Medicaid—diverted some responsibility from the states to the federal government.

The executive branches

The executive branches share with the legislatures the perceptions that the public is not interested in the needs and welfare of the mentally ill, thus contributing to a lack of initiative on their part. An additional impediment to proactive and creative policy development lies in the nature of bureaucratic systems whose major concern often is to avoid ever being embarrassed by the acts or omissions of a constituent department. A state governor has little hope of being bathed in glory by a mental health department. Often, what leaders most want from their mental health departments is silence, a purpose easier to achieve with a narrow mandate. When homelessness of the psychiatrically ill became such a prominent concern in the 1980s, for example, it was a rare public official who assumed responsibility.

Compounding the executive branch's interest in narrowing their responsibilities is the phenomenon of departmentalization.[9] A government department has limited resources. Therefore, it is easier to attain quality care if the department is accountable for a smaller number of citizens. Further, avoiding mistakes can become a major goal, achieved through narrowing responsibilities.[9] This affects the ethics of involuntary treatment and deinstitutionalization in two ways. First, it motivates departments to avoid serving large numbers of the psychiatrically ill by discouraging involuntary hospitalization. Second, while state public institutions previously had been responsible for all the board, housing, social, vocational, recreational, and health care, including psychiatric treatment of the psychiatric patient in the hospital, the transfer of account-ability to the community sharply confused and fragmented the situation. Restated, when the disabled psychiatric patient moved from the public state mental hospital to the community, the responsibility for that patient, at best, moved from one agency to many: departments of housing, welfare, vocational rehabilitation, recreation, etc., all striving to narrow their accountability, with predictable unfortunate results for discharged patients, many of whom fall between the cracks.

An additional consequence of departmentalization of public accountability is the federal–state–city–county split that leads to further fragmentation of responsibility for the psychiatrically ill. Until the early 1960s, mental health was the state's responsibility. When, in addition to SSI, Medicare, and Medicaid, the federal government began to see itself as a major player through stimulating the roles, via grants, of the counties and cities, often labeled 'communities', the states were seen as the bad guys, who could no longer be entrusted with the care and treatment of the mentally ill. When the federal government changed its tune in 1981 and withdrew, a vacuum in responsibility was created. Today, there is no consensus on who is ultimately responsi-ble—the federal, state, city, or county government, and, even if such responsibility were fixed, it would be split among several agencies.

Police

The values of the police are, of course, those of a government department, but their primary interest in safety makes them eager to get the psychiatrically ill off the street, and, in fact, they are major initiators of psychiatric hospitalization. Seeing the mentally ill as potential harm-doers has made the police eager to narrow the criteria for involuntary hospitalization to dangerousness alone. For example, in the District of Columbia, although dangerousness includes an inability to take care of oneself, the police avoided that interpretation of the law for years in claiming that they were only able to hospitalize the homicidal or the suicidal. Even when they do decide to act, the tendency to limit their efforts can lead the police to criminalize rather than hospitalize the mentally ill person since the latter process can be more time-consuming and feels more foreign to a policeman. The result, the substitution of correctional system justice for the hospital system, contributes to a major ethical problem for psychiatrists.

Accrediting bodies—standard setters

Accrediting bodies in the United States have an important role in the debates on involuntary hospitalization. Advocates of involuntary hospitalization could argue, as has the American Psychiatric Association, that hospitals receiving involuntary patients be accredited to assure that the psychiatrically ill will be well treated in well-functioning facilities. On the other hand, those supporting involuntary hospitalization rarely advance this argument, a possible ethical lapse on their part. In spite of good intentions, accreditation bodies have had difficulty convincing the public or the profession that their requirements are really meaningful. For public hospitals the phenomenon of departmentalization creeps in: it is easier to reach accreditation standards if one has few patients—and no difficult ones. A Georgia governor once said that he could improve his prisons if they would imprison more good inmates. So, in mental health institutions, it is far easier to create good programs if one limits admissions to 'good' patients. The ethical issue is obvious. What has the higher value, an excellent program serving relatively few patients or a more open one with less to offer?

Since the 1980s, accrediting bodies have been emphasizing the need for adequate discharge planning. Thus, they address 'back-door' issues of discharge, but not 'front-door' admissions issues. The death of a hundred psychiatrically ill persons on a city's streets would not affect that city's hospital accreditation status, whereas one suspicious death inside the institution would bring in Joint Commission of Accreditation and Medicare surveyors within weeks for a special look. Accrediting bodies probably need to be part of any debate concerning the involuntary treatment of the psychiatrically ill, but as long as those bodies neglect the responsiveness of an institution to public need, their effects may be harmful.

Managed-care organizations

The values of these organizations, which are the values of corporate culture and the business marketplace, are becoming a major part of health care in the United States. In the case of private patients, their stated primary goal is simple enough: achieve quality care at minimal cost. For the mentally ill, quality care could be defined by such organizations in a manner that serves their business interests, i.e. treatment that is brief, medication-centric, and hospitalization-avoidant. Through the application of restrictive utilization review methodology, this model serves to maximize earnings, arguably a compelling business value. This is not to deny that it may also, with varying degrees of efficacy, serve the mental health treatment needs of the sizeable number of insured not suffering severe and persisting psychiatric illnesses.

In view of their governing profit motive, the care of the 'expensive' patient is a responsibility to be avoided by these organizations. The health maintenance organizations (HMOs) of the 1970s, and some even later, often took the position that they did not provide care for the 'chronically' mentally ill. Since they defined 'chronically' as they wished, they were able to assume limited responsibility for the psychiatrically ill—and thus profit. Involuntary treatment was not an issue in itself as long as they had an 'out' when the patient became expensive. In the 1990s, however, HMOs began to contract for public patients. While sufficient evidence has not yet accumulated to render judgments, one would assume that HMOs will be another force limiting involuntary treatment.

Lay advocacy groups

For most of this century, advocates pressed for improvements in the resources that the states were providing for the psychiatrically ill. Since the 1960s, however, advocacy voices have become discordant. Some groups continue to work for improved services and to support involuntary treatment. Others, in the spirit of the late 1960s, see involuntary treatment as abhorrent in principle and cite examples of abuse.

The major new advocacy group in the United States is the National Alliance for the Mentally Ill (NAMI). NAMI's major focus is on the adequacy of care and treatment. They see the value of involuntary hospitalization and have opposed aspects of deinstitutionalization. NAMI's concern, however, is limited to certain groups of patients, especially people with 'brain diseases', principally schizophrenia and bipolar illnesses, not those suffering from substance dependence and personality disorders.

Ethical issues of involuntary treatment

In this section we will review: the basic ethical issue; the specific arguments against involuntary treatment; the specific counter-arguments in its favor; the differences among the advocates of involuntary treatment; the issue of informed consent; and the issues of abuse.

Basic ethical issues

One of the authors has written:[1]

Each side hurls its thunderbolts of horrible examples at the other. The civil libertarians attack with Donaldsons incarcerated for years without treatment in a gulag of warehouses or 'treated' by powerful drugs with irremediable side effects ... The psychiatrists fire back with the multiple dislocations and misery caused by the fiasco of deinstitutionalization.

Some, among those opposed to involuntary hospitalization under any circumstances, argue that liberty 'is so important a value to society that it transcends other values'. Those favoring involuntary treatment are likely to maintain the utilitarian view that removing or diminishing the barriers that mental illness imposes on the health functioning of their patient is the right thing to do and justifies temporary deprivation of physical liberty.

Specific arguments against involuntary treatment

Specific arguments are held by:

1. Those who maintain that mental illness is a myth, that there are problems in living that deserve counseling and education, but such problems should not be seen as part of medical illness.[10] That being the case, obviously people with these problems should not be subjected to involuntary treatment for a non-existent entity.

2. Those who grant that mental illness exists, but believe that the mentally ill should never be subjected to involuntary treatment. For some of these, involuntary treatment is so horrible that it should never be imposed on anyone. This view is often tied to a more general attitude that psychiatry is misguided at best, evil at worst.

3. Those who argue that mental illness exists and agree that psychiatric treatment can sometimes be humane and effective, but only with the cooperation of the patient, and that coerced treatment cannot be effective.

4. Those who grant that mental illness exists, agree that psychiatric treatment can be humane and effective, and that coerced treatment may benefit the patient, but take the position that society should first work to make psychiatric treatment in clinics and hospitals attractive and accessible before expending any resources on involuntary treatment.[11] Clean, attractive settings, open 24 hours a day with skilled clinicians always available should be provided rather than relying on unattractive, inaccessible centers which most people, ill or not, would find uninviting. This position asserts that the number of those who would 'need' involuntary treatment would shrink if all psychiatric hospitals and clinics were attractive and easily accessible.

Specific counter-arguments in favor of involuntary treatment

In opposition to these arguments, advocates of involuntary treatment believe psychiatric illness exists, that psychiatric treatment can be beneficial, that coercion is often humane and effective, and that attractiveness and accessibility cannot always replace the need for coercion.

The argument that mental illnesses are a myth[10] has become increasingly tenuous over the past three decades with the impact of modern medications and with impressive evidence demonstrating biological factors in the aetiology of psychiatric disorders. As stated above in describing NAMI's position, the argument now is about which mental illnesses society will recognize as 'biological' and thus treat like other medical and surgical diseases. Thus, the Szaszian[10] assertion, at least about the major mental disorders that may necessitate involuntary hospitalization, has become a 'non' issue, outside the area of ethical concern.

Whether coercion has any place in medicine, psychiatric or otherwise, is a key issue. Those arguing the negative view on a purely ideological basis, are ignoring a great deal of evidence to the contrary that coercion plays a major role in human development and effective treatment. 'Coercion, persuasion, suggestions, and direction are legitimate dimensions of both parenting and treatment, but they require careful scrutiny, and their use demands that the clinician be scrupulously reflective' (see ref. 12, p. 2). Hospitalizing a 52-year-old depressed man who is not eating, not sleeping, and contemplating suicide over his strenuous objections, for treatment, is no more immoral, many think, than taking a 16-year-old girl with a temperature of 103 °F and stiff neck to a hospital over her strenuous objections. Psychiatric illness puts some people in a child-like state, thus, incidentally, affording a justification for *parens patriae* criteria for involuntary hospitalization. Despite this persuasive reasoning, there persists an ethical discomfort with ever coercing patients, even more so now that informed consent has become part of the core of medical ethics.

The argument that involuntary treatment can be effective even when coercive is supported by the following lines of evidence (see ref 12, p. 13):

- the successful coercion which commonly takes place in the treatment of children and adolescents, especially in the early stages of treatment;
- the effectiveness of treatment when people are given a choice of prison or treatment;
- the success of threats to one's job if one does not accept treatment, as, for instance, in the case of medical societies and state licensing boards that insist that ill physicians get treatment, the military in threatening to discharge persons who do not agree to treatment, and employers who threaten to fire an alcoholic patient who refuses treatment;
- follow-up studies of patients who, after their involuntary experience, are grateful for having been coerced into treatment.

After reviewing the place of coercion in the treatment of the psychiatrically ill, the Group for Advancement of Psychiatry concluded (ref. 12, pp. 99–101):

As we examined these forced-treatment situations, we found repeatedly that initial coercion can lead to greater freedom ... As we researched and studied the exceptions to the original premise that coercion is antithetical to treatment, we began to view coercion not in terms of presence or absence, but in terms of degree and source ... Voluntary and forced treatments lie on a continuum, with different elements working to strengthen motivation. We believe that optimism in these forced-treatment situations can be justified. We encourage psychiatrists to provide such treatment when appropriate to help the patient progress from a posture of defiance, to compliance, to alliance.

As for the argument that we should first apply our resources to provide an attractive environment so that disturbed people will agree to treatment, before putting any effort into involuntary settings, clinical experience suggests that this is unlikely to be effective with some of the severely mentally ill in whom denial of illness is often so strong that no amount of attractiveness and accessibility is likely to induce compliance. The attractive-and-accessible-use-of-resources concept, although certainly positive, is limited by the inability to talk a person with mania, paranoid schizophrenia, or phencyclidine delerium into treatment.

Even though we believe that Morse's[11] proposal means the abandonment of the most severely mentally ill people to jails and prisons, this does not ethically condone the consigning of severely ill people to unsafe, uncomfortable, and poorly staffed institutions.

In summary, some of the heat about the ethical legitimacy of involuntary treatment of the mentally ill has been cooled by clinical data, leaving the debate now focused on this question: Under what circumstances should involuntary treatment be allowed?

Differences among advocates of involuntary treatment

Although there are a number of complicated formulations, they boil down to two basic views. Both stipulate a diagnosis of mental illness but differ in that one requires a need for treatment, the other the presence or risk of danger-ousness. The former was dominant in the United States from the early part of the nineteenth century until the 1960s. While concerns about abuse arose periodically over those 150 years, they were addressed through increased resort to due process, not through a change in the criterion. Since the 1960s, the dangerousness criterion of involuntary hospitalization increasingly has dominated judicial decisions and legislation. Dangerousness has taken vari-ous forms and patterns of implementation, but basically is defined as the likelihood of harming others or oneself as a result of mental illness. When the former criterion includes an inability to care for oneself, as it often does, the distinction from need for treatment is attenuated. However, even with this expansion, which is not universal, three groups of potential patients are still not reached:

1. Those with mental illnesses that keep the individuals living very marginal existences, but without clear indications that they are putting themselves in harm's way.

2. Those whose mental illnesses make them a public nuisance, irritating but not dangerous. Too often these people are charged and enter the criminal system in the United States. Before the 1960s they would have been subjects for the mental health system.

3. While substance abusers are among those who can benefit greatly from involuntary treatment,[12] they are often excluded from the process that might lead to involuntary treatment of their addiction and often become criminalized.

The focus on dangerousness as the principal or sole determinant for involuntary hospitalization also prevails in other countries, including Austria, Belgium, Germany, Israel, the Netherlands, Northern Ireland, Russia, Taiwan, and Ontario, but this emphasis has been softened by due process procedures.[2] For example, Israel, and New South Wales in Australia, have broadened the dangerousness criteria by allowing involuntary treatment for mentally ill people whose capacity for reality testing or judgment is considerably impaired, or who cause severe mental suffering to others.

However, in spite of these trends towards dangerousness in the above countries, the need-for-treatment criterion is still dominant in most. Some examples from Appelbaum's review:[2]

- *Great Britain*: mental illness and the need to receive treatment necessary for the health and safety of the person;
- *Finland and Denmark*: mental illness and dangerousness, or mentally ill persons who would deteriorate if not treated;
- *Switzerland*: mental illness and detention in the interest of the patient's welfare if necessary personal care is not otherwise guaranteed;
- *Italy*: mental illness and urgent intervention is required, treatment is being refused, and there is no less restrictive alternative;
- *Japan*: mental illness and need of hospitalization;
- *India*: mental illness and a relative or friend and two physicians concur that psychiatric hospitalization is indicated.

One issue of interest, as this century comes to a close, is a reversal of values about 'sexual psychopaths' in the United States. For the first six decades of the twentieth century, many states had sexual psychopathic laws that led to the indefinite involuntary hospitalization of patient with sexual disorders. In the 1960s the objection was raised that one cannot hold these sexual psychopaths in hospital without providing them with psychiatric treatment; the Sexual Psychopaths Laws fell by the wayside or were never enforced. Then, in 1997, Kansas passed a law that called for the indefinite, involuntary hospitalization of dangerous pedophiles. The American Psychiatric Association and other mental health professions spoke out against such laws, but the Supreme Court ruled them not unconstitutional.[13] Why would the profession be opposed? Psychiatrists objected, on ethical grounds, to returning to the role of being *only* custodians and jailers for individuals not suffering from a treatable mental disorder. Also, pragmatically, psychiatrists in the public sector have adopted some of the values of government departments, of which they are a part, in wanting to avoid disastrous mistakes by having to predict the dangerousness of such patients.

Informed consent issues

Informed consent may be becoming the fulcrum on which legal and ethical issues of involuntary treatment are balanced. If the patient, even though psychotic, has the capacity to make rational treatment decisions, is it ethical to force treatment since physicians operate under the ethical obligation to inform the patient fully and not to use coercion. Both of these ramifications deserve comment.

It is not always easy to determine when one has discharged the duty adequately to inform the patient before a decision can be made. Does one inform the patients about all of the two dozen or so antipsychotic agents or only those one prefers to use? Does one list all the side-effects or only the most relevant? Is it really possible to inform adequately about benefit versus harm of treatment? Here, practical considerations may be in conflict with ethical ones.

As to coercion (aspects of which have been previously addressed), it cannot always be avoided with incompetent patients who are unable to consent to necessary treatment. What to do about a patient who consents to treatment but is incompetent? In dealing with this dilemma, some take the position that the ethical clean procedure is first to determine if the patient has the capacity to make the decision. If not, then, in theory, one goes ahead with the commitment process even if the patient 'agrees' to treatment. But many clinicians prefer voluntary to involuntary admission and are not inclined to initiate involuntary procedures when dealing with an incompetent patient who is giving at least lip service to voluntary admission. Legal jurisdiction makes a difference, however. Some judges will not commit a patient who accepts voluntary admission, regardless of how sick he may be. When the patient does not refuse but also does not agree, some states have laws that allow for the admission to hospitals of such 'non-protesting' patients, again raising the ethical question about the bases for involuntary treatment.

It is not always wise to define a question in an ethical context. Sometimes a clinician is better served to frame a question in legal rather than in ethical terms, as in clinical situations where both treatment or non-treatment can have dire consequences; it may be best to move for a guardian or a court to decide, for example, if one has to decide on a risky brain operation for an incompetent patient. A consideration here is that informed consent disputes may end up with the patient and clinicians on the sideline while the lawyers hold center stage.[14]

Abuses of involuntary treatment

Abuses come in two forms. One is involuntary hospitalization of someone who does not meet the criteria, and the other is mistreatment during hospitalization.

The inappropriate use of psychiatric hospitals has been a concern for over a hundred years. In the nineteenth century, a few questionable commitments initiated by relatives were responsible for corrective judicial action. One hears of very few such blatant misuses in the United States today; it is our contention that the ethical pendulum has swung to the other extreme, in the form of legal obstacles to the hospitalization of severely disturbed persons in urgent need of inpatient psychiatric care. In recent decades, inappropriate hospitalization was initiated not by relatives but by governments. This practice in the former USSR was a major issue for psychiatrists and the World Psychiatric Association during the 1970s and 1980s. (See Chapter 4.) Alan Stone, in reviewing the cases of two generals, one Soviet, one American, both seen as paranoid, and involuntarily hospitalized, concluded that in both cases a person expressing vociferous anti-government positions[14] may be seen as mentally ill. In the Soviet Union, during the period in question, such a political dissident who otherwise would have ended up in the criminal system was likely to be hospitalized as mentally ill. It could be claimed that such an action was no different than that of the United States psychiatrist who found Ezra Pound mentally ill and saved from the criminal system, but such miscarriages have been rare in the United States and in the West generally for a number of reasons, particularly due process.

The second concern is a vast one. While *One flew over the cuckoo's nest*[15] is a fictitious nightmare, the less-than-humane care and punishment-as-treatment of both involuntary and voluntary patients remain a concern in many a psychiatric unit.[16] Where to draw the line between treatment as control and punishment as opposed to appropriate therapeutic action is not always clear. The Joint Commission on Accreditation of Healthcare Organizations (JCAHO) in the United States is very sensitive to this concern. JCAHO approval is a positive sign, but such approval cannot assure the elimination of perversion of treatment into punishment.

Consequences of the dangerousness criteria

At first blush, one might attribute the huge increase in homelessness and imprisonment of the psychiatrically ill over the past three decades in the United States to the change in criteria towards exclusive reliance on dangerousness and the consequent decrease in hospital admissions. However, the number of people with mental illness being admitted involuntarily to hospitals in the United States has not decreased.[2] In 1960, Saint Elizabeth's Hospital, in Washington, DC, the main public psychiatric hospital, had about 6000 filled beds and about 1000 admissions a year, mostly involuntary, while in 1997, about 800 beds were occupied although there were more than 2000 admissions a year—again, mostly involuntary. The huge change in bed size is the result, not of fewer admissions, but of a drastic shortening of time spent in hospital.

In Austria, another country in which dangerousness criteria prevail, there was also no change in the rate of involuntary hospitalization.[2] How to explain this phenomenon in the United States and Austria? It appears that judges and juries base decisions about commitment on what they think is best for the person, regardless of formal criteria. As one civil-libertarian attorney complained, 'the jury, in its wisdom, always commits'. After an international review, Appelbaum[2] concluded, 'Insofar as law fails to reflect widely held moral sentiments, it is subject to being moulded in practice to conform more closely to those sentiments'.

One cannot quite say, however, that with the triumph of dangerousness, civil libertarians won the battle in the legislatures and courts but lost the war. The vast changes in hospital censuses and increased homelessness over the past 30 years are a result of other cultural shifts addressed earlier in this chapter. That is not to say that the establishment of the dangerousness criterion has not had an impact. Its influence is felt not only by what has happened in the courtroom, but by the way it has fed into the values of other players discussed at the beginning of this chapter. How these values produced deinstitutionalization is our next question.

Ethical issues inherent in deinstitutionalization

In the early nineteenth century in Europe and the United States, those assuming responsibility for the psychiatrically ill had a vision, embodied in what was called 'moral therapy', that these people suffered from disorders caused by exposure to immoral conditions in the community such as crime, alcoholism, prostitution, gambling, and so forth. It followed that treatment for these unfortunate souls lay in placing them in a setting where moral values predominated, where they would be treated in a kindly fashion, and protected from corrupting influences. It is important to point out that this approach was seen as treatment, not humanism for its own sake. In the first half of the nineteenth century 'moral therapy' was said to have 'cured' the majority of patients, but by the second half these claims were proven exaggerated and moral therapy was abandoned. Hospitals caring for these patients became huge, regimented institutions—not treatment centers. The profession, in an effort to parallel the rest of medicine's scientific progress, became more 'scientific', and adopted the hypothesis that the psychiatrically ill suffered from brain diseases,[16] not from the malignant influences of the community. Since there were no effective treatments for brain diseases, nihilism took over, and the asylum became a snake pit.

The inhuman conditions in these institutions lead to periodic calls for reform from the 1930s through the 1940s,[17] escalating in the 1950s to a call for abolishing the public mental hospital.[18] This new attitude stemmed from a position opposite to the early nineteenth-century view: instead of conceiving the mentally ill as suffering from the corrupting influences of the community, with the cure being placement in institutions with a corrective moral setting, it was held that the mentally ill suffered from the institutional environment itself, from which they should be removed and placed in the warm, welcoming bosom of the community. Medications discovered in the 1950s facilitated this transfer. The number of people in public psychiatric hospitals (550 000 in 1955) had shrunk to less than 90 000 by the mid-1990s. The effectiveness of this new policy in benefiting the mentally ill, however, was never subjected to empirical scrutiny.[19]

The result of these revolutionary changes has been a huge deinstitutionalization and transinstitutionalization of the mentally ill. State hospital populations in the United States have shrunk by more than 400 000 even though the US population has grown by 60 per cent. Many former patients have been transinstitutionalized into nursing homes and prisons, or treated in general hospitals. Four decades ago, a general hospital with a psychiatric unit was rare. Now it is unusual for major general hospitals to be without one. The number of private psychiatric hospital beds has also grown over the past four decades. Yet, all these bed increases have not compensated for the loss of state hospital beds and there are still hundreds of thousands of the psychiatrically ill[4] on the streets of cities all over the country.

Deinstitutionalization has evoked a variety of responses among different segments of our society but seems to have met the approval of many, for example:

- Deinstitutionalization is championed by those mental health professionals who believe that hospitalization leads to dependency, to 'institutionalitis'.[20] Further, even if the clinician does not believe in 'institutionalitis', there are other pressures to keep the hospitalization short, e.g. the desire to do quality work requires limits on the size of the workload. Because modern treatments often can stabilize a patient in weeks, if not days, clinicians can use the dangerousness criterion as a rationale to conclude that the no longer dangerous patient does not require further hospitalization. While discharge to the streets would have been unthinkable three decades ago, the dangerousness criterion can justify the conclusion. 'The patient needs treatment, but we can't hold him because he is not dangerous.'

- Because resources in public hospitals are limited, clinicians may find themselves 'treating the census' rather than treating the patients. On a Friday, for example, the psychiatrist in charge of a ward of 21 beds, 20 of which are filled, and who expects five admissions over the weekend, has little recourse except to review the 20 patients to decide which four can be discharged. 'Lack of dangerousness' is likely to be the deciding factor. It is not unheard of for a mental health professional to complain about the dangerousness criterion and yet to use it to meet census goals. The ethical hazard here is unmistakable as people who have the misfortune of not being dangerous are abandoned to the streets.

- Deinstitutionalization meets the values of the law in their belief that due process is the route to truth, that a very high burden should be placed upon any agent that would deprive a person of liberty, and that a positive goal can be expressed in negative terms, that is a lack of restrictions is equivalent to an increase in liberty. While the courts are quite willing to commit patients, the constraints of judicial due process discourage clinicians, and the 'least restrictive setting' conception provides a rationale to keep hospitalization short. Restated, the irony is that the courts contributed to the domination of dangerousness, but they seem the least interested party in enforcing it.

- Deinstitutionalization meets the values of legislatures in that they allot fewer funds to a population with little political power.

- Deinstitutionalization meets the values of the executive branch and its departments in that they can narrow their responsibilities and do better work in the area for which they are accountable.

- Deinstitutionalization meets the values of hospitals focusing on their accreditation objectives. Too many patients, particularly involuntary ones, jeopardize accreditation.

- Deinstitutionalization meets the values of managed-care organizations to keep their costs down to maintain profitability.

- Deinstitutionalization has the support of antipsychiatry organizations.

It is difficult to estimate how many of the mentally ill have benefited or been harmed by deinstitutionalization, but the numbers in each category are considerable. Tens of thousands of patients are living lives with far greater independence and productivity, and tens of thousands of patients are living barren, dangerous lives on the city's streets. There are also tens of thousands in jails and prisons.[4] In the United States, the largest 'mental health institution' is the Los Angeles County Jail with 2000 mentally ill inmates (personal communication, 1998). Over the past four decades we have moved from a major model of care and treatment to many models. Ethically, the goal to move towards individuality of care and treatment is met by the presence of more options. Any statement, however, that 'the mentally ill need . . .' is suspect because the mentally ill are such a varied group. Even those who believe in hospitals, for example, can cite a success story or two of patients being dragged out of psychiatric hospitals against their will and becoming more independent and productive. If the goal is concern for the individual, blanket statements about what the psychiatrically ill need in terms of care or treatment are not very meaningful.

When considering the ethical principles that should underlie the quest to provide a nation's psychiatrically ill with humane care and effective treatment, the question is not so much 'Whose ethic is right?' but 'Who is to be responsible?' It may be granted that everyone involved in this complicated issue is acting in a manner consistent with their particular values and moral contexts. Can the courts, the legislatures, the governments, the accrediting bodies, or the professions all be required to adjust their values so that the psychiatrically ill receive more humane care and better treatment? Basically, we feel that if one agent is given the primary responsibility, ethical concerns about the various issues we have raised will become more clearly focused. We believe that this role should be undertaken by the state. States operate at the governmental level where all the key contributions to care—psychiatric hospitalization, food, housing, vocational support, and social support—are concentrated, and many states are in a position to provide direction to cities and counties, just as the state does with education.

The ethical debates over the past 30 years have produced a certain level of consensus. There is agreement that the extreme views of the late 1960s and early 1970s in the United States have led far too many of the psychiatrically ill into the streets, into jails, and prisons. But until it is clear who has the burden to assure humane care and effective treatment, this knowledge will have little impact, and discussions about what is the right thing to do will continue to be academic rather than practical.

If empowered, what ethical positions should states adopt? If there is agreement on the simple but important principle that the state is responsible for the psychiatrically ill within its borders, discussion could then move from the legitimacy of involuntary treatment to the broader question of how to reach all the psychiatrically ill in need of humane care and effective treatment and assure that care is humane and treatment is effective. It is within such a framework that differing views about the morality of involuntary hospitalization can continue to move from debate to data. Hopefully, such a process will encourage a consensus benefitting all the concerned participants, especially the severely mentally ill who are now the victims of a fragmented system with no one in firm control.

References

1. Chodoff, P.: Involuntary hospitalization of the mentally ill as a moral issue. *American Journal of Psychiatry* **141**:384–9, 1984.
2. Appelbaum, P. S.: Almost a revolution: an international perspective on involuntary commitment. *Journal of the Academy of Psychiatry and Law* **25**:135–48, 1997.
3. Chodoff, P.: Paternalism vs. autonomy in medicine and psychiatry. *Psychiatric Annals* **13**:318–20, 1983.
4. Torrey, E. F.: *Nowhere to go: the tragic odyssey of the homeless mentally ill*. New York, Harper and Row, 1988.
5. Felder, R. L.: I'm paid to be rude. *New York Times* July 1997, p. 24.
6. Galie, L. P.: An essay on the civil commitment lawyer: or how I learned to hate the adversary system. *Journal of Psychiatry and Law* **6**:71–8, 1968.
7. *Shelton* v. *Tucker*, 374US479, 81SCT257, 5LED2ND 231 (1960).
8. *O'Connor* v. *Donaldson*, 95 S.CT.2486 (U.P.SUP.CT, June 26, 1975).
9. Koontz, H. and O'Donnell, C.: *Principles of management*. New York, McGraw-Hill, 1968, p. 215.

10. Szasz, T. S.: *The myth of mental illness: foundations of a theory of personal conduct.* New York, Dell, 1961.
11. Morse, S. J.: A preference for liberty: a case against involuntary commitment of a mentally disordered. *California Law Review* **70**:54–106, 1982.
12. Group for the advancement of psychiatry: *Focused into treatment: the role of coercion in clinical practices.* Washington DC, American Psychiatric Press, 1994.
13. *Kansas v. Hendrickson*, ST.S.CT. (1997).
14. Stone, A. A.: *Psychiatry and morality.* Washington DC, American Psychiatric Press, 1984.
15. Kesey, K.: *One flew over the cuckoo's nest.* New York, Penguin, 1977.
16. Braslow, J.: *Mental ills, bodily cures.* Berkeley, CA, University of California Press, 1997.
17. Deutsch, A.: *The shame of the states.* New York, Harcourt Brace, 1948.
18. Goffman, E.: *Asylums: essays on the social situation of mental patients and other inmates.* New York, Doubleday, 1967.
19. Wyatt, R. J. and DeRenzo, E. G.: Scienceless to homeless. *Science* **234**:1309, 1986.
20. Barton, R.: *Institutional neurosis.* Bristol, Wright, 1959.

21

The ethics of suicide

David Heyd and Sidney Bloch

The special status of the problem of suicide

Suicide is the most demanding clinical situation psychiatrists have to face. At annual rates of 5000 suicides in England, 2200 in Australia, and 30 000 in the United States for example, and with an alarming increase in males in the 15–30 year age-group since the 1960s,[1] no psychiatrist can deny the gravity of the problem. And as the number of attempted suicides is 10 times the number of fatal suicides, all psychiatrists inevitably deal with suicidal patients and their families.[2] While the incidence makes suicide impossible to ignore, its nature makes it difficult to confront—psychologically and ethically.

Suicide differs in four important respects from other clinical circumstances that involve ethical dilemmas. First, most medical and psychiatric problems are concerned with the adjustment of the right means to a given end that is shared by doctor and patient; suicide however focuses on the end itself, about which the two parties may hold polarly opposite views. The psychiatrist's task extends beyond technically assisting the patient in attaining his own goals; he/she is required to persuade the patient to change his most basic desires and attitude to life.

Second, the conflict between the psychiatrist's values and his patient's goals is deeper than an incidental disagreement. The value of life as an end in itself is not only shared by most people, but also considered the most important value. Accordingly, the phenomenon of suicide is regarded as a threat to our deepest convictions about the 'sanctity of life'.

Third, it is difficult for us to rid ourselves of this sense of threat, because the dilemma of suicide is logically and ethically puzzling. As we shall see, there are problems in justifying the value of life and the alleged moral duty to go on living. Our belief in the obvious value of life is further offended by the relative failure to prevent suicide, either through psychiatric treatment or social engineering; the rate remains constant. And the optimism raised by successful prevention in individual cases is offset by the people under psychiatric care who nevertheless take their own lives. Suicide is disturbingly ubiquitous—across cultures and ages.

Finally, the suicide rate among physicians including psychiatrists is substantially higher than that in the general population.[3] This proneness places them in a vulnerable position when they treat a suicidal patient. In other spheres of treatment the doctor can more readily remain detached. But since the possibility of suicide is considered by almost every human being at some stage this makes it harder for the doctor to take a balanced and objective view.

Beyond these concrete problems facing the clinician, methodological difficulties abound. Although suicide could be thought to be easily definable, a range of definitions and a plethora of synonymous terms pervades the field ('suicide', 'self-killing', 'self-poisoning', 'deliberate self-harm', 'attempted suicide', 'para-suicide', etc.). The fact that suicide is the denial of a value, and not just a physical act of terminating life, makes its definition *value-laden,* that is to say not purely descriptive. The language of suicide reflects this: for example, the lack of a specific Biblical term, Augustine's emotive phrase 'self-murder', the attempt to neutralize the concept by using scientific terms. 'Suicide' itself is a relatively new (seventeenth-century) term whose function was to replace the more incriminatory 'self-homicide'.[4]

On the other hand, ethical analysis cannot ignore scientific theories about the nature of suicide, namely *descriptive* studies of psychiatry, psychology and sociology. Both the way suicide is conceptualized and our approach to the question of the right to intervene depend on these studies, especially on the questions whether suicide is a form of mental illness or a rational choice, and whether it reflects a pure intention to die or a 'cry for help'. Furthermore, the analysis of voluntariness—one condition of suicide—partly depends on our theory of human behaviour, including criteria to distinguish between an impulsive act under conditions of stress and a rational choice based on consideration of alternative courses of action.

This 'circular' nature of definition and theory (the interdependence of descriptive and normative factors) is both theoretically and clinically important; it will become clearer when we cover major views about suicide in Western thought and clinical aspects. In the philosophical discussion we suggest that difficulties in refuting the 'rationality' of suicide are considerable, but leave room for morally justifiable intervention. The ethical basis of intervention is spelled out in pp. 450–8.

The philosophical point of view: the value of life

That life has value, indeed is the greatest value, is taken for granted. Being such an obvious 'good', it requires no justification. Being held as a primary value, it needs no inculcation. Not surprisingly, questioning of life's value is taken by many as a sign of crisis, or even of 'illness'.

Yet, the persistent occurrence of suicide challenges the obviousness of life's value. On the one hand, it proves that the drive to preserve life is not always powerful enough to override other drives. On the other hand, it casts doubt on the possibility of rationally justifying the value of life because it forces us to admit that most people go on living not as a result of a well-grounded conclusion of reasoning. This may not disturb as long as we are not confronted by a person's preference for death over life. Besides the tragedy of death itself, the absence of rational justification is perhaps the main cause of the shattering impression suicide leaves on us. In a more existentialistic vein we can say that the tragedy of suicide is not only the victim's but also that of the survivors, since the act lays bare the absurdity of life. As Camus put it: 'There is but one truly serious philosophical problem and that is suicide. Judging whether life is or is not worth living amounts to answering the fundamental question of philosophy.'[5]

Most cultures have recourse to linguistically powerful tools for expressing the special value of life: the inalienable right to life, respect for life, its sanctity, reverence for life, and its dignity. These terms are typically vague and difficult to unpack, often expressing deep beliefs, fears, and taboos rather than rationally formulated conceptions.[6] But beyond the awesome terminology, the main source of philosophical difficulty in justifying the value of life lies in a symmetry between the choices of life and death. The prolongation of life does not mean the shortening of death, and cutting life short does not imply having more of the other state (death).[7] Therefore, even if we could assign 'values' to life and death they would be incommensurable. How can we compare the state of conscious experience with the complete loss of consciousness and personal identity? We are reminded of the Epicurean argument: we should never fear death or regard it as an evil, because as long as we live it is not with us, and when we die we are not there to suffer it. We have no scale of values, no 'parameter', by which we could choose between existence and non-existence. This perplexity is reflected in the difficulty to conceive one's own death. Indeed, Freud was convinced that we can never imagine ourselves dead, and that if we try, we always remain as spectators.[8]

A possible attempt to avoid the puzzling logical asymmetry of the values of life and death consists in shifting the emphasis from life *as such* to the *good life*. It is often argued that what carries value is the good life—pleasant, happy, honourable, virtuous, and so forth—not sheer biological life. Thus, assuming any scale of values, not only can we compare the value of different lives, but we can also declare certain lives as not worth living at all. This argument underlies the more 'rational' cases of suicide: Saul kills himself to avoid shame; the terminally ill patient opts for voluntary euthanasia to spare herself pain; Socrates refuses to escape from prison and drinks the poison to avoid the immoral life of an outlaw; Captain Oates sees no value in his life if it risks that of his companions; the ideologically driven terrorist blows himself up to promote his cause; and the religious martyr dies in order not to violate divine command. In all these examples, consideration of quality of life rather than the comparative value of life versus death lead to the suicidal conclusion.

The problem of the incommensurability of the values of life and death is circumvented only at the price of introducing other controversial moral or theological values. Ascribing value to life rather than to life of a certain quality has the advantage of universality and independence of subjective belief. More-over, proponents of the quality-of-life theory have to concede that life as such is a necessary condition to the worthwhile life, and therefore has indirect value. These remarks are relevant to our approach to suicidal behaviour because they have far-reaching ethical implications. As we shall see in the section on psychiatric intervention and suicide (pp. 450–8), there are good reasons to prevent a person from committing suicide even if he sincerely believes at a certain moment that his life has lost all value. These reasons appeal to the value of life itself, from which a new meaning might be created. In other words, even if philosophically speaking only the meaningful life is valuable, life should be morally respected and enhanced as the only way to attain that mean-ingfulness.

This last point suggests that the person considering suicide and the psychi-atrist do not share the same outlook. For the person, the question is that of the meaning of life, the subjective assessment of its value *for him*. For those who judge his decision to take his life, the question is whether it is right or wrong to do so, rational or irrational. Thus far we have considered suicide mainly from the point of view of the agent. On this level suicide has no specifically moral meaning because morality is concerned with the rules and guiding principles of 'the game of life', whereas suicide is a decision to opt out of the game. The decision to die lies beyond the reach of moral arguments. But the view of others is the ethical one on which we should focus—by considering the major ethical approaches to suicide in the history of Western thought and then by examining the moral dilemma of those who are in a position of responsibility in the face of a person's intent to kill himself.

Major ethical approaches towards suicide in Western thought

The Biblical approach to suicide is mentioned only as a curious exception and indeed there is no specific term for it. Throughout the Old Testament there are only five cases—Saul, his slave, Samson, Achitofel, and Zimri—and in their stories any moral condemnation (or praise) is conspicuously absent. Death by one's own hand is described as a natural concomitant to another legitimate intention such as avoiding torture by the enemy, loyalty to the King, and wreaking revenge. In the same neutral manner the New Testament describes Judas hanging himself.

Suicide played a more prominent role in Greek and Roman culture. Under certain conditions it was approved, even praised. Aristotle,[9] however, claims that killing oneself is 'contrary to the right rule of life' and unjust to the state; the state consequently is justified in taking punitive measures against the suicidal person and her family. A similar extension of the meaning of suicide can be traced in Socrates'[10] argument that self-annihilation may be viewed as unjust towards some 'person' other than the agent, but it is the gods rather than the state who are wronged. For a person is not the owner but only the custodian of life given to her by the gods.

The Romans considered suicide mainly from the agent's point of view concluding that it was not morally wrong. In Seneca's words, 'mere living is not a good, but living well. Accordingly, the wise man will live as long as he ought, not as long as he can.'[11] Trouble, lack of peace of mind, or a bad turn of fortune are for Seneca sufficient reasons for suicide. Like other Stoics he also values the ultimate exercise of freedom which characterizes our choice of one of the 'many exits' from life. Dying is typically described as a liberating event. In this kind of freedom, says Pliny, we are superior even to the gods. And indeed the incidence of suicide in Imperial Rome was widespread, with no legal sanction against it.

The rise of Christianity as a persecuted religion led to acts of suicide which were justified as martyrdom. The Church responded by banning it formally in the sixth century. St Augustine[12] interpreted the sixth commandment prohibiting murder as applicable to self-killing no less than to the killing of others. Countering the thesis that suicide was a legitimate way of avoiding sin, Augustine states that suicide is itself the gravest sin and wrong under all circumstances (with the exception of a definite command of God as in Samson's case). The most systematic argument against suicide in medieval Christianity is that of Thomas Aquinas (thirteenth century). Thomas[13] presents three reasons:

1. Suicide is a violation of the natural law according to which 'everything naturally keeps itself in being' and which prescribes self-love.
2. It is a violation of the moral law, being an injury to the community of which the suicide is a part.
3. It is a violation of the divine law, which subjects man to God's power and leaves to God the right to take life.

The first reason is self-regarding; the second and third regard others and are typically moral. The second reason is utilitarian, conditioned by the assumption that suicide has bad consequences for society. The first and third reasons are absolutist or deontological, that is to say derived from general rules in an a priori manner. Suicide is declared as a triple sin—against oneself, society, and God.

This condemnation of suicide had a long-range effect on European attitudes. A more tolerant view emerged from the time of the Renaissance (for example in Montaigne and later in the poet John Donne). A liberal position can be found in the writings of the eighteenth-century philosopher, Montesquieu[14] who sharply criticizes the anti-suicide laws in Europe as unjust. No person is obliged to work for society when he has become weary of life, since the relationship between the individual and society is based on reciprocity, and the laws of the state have authority only on those who decide to go on living. The first bold and systematic challenge to Thomas's reasoning came only after half a millennium; the Scottish philosopher David Hume[15] critically considers the three reasons against suicide, although in reverse order to that of Thomas:

1. If God governs the world down to the minutest detail, then suicide must also conform to his laws and not encroach on his power. And if suicide is a disturbance of the natural order, so must be any act of saving life from natural destruction, and this is absurd.

2. Suicide does no harm to society because death absolves man from all duties, which are reciprocal and binding only as long as the individual benefits from society. Indeed, an act of suicide may reduce the burden borne by society and even be laudable.

3. Suicide is not necessarily against the agent's interests. Misery, sickness, and misfortune can make life not worth living. The fact that people commit suicide despite the 'natural horror of death' proves that in some cases it is not unnatural.

Kant,[16] however, tried at about the same time to support the absolute prohibition of suicide using rational argument. He does not appeal to the unnaturalness of the act but to its inherent inconsistency: we cannot attempt to improve our lot by destroying ourselves; suicide is egoistic and therefore self-defeating. We have a duty to ourselves to choose life rather than death. Kant shows by means of his Categorical Imperative that the maxim 'from self-love I make it my principle to shorten my life if its continuance threatens more evil than it promises pleasure' can never become a 'universal law of nature'. This is due to the fact that the function of the feeling of self-love is 'the furtherance of life', and it would contradict itself if it led to its destruction.

Both Hume and Kant, although holding opposite views on suicide, reflect the modern tendency, starting from the Renaissance, to discuss it on a purely moral level, and not as a religious sin. This change allowed on the one hand the introduction of state laws in which suicide and attempted suicide came to be regarded as crimes, and on the other hand also paved the way for a growing interest in their scientific study and a more tolerant approach. In a seventeenth-century study, Robert Burton suggests a clear causal link between depression ('melancholy') and suicide, and interestingly regards it as a mitigating factor in our moral judgement of those persons who are 'mad, beside themselves for the time ... deprived of reason, judgement'.[17] This attempt at scientific understanding was crowned in 1897 by the study of the French sociologist Emil Durkheim. This is a descriptive account of a social phenomenon which avoids value judgement either by way of assumption or conclusion. Although Durkheim uses the terms 'altruistic' and 'egoistic' to characterise suicides of different types, he does not mean to praise or condone the first and to condemn the second. He is merely analysing motives and their relation to social forces.[18] If there are any normative implications, they consist of a criticism of society rather than blame of the individual, who is regarded as a victim of social change or the loss of religious affiliation (what Durkheim called 'anomie').

Developments in psychiatry in the twentieth century contributed to the 'demoralization' of attitudes to suicide. In the light of his belief in a strong life instinct, Freud found the phenomenon of suicide puzzling. In the earlier stages of his theory he claimed that thoughts of suicide are 'murderous impulses against others' turned upon the self.[19] This notion was later supplemented by the concept of the 'death instinct'. Beyond that attempt to explain the dynamics of suicide, psychiatry has sought to develop effective treatment of potential suicides and to care for survivors of bereaved families of completed cases.

Historically, this is a radical shift. Instead of a *post hoc* judgement—whether it is theological, moral, or legal—there is an effort to diagnose and prevent: rather than trying to discourage suicide by means of threat (of worldly or divine punishment), there is an attempt to eradicate its causes. Treating replaces preaching! Like many other phenomena (madness is a good example) suicide has been medicalized. This process has ethical implications as we shall see in the section on psychiatric intervention and suicide and it is by no means agreed that it has created a more humane moral approach. At this stage we may note that in both psychological and sociological attitudes to suicide, the subject is regarded as a victim of external forces or as a patient; he is thus absolved from any moral responsibility for the act.

This more 'liberal' view is not only a function of the rise of medical interest. Our attitude to the value of life and to the valuable life has changed. With the weakening of religious belief scepticism prevails about the possibility of justifying the value of life and about the traditional criteria of the valuable life. According to the Existentialists the meaning of life is derived from a purely subjective choice rather than from any objective norms. More value is placed on autonomy than in previous times, and as—according to many—a woman has a right over her body in the case of abortion, so must we respect the right to opt out of life.

This view is not easily applied to cases in the clinic and is incompatible with views held by most psychiatrists. Moreover, the search for scientific causes of suicide paradoxically leaves us in a more ignorant and psychologically vulnerable state. For it is easier for society to declare an act of suicide as, for example, moral cowardice, virtuous heroism, or mortal sin than to face it as a social or psychological problem. It is therefore not surprising that the law's view of suicide has changed slowly; for example the offence of suicide was abolished in Britain only in 1961.

Finally, modern advances in medicine, particularly in geriatric and oncological treatment that extend the life expectancy of terminal patients, have triggered an intense public debate on the ethics of physician-assisted suicide (PAS). Unlike 'voluntary euthanasia', in which the patient asks the doctor to kill her, in PAS the patient is the direct agent of the act which can accordingly be categorized as suicide. The ethical challenge underlying this practice is especially acute, since PAS is typically sought in circumstances in which suicide appears to be indeed the *rational* solution. 'Death machines', such as the device offered by Dr Kevorkian, have attracted much public attention and drawn opposite responses among both lay people and legal and medical professionals. Starting from the 1970s some societies like Holland, Oregon State, and the Northern Territory in Australia have taken preliminary steps to legalize PAS and some theoreticians regard it as a 'constitutional right' of individuals.[20]

However, legalizing PAS would impose a new and heavy burden on the psychiatrist who will inevitably become the ultimate arbiter of the question whether the strict conditions of a rational suicide are satisfied. The decision, as we have seen, is marred by many difficulties, such as the characterization of autonomy, persistence of intention, quality of life, and authenticity of choice. This would also force the psychiatrist to assume yet another 'judgemental' (rather than therapeutic) role, which to many practitioners contradicts the basic ethos of the profession.[21] In that respect, the reluctance of many psychiatrists to assume responsibility in otherwise justified cases of PAS is reminiscent of the opposition many physicians feel regarding the public expectation that they play the crucial role in active euthanasia.

Clinical aspects

As we suggested above, the clinical view of suicide is a link in the history of its social evaluation. The attempt to strip the concept of moral overtones is reflected in modern definitions, a necessary starting-point to consider clinical aspects. According to Durkheim:

The term suicide is applied to all cases of death resulting directly from a positive or negative act of the victim himself, which he knows will produce this result.[22]

This definition covers cases that we do not ordinarily label 'suicide', such as religious martyrdom, self-sacrifice of soldiers in war, and hunger-strikes as a political protest. Durkheim's definition requires only the agent's *knowledge* of his resulting death and only an indirect causal link with his action. Yet, we usually describe as suicide only cases involving a *wish* to die, carried out *actively* by the agent as the result of a specific *decision*. Beauchamp's[23] definition is useful in the clinicoethical context. A person commits suicide if: she intentionally brings about her own death; others do not coerce her; and death is caused by conditions arranged by the person to bring about her own death.

But philosophers have known only too well how difficult it is to assess intention. As in the doctrine of 'Double Effect', an intentional act may have two effects—one intended, the other unintended, though foreseen. For example termination of pregnancy may result both in saving the woman's life and in the death of the fetus: only the first outcome is desired, whereas the second is seen as a necessary and undesirable means. But we should be careful in applying this distinction between intended result and reluctant acceptance of secondary effects, because direct intentions may lie beyond conscious awareness and intentions explicitly claimed as primary may not be so. For example 'suicidal' intention may lie behind some cases of heavy smoking or drinking, dangerous sports like motor-racing, and heroic altruistic actions. No less clear is the observation that expression of suicidal intent is, in many cases, a cry for help, a wish to gain sympathy, a desire to take revenge, or a hope to be relieved from distress, and so forth. The distinction therefore between direct and oblique intention is not an academic exercise but important to the clinician, who assumes a parallel distinction between overt expression of intention and covert motivating forces. It determines whether a case should be classified as 'suicide' and the ethical criteria to intervene.

Most people label as suicide: active rather than passive acts; egoistic rather than altruistic motivation; a conscious rather than unconscious decision; and action leading to certain death rather than gambling with life. However, the active–passive distinction is criticized as morally and psychologically irrelevant.[24] Durkheim's inclusion of both egoistic and altruistic forms of suicide seems valid psychiatrically, at least in some cases; unconsciously intended death may be more effective in causing death than expressed suicidal intention; finally, the 'suicidal attempt' commonly referred to since the 1990s as 'deliberate self-harm' is no less meaningful a suicidal behaviour than the case of completed suicide, although there are reasons to distinguish between them.[25] Theoretical and clinical studies therefore cast doubt on a view of suicide as only the first sort of case in each of the above pairs. Yet, our moral intuition about the right to intervene in a potentially suicidal act is still based on that natural tendency rather than on sophisticated philosophical and clinical views: we do not usually feel morally bound to intervene in the case of a patient who refuses to comply with treatment (passive suicide), or in an extravagant and 'irrational' act of heroism or hunger-strike (altruistic suicide), in a heavy drinker's life-threatening habit (unconscious suicide), or in a game of Russian roulette ('probable' suicide).

The crucial issue clinically is the relation between suicide and mental illness: is suicide itself a disorder? Is it always associated with mental illness? There are theoretical difficulties in defining both mental illness and suicide, and there are obstacles to empirical research in the form of unreliable sources of information and the methodology used in psychological autopsies (reports of failed suicides, of surviving relatives, of doctors, of coroners, etc.). Then, suicide is linked with other factors such as age, sex, marital status, place of residence, physical condition, family history, social class, and even with 'cosmological' factors such as the season. Methodologically, if we take cases of suicide in a suicide-prone group (elderly men living on their own in big cities), we might end up with different results regarding the weight of mental illness than if we studied another group in a different context.

Despite the complexities, the data are persuasive. Barraclough and his colleagues[26] in their thorough examination of suicide in England found that of 100 cases 93 were judged to be mentally ill by a panel of three psychiatrists, each of whom independently reviewed all the available evidence. A similar level of disorder was found in a noted American study of 134 completed suicides.[27–28]

In the British study patients (64 per cent) were diagnosed as suffering from depressive illness; the next sizeable group were cases of alcoholism (15 per cent). The strong link between suicide and depression has been found by several investigators. In follow-up studies there is a consistent finding that about 15 per cent of people with moderate to severe depression will die by suicide.

Other findings pertinent to this are that: completed suicide is frequently preceded by one or more attempts; the risk is high in patients immediately following discharge from hospital; suicide occurs among inpatients of psychiatric hospitals;[29] most suicides give warning signals; and a sizeable proportion consult their family doctor or psychiatrist in the weeks preceding the act.

These findings support the notion that suicide-proneness can be identified, and predicted with a degree of confidence in individual cases.[30] This is important in the ethics of prevention since it is a well-known principle that we ought to do only what we can do: intervene only when we know we can identify those at risk and stand a good chance of preventing the death.

Prevention can assume various forms. The family doctor's recognition of early signs of serious depression, the Samaritans and other lay organisations' response to crisis,[31] effective psychiatric treatment and social measures to promote emotional health are means to reduce the suicide-rate.[32–36] However, it remains a question whether these measures can prevent suicide in the long run and on a large scale, or whether the basic cause, and hence also cure, lies on a social rather than psychological level.[37]

If we accept that the ability to prevent suicide is feasible and a clear association between suicide and mental illness exists, at least in a proportion of cases, are there still moral grounds to intervene? This may require involuntary hospitalization and forced drug or electroconvulsive treatment, particularly in psychotically depressed patients; it also involves the risk of erroneously imposing treatment on a person who is not in fact contemplating suicide, or on someone who wishes to die but is definitely not mentally ill.

Moreover, as we shall see below, it is by no means obvious whether intervention is justified, even if we assume that suicide virtually always points to mental illness; or that intervention is always wrong, even if suicide is considered as the rational, voluntary act of a 'healthy' person.

The ethics of psychiatric intervention and suicide

For psychiatrists the ethics of suicide centres around the justification of an intervention policy: general prevention of potential suicidal acts and life-saving measures applied to a person who has made an attempt on his life, as well as the potentially new role of the psychiatrist in assisting suicide in special circumstances.

The dilemma of whether to intervene preventively is intensified by the fact that whatever we do, a price must be paid. This dilemma is presented schematically in Table 21.1.

Let us consider four clinical cases to take the issue of intervention further:

Case A

A 65-year-old widower insists on learning the truth about his prognosis. Two years have passed since his first symptoms led to the discovery of cancer of the colon. Now, with widespread secondaries, he is fully aware that the prognosis is grave. He has a few weeks or months left to live. Throughout his life he has been an advocate of voluntary euthanasia, and concludes now that he does not wish to battle futilely; he would rather die 'with dignity' and in his full senses than in excruciating pain which calls for massive

Table 21.1

Intervention	*Non-intervention*
Taking the *patient's* decision as irrational, impulsive, distorted by mental illness.	Take the *patient's* decision as authentic, deliberate, clear-headed, and rational.
On the assumption that her decision is reversible, (that is, she may change her mind about killing herself), certain steps, which are also reversible (for example the psychiatrist ends what appears to be unhelpful treatment), are taken to prolong her life.	On the assumption that her decision is irreversible, (that is, there is no evidence that she will change her mind) no steps are taken, thus irreversibly letting her commit suicide (the psychiatrist takes no action).
Paternalism: forcing the patient to act rationally as an expression of care for her real interests.	Respect for the *patient's* autonomy and liberty to kill herself as to take any other decision, even if it seems irrational to us.
Care for the patient's family, who usually ask for intervention.	Take the *patient's* side rather than that of her family. Priority of her freedom over the family's interests.
The price: forcing her to act against her will, prolongation of her mental and physical misery, serious loss of liberty.	The price: missed opportunities, the infinite loss involved in death, possibility of the most 'tragic mistake'.
Underlying assumption: the instinctive drive to save other people's lives plus the professional duty and practice of doctors to do so.	Underlying assumption: 'nothing in life is as much under the direct jurisdiction of each individual as are her own person and life' (Arthur Schopenhauer)

doses of opiate drugs. He is also steadfast in his conviction that it would be unfair to saddle his only daughter with his problems. He knows he can no longer fend for himself and that his only options are to be hospitalized or to move in with his daughter's family. Both prospects are unacceptable to him. He has always been proud of his self-reliance, and will not easily forgo it now. He talks candidly about his wish to die—through his own hand. His plan is to collect a sufficient number of pills to enable him to die in what he avows to be a decent fashion.

Case B

A 35-year-old married woman and mother of three small children has been feeling utter despair since the tragic death in a domestic fire of her youngest child eight months earlier. During this period, her feeling of loss has increased to the point where she now believes that she must join 'the kiddy in heaven'. She has always been a devout Roman Catholic, now more so than ever. Her belief is strong that the deceased child needs her while the three living children can be cared for by her husband and relatives. She is convinced that she is to blame for the tragedy—she should not have left the child unattended. There is absolutely no point in continuing to live her life when 'Paul needs me'. She tried to hang herself on the day of consultation but her husband, close to breaking point because of his wife's insistence on being reunited with Paul, managed to intercede. He has no doubt that she will kill herself unless help can be provided. On the other hand, as a devout Catholic himself, he can appreciate his wife's wish to 'join Paul in heaven'.

Case C

A 40-year-old housewife and mother of three teenage children presents with apathy, withdrawal, and self-neglect over several weeks. She has lost interest in her family and friends, wakes at about 2 a.m. each morning and cannot return to sleep, and has lost 5 kg in weight. She has developed the unshakeable belief that she is worthless, has let her husband and children down, and deserves to die. She feels quite helpless and sees no future for herself. She suffered a similar episode three years previously for which she was treated as an inpatient with antidepressant medication. She made a good recovery then and had felt content and cheerful until the onset of her present state.

Case D

A 60-year-old retired teacher and mother of two children feels physically unwell and is diagnosed as suffering from the side-effects of long-term treatment with lithium. During the course of her admission to a general hospital to investigate the physical problem she shows features of depressed mood; these become so severe as to require her transfer to a psychiatric unit. There, her pessimism, anergia, insomnia, and more particularly her intense suicidal thoughts, lead to a decision to apply electroconvulsive therapy (ECT). She responds reasonably well but the improvement is short-lived. ECT is resumed, again with evidently good results. Periods of home leave follow, with the anticipation that recovery is almost complete and full discharge imminent. By this time she has spent six months in a hospital. The depression however, soon recurs, this time more severely and also more frustratingly to herself, her family, and the staff. A doubt develops as to whether the condition is treatable. A third course of ECT is instituted, in conjunction with antidepressants. And, because the patient is constantly preoccupied with ways of 'ending it all', her status of voluntary admission is converted into a compulsory one. Not only is this drastic step taken, but also the practice of 'constant observation', even to the point of supervising her toiletries. Immense concern prevails about the patient's safety following her disappearance for 36 hours. Found by the police, she explains how she is 'longing for death' and feels 'utterly desperate'. Yet another course of ECT begins, although the staff feel confused about persevering when after nine months it is obvious that their patient is determined to die. They are all the more bewildered in the face of her repeated requests for advice on how she can accomplish her wish, and her spurning of her family's concern.

Two months later sees a mounting desperation in all the protagonists, culminating in the patient's attempt to asphyxiate herself. Saved from death, she repeatedly expresses the wish to die, but also joins in ward activities and even exhibits a dry humour. Exactly one week later she is discovered in the bathroom with a plastic bag over her head. A determined effort to resuscitate her proves to no avail. The one-year saga is at an end, save for the profound feelings of the bereaved family and of the medical and nursing staff.

One final point needs to be made. The patient had been successfully treated for bouts of depression 32, 26, and 20 years previously, and in the intervening periods had led a reasonably contented life in her various roles of wife, mother, and teacher.

Let us now analyse these four cases.

Case A can be confidently classified as an example of 'rational suicide'. Most doctors would respect the patient's wish 'to die with dignity', although they might find it psychologically (and legally) difficult to cooperate actively in his suicide. No psychiatrist would consider forced hospitalization for such a person. In terms of our scheme, we can assume that the patient's decision to die is deliberate, authentic, and, in all likelihood, irreversible. The family might well be relieved rather than distressed. Forcing him to continue to live means prolongation of despair, pain, and loss of dignity.

Case C is common in practice and characterizes a class of suicides caused by depression. Psychiatrists would suspect that her wish to die is not rational and sincere, but that her thinking has been distorted by reversible causes. Previous treatment proved helpful, and it can be assumed that therapy for the present state might be equally effective. Unlike the widower of case A, whose liberty is to all intents and purposes lost until his natural death if life is forced on him, deprivation of liberty will be temporary and reasonably short. There is much hope of applying therapy which will relieve her sense of helplessness and enable her to see that her interests and those of her family are better served by her continuing to live.

It is case B which is baffling to decide about. Her wish to die can be labelled as irrational only on the grounds of our rejection of her religious convictions. Her suicidal wish is not irrational in being impulsive, lacking deliberation, ambiguous, or distorted by mental illness. Even her close relatives, who stand to 'lose' from her decision, sympathize with her reasoning. On the other hand, the psychologically sensitive observer would ascribe her desperate decision to intense grief over the death of her child, and conclude that her despair can be relieved with treatment. How far should the psychiatrist intervene?

Psychiatric ethics

Case B shows that blend of sound reasoning (at least from the agent's point of view) and non-rational motives; it is a complex which resists disentanglement. The area in the spectrum of cases lying between type-A and type-C is 'grey' and ethically indeterminate; and no recipe for solving the dilemma of intervention can be readily offered. A methodological remark may however prove useful.

There is an asymmetry between the two horns of the dilemma of intervention, because of the irreversibility of the act of suicide, and correspondingly of the decision not to intervene. This source of asymmetry—temporal in nature—is not often considered by philosophers who discuss the ethics of suicide on an abstract level. But it is crucial clinically, such as in case D. The irreversibility of non-intervention places a burden of moral responsibility on the psychiatrist. By contrast, a decision to intervene can always be reversed, if shown to be erroneous. The responsibility for an irreversible act is even more serious because the decision is often taken under conditions of uncertainty: is the suicidal intention final, authentic, rational, and will the person be grateful if saved?

Case D is particularly challenging to the treating psychiatrist in this context, for unlike cases A and C, the issue is not the rationality and authenticity of the suicidal person's *choice*, but rather the chance of success of intervention. The moral dilemma is not whether to force treatment on someone who does not want it, but whether to force treatment on someone who is for all practical purposes, untreatable. If the suicidal condition is indeed incurable, the only point in hospitalizing, that is, detaining, the patient is to compel her to live.

On the basis of our remarks regarding the dependence of the value of life on the idea of a valuable life, we can seriously doubt the legitimacy of compulsion. However, the question whether a condition is untreatable is a matter of professional judgement rather than of moral judgement. And as all clinical judgement is prone to error, the psychiatrist wards off responsibility by continuing to apply treatment despite her belief in its inefficacy. Although this strategy is understandable, we should recognize the vast difference between an heroic effort to save the life of a 'hopeless' case (such as a victim of a serious accident) and the struggle against an 'untreatable' patient with a mental illness set on a suicidal course. The slightest chance of a 'miraculous' cure in the first case justifies the policy of 'never giving up'. A similarly slender chance in the second cannot justify the violation of the patient's autonomy and the creation of distress involved in enforced treatment.

However, in cases such as A, B, and C this responsibility over a potentially irreversible decision under conditions of uncertainty suggests a 'policy of postponement'. We are justified in asking or even forcing potential suicides to reconsider, to give themselves a second chance, or to defer a final decision lest there be changed circumstances. This policy is sounder than non-intervention because intervention itself is reversible. If further study shows that suicide is 'rational' and authentic, or treatment fails to alter the person's frame of mind, or the person persists in his wish to kill himself regardless of change of circumstances—then there is always the option of letting him carry out his intentions. Although there is no good reason to argue that paternalistic regard for the person's interests, and those of his family, is in principle more important than respect for his autonomy and liberty, the reversibility of the decision to intervene makes violation of autonomy less weighty. Only in extreme cases such as a paraplegic who can be technically prevented from killing himself indefinitely, can we question the moral legitimacy of prevention. The freedom to end one's own life remains a basic consolation to human beings. Beyond temporary measures we may take to save life, we must respect this freedom.

Throughout this section the focus has been on the question of the moral justification of *preventing* suicide. Although our remit does not extend to the subject of euthanasia (see Rachels[38] for a clear account of this topic), the controversial issue of the psychiatrist's role to assist or at least abet a patient to commit suicide requires earnest attention. The circumstances of Case D point to the potential relevance of the issue, while the cases of Elizabeth Bouvia and Dr Chabot demonstrate its complexity.

Ms Bouvia, a 26-year-old woman with incapacitating cerebral palsy, declared herself as suicidal on her voluntary admission to the psychiatric service of a Californian general hospital in September 1983. She both refused nourishment and sought a court order preventing the staff from force-feeding her. Her wish to die was the result of a belief that her future prospects were bleak.

The Court ruled in favour of the hospital on the grounds that while Ms Bouvia was competent to decide, the requirement of the common good overrode respect for her autonomy. Concluding that: '... society's interest in preserving life and the medical profession's obligation to do so outweighed her right to self-determination', the judge referred to the 'devastating' effects that assisting suicide would have on other patients and others afflicted with handicaps.[39]

Most commentators concur with the decision (as we do) although arguments differ. For example, Bursztajn *et al.*[40] adopt an empirical approach, namely that 'physical illness alone, *per se*, is rarely a cause of suicidality'. Rather, it is the associated swirl of emotional feelings, especially depression, which clouds judgement. Intervention in the form of a 'therapeutic cooling-off period' (at least six months) provides an opportunity to alleviate or ameliorate the depression. This position resembles our policy of postponement. Bursztajn and his colleagues also contend that the autonomous patient is a myth, and that a person, like Ms Bouvia, who presents to the hospital in a distressed state is likely to be calling for professional help because she is ambivalent about her decision to die.

Alan Stone[41] has criticized this analysis, claiming that the patient's mental state is irrelevant. Following the Bursztajn argument, the Court should have found Bouvia incompetent and forced her doctors to intervene. For Stone, hospitals and doctors are not duty-bound to passively abet the suicide of a patient, competent or incompetent, who is not terminally ill; and, conversely, patients have no right to compel their doctors to participate, even passively, in their suicide. He would wish to dispel a double myth by adding to the original myth of the autonomous patient the one of the 'omniscient and omnipotent psychiatrist'.

A third argument concerns the common good, and comes closest to the gist of the Court's decision in the Bouvia case. Kane[42] has asserted that her plea could not be based merely on an appeal to the right to self-determination. Even if a person should have the freedom to commit suicide, '... it does not follow that the civic community has the responsibility to assist anyone in that act of suicide'. Kane asked rhetorically about the freedom of the doctors, nurses, and hospital staff, if the judge had ordered their collaboration in Ms Bouvia's suicide. Most of them would have been forced to violate their codes of ethics and to act against their conscience. We end up in the dilemma of having to respect the liberty of both the patient and the professional staff. Even if personnel could have been found to assist in the suicide, their collaboration would still have had detrimental effects on the broader community, including the rest of the professional staff, other patients, and society as a whole. In the final analysis, Kane argues for the primacy of the common good, which must override private interest.

Even more ethically intriguing is the Chabot case.[43] In 1991, Dr Boudewijn Chabot, a Dutch psychiatrist, was consulted by a 50-year-old retired social worker, Hilly Bosscher. This consultation was quite extraordinary: Mrs Bosscher wanted Dr Chabot to assist her to commit suicide. Her story was tragic. Three men had played a role in her life: her ex-husband had abused her physically, a feature of his dependency on alcohol, one son had died by his own hand, the other had lost a battle against cancer.

Dr Chabot got to know his patient well over several months and concluded that she was not suffering from any diagnosable psychiatric disorder. Moreover, her contact with reality was consistently intact. Notwithstanding, he recommended antidepressants and psychotherapy. Her response was emphatic: life had no meaning for her, she sought help to achieve a foolproof and painless suicidal death. Having consulted several professional colleagues, Dr Chabot gave his 'patient' a lethal drink in her own home.

The legal repercussions are noteworthy. In view of the significance of the case, the Dutch Supreme Court became involved and ruled that Dr Chabot was guilty of assisting in a suicide, but also concluded that he had adhered to the guidelines on euthanasia and assisted suicide set by the country's Medical Association by judging Mrs Bosscher to be a suitable candidate: she had suffered dreadfully, been mentally competent, and sought to die without any sign of external duress or coercion. Given these circumstances, Dr Chabot was permitted to continue his psychiatric career.

The Chabot case raises new issues in physician-assisted suicide. One factor which usually serves as part of the justification for professional cooperation with suicidal plans (as well as with requests for euthanasia) is the irreversibility of the condition from which the patient is suffering. In the present case the woman is experiencing very intense grief, which can be expected to last for quite some time; yet, it is not necessarily an irreversible (let alone deteriorating) condition, and one cannot judge the woman's situation as 'hopeless'. This by no means implies that there is no rational basis for suicidal choice, since the severe pain of the present may outweigh the prospects of a better future; but it does impose a special ethical constraint on the behaviour of the physician who is expected to take the broad view of the overall and long-term interests of his patients.

Another (related) intriguing element in the Chabot case is the absence of any medically defined syndrome or pathology which is usually the ultimate grounds for the intervention of a physician. Unlike all the cases discussed here, the present one consists of a woman whose pain is not associated in any way with either a physical or a mental *illness*. It is noteworthy that Dr Chabot himself emphasizes in his report that he did not consider himself as a doctor and the woman as a 'patient' in that particular case. But if that is indeed true, it is not clear why of all people should it be the doctor/psychiatrist who should serve as the assistant in the act of suicide? Should not physician-assisted suicides be limited, by their very definition, to circumstances in which the relationship between the two parties is of a 'medical' nature, that is involving the attempt of a professional physician to help a patient suffering from a medically defined syndrome?

One could argue (as often has been argued in the debate over both abortion and euthanasia) that even if the practice of the active causation of death of human beings is under certain conditions morally justified, it should not be the business of physicians, whose primary professional role consists of giving and saving life.[44,45] Psychiatrists, according to this view, should not be expected to serve as 'executioners', mercy killers, sympathetic relievers of intolerable pain. They should cooperate with people's requests for help in suicide only when the basis for these requests is associated with a pathological (non-curable and irreversible) condition. Although many of the warnings of the threat of a 'slippery slope' are overstated it seems that the Chabot case, due to its qualitative distinction from other cases of PAS, calls for particular ethical caution.

All these positions have been associated with the long-standing acceptance by legal jurisdictions that to aid, abet, or counsel suicide is an offence. Thus, the medical profession is legally bound to act in a specific fashion. But the advent in the Netherlands from the mid-1970s of a series of guidelines[46] (although they are not enshrined in law) dealing with the active euthanasia of terminally ill patients is challenging our customary notions. Although these guidelines are confined to terminally ill patients who are afflicted with intolerable pain and other physical symptoms, and who freely, competently and repeatedly request that their lives be ended because of suffering, they do facilitate the assisting of a form of suicide. These circumstances differ in fundamental respects from those obtaining in the psychiatric context dealt with in this chapter, and arguments advanced against assisting a 'psychiatric suicide' are likely to prevail.[47-51] The Chabot case however does constitute a notable precedent.

In turning to the question of suicide within a psychiatric framework, we may conclude by saying the following—that it is better to err on the side of preserving life than on the side of letting it be lost. Although philosophical considerations may show that there is no valid argument to prefer life over death and that our bias for life is irrational, we should remember that the potential suicide may, deep in his heart, harbour that irrational preference.

References

1. Diekstra, R.: The epidemiology of suicide and parasuicide. *Acta Psychiatrica Scandinavica* (Suppl.) **371**:9–20, 1993.
2. Asnis, G., Friedman, T., Sanderson, W., *et al.*: Suicidal behaviours in adult psychiatric outpatients, I: description and prevalence. *American Journal of Psychiatry* **150**:108–12, 1993.
3. Lindeman, S., Laara, E., Hirvonen, J., and Lonnquist, J.: Suicide mortality among medical doctors in Finland: are females more prone to suicide than their male colleagues? *Psychological Medicine* **27**:1219–22, 1997.
4. Daube, D.: The linguistics of suicide. *Philosophy and Public Affairs* **1**:415–17, 1972.
5. Camus, A.: *The myth of Sisyphus*. Harmondsworth, Penguin, 1975, pp. 11–12.
6. For a detailed analysis of the various aspects of the valuation of life, see Kleinig, J. *Valuing life*. Princeton, N.J., Princeton University Press, 1991.
7. Nagel, T.: Death, in *Mortal problems,* ed. J. Rachels. New York, Harper and Row, 1975, p. 403.
8. Freud, S.: *Thoughts on war and death,* Standard Edition. London, Hogarth, 14: 289–90.
9. Aristotle: *Ethica Nicomachea*. Oxford, Oxford University Press, 1925, 1138a.
10. Plato: Phaedo, in *The dialogues of Plato*. Oxford, Clarendon Press, 1953, Vol. 1, 62b–c.
11. Seneca: Epistle 70, in *Epistulae morales,* ed. Loeb. London, Heinemann, 1925, Vol. II.
12. Augustine: *The city of God*. Harmondsworth, Penguin, 1972, Book I, Chapters 17–27.
13. Thomas Aquinas: *Summa Theologica*. New York, Benziger, 1947, II, ii, Q. 64, Art. 5.
14. Montesquieu, Baron de.: *Persian letters,* No. 76. Harmondsworth, Penguin, 1973.
15. Hume, D.: On suicide. In *Essays,* ed. T. H. Green and T. H. Grose. London, Longman, 1882, Vol. 4, pp. 406–14.
16. Kant, I.: Groundwork of the metaphysic of morals, in *The moral law,* ed. J. Paton. London, Hutchinson, 1948, p. 89. Cf *Lectures on ethics*. New York, Harper and Row, 1963, pp. 148–54.

17. Burton, R.: *Anatomy of melancholy*. London, Nonesuch Press, 1925, pp. 224–6.

18. Durkheim, E.: *Suicide*. London, Routledge and Kegan Paul, 1952, Chapter 1.

19. Freud, S.: *Mourning and melancholia,* Standard Edition. London, Hogarth, 1957, 14:239–60.

20. Dworkin, R. *et al.*: Assisted suicide: the philosophers' brief. *New York Review of Books* (March 27, 1997). This is a text, presented as an '*amicus curiae*', to the US Supreme Court by six prominent moral philosophers.

21. Zaubler, T. S. and Sullivan, M. D.: Psychiatry and physician-assisted suicide. *Psychiatric Clinics of North America* **19**:413–27, 1996.

22. Durkheim, E.:*Suicide*. London, Routledge and Kegan Paul, 1952, p. 44.

23. Quoted in Rachels, J.: *The end of life*. Oxford, Oxford University Press, 1986, p. 81.

24. Glover, J.: *Causing death and saving life*. Harmondsworth, Penguin, 1977, pp. 176–81.

25. Bloch, S. and Singh, B.:*Understanding troubled minds*. Melbourne, Melbourne University Press, 1997, pp. 253–65.

26. Barraclough, B., Bunch, L., Nelson, B., and Sainsbury, B.: A hundred cases of suicide: clinical aspects. *British Journal of Psychiatry* **125**:355–73, 1974.

27. Robins, E., Murphy, G.E., Wilkinson, R.H., *et al.*: Some clinical considerations in the prevention of suicide based on a study of 134 successful suicides. *American Journal of Public Health* **49**:888–98, 1959.

28. Robins, E.:*The final months: a study of the lives of 134 persons who committed suicide*. New York, Oxford University Press, 1981.

29. Morgan, H. and Priest, P.: Suicide and other unexpected deaths among psychiatric in-patients. *British Journal of Psychiatry* **158**:369–74, 1991.

30. Martin, G., Rozanes, P., Pearce, C., and Allison, S.: Adolescent suicide, depression and family dysfunction. *Acta Psychiatrica Scandinavica* **92**:336–44, 1995.

31. Bagley, C.: Social policy and the prevention of suicidal behaviour. *British Journal of Social Work* **3**:473–95, 1973.

32. Isometsa, E., Henriksson, M., Hillevi, M., *et al.*: Suicide in major depression. *Acta Psychiatrica Scandinavica* **151**:530–36, 1994.

33. Morgan, H.: Suicide prevention and 'The Health of the Nation'. *Psychiatric Bulletin* **17**:135–36, 1993.

34. Depression and suicide:are they preventable? *Lancet* **340**:700–1, 1992.

35. Garland, A. and Zigler, E.: Adolescent suicide prevention. *American Psychologist* **48**:169–82, 1993.

36. *Support in suicidal crises: the Swedish programme to develop suicide prevention.* Stockholm, National Council for Suicide Prevention, 1996.

37. Dew, M. A., Bromet, E. J., Brent, D., and Greenhouse, J. B.: A quantitative literature review of the effectiveness of suicide prevention centers. *Journal of Consulting and Clinical Psychology* **55**:239–44, 1987.

38. Rachels, J.: *The end of life*. Oxford, Oxford University Press, 1986.

39. *Bouvia* v. *County of Riverside*. No. 159780, Supreme Court, Riverside County, CA, Tr. 1238-1250, 16 December 1983.

40. Bursztajn, H., Gutheil, T. G., Warren, M. J., and Brodsky, A.: Depression, self-love, time and the 'right' to suicide. *General Hospital Psychiatry* **8**:91–5, 1986.

41. Stone, A.: Response to the article 'Depression, self-love, time and the 'right to suicide', by Bursztajn, H. *et al. General Hospital Psychiatry* **8**:97–9, 1986.

42. Kane, F. I.: Keeping Elizabeth Bouvia alive for the public good. *Hastings Center Report* **15**:5–8, 1985.

43. Sheldon, T.: Judges make historic ruling on euthanasia. *British Medical Journal*. **309**:7–8, 1994; Dutch argue that mental torment justifies euthanasia. *British*

Medical Journal **308**:431–2, 1994. Also see: Hendin, H.: Assisted suicide, euthanasia, and suicide prevention: the implications of the Dutch experience. *Suicide and Life-Threatening Behaviour* **25**:193–204, 1995.

44. Battin, M.: Assisted suicide: can we learn from Germany? *Hastings Center Report* **22**:44–9, 1992. (Battin provides an account of the role of the non-medical German Society for Humane Dying in facilitating suicide; founded in 1980, it has some 50 000 members, many of them elderly and terminally ill.)

45. Zaubler, T. and Sullivan, M.: Psychiatry and physician-assisted suicide. *Psychiatric Clinics of North America* **19**:413–27, 1996.

46. Van der Maas, P., Van der Wal, G., Haverkate, I., *et al.*: Euthanasia, physician assisted suicide, and other medical practices involving the end of life in the Netherlands, 1900–1995. *New England Journal of Medicine* **335**:1699–705, 1996.

47. Stone, A.: Psychiatry's undiscovered country. *American Journal of Psychiatry* **151**: 953-955, 1994.

48. Hendin, H. and Klerman, G.: Physician-assisted suicide:the dangers of legalisation. *American Journal of Psychiatry* **150**:143–5, 1993.

49. *Report of the House of Lords Select Committee on medical ethics*. London, HMSO, 1994.

50. Report of the Committee on physician-assisted suicide and euthanasia. *Suicide and Life-Threatening Behaviour* **26**:1–19, 1996 (Supplement).

51. Gostin, L.: Deciding life and death in the courtroom. *Journal of the American Medical Association* **278**:1523–8, 1997.

22

Ethics and psychiatric research

John Wing

Introduction

Changes since the earlier editions

The basic principles of ethics as applied in medicine, and more particularly as they affect psychiatric research, are well established and unlikely to change within the time span of the three editions of this book. However, the context for application has been changing rapidly and codes of practice have become increasingly focused and precise. The field of clinical informatics, in particular, has contributed to a widening of focus. Shared responsibility within the clinical team is accompanied by extended responsibility for the quality, security and proper use of clinical data. This 'bottom-up' responsibility is strengthened and supported by concepts such as clinical audit and evidence-based medicine, which have a strong ethical basis. Both procedures are beginning to be extended to the use of clinical data when used 'top-down', following anonymization and aggregation, for wider public health, administrative, and scientific purposes. The enormously increased power of computers to facilitate these processes has emphasized the need for quality control. Thus, although basic ethical principles have not changed, the contexts in which they are being applied do warrant detailed consideration. For all these reasons, it is necessary to take a broad view of what constitutes the ethics of 'research'. Examples in the following text are chiefly based on UK practice and rules.

The ethical background

In the last chapter of his intellectual autobiography, Karl Popper explained, paraphrasing Wolfgang Köhler, why few scientists care to write about values: 'The reason is simply that so much of the talk about values is hot air'.[1] A value is involved every time a practical and immediate problem has to be solved or a decision made. There is no satisfactory substitute for rational consideration of the pros and cons of each issue. Although we have to evolve general ethical guidelines in order to avoid having to think out the rights and wrongs of every possible alternative before taking everyday decisions, each one must be a matter for individual responsibility, open to challenge and rational argument.

Some famous ethical theorists have rejected this common-sense approach. Comte, who created positivism and Marx, who created dialectical materialism, are prime examples. They thought, though for quite different reasons, that they could forecast, far ahead of events, the way that human society would evolve. Once the predictions had been made, the task of the politician was to ensure a smooth transition towards the inevitable future. The criterion for morality, therefore, was whether an action was or was not likely to bring forward the golden age; the end justified the means.[2]

Plato, who was a historicist of another kind, created a system of ethics that has been much admired; but he was able to propose the establishment of a correctional institution where those with atheistic views would be incarcerated for a period of five years in order to be given appropriate instruction. 'And when the time of their imprisonment has expired, if any of them be of sound mind let him be restored to sane company, but if not, and if he be condemned a second time, let him be punished with death.' The idea that the state should designate what is healthy and what is sick is part of what the author who has brought this platonic equation of insanity and dissent to our notice calls 'social psychiatry'.[3] Although this concept of social psychiatry is unrecognizable to most of those who use the designation[4] it is important to understand the nature of the claims that can be and often are made in their name. One such, now thankfully forgotten, stated that radical social reconstruction, based on freeing the people from 'surplus repression' would solve the ills of Western society.[5] If such theories were to be seriously applied the outcome could not be guaranteed to be more democratic than Plato's *Republic* would have been. Another example of historicist morality applied to psychiatry was the manipulation of medical concepts, in the former Soviet Union and elsewhere, in order to label political dissent as madness.[6]

Robert Neville once made an attempt to look at the recommendations of a modern commission of enquiry into ethical issues through the eyes of a modern equivalent of a seventeenth-century Puritan divine.[7,8] The exercise is not wholly convincing, but the notion that each individual is flawed and in order to achieve grace has to seek the common good rather than his own necessarily incomplete personal fulfilment, is indeed still latent in modern Western societies. Such a sense of responsibility is shown by those who give blood, carry kidney donor cards, or regard it as their duty to take part in research projects if satisfied that the design is likely to lead to a useful advance in knowledge. The potential for such individual responsibility may be underestimated in debates on the ethics of clinical and research practice.

Clinical practice and clinical research

The ethics of clinical research depend almost completely on the ethics of clinical practice. Practice focuses on one patient at a time, but the physician is, and should always be, trying to learn something that will benefit others. Every diagnosis and every prescription for treatment provides an opportunity for an experiment; putting forward and testing a hypothesis. Current methods of treatment depend on experience of past methods. In this sense, research is a normal part of practice and a value to be preserved. Ethical problems are most likely to occur when treatment is based on theories that have been insufficiently tested or, worse, are virtually untestable because they are stated with insufficient clarity and detail. The scientific testing of diagnostic and therapeutic claims is therefore itself a moral imperative.

The reverse side of this coin is that patients whose cognitive ability to understand the issues involved in a proposal (for example, to take medications such as antipsychotics) is limited, need special consideration as to their abilility to give informed consent whether research is involved or not. Such questions will therefore be considered together.

The general agreement that new medications must be tested according to strictly defined principles has no parallel consensus in respect of social or 'community' treatments, which can be firmly adopted without any attempt at thorough examination. The harm that may come through the application of misguided social theories can be as great as any harm that follows the prescription of an untested medication. It can also be more lasting, since such practices can be institutionalized into the structure of a psychiatric service. The 'custodial era' in psychiatry, although redeemed to some extent by examples of very good practice, illustrates how regimens inherent in the concept of the 'total institution' can become generally and uncritically accepted. It is not clear that those lessons have been learned and incorporated into the clinical and social structures that serve what is now called 'care in the community'.[9]

The structure of the chapter

The following text is divided into two major parts. In the first, the controls exercised by legislation and by ethical committees to ensure that research projects follow ethical rules will be examined in three sections: the balance of good and harm to which a patient may be exposed during a formal experiment, what constitutes informed consent to any procedure, and ethical committees. The second part is concerned with the use of routinely collected clinical data for administrative and research purposes. In particular, the ethical problems posed by the widespread use of linked computers, and the consequent issues of security, quality and use or misuse of data, which tend to blur the ethical borderlines between practice and research still further.

The ethics of formal research

The balance of good and harm

The principle of least harm

The central principle in clinical practice is that doctors must not knowingly act against the interests of their patients and must take all reasonable steps to ensure that they do not do so unwittingly. Doctors have to decide, first of all, whether their specific expertise can be applied to any of the problems brought to them by a patient. If one of the problems does seem to be explicable in terms of some medical concept or theory ('diagnosis') they have to weigh the consequences of advising the patient to accept investigation or treatment based on predictions derived from this theory. This means balancing the consequences of giving the advice against those of not giving it, in the light of knowledge that is rarely complete and may be conflicting. This uncertainty is particularly great in psychiatry because disease theories are not as well developed as in other branches of medicine, and also because many of the problems brought by patients arise out of difficulties in everyday life to which disease theories have almost no relevance. Some of the most reasonable criticisms of psychiatric practice have arisen because pseudomedical 'expertise' has been applied to people whose problems were untouched or made worse by it, or because treatments that could be useful for some conditions (physical, psychological or social) were applied indiscriminately, without consideration of potentially harmful effects. The history of medicine is full of examples of ingenious but almost completely false theories about various ills and their treatments. 'One of these ideas was the very simple one of John Brown of Edinburgh, that all ills are either depressions or excitements; to be treated, respectively, with alcohol or opium. His own ills were depressions and he died of the cure.'[10] The more theories are subjected to rigorous testing, the better informed the doctor and the less likely the harm to patients.

Apart from the ethical obligation on any doctor to be as well equipped as possible for clinical practice, no special ethical issue is raised by accidental or unforeseeable damage. In any case, there is provision through the courts for deciding issues of negligence. There are circumstances in which the possibility of doing damage may be accepted by patient and doctor because of the likelihood of a greater good. The amputation of a gangrenous foot is a case in point; by losing the foot the patient may save the rest of the limb. The fact that medication may help to ameliorate symptoms and prevent relapse in schizophrenia is a factor to weigh against the possibility that side-effects may occur if medication is continued in the longer term.

However, psychiatry *is* at the growing point of practice, and the balance between good and harm is not always precisely calculable. As in the case of the first heart transplants, and the first introduction of medication that turned out to be helpful for schizophrenia, the decision should be made by physician and patient together, each trusting the other's judgement after a consideration of the risks and possible benefits. Thus even without the framework of a formal trial, it is wise to assume that every decision to provide a treatment may be, in effect, an experiment. Problems that may arise if this principle is neglected have been discussed in the context of medications for schizophrenia, given the fact that it may be cognitively difficult for some patients, either because of the presence of acute symptoms or of longer term 'negative deficits', to weigh up the issues involved in consent to treatment.[11,12] The issues involved are the same as those that arise in controlled trials (see below).

The balance of risk and benefit

The majority of research projects do not involve any probability of serious harm coming to those involved. There is no risk at all in many projects and a very low risk in most of the rest. Fewer than 5 per cent of projects present more problems than this.[8] Examples of low risk include the collection of a sample of urine (possible embarrassment), taking a single venous sample from an adult (possible bruising), or a transitory headache or feeling of lethargy. However, the situation 'where there is a very remote chance of serious injury or death, analogous to that of travelling as a passenger on public transport'[13] must also be considered. Any benefit to knowledge may be converted into an advantage to the individual patient in the short term. It may also result in longer term benefit because new information about that patient's condition is likely to result from a pooling of results from all those taking part. In practice, benefit 'stands for the combined probabilities and magnitudes of several possible favourable effects'.

A distinction is often drawn between 'therapeutic' and 'non-therapeutic' research, depending on whether or not a patient stands to benefit directly from a proposed intervention. The principles of analysis of risks and benefits considered above also apply to these cases, as does the requirement to obtain informed consent and to preserve confidentiality. But ethical committees would reasonably conclude that the benefit would have to be very substantial to justify more than minimal risk in the case of non-therapeutic research.

The ethics of clinical trials

The British Medical Research Council more than 30 years ago specified principles that should guide medical research workers setting up trials of treatments or methods of prevention that require control groups.[14] The value of controlled designs is that they speed up the acquisition of knowledge concerning the advantages and disadvantages of new methods. The more representative the group of patients selected for the trial, and the more random the allocation to experimental or control groups, the more useful will be the information gained.

As part of an ethical responsibility, research workers must be concerned to ensure that trials are conducted in accordance with strict scientific principles. The design and conduct of research projects has been the subject of much discussion.[15] A poor design means a wasted and unnecessary project. In a recent search for well-conducted quantitative studies of methods for preventing or coping with violent behaviour on acute psychiatric wards there was a dearth of papers presenting an adequate hypothesis-based design, with clear method-olgy and analysis and disinterested discussion and recommendations.[16] But even when the project is satisfactory in these respects it must be asked whether the motivation (excellent in itself) to solve a key problem is compatible with the overriding necessity to assess the balance of good and harm and to inform the patient accordingly. It is not suggested that research workers will knowingly give inaccurate information in order to persuade patients to enter a trial; but the possibility of unconscious bias cannot be discounted. The safest procedure is that the patient's own clinician should not be involved in the research but should act independently in the patient's interest. If this is not possible, for example in a small university department, there should always be an independent clinician who can undertake this important responsibility.

The issues involved in deciding whether and how to obtain 'true consent' are discussed below, but they are nowhere clearer than when procedures are involved that are not of direct benefit to the individual who is asked to take part in the project. The possibility or probability that an investigation will be of benefit to humanity or posterity is no defence in the event of legal proceedings. Nor can an individual consent to be harmed. 'The individual has rights that the law protects and nobody can infringe those rights for the public good.'[14]

Informed consent

How informed is 'informed'?

There is no disagreement with the general rule that people chosen to participate in research projects should be told frankly what the risks and benefits are likely to be and what the purpose of the research is. However, there can be difficulties in the way of obtaining consent or providing sufficient information.

First, it is impossible for a clinician to tell 'everything'; there must be selection. Second, the patient can only rarely be as well informed as the clinician. Even when the patient *is* a clinician, has taken a second opinion, looked up the textbooks, consulted the original papers, obtained the best statistics as to cure rates, side-effects, and so on, there may well still be an understandable need for advice as to the best course of action overall. Most patients would not wish to go to such lengths but would appreciate a statement about 'the aims, methods, anticipated benefits, and potential hazards of the study and the discomfort it might entail'.[17] This raises the third problem: gauging how far the patient can understand an explanation of why a particular treatment or course of action is recommended rather than one of the other options available to the clinician. In the last resort, the matter is one of whether the patient can trust the medical team. That leaves the ethical responsibility for providing appropriate information before seeking consent to take part in an experiment firmly with the doctor.

Is fully informed consent always required?

It can be argued that informing patients of every detail of a trial when asking their consent to take part may occasionally be contraindicated. 'For example, to awaken patients with a possibly fatal illness to the existence of doubts about the effectiveness of treatments may not always be in their best interest; or suspicion may have arisen as to whether a particular treatment has any effect apart from suggestion and it may be necessary to introduce a placebo into part of the trial to determine this.'[14] The *Declaration of Helsinki*[17] states that adequate information must be given about 'the aims, methods, anticipated benefits and potential hazards of the study and the discomforts it may entail'. Freely given informed consent should be documented and the patient can withdraw at any time. However, there is a let-out clause which states: 'If the clinician considers it essential not to obtain informed consent, the specific reasons for this proposal should be stated in the experimental protocol' for submission to an ethics committee. The problems have been discussed in detail in the context of two controlled studies, in which a decision not to seek full consent *was* agreed by local ethical committees. Each paper is followed by a commentary and the issues are discussed in full in an editorial in the same issue of the journal.[18]

In the study of methods of coping with violence referred to earlier,[16] the lack of studies in which methods of restraint and seclusion were evaluated was due in part to the fact that obtaining informed consent was not feasible in the circumstances. Similarly, although the clinician could be blind in a trial of medication for rapid tranquillization, an adequately informed double-blind experiment was out of the question.

It should be understood that such issues do not arise in the vast majority of trials. In general, the underlying principle should be to provide information that will promote the fullest possible understanding of the issues so that patients can make their own balanced judgement whether to participate. Scientific journals have a duty to reject trials that do not meet high standards in this respect.[19,20]

Consent by children

In many countries, children below the age of 18 years are regarded as incompetent to give consent to treatment. Judgments in English courts have modified the situation somewhat, particularly above the age of 16 years, and even below that age if the child is able to understand what is proposed. In such circumstances the consent of parent or guardian is not essential.[21] For example, the child might be away from home or there might be a conflict of interest between parent or child. Nevertheless, it would be very unusual for a doctor to treat a child under 16 years of age without the consent of a parent or guardian, particularly in the case of a clinical trial.

In the case of children who are unable to make valid decisions, the parent's duty to act in the best interests of the child can reasonably be interpreted to mean that the investigator can properly rely on the consent of a parent or guardian. Nevertheless, behavioural refusal by the child should lead to reconsideration by all parties as to whether to proceed.

Other important precautions are that no research should be undertaken on children that can as readily be carried out with adults, and that research should only be concerned with risks or problems that are of relevance to the children taking part.

Consent in the mentally incapacitated

In the case of people who are unable to make valid decisions by reason of severe mental handicap (severe learning disability), mental illness, coma, or dementia there is no provision in English law that allows a proxy to give consent on their behalf. In many countries the *parens patriae* jurisdiction still operates. This originated in the power and duty of the Crown to protect the persons and property of those unable to do so for themselves, including children and 'persons of unsound mind'. It has been superseded by other provisions in English law. Possible ethical problems are illustrated by the case of a severely mentally handicapped woman who had formed a seemingly satisfactory sexual relationship but for whom, in the opinion of her relatives and doctors, pregnancy would be disastrous. Application was made to the High Court for permission to proceed with sterilization. This was granted but, in order to test the law, the case was referred to the Appeal Court and then to the Law Lords. All agreed.

The principle involved is whether the proposed operation would be in the person's best interest. If it was it would be lawful. One of the judges put it particularly clearly, emphasizing 'the importance of not erecting such legal barriers against the provision of medical treatment for incompetents that they are deprived of treatment which competent persons could reasonably expect to receive in similar circumstances. The law must not convert incompetents into second class citizens for the purposes of health care.'[22]

This is helpful in the case of therapeutic research. It may also be helpful in the case of controlled therapeutic trials conducted in order to discover whether a seemingly promising but untested intervention actually does have value for the people involved. The position of non-therapeutic trials, however, is less clear. Suggested safeguards require that there should be:

- no more than minimal risk;
- the research is concerned only with the health problem of the people concerned and cannot be carried out with competent patients;
- those involved do not indicate objection either verbally or behaviourally;
- their relatives agree after being fully informed;
- an Ethical Committee gives its sanction;
- a 'patient's friend' is appointed with the approval of the ethical committee to provide a decision on whether inclusion in the trial should go ahead.

Research in circumstances where consent might not be freely given

When research is proposed with individuals who are under some form of constraint, including for example prisoners, employees, or people detained under Mental Health Act legislation, the necessity for truly informed and free consent is particularly crucial. There should be no hidden pressures, as in the promise of some form of reward from which people who refuse are excluded, no victimization of those who do not participate, and no relaxation of any of the usual ethical procedures. The responsibility of an ethical committee is particularly important in such cases.

Ethical committees

It is fitting that ethical committees should themselves be the subjects of research. In a survey published in 1996,[23] there was substantial variation in almost every aspect of procedure between 24 district research ethics committees responding to identical submissions concerning a multicentre research project into neonatal care. There was differing practice in regard to lay and non-medical participation, in relationship to the examination of purely scientific aspects of the proposal, and in requirements for scrutiny of the application and varied degrees of usefulness in the eventual replies. The Royal College of Psychiatrists[24] and Royal College of Physicians[25] have considered the issues in detail. They favour a broad definition of research, and provide guidance under the headings of risk/benefit, confidentiality, consent, information given, information understood by patients, and problems of patients in special circumstances, such as detained under the Mental Health Act, children, and people without the ability to give informed consent. The issues raised have been dealt with in earlier sections. Guidelines of these kinds, if the opportunity is taken to monitor the practice of committees, offer an opportunity to standardize decision-making, or at least to reduce variation in practice. A useful addition would be a follow-up of any resulting studies to discover how far any guidance had been followed and whether lessons had been learned that would improve the process of scrutiny in future.

Ethics and health services research

Confidentiality

Confidentiality in modern clinical practice

A basic ethical principle in medicine is that doctors should take all reasonable precautions to ensure that private information provided by patients is not disclosed to other parties. This is the duty of confidentiality. Increasingly, however, circumstances arise when such information cannot and should not be used only within the context of the personal patient–doctor relationship. The evidence given on behalf of the British Medical Association to a government Committee on Privacy[26] included the following statement: 'It is no longer practicable to look upon the single physician as the patient's sole confidant in any serious illness and it is assumed by public and profession alike that any

Psychiatric ethics

contact with the complex medical machinery of today implies acquiescence in some degree of extended confidence.' This concept of extended confidence is essential to a discussion of privacy.

It is taken for granted that immediate members of a clinical team must have access to confidential information and that they must not abuse this trust. In Britain, doctors would be responsible to the General Medical Council if a lapse occurred. But doctors and nurses and other staff must share information to various degrees and often have easy access to each other's case records. How much is disclosed to the patient involves issues briefly discussed above in the context of consent for treatment. The implied bond of trust between patient and doctor (and, on a wider scale, between the public and the medical profession) is based on an assumption that doctors' actions are intended to be beneficial and that no harm will come from them. These actions include the passing of confidential information to other people who will in turn act with the same responsibility. Specific permission from patients cannot be sought every time private information is transferred.

Even if it were possible for a patient to give blanket permission for all such acts of transfer of information, the agreement would not protect the doctor from legal action if harm should result. A patient cannot, in law, consent to be damaged. The question therefore becomes one, not of whether but of how far, a doctor can reasonably pass on private information without asking permission. The most likely source of a leak to unauthorized persons is a lack of security in the clinical records system. Attention at this level is probably as important as at any other. However, public concern has mainly been aroused by the possibility of unauthorized access to medical information systems with a facility for computer linking. Data are routinely collected, analysed and used for managerial and administrative purposes. In ordinary clinical practice the chief ethical issues have to do with anonymity, quality, adequacy of analysis and integrity of use of data. Increasingly, however, the same data can be used for research purposes as well. Indeed, a strong case can be made that routine data *should* be used in this way. There are two main categories of use of medical records for research purposes:

- small projects in which information is collected directly from patients and augmented by access to medical records and death or birth or other registers;
- moderately sized data-collection systems that require an *ad hoc* register to be set up.

Small-scale research projects

In small-scale projects the main problem is likely to be carelessness. Documents might be left lying around and seen by unauthorized people. However, a well-trained research group would not be likely to be so slapdash, and it is routine practice for applicants to ethical committees to spell out their procedures for ensuring the confidentiality of the data collected, in line with the strict rules of the British Data Protection Act. Larger scale collaborative projects, in which information about identified individuals is collected at or from a number of centres, pose more complicated problems but the precautions taken locally should be the same:

- security of the name–number list;
- restriction of access to specified people;
- licence by an ethical committee;
- statement of how long the data will be stored after the project ends;
- what will then happen to the archive.

It should not be necessary to hold names or other identifiable information on such a computer file.

Local research registers

The early case registers were set up principally for research purposes.[27] There has been little complaint about this kind of use. Confidentiality and security have been good. Most are now thoroughly computerized. It is necessary to collect identifying data, such as name, address, date of birth, etc., for two kinds of reason. First, these items are needed to link records from different agencies on different occasions so that cohort studies can be undertaken and individual patients tracked for clinical purposes. Thus, for example, it is possible to make the vital distinction between person and event statistics; e.g. between one person being in hospital ten times during a given period and ten people being in hospital once. Without this, statistics of first admissions to psychiatric hospitals, the raw data required for epidemiological and administrative purposes, could not be produced. Second, the register can be used as a sampling frame for more detailed epidemiological studies, such as a survey in contrasting districts of the outcome of a particular disorder. Background information from the registers would also allow confounding factors to be eliminated.

Such systems have in common that the more complex and long-lasting they are the more difficult it is to get informed consent for each item of data collected. What clinicians and informed patients (including potential patients) will be concerned with, therefore, is the likelihood of public benefit accruing from each transfer of information balanced against the possibility of harm to the patient.

National and regional registers

More recently, psychiatric case registers under local control have been developed in most Western countries for clinical and administrative rather than, or as well as, research purposes. It is now almost routine to collect electronically the core working information needed to record a patient's medical progress throughout a spell of care, to link that record to other spells of care that the patient has had or will have, and to store these records with those of other patients. It is possible to distinguish between clinical, administrative, and research uses of such records but the basic ethical implications are similar for all three.[28,29]

When used by mental health teams purely for local clinical purposes, without data linkage to other systems, they are unlikely to give rise to new problems, though the discipline imposed on research teams is more difficult to impose in the clinical than in the research setting. The boundaries between the two tend to become blurred because such registers can be, and if of sufficiently good quality probably should be, used for local research purposes as well. However, the potential for linking means that a distinction between local and large-scale regional and national registers is becoming blurred.

Privacy regulations: unduly restrictive or reasonably helpful?

During the 1980s there was a clear perception among many epidemiologists that restrictive regulations, requiring the explicit consent of individual patients before information from their records could be used, were making the scientific use of data from case registers difficult or impossible. Examples given in the second edition of this book included:

- complaints by Swedish epidemiologists that research was made tedious, time-consuming, and ineffective by imposed regulations;[30]
- access to records had been severely curtailed by the US Privacy Act of 1974 and the Family Educational Act of the same year;[31]
- the data protection laws had had a devastating effect on research in Iceland;[32]
- closure of the Mannheim register followed the law introduced in Baden-Wurtemberg.[33]

The British Data Protection Act[34] has worked reasonably well without attracting similar criticisms from research workers. The Act provides for the creation of a public register of data-users supervised by a Data Protection Registrar and Tribunal. All data-users holding personal data are required to:

- state the purpose of their registers;
- give details of the data-sets held and their sources;
- ensure security;
- allow individuals the right to access and correct them;
- provide a list of everyone to whom named data are disclosed.

Once registered, no other kind of purpose, data-set, or disclosure is allowed without further permission.

The rights of a 'data-subject' to see a copy of any personal record and to receive compensation if any damage is incurred are set out in detail. Certain limitations are placed on the rights of access to personal data concerning physical or mental health, and on data held only for the purpose of preparing statistics or carrying out research. Sensibly applied, the Act and Code of Practice appear to provide adequate safeguards for personal information without unduly impeding epidemiological research. The code is consistent with the statement by the Medical Research Council[14] and preserves a base for research that is fully compatible with human rights.

The main criticism until recently has come from patients who found difficulty accessing their own personal information, particularly comments written about them. These are dealt with in the last resort by the registrar. However, safeguarding the interests of patients whose data are included on computerized registers requires consideration of a wider range of issues. Interestingly, techniques familiar to epidemiologists can be used to avoid some of these problems.

Ensuring the integrity of data

Based on the experience of administering the provisions of the Data Protection Act, the Department of Health has issued guidance on the way that information must be protected and handled within the National Health Service.[35] This covers:

- basic principles governing the use of patient information;
- telling patients why information is needed, how it is used, and their own rights of access to it;
- the safeguarding of information required for NHS and related purposes;
- the circumstances in which information may be passed on for other purposes or as a legal requirement.

More detailed guidance is obtainable on topics such as security measures, public health issues, coordination with other agencies, and legal matters.

The threat to the privacy of data in automated systems stems largely from their increased efficiency in retrieving patient information. Within the relatively new conditions of the 'internal market' problems have arisen whereby, for example, a bill for an identified patient can be sent by a provider to a purchaser, thus bypassing the ethical responsibility of the clinician. 'The creation of standards to which all individuals involved in the storage, retrieval, manipulation and transfer of patient information can adhere, is thus of paramount importance.'[29] The issues involve not only confidentiality but the quality of the information recorded, its security (including all aspects of access), and the integrity of the uses to which it is put.

An example of the issues now arising for research, for practice, and for administration is provided by the construction of the Health of the Nation Outcome Scales (HoNOS).[36] An instrument was commissioned that could be used to evaluate progress towards the achievement of a target set by the

Department of Health: 'to improve significantly the health and social functioning of mentally ill people'. This remit required a new instrument with the
following characteristics:

- short, easy to use and repeat
- acceptable to clinicians (mostly nurses)
- adequate cover of symptoms and social functioning
- able to measure change or the lack of it
- known reliability and relationship to more established scales
- one or two derived indicators for administrative and epidemiological
  purposes, and for measuring success against a national target.

   Over a period of two and a half years, four successive versions were created
and thoroughly tested and the final instrument was accepted by the Department for wide field testing within the NHS. A further intention from the
beginning had been to use HoNOS as a central clinical component in a
minimum data-set, also for eventual routine use.[37]
   The lessons learned from the exercise to date have illuminated several problems, clinical, technical, and administrative, about the use of data in a modern
health service. The first is that clinicians must be trained to collect data if
accuracy and comparability are to be assured; also that this training must be
maintained over time by skilled supervisors. The second is that data must be
anonymized before being made available for use by providers and purchasers.
The third is that data should be aggregated for use in planning and administration.
   Ensuring the integrity of data in these ways also provides a mechanism for
monitoring and preventing perverse incentives and misuse of data. Such quality
control is a public health function and it is also an ethical one. Careful
attention to detail in order to ensure high-quality data, collected for specified
purposes, analysed efficiently, and used in accordance with ethical guidelines, is
easier to achieve with dedicated research registers. But similar monitored
standards should now be the aim of the routine data collection systems
required by modern health services.

Conclusions

Research committees are now well established and have had long experience
of the problems that can arise when vetting applications. New issues are
constantly coming to attention but the principles considered in this chapter can
usually be applied in order to reach a conclusion. There are exceptions. Even
a familiar issue, such as the necessity to obtain full consent by a patient to
participate in a controlled trial, can occasionally present a new facet for
consideration and controversy, as discussed above.[18]

Another issue, broad enough to cover most of the chapters in this volume, should be mentioned; that is the participation of consumers. This is gradually being transformed from a paper or token presence at an occasional meeting to full membership of working committees.[38] For example, the guideline on violence mentioned earlier[16] has a service user as full member and groups of users and carers have been convened in order to put forward their own comments, which are published as appendices to the report.

Perhaps the chief challenge to medical ethics today is the near-universal use of electronic data-linkage. While case registers were relatively small, and run for specific purposes by dedicated research workers, criticism was relatively mild. Ethical standards were fairly easy to apply and maintain. Nowadays, the collection of personal data is so simple, and the facilities for transfer so freely available, that control of accuracy, access, transfer, and use has become very complicated. These are predominantly matters for health service clinicians and managers, but the way they are handled will also affect the use of data for research purposes. A key figure should be explicitly responsible for the integrity of data; for example the physician in charge of public health issues in each health district. If this can be guaranteed the opportunities for epidemiological and health services research are tremendous.

Karl Popper's comment on personal responsibility for one's ethical decisions applies perfectly to clinicians in their role as researchers: 'the responsibility for our ethical decisions is entirely ours and can be shifted on to nobody else; neither to God, nor to nature, nor to society, nor to history. Whatever authority we may accept it is we who accept it. We only deceive ourselves if we do not realize this simple point.'[39]

References

1. Popper, K.: *Unended quest: an intellectual autobiography.* Glasgow, Fontana/Collins, 1976, p. 193.
2. Wing, J. K.: *Reasoning about madness.* London, Oxford University Press, 1978, pp. 5–7.
3. Simon, B.: *Mind and madness in ancient Greece: the classical roots of modern psychiatry.* Ithaca, Cornell University Press, 1978, p. 187.
4. Wing, J. K.: Social psychiatry, in *Social psychiatry: Theory, methodology and practice*, ed. P. E. Bebbington. New Brunswick, Transaction, 1978, pp. 3–22.
5. Marcuse, H.: *Negations: Essays in critical theory.* Harmondsworth, Penguin, 1968.
6. Wing, J. K.: Psychiatry and political dissent, in *Reasoning about madness.* Oxford, Oxford University Press, 1978, pp. 167–93.
7. Neville, R.: On the national commission: a Puritan critique of consensus ethics. *Hastings Center Report*, April 1979, p. 22.
8. National Commission for the Protection of Human Subjects of Biomedical and Behavior Research: *Report and recommendations.* Bethesda, Department of Health, Education and Welfare, Publication No. (OS) 78-006, 1978.
9. Wing, J. K. and Brown, G. W.: *Institutionalism and schizophrenia.* London, Cambridge University Press, 1970, pp. 189–94.

10. Pledge, H. T.: *Science since 1500*. London, H.M.S.O., 1939, p. 100.
11. Jones, G. H.: Informed consent in chronic schizophrenia? *British Journal of Psychiatry* **167**:565–8, 1995.
12. Brabbins, C.,Butler, J. and Bentall, R.: Consent to neuroleptic medication for schizophrenia: clinical ethical and legal issues. *British Journal of Psychiatry* **168**:540–4, 1996.
13. *Research on patients*. London, Royal College of Physicians, 1989.
14. Medical Research Council: *Responsibility in investigations on human subjects*. Cmnd. 2382. London, HMSO, 1962–63.
15. Lieberman, J. A.: Ethical dilemmas in clinical research with human subjects. An investigator's perspective. *Psychopharmacology Bulletin* **32**:19–25, 1996.
16. *The management of imminent violence in clinical settings. A clinical practice guideline*. London, Royal College of Psychiatrists, 1998.
17. Declaration of Helsinki. *British Medical Journal* **313**:1448–9, 1996.
18. Informed consent: the intricacies. *British Medical Journal* **314**:1059–60, 1997.
19. Amdur, R. J. and Biddle, C.: Institutional review board approval and publication of human research results. *Journal of the American Medical Association* **277**:909–14, 1997.
20. Rennie, D. and Yank, V.: Disclosure to the reader of institutional review board approval and informed consent. *Journal of the American Medical Association* **277**:922–3, 1997.
21. *Gillick* v. *West Norfolk and Wisbech Area Health Authority* and the Department of Health and Social Security: House of Lords, 1985 3 All ER 402.
22. Judgment re *'F'*: Court of Appeal (Civil Division): 3 February 1989.
23. Redshaw, M. E., Harris, A., and Baum, J. D.: Research ethics committee audit; differences between committees. *Journal of Medical Ethics* **22**:78–82, 1996.
24. Royal College of Psychiatrists: Guidelines for research ethics committees on psychiatric research involving human subjects. *Psychiatric Bulletin* **14**:48–61, 1990.
25. *Guidelines on the practice of ethical committees in research involving human subjects*. London, Royal College of Physicians, 1990.
26. Home Office: *Computers and privacy*. Cmnd. 6353. London, HMSO, 1975.
27. Wing, J. K. and Hailey, A., M. (ed.): *Evaluating a community psychiatric service, the Camberwell Register 1964–1971*. Oxford, Oxford University Press, 1972.
28. Baldwin, J., A., Leff, J. and Wing, J., K.: Confidentiality of psychiatric data in medical information systems. *British Journal of Psychiatry* **128**:417–27, 1976.
29. Andrews, G. and Morris-Yates A.: The ethical implications of the electronic storage of electronic data, in *Computers in mental health*, ed. T. Üstün, G. Andrews, H. Dilling, and M. Briscoe. Geneva, WHO, 1994, pp. 129–35.
30. Vuori, H: Privacy, confidentiality and automated health information systems. *Journal of Medical Ethics* **3**:174–8, 1977.
31. *Privacy Protection Study Commission: Personal privacy in an information society*. Washington DC, US Government Printing Office, 1977.
32. Helgason T.: Data protection and problems of data confidentiality. The Icelandic experience, in *Psychiatric case registers in public health*, ed. G. ten Horn, R. Giel, W. Gulbinat, and J. Henderson. Amsterdam, Elsevier, 1986, pp. 372–5.
33. Häfner, H. and Pfeiffer-Kurda, M.: The impact of data protection laws on the Mannheim case register, in *Psychiatric case registers in public health*, ed. G. ten Horn, R. Giel, W. Gulbinat, and J. Henderson. Amsterdam, Elsevier, 1986, pp. 366–71.
34. *Data Protection Act*. London, HMSO, 1984.

35. *The protection and use of patient information.* London, Department of Health, 1996.
36. Wing, J. K., Beevor, A. S., Curtis, R. H., Park S. P. G., Hadden S., and Burns, A.: HoNOS. Health of the Nation Outcome Scales. Research and development. *British Journal of Psychiatry* **172**:11–18, 1998.
37. Glover, G.: The public health perspective, in *Measurement for mental health*, ed. J. Wing. London, Royal College of Psychiatrists Research Unit, 1995, pp. 71–80.
38. Liberati, A.: Consumer participation in research and health care. Making it a reality. *British Medical Journal* **315**:499, 1997.
39. Popper, K. R.: *The open society and its enemies*, vol. 1. London, Routledge, 1945, p. 62.

23

Ethics and psychiatric genetics

Anne Farmer and Peter McGuffin

Introduction

Although now often viewed as one of the most exciting and rapidly expanding areas of psychiatric research, with real potential for biological understanding and therapeutic advance,[1] psychiatric genetics has had a difficult and often controversial history. It came into being at the beginning of the twentieth century when the development of a workable psychiatric classification scheme, largely due to Kraepelin, coincided with the rediscovery of Mendel's Laws. These had been ignored for over 30 years after they were first put forward in 1866, but their rediscovery signalled the birth of a new branch of science which in 1905 Bateson called 'genetics'. However, psychiatric genetics had become decidedly unfashionable by the third quarter of the twentieth century and was not much talked about except in a few eccentric enclaves until regaining popular academic footing again in the last quarter of this century. This renaissance of interest in psychiatric genetics has coincided with the rapid expansion of human molecular genetic research and its widespread influence on medicine as a whole. At the same time concern about ethical aspects of genetic research has been a major interest for a flourishing 'bioethics industry'.[2]

Studies of normal or abnormal behaviour form a comparatively small portion of the total global investment of money and manpower in genetic research, but they have thrown up more than their share of ethical concern and debate. Consequently genetic research to do with behaviour must be seen as one of the main catalysts in the recent growth of bioethics as an academic discipline. In this chapter we will first describe and consider the current state of the 'bioethics industry' and then take a brief look at the history of psychiatric genetics and its 'ugly sister'—eugenics. We will then describe current ethical issues in research and those deriving from psychiatric genetics in future clinical practice.

Dolly, ELSI and the rise of bioethics

It is now not uncommon for advances in genetic research to feature in newspaper headlines. A striking example was the media response to a paper published in *Nature* by Wilmut *et al.* on the 27th February 1997 giving an account of 'viable offspring derived from fetal and adult mammalian cells'. The story of 'Dolly' the first cloned lamb, the work of a Medical Research Council-funded group in Edinburgh, made front page news nationally in the UK and internationally. Indeed the initial press reports based upon a media release were on the newsstands before most scientists had seen copies of the scientific account in *Nature*. Initial reporting emphasized the landmark significance of the scientific breakthrough, e.g. 'In the past few days we have been through a change in our condition as momentous as the Copernican revolution or the splitting of the atom'.[4] Subsequently however, the possibility of human cloning inevitably provoked some journalists to mix fantasy, artistic licence and scientific fact: 'Clone cologne—for men who want to smell like themselves'.[5] On the whole, press accounts particularly in the serious 'broadsheets', attempted to allay public concerns 'Cloning provides an opportunity not a threat'[6] but suggested that scientific advances had already left ethical considerations lagging behind: 'Dolly's already here—ethics will have to cope'.[7]

Thus in a few short days a technological advance had captured the public imagination in a sensational and, for some, shocking and frightening way. What was now abundantly clear was that the debate about ethical aspects of genetic research was firmly in the public arena. The debate about ethics and genetics had of course already been going on for some years, albeit often behind the closed doors of the laboratory or the seminar room, but the emergence of the debate into more public areas had already happened before the birth of Dolly in the United Kingdom. It occurred with the birth of ELSI in the United States nine years earlier.

In October 1988, the director of the United States National Institutes of Health component of the human genome project, Nobel Laureate James D. Watson, announced that 3 per cent of his budget would be devoted to supporting a program of research and discussion on the ethical, legal, and social implications (ELSI) of new genetic knowledge. This meant that in the first year of its existence the ELSI program had a budget of around 1.5 million US dollars. In subsequent years this increased to 5 per cent of the total US human genome project spend, so that by 1996 the annual ELSI budget was approximately 7 million dollars. This makes ELSI by far the largest single source of funding of activities in ethics in the world.[8] The program of course covers a wide range of activities, most of which do not have a direct bearing on psychiatric genetics. Nevertheless, it is clear from Watson's own account[9] that he was well aware that studies of the genetics of behaviour constitute a particularly sensitive area and that this provided one of the springs of action for his early establishment of the genome ethics program. Watson explained that he was at pains to discount the idea that 'I was a closet eugenicist, having as my real long term goal the unambiguous identification of genes that lead to social and occupational stratification as well as to genes justifying racial discrimination'.[9]

The ELSI program has certainly contributed to the 'business boom' in bioethics in the United States,[10] but elsewhere similar if more modestly funded initiatives have taken place. In the UK the major medical research funding bodies have become acutely aware of ethical issues linked to genetics. As one of its activities in this field during 1997 the Wellcome Trust staged a public debate on genetics while the Medical Research Council mounted a public consultation exercise focused directly on behaviour genetics. Both bodies contribute to funding of the independent organization, the Nuffield Council in Bioethics, which, also in 1997, set up a working party on ethical aspects of the genetics of psychiatric disorders. Meanwhile, in France, which has had a National Bioethics Committee since 1983,[11] there is, characteristically, greater emphasis on legislation than on public debate, and in Germany the setting up of a National Bioethics Advisory Group is being proposed with pressures coming particularly from the opposition Social Democrat party.[12]

In the midst of all this activity in Western Europe and North America a voice of disquiet has come, as we have already noted, from a leading medical journal, *The Lancet*.[2] *The Lancet's* term 'the bioethics industry' has also been used by *Nature* in an editorial which pointed out that perceptions about new moral concepts resulting from medical developments in biology are often misconceived.[13] Nevertheless, independent consideration of ethical implications (i.e. not just by scientists) is in the long run beneficial. We will return to this theme later. However, since much of the ethical debates in psychiatric genetics are impinged on by the legacy of its history, we will first take a brief, and necessarily superficial, look at the history of psychiatric and behaviour genetics and its frequent, but usually unfortunate, entanglement with the history of eugenics.

Behaviour, psychiatry, and eugenics

Both eugenics and behaviour genetics are usually considered to have originated from the work of Francis Galton, the English Victorian polymath. A cousin of Charles Darwin, Galton contributed much to the foundations of modern statistics, population biology, and genetics. Apparently completely unaware of the work of his contemporary Gregor Mendel, Galton published his monograph on 'Hereditary Genius' in 1869, representing the first attempt to explore the inheritance of intellectual ability. Galton subsequently coined the term *eugenics* derived from the Greek for well-born. Eugenics as Galton perceived it, was to be a branch of biology devoted to improvements in the human race by attention to optimal reproductive practices. Following Galton, the basic tenets of eugenics were the rational sounding ideas that reducing reproduction of people suffering from inherited defects could allow certain diseases to be abolished (negative eugenics), while encouraging fecundity among those with desirable attributes should lead to improvement in the human stock (positive eugenics). Such notions became prevalent and popular in intellectual circles, and later in not so intellectual circles, in the first half of the twentieth century. Although sometimes spoken of as the 'eugenics movement', eugenic ideas were in fact taken up by a whole series of movements. Thus despite often being thought of as associated with politics of the right, eugenic ideas were espoused by George Bernard Shaw and other members of the socialist Fabian movement, as well as by other more down-to-earth socialist thinkers who found it quite reasonable that the 'feeble minded' should be prevented from having children because otherwise they could 'cost other people a lot of money'.[14]

What Galton bequeathed to psychiatric genetics was the idea that studies of the familial clustering of disorders could throw light on their aetiology. Furthermore, although he put forward his proposals only in broad outline, Galton was also the first to suggest that studies of twins could provide a method of teasing apart the effects of genes and shared environment then the causation of familial traits.[15] It was left to the German researcher Siemens and psychiatric geneticists of the Munich School, such as Luxemberger, to fully expound on and apply the, now classic, twin method.[15] The first systematic family studies of dementia praecox (schizophrenia) were carried out by Ernst Rüdin.[16] Although such work was in many respects seminal, Rüdin's subsequent involvement with the Nazi party[17] and his possible contributions to their view on how eugenic principles might be implemented, has led to heated debate. An attempt to reassess Rüdin's work and present some of it in English translation for a modern audience[18] resulted in outraged correspondence in letters to the editor of one of our leading psychiatric genetics journals.[19-22]

As it turned out Rüdin was arrested at the cessation of World War II and appeared at a local Denazification court in 1947, but was judged to have been a 'fellow traveller' and as such not a major contributor to Nazi crimes. Whether this view was justified or overlenient remains a contentious issue. What is not contentious is that the Nazi regime adopted a simplistic and ruthless set of eugenic policies that now seem as astonishingly naïve as they were unbelievably repugnant. This included first the forcible sterilization of the mentally ill (a broad sweep from Huntington's disease to manic depression, schizophrenia, and alcoholism) and subsequently progressed to 'euthanasia' of psychiatric patients along with the extermination of other undesirables including allegedly genetically inferior ethnic groups such as Jews and gypsies.[23] There can be little doubt that several leading scientists not only accepted these policies but encouraged their adoption. It was as if the arrival of Mendelian genetics finally settled the question in the minds of anti-semitic Germans of 'whether their enemy was the Jews themselves or their religion'.[9] Despite this it is also clear that some leading German psychiatric geneticists were appalled at what they saw, for example, Bruno Schulz abhored Nazism and refused, to the detriment of his career, to join the party,[24] while Luxemberger ridiculed some of the more extraordinary Nazi 'scientific facts'. For example, he pointed out the absurdity of the view put forward by the leading Nazi medical examiner, Streicher, that an Aryan woman who had a child fathered by a Jew would later give birth to half-Jewish children even if these were fathered by an Aryan. This led to Luxemberger, another non-Nazi party member, being banned from public lecturing.

Although nowhere else did the application of eugenics result in such florid cruelty, harsh principles have certainly been applied elsewhere, as reflected in policies on sterilization, immigration, and assimilation of ethnic minorities. In the United States, an early advocate of eugenics was Charles B. Davenport who held an influential position as director of the Cold Spring Harbor Laboratories. Unlike his near contemporaries in the Munich School of Psychiatry, who were commencing systematic family and twin studies, Davenport was untroubled by a lack of scientific evidence and simply assumed that much of insanity, feeble-mindedness, and other forms of undesirable behaviour were genetically determined. In 1910 he set up a eugenics record office and his views were pursuasive in forming United States immigration policies that favoured certain groups (e.g. from the British Isles, Germany, and Scandinavia) over others (e.g. from Southern and Eastern Europe).[9]

The introduction of psychometric testing in the United States, which began on a large scale with World War I army conscripts, provided the beginning of another controversial area that remains provocative to the present day. The development of intelligence quotient (IQ tests) by the Stanford psychologist Terman, based on the earlier model of the French psychologist Binet, provided a novel measure that was widely and enthusiastically adopted. It was assumed by most from the beginning that IQ scores provided a measure of innate ability and, although it is now accepted that certain aspects of conventional IQ tests are culturally influenced, this was initially overlooked. Thus the poorer average scores of non-English speaking immigrants or of black army recruits compared with white Americans were interpreted as genetically based and were effectively used as a justification for discrimination.[25]

Although eugenic philosophies never entirely disappeared (for example, until the 1960s, they influenced Swedish policies on sterilization of the mentally handicapped and Australian government practice on attempting to eliminate Aborigines as a distinct ethnic group), they became decidedly unfashionable in the aftermath of World War II and the downfall of the Third Reich. There is little doubt that psychiatric genetics suffered from a sort of guilt by association. The Munich School, in most respects its birthplace, was no longer a centre for psychiatric genetics. Foreigners who had visited Munich or studied there as research fellows in the pre-war years kept the subject alive in their own countries. These include Slater in the UK[26] and Stromgren and Essen-Moller in Scandinavia. In the United States Franz Kallmann, a part Jewish German who had fled the country in the pre-war years, was a leading proponent of psychiatric genetics and a founding member of the American Society for Human Genetics.

Psychiatric genetics was therefore by no means dead, but neither was it fully part of mainstream academic psychiatry which in North America was dominated by psychoanalysis, while in Europe epidemiological and social psychiatry largely held sway. Despite its status as a minority interest real progress was made in psychiatric genetics during the third quarter of the twentieth century in refining and implementing the methods of family, twin and adoption studies. Thus nearly all of the important evidence favouring a substantial genetic contribution to schizophrenia and manic depression comes from studies published during the 1960s and 1970s.[27,28] Such studies demonstrated that genetic factors exist but that they are complicated, and that with rare exceptions, such as Huntington's disease, disorders presenting with psychiatric symptoms do not have straightforward Mendelian patterns of inheritance. For many, therefore, the subject matter of psychiatric genetics seemed remote, somewhat abstract, and to have little bearing on clinical practice. What changed this was the advent of molecular genetics and the knowledge that genes could be localized and identified even in diseases where the aetiology is complex and multi-factorial. Psychiatric genetics is now one of the 'hot' areas of psychiatric research probably rivalled only by brain imaging research. However, unlike brain imaging it carries with it, as we have seen, an historical burden as well as an ethical burden of new dilemmas that may be posed by an ability to dissect out susceptibility to psychiatric disease at a molecular level.

Ethics and research in modern psychiatric genetics

Two broad questions are posed by current research. Should it be done at all? If it is to be done, what ethical safeguards should be put in place? The first question may seem odd given that, as we have discussed, psychiatric genetics is being researched on a scale far greater than at any time in its history. Nevertheless there remain those who are fundamentally opposed to research that touches upon the genetic basis of normal or abnormal behaviour.[29] Part of this arises from suspicion about what psychiatric genetic research is 'for' (is it, for example, to 'label' people or to discriminate against them?). There is also a belief that genetic research promotes notions of biological determinism and negation of free will, and supports the idea that an inherited disorder is fixed, immutable, and effectively untreatable.

Some of the common fallacies surrounding psychiatric genetic research have been succinctly reviewed and effectively refuted by Rutter and Plomin.[1] The general point is well made that although psychiatric genetic research is *reductionist* (i.e. the ultimate aim is an understanding of mechanisms at a molecular level) it is by no means *deterministic* in the sense that for most disorders seen in psychiatry there is not a direct correspondence between genotype and phenotype. For example, even in identical twins, concordance for disorders such as schizophrenia or manic depression fall well short of 100 per cent. Furthermore, even in the case of rare, single gene disorders that affect behaviour, an understanding of the biochemical defect provides a basis for prevention (the classic example being phenylketonuria), or the development of new treatments where none previously existed. Here the cloning of the Huntington's disease gene and the discovery of the mutations that cause early-onset, autosomal-dominant Alzheimer's disease are examples of promising developments. In both cases we have brain disorders where previously little was known about aetiology other than the fact that there is a genetic basis. The ability to identify the genes, to uncover their sequence and structure and to study the nature of the gene products and how they behave differently in the mutated and non-mutated forms, provides totally new insights and opens a pathway for the development of specific treatments.

We will return to this in our final section on clinical matters, but assuming for now that the outcomes of psychiatric genetic research are predominantly beneficial, and that there are no substantive ethical objections to such research continuing, we can address our second question regarding what should be the necessary ethical constraints upon such research. Meslin[8] has listed these in the context of the ELSI program. As we have discussed, this program is not confined to psychiatry and is conducted in the United States. Nevertheless, ELSI aims are relevant to psychiatric genetic research universally. The topics of concern of the ELSI program are informed consent, the role of institutional review boards (IRBs) (otherwise called ethics committees), the role of individuals and families as participants, privacy and confidentiality, and commercialization of products. We will deal with these in turn.

Informed consent

Informed consent in psychiatric genetic research has been commented on by Shore;[30] he points out straightforwardly that subjects need to understand any likely benefit, foreseeable risks, and alternatives to participation in research. In psychiatric genetic research the physical risk is usually minimal or small. Participation usually entails a standard diagnostic interview, completion of questionnaires or other psychometric tests, and provision of a sample of venous blood for extraction of DNA. Venepuncture is therefore the only physical hazard; even this can be avoided if necessary where the quantity of DNA required is small, by obtaining a sample of buccal mucosa cells by mouthwash or swabbing the inside of the cheek. What may be less tangible and easier to quantify is the degree of *non-physical* harm. This could occur if, for example, research subjects fail to understand the difference between clinical diagnosis or treatment and participation in a research study designed purely to generate scientific data. Thus people may agree to participate because they believe they will learn about their own risk for particular genetic disorders. Thus far, for certain psychiatric disorders such as schizophrenia or manic depression, promising candidate genes are under investigation; there are also promising genetic linkage findings.[31] However, none are yet definite. Therefore revealing the results of DNA testing to subjects would be of no tangible benefit.

However, what should be the practice once genes are identified, as is the case in rare psychiatric disorders such as Huntington's disease and autosomal dominant forms of Alzheimer's disease? Following test results we can tell a subject who is currently well whether they are at risk or not with virtual certainty. Most ethics committees, and probably most researchers in the field, advocate a clear distinction between research and predictive, clinical testing. We would advocate that it is made clear to subjects that results of DNA tests will not be revealed and that any benefits that accrue are purely those of advancing medical and scientific knowledge.

Ethics committees

The role of ethics committees, or IRBs, is accepted in most industrialized countries regarding research involving human subjects. The guiding principles are those embodied in the Nuremberg code[32] (see Appendix) and include such basic safeguards as ensuring that the research subject gives voluntary consent and is not subjected to suffering and that the experiment is likely to yield 'fruitful results for the good of society, unprocurable by other methods or means of study'.

The question arises as to whether psychiatric genetic research differs from any other form of research in respect of the role of the ethics committee. We believe the answer is no. There are, however, three areas worthy of consideration. The first, common to any branch of science that depends on rapidly advancing technologies, relates to the extent to which any ethics committee is competent to judge the scientific merit of a research proposal. As we have noted, one basic tenet of the Nuremberg code is that ethical research is scientifically sound. Increasingly, locally based ethics committees, faced with assessing research in novel areas using new techniques, have the dilemma of either needing to take investigators' proposals 'on trust' or using external referees. Sound judgement is required combined with sound local knowledge. It makes no sense for an ethics committee to duplicate the work of a grants committee in assessing the scientific merit of a proposal from an established researcher or from a relatively inexperienced researcher carrying out an orthodox piece of work. However, when research is highly novel and when there has been no peer review from funding bodies closer scrutiny is indicated.

The second question, a particular one for genetic research, relates to the fact that subjects may have to be drawn from a wide geographical area in order to fulfil sample requirements. There is, however, an increasing trend both in Europe and North America for ethics committees to be locally based and to exercise local autonomy. Thus the situation has arisen whereby a project is deemed ethically sound in, for example, one Welsh county but not in an adjacent one. Within the UK, the Medical Research Council and other funding bodies are seeking mechanisms whereby genetic research or other multicentre studies, for example drug trials, receive ethical scrutiny from bodies with a wider geographical jurisdiction.

The role of individuals and their families

The third problem for genetic research is that it involves not just persons affected by a particular disorder but also unaffected relatives. This poses the problem of recruitment. Can relatives be recruited in their own right or only via the affected person through whom they have been identified? We do not feel it defensible to approach relatives when the index subject withholds permission. On the other hand, it is more debatable whether one should take the view, as some ethics committees do, that once permission is given to approach relatives the approach can *only* be made via the index subject and not directly to relatives themselves.

A more fundamental ethical issue relates to whether a family's perception of the illness suffered by one or more of its members is altered by the family becoming involved in a genetic study. The potential dangers are again in the area of 'non-physical' harm. For example, unaffected family members may have been previously unaware that a disorder such as depression has a familial component; their involvement in a family study may bring this home to them for the first time. A genetic study may also raise old-fashioned, but still prevalent, notions about 'hereditary taint'. For example, one occasionally comes across a parent of an affected offspring who is at pains to explain that the disorder comes from their spouse's side of the family, not their side. Fortunately, this is being replaced by a different and exculpatory view of genetics where families, particularly parents, view with relief the idea that a severe psychiatric disorder such as autism or schizophrenia results largely from faulty DNA rather than a faulty upbringing.

Confidentiality

Questions of privacy and confidentiality arise in genetic research in ways not seen elsewhere in psychiatry. Thus family members may be prepared to reveal symptoms to the researcher that they have concealed from their relatives; in such circumstances, they should expect to have confidentiality strictly respected. A more general issue is that information uncovered by genetic research may be of potential interest to other agencies, such as employers or insurance companies. Experience with single gene disorders such as Huntington's disease has provided a useful test ground; few would argue with the view that there should be a strict embargo on divulging any information derived from genetic research to a third party.[33]

Commercialization of products

The final concern regarding research into psychiatric genetics are potential commercial outcomes. There has been considerable debate about the rights and wrongs of patenting genes responsible for Mendelian disorders. Well-known (some would say notorious) examples include cystic fibrosis and a comparatively uncommon form of a common condition, breast cancer, caused by an autosomal-dominant mutation in the *BRCA1* gene. A less well-known example—but highly relevant to psychiatry—is Alzheimer's disease where early-onset Mendelian subforms occur, one of which results from mutations in the amyloid precursor protein (*APP*) gene; a patent has been granted to the discoverers of the first of these mutations.[34] The ethical debate centres on two issues. The first is whether it is justifiable to patent something which is not an invention but a spontaneously occurring biological anomaly. The argument in favour of allowing patenting is that isolating a gene and finding a particular mutation is a form of discovery where the endeavour has the same elements of originality as invention, even if the discovery happens to have occurred in another person's DNA. The second dilemma has to do with profit. Is it acceptable that the discoverer of a gene should profit when the research subjects on whom their discovery was made obtain no reward? One view that has been taken on patenting as practised in North America is that the discoverer of a mutation is its sole owner. (Interestingly this is not the usual view taken in the case of a prospector who discovers a valuable commodity, say oil or gold, on someone else's land!).

A more remote issue is the influence of genetic research on drug discovery. We will return to this issue in considering the likely impact of genetics on clinical practice, but here the issue is one of profit. Pharmaceutical companies have become interested in the genetic basis of common diseases since they see it as a route to identify novel targets for which they hope to develop therapeutic compounds.[35] For this reason several major companies have begun to invest in genetic research including psychiatric genetics. What information or inducements should be given to the human subjects involved in such research? At the very least it would seem necessary that in obtaining informed consent subjects should be told that their relevant clinical details and information derived from studying their DNA (or even the DNA itself) will be supplied by the researcher to the pharmaceutical company, but that this will be safeguarded by anonymity and confidentiality.

How psychiatric practice will be affected by genetics

We have noted that psychiatric genetics has had little direct impact on clinical practice. However, it has been predicted[1,36] that this will change and that some results of genetic research will have a marked or even revolutionary effect.

Some such effects will have little or no ethical implications whereas in others the ethical issues could be large.

The first area in which genetic knowledge is relevant to clinicians is that it improves understanding of the neurobiology of the conditions they treat. The essential paradigm of most modern molecular genetic studies of disease is positional cloning,[37,38] that is the existence of a detailed map of genetic markers spread throughout the genome (all 23 pairs of chromosomes) allows detection of linkage in families containing more than one affected individual. Linkage is the phenomenon where a particular marker assorts with the disease and indicates that the marker and a gene causing (or contributing to) the disease are close together on the same chromosome. Linkage therefore provides the location of the gene; using various techniques the task is then to isolate the gene itself. This can prove complicated and time-consuming but techniques are well established and can be relied upon to deliver. Having done this the sequence and structure of the gene can be studied and the gene product, the protein that it encodes for, can be identified. Subsequently, if it is not a known protein, its distribution and likely function need to be discovered.

In summary, although it may entail complicated technology and a great deal of time, positional cloning has a ruthless logic that should solve the aetiological puzzles of all single gene diseases and, with a degree of adaptation, also uncover the causes of multifactorial or polygenic disorders.

A better understanding of the neurobiology of conditions like schizophrenia or affective disorders might seem ethically neutral. However, a number of consequential effects are not neutral. Thus a second area in which genetics will impact upon clinical practice is in altering both public and professional perception of psychiatric disorders. We have already touched upon two examples, childhood autism and schizophrenia, where even in the absence of firm, molecular genetic findings, classic family, twin, and adoption methods point to a substantial genetic contribution. The acceptance of this by most clinicians has meant a move away from explanations involving concepts such as the 'schizophrenogenic mother' or 'refrigerator' parents which are inevitably seen as carrying blame. The societal equivalent of family blame is stigma and here genetic knowledge is also likely to have a large effect.

Concern is sometimes expressed by patients or their relatives that exploring the genetic basis of psychiatric disorders will increase 'labelling' at-risk people and the associated stigma. History suggests the opposite. In the eyes of most members of the public uncovering a 'physical' cause of mental disturbance tends to turn it into a 'real' disease, one worthy of care and treatment rather than shame and stigma. A nice illustration of this, even among what may be regarded as more cultured members of the lay public, is in Alan Bennett's play *The Madness of King George* (also a successful film). In the closing moments it is explained that the King probably suffered from acute intermittent porphyria (an autosomal-dominant metabolic disorder) and was therefore not 'really' mad. Thus even if a person's behaviour is floridly psychotic, the perception goes, a biochemical explanation indicates that the disorder is no longer 'psychiatric'.

Another example of this phenomenon is seen in the changed public attitude to Alzheimer's disease. This is a disorder where great strides have been made in understanding its molecular neurobiology and molecular genetics;[39] although most people have not the sketchiest idea of the details, they will at least have heard about Alzheimer's disease and identified it as a type of illness rather than moral failure. Thus it is acceptable for public figures such as a past President of the United States to be identified as suffering from the early stages of Alzheimer's disease. The public perception of other forms of mental illness, particularly schizophrenia and manic depression, is changing similarly; this development will accelerate as molecular genetic research advances. (Incidentally, although this may benefit sufferers, psychiatrists might beware that the end of their speciality is nigh; a clinical geneticist has remarked that Alzheimer's disease is no longer a psychiatric disorder but a neurological one!)

Two associated areas of clinical practice likely to alter as a result of genetic research are psychiatric diagnosis and predictive testing. Most of the diagnostic concepts used in psychiatry are working hypotheses rather than clear-cut diagnostic entities.[40] The benefits of genetic research in other common disorders such as diabetes has led to a variety of emerging diagnostic entities: oligogenic types 1 and 2 diabetes and rarer, single gene forms like the oddly named, maturity onset diabetes of the young (MODY). Similarly, three different single gene forms of early-onset familial Alzheimer's disease have been identified resulting from gene mutations on Chromosomes 1, 14, and 21; in the later onset forms the presence of the *e4* allele of apolipoprotein E is associated with an increased risk, but several other as yet unidentified genes are probably also involved. Most other psychiatric disorders are likely to be oligogenic (involving a handful of genes) or polygenic (involving many genes of small effect) but it seems likely that once these are identified our classifications will need to change. This may be seen as ethically neutral, but the allied issue of applying genetic tests to predict who will become ill raises salient problems.

Fortunately, experience with the rare, single gene cause of a psychiatric disturbance, Huntington's disease, has allowed many of these issues to be explored.[33] Huntington's disease typically shows its first symptoms when patients are in their thirties or forties. Behavioural change is inevitably followed by movement disorder, dementia and premature death. Although symptomatic treatment may be offered there is no cure or treatment to slow the progress of the disorder. Therefore, and perhaps not surprisingly, the uptake of predictive testing among people at risk, usually those with a parent affected, is low (predictive testing in the UK is restricted to specialist units that offer education, counselling, and follow-up support.[41] Disorders such as schizophrenia or manic depression differ from Huntington's disease in that there is no simple one-to-one correspondence between genotype and phenotype but also in that useful symptomatic treatments are available. There is also evidence that early treatment of schizophrenia may be associated with a more favourable outcome. Predictive testing for such conditions is likely to be less precise and less threatening than for single gene disorders. Nevertheless, it would seem prudent to advocate that when tests that usefully predict the risk of schizophrenia in high-risk persons become available, they should be offered in specialist centres with expertise in the performance and interpretation of tests and resources to provide education, counselling and support. Genetic counselling for disorders like schizophrenia and manic depression has been offered by specialist centres, but the information imparted is at the level of providing empirical risks derived from published data in various categories of relatives.[38] It is important to realize that for complex (oligogenic or polygenic) disorders the accuracy of predictive testing will never achieve 100 per cent; indeed, the upper limits of predictive accuracy are probably indicated by monozygotic twin concordance rates (which for schizophrenia and manic depression are about 50 and 70 per cent respectively).

The ethical spectre of population screening for susceptibility to common diseases including psychiatric disorders is unlikely to become a reality because a corollary of a disease having a polygenic or even oligogenic basis is that susceptibility loci are likely to show alleles (or genetic variants) of high frequency in the general population. For example, a putative risk factor for schizophrenia is an allelic variant at the gene encoding for the 5-HT$_{2A}$ serotonin receptor.[42] However, the 'high risk' allele is found in 60–70 per cent of the population. Those with this variant, compared with those who do not appear to have a modestly increased risk, that is they are 1.5 times as likely to develop the disorder as those who do not carry the variant.[43] Most susceptibility loci in schizophrenia are likely to be of this type, i.e. common genes each, on their own, confirming only modest risk. Even when the risks associated with susceptibility loci are much greater they may be of only limited use or no use at all for population screening. For example, ankylosing spondylitis, an inflammatory arthritis of the spine predominantly affecting young men, has long been known to be associated with unlocking of a particular histocompatibility antigen HLA-B27 such that B27-positive individuals have a risk which is more than 80 fold that of B27-negative individuals. Nevertheless, possessing B27 is neither necessary nor sufficient to cause the disorder and the vast majority of B27-positive members of the general population never develop it.

The final area where genetic research will affect clinical psychiatry is that it should lead to the development of targeted treatments. At present, the limited number of targets for effective treatment reflects our poor understanding of the pathophysiology of psychiatric disorders. The whole area of genomics-led drug development is seen as of enormous potential by the pharmaceutical industry.[35] That genetic research may lead to the development of safer, more specific treatments with less side-effects should again not in itself raise ethical difficulties. In fact, such development is a realistic prize which will provide benefits that far outweigh the ethical difficulties raised by psychiatric genetic research.

References

1. Rutter, M. and Plomin, R.: Opportunities for psychiatry from genetic findings. *British Journal of Psychiatry* **17**:209–19, 1997.
2. Editorial: The ethics industry. *Lancet* **350**:897, 1997.
3. Wilmut, T., Schnieke, A. K., McWhir, J., Kind, A. J., and Campbell, K. H. S.: Viable offspring derived from fetal and adult mammalian cells. *Nature* **385**:810–13, 1997.
4. Galileo, Copernicus—and now Dolly! *Independent* 26th February 1997, p. 17; see also: The spectre of a human clone, ibid., p. 1.
5. Clone cologne—for men who want to smell like themselves. *Daily Telegraph* 1st March 1997, p. 14.
6. Cloning presents an opportunity, not a threat. *Independent* 28th February 1997, p. 17.
7. Dolly's already here—ethics will have to cope. *Daily Telegraph* 5th March 1997, p. 22.
8. Meslin, E.: *Plenary address.* 5th World Congress of Psychiatric Genetics, Santa Fe, USA, 1997.
9. Watson, J. D.: Genes and politics. *Journal of Molecular Medicine* **75**:624–36, 1997.
10. Wadman, M., Levitin, C., Abbott, A, *et al.*: Business booms for guides to biology's moral maze. *Nature* **389**:658–9, 1997.
11. Butler, D.: France reaps benefits and costs of going by the book. *Nature* **389**:661–2, 1997.
12. Abbott, A.: Germany's past still casts a long shadow. *Nature* **389**:660, 1997.
13. Editorial: Trust and the bioethics industry. *Nature* **389**:647, 1997.
14. Mitchison, N.: An outline for boys and girls. Cited in 'When Britain was for good breeding'. *The Sunday Times* 31 August 1997.
15. Plomin, R. De Fries, J. C., McClearn, G. E., and Rutter, M.: *Behaviour genetics*, 3rd edn. New York, Freeman, 1997.
16. Slater, E. and Cowie, V.: *The genetics of mental disorders.* Oxford, Oxford University Press, 1971.
17. Gottesman, I. I. and Bertelsen, A.: Legacy of German psychiatric genetics: hindsight is always 20/20. *American Journal of Medical Genetics* (*Neuropsychiatric Genetics*) **67**:343–6, 1996.
18. Kendler, K. and Zerbin-Rüdin, E. (1996). Abstract and review of 'Zur Erb-pathologie der Schizophrenie' (Contribution to the genetics of schizophrenia) 1916. *American Journal of Medical Genetics* (*Neuropsychiatric Genetics*) **67**:338–42, 1996.
19. Gejman, P. V.: Ernst Rüdin and Nazi euthanasia: another stain on his career. *American Journal of Medical Genetics* (*Psychiatric Genetics*) **74**:455–6, 1997.
20. Gershon, E. S.: Ernst Rüdin, a Nazi psychiatrist and geneticist. *American Journal of Medical Genetics* (*Neuropsychiatric Genetics*) **74**:457–8, 1997.
21. Lerer, B. and Segman, R. H.: Correspondence regarding German psychiatric genetics and Ernst Rüdin. *American Journal of Medical Genetics* (*Neuropsychiatric Genetics*) **74**:459–60, 1997.

22. Kendler, K.: Reply to Gejman, Gershon, and Lerer and Segman. *American Journal of Medical Genetics* (*Neuropsychiatric Genetics*) **74**:461–3, 1997.
23. Muller-Hill, B.: *Murderous science.* Oxford, Oxford University Press, 1988.
24. Slater, E.: Autobiographical sketch: the road to psychiatry, in *Man, mind and heredity,* ed. J. Shields and I. I. Gottesman. Baltimore, Johns Hopkins Press, 1971, pp. 1–23.
25. Kamin, L. J.: *The science and politics of IQ.* Chichester, Wiley, 1974.
26. Gottesman, I. I. and McGuffin, P.: Eliot Slater and the birth of psychiatric genetics in Great Britain, in *150 years of British psychiatry II,* ed. H. Freeman and G. E. Berrios. London, Athlone, 1996, pp. 537–48.
27. Tsuang, M. T. and Faraone, S. V.: *The genetics of mood disorder.* Baltimore, Johns Hopkins Press, 1991.
28. Gottesman, I. I.: *Schizophrenia genetics.* San Francisco, Freeman, 1991.
29. Rose, S., Kamin, L. J., and Lewontin, R. C.: *Not in our genes: biology, ideology and human nature.* London, Penguin, 1990.
30. Shore, D.: Ethical issues and informed consent in psychiatric genetic research. *American Journal of Medical Genetics* (*Neuropsychiatric Genetics*) **74**:593, 1997.
31. Owen, M. J. and McGuffin, P.: Genetics and psychiatry. *British Journal of Psychiatry* **171**:201–2, 1997.
32. Faraone, S. V., Gottesman, I. I., and Tsuang, M. T.: Fifty years of the Nuremberg Code: a time for retrospection and introspection (editorial). *American Journal of Medical Genetics* (*Neuropsychiatric Genetics*) **74**:345–7, 1997.
33. Harper, P. S. and Clarke, A. J.: *Genetics, society and clinical practice.* Oxford, Bios Scientific, 1997.
34. Goate, A., Chartier-Harlin, M., Mullan, M., *et al.*: Segregation of a missense mutation in the amyloid precursor protein gene with familial Alzheimer's disease. *Nature* **349**:704–6, 1991.
35. Knowles, J.: Hunting down diseases. *Odyssey* **3**:18–24, 1997.
36. Farmer, A. E. and Owen, M. J.: Genomics: the next psychiatric revolution? *British Journal of Psychiatry* **169**:135–8, 1996.
37. Collins, F.: Positional cloning: let's not call it reverse any more. *Nature Genetics* **1**:36, 1992.
38. McGuffin, P., Owen, M., O'Donovan, M., Thapar, A., and Gottesman, I. I.: *Seminars in psychiatric genetics.* London, Gaskell, 1994.
39. Sandbrink, R., Hartmann, T., Master, C. L., and Beyreuther, K.: Genes contributing to Alzheimer's disease. *Molecular Psychiatry* **1**:27–40, 1996.
40. Farmer, A. E.: Current approaches to classification, in *Essentials of postgraduate psychiatry,* 3rd edn, ed. R. Murray, P. Hill, and P. McGuffin. Cambridge, Cambridge University Press, 1997, pp. 53–64.
41. Scourfield, J., Soldan, J., Gray, J., Houlihan, G., and Harper, P. S.: Huntington's disease: psychiatric practice in molecular genetic prediction and diagnosis. *British Journal of Psychiatry* **170**:146–9, 1997.
42. Williams, J., Spurlock, G., McGuffin, P., *et al.*: Association between schizophrenia and the T102C polymorphism of the 5-hydroxytryptamine type 2a-receptor gene. *Lancet* **347**:1294–6, 1996.
43. Williams, J., McGuffin, P., Nöthen, M., Owen, M. J., and EMASS Collaborative Group: A meta analysis of association between the 5-HT2a receptor T102C polymorphism and schizophrenia. *Lancet* **349**:1221, 1997.

24

Teaching psychiatric ethics

Robert Michels and Kevin V. Kelly

Psychiatrists, ethicists, and social theorists have shown increasing interest in the ethical aspects of psychiatry over the past few decades. Such issues as involuntary treatment, the control of social deviance, the right to treatment, informed consent, and confidentiality captured the imagination of the public and the profession, since they presented both painful dilemmas and the possibility for serious abuses. Since the 1980s, even greater attention has been devoted to psychiatric ethics, largely because of concerns about the consequences of dramatic changes in the health-care delivery system, and about sexual misconduct in the professions.

Discussions of such issues frequently confuse ethics with morals. Ethics has to do with the way in which one thinks about and discusses moral problems. A good person may not understand ethics, while a bad person may be quite sophisticated about it. Certainly we would like psychiatrists to be good people, but in addition to this, we would like them to understand the ethical aspects of psychiatric issues. Training programs in ethics often suffer from an unrecognized confusion between these two goals.

The effort to develop training programs for psychiatric ethics, particularly in consultation–liaison settings, has furthered the discussion of psychiatry's special relationship to ethics.[1–4] The philosophical background of the issue is discussed in Chapter 3; in its clinical form, the question commonly arises when the consulting psychiatrist is asked to assume the role of moral arbiter. Psychiatry's uncertainty about how to respond to this situation underscores the need to train psychiatrists more thoroughly in ethical reasoning, as well as in moral behavior.

Can psychiatric ethics be taught?

There are several points of view about the teaching of ethics in psychiatry. Perhaps the oldest and most widespread is that ethics cannot be taught. Proponents of this view argue that certainly psychiatrists should be 'ethical' (by which they mean 'virtuous'), but that the only way this can be assured is to select 'ethical' individuals and train them to be psychiatrists. The general structure of this argument is familiar to psychiatrists, since it is analogous to the view held by many physicians concerning the skills involved in the doctor–patient relationship. At least three counter-arguments are important for consideration. The first is that this position applies to morality, rather than to ethics, and exemplifies the common confusion between the two. Secondly, a trait may have a basis in temperament, talent, or character, and yet be enhanced, developed, or refined through education; musical skill, athletic ability, and the conduct of psychotherapy are all examples. Finally, scholars have devoted considerable effort to the study and analysis of ethical problems in general, and of psychiatric ethics in particular, and it would be unfortunate if we expected each student of the field to explore these issues anew, without access to the wisdom that has already been collected.

Teaching by modeling

The second view of the teaching of ethics in psychiatry is that ethics can be taught, but only through modeling. This view would suggest that the critical problem is not selecting students, but selecting teachers. The importance of education through modeling is a prominent theme in psychiatry in general, emphasized in psychodynamic, psychobiological, behavioural, and developmental approaches to psychiatry. Some psychiatrists believe that most psychiatric education occurs through modeling, and almost all believe it to be important. This kind of teaching may be seen in a wide variety of clinical and pedagogic settings. It occurs most overtly and most powerfully in the individual supervision by an experienced psychiatrist of a trainee's clinical work, and ethical positions and attitudes are often communicated, implicitly or explicitly, in this setting. However, accepting the importance of modeling shifts or broadens our problem rather than solving it; we must consider how to teach the supervisors as well as how to teach the students.

Teaching by cases

The third approach considers psychiatric ethics to be an aspect of practical wisdom, taught by the case-method in the discussion of specific clinical situations and practical decisions. Rounds and case conferences, in addition to the supervision of specific treatments, form the core of most psychiatric training programs, and ethical aspects of the psychiatrist's work can be studied in the same way as psychodynamic or psychopharmacologic aspects.[5–7] This approach has the virtue of bringing the teaching of psychiatric ethics into the pedagogic setting that has the trainee's greatest attention and emotional investment. One disadvantage is that ethical issues are often set aside because of the urgency of specific therapeutic problems, and there is a tendency to associate psychiatric ethics with unusual or 'tough' cases, rather than to recognize the universality of ethics as a framework for understanding professional functioning. Furthermore, this method of teaching focuses on issues related to specific patients, rather than those that emerge in consideration of broader questions of professional functioning. Ethical aspects of the relationship between the psychiatric profession and society, economic decisions involving the distribution of limited resources, the role of the public in professional decisions, and similar matters will rarely be discussed in the context of specific cases, but they should be discussed in the course of psychiatric education. Finally, psychiatric educators who are excellent teachers of clinical psychiatry may not have the knowledge or interest required to teach ethics, while moral philosophers who could enrich the experience of psychiatric trainees might not be competent or appropriate as general psychiatric supervisors. It would be unfortunate if the structure of the curriculum in psychiatric ethics precluded participation by those who were the most competent to teach it.

Teaching by seminars

The most ambitious, but most rewarding, approach to the teaching of ethics in psychiatry regards ethics as one of the themes of a core curriculum. A fundamental body of knowledge is taught in seminars and courses, while applications to specific problems occur in the discussion during ward rounds and supervision. This method provides exposure to the philosophical or theoretical aspects of ethics—theories of justice, concepts of right and duty, and so on; the application of these principles to the major problems of psychiatry; and experience with evaluating decisions in concrete situations. This more comprehensive approach has been recommended for the teaching of general medical ethics,[8,9] and has been employed in the few structured teaching programs in psychiatric ethics which have appeared in the literature (cf. ref. 1).[10–13]

When to teach?

Teaching in college and medical school

Turning from how to teach psychiatric ethics to when the teaching should occur, we have the choice of pre-professional education, medical school training, psychiatric training, or continuing education. The undergraduate period would seem to be the obvious time to develop a basis in the philosophical underpinnings of ethics. However, pre-medical preparation is so heterogeneous that courses on medical ethics in medical schools, whether required or elective, have become widespread (cf. ref. 9). Investigators have, interestingly, used an instrument to measure skills in moral reasoning in order to demonstrate that medical students can learn and retain the ability to apply ethical principles.[14]

Since the 1970s, medical educators have responded to a widely held perception that the practice of medicine has become 'dehumanized', especially as a result of economic factors and the increasing use of elaborate technology, by designing programs to cultivate greater 'humanism' among medical students. The growth in number and variety of such programs has been enormous,[15–18] and some have employed innovative teaching techniques.[19] In these programs, ethics tends to be subsumed under the larger category of 'humanism', and psychiatry usually plays no special role. Thus these efforts, while laudable in general, may not advance the teaching of psychiatric ethics in particular, because they tend to concentrate on cultivating good (that is, moral) attitudes and practices, rather than on cultivating critical thinking about ethical problems, and fail to address the important and complex relationships among psychiatry, medical humanism, and ethics.

Traditionally, psychiatrists have viewed themselves, and have been viewed by their colleagues in other branches of medicine, as having special interests and expertise in both humanism and ethics (cf. ref. 2).[20] This perception is, to some extent, appropriate and useful, since that branch of medicine which deals primarily with the mind should be based on a broadly inclusive view of what it means to be 'human', and since disorders of the mind frequently compromise an individual's autonomy, a category central to ethical arguments. However, the association of psychiatry with ethics contains dangers for both fields. One danger is that both fields are often treated with the same subtle disparagement by medical school faculty members and students. Many believe that there is no real expertise in these areas, and therefore no need for any specially trained faculty; they are seen as part of the 'art' of medicine rather than the 'science', part of the tradition shared by all physicians. Another danger is that linking psychiatry and ethics may contribute to the common confusion in clinical practice between ethical dilemmas and psychiatric problems; situations that are emotionally troubling because they embody difficult moral problems may be misidentified as presenting psychiatric questions,[21] while the medico-legal necessity of obtaining psychiatric consultation in cases of treatment-refusal contributes further to this blurring. Finally, there is a risk that psychiatry, eager to secure a place among the medical specialties and to be seen as 'scientific', will subscribe to the general distortion that ethics is intellectually 'soft', and will, for political reasons, renounce its special connection to ethics.

Teaching in psychiatric training programs

The most natural setting for teaching the ethical aspects of psychiatry would seem to be during psychiatric training programs, and surveys of training directors have found the vast majority in agreement that ethics should be part of the core curriculum in psychiatric training.[22,23] However, the same surveys show a sharp discrepancy between what these educators believe the curriculum should contain, and what their trainees are actually offered; only 60 per cent of the programs in the US offered any formal instruction in psychiatric ethics, and less than half of these covered the central issues of involuntary treatment, confidentiality, and sexual misconduct. In another survey, 76 per cent of psychiatric trainees reported feeling unprepared to handle ethical dilemmas.[24] These findings are especially striking in view of the facts that a number of prominent psychiatric educators have a strong interest in ethical issues, and that the American Psychiatric Association's *Principles of medical ethics, with annotations especially applicable to psychiatry* is intended to be understood and used not only by practicing psychiatrists, but by trainees as well.[25] The dramatic expansion of interest in the ethical aspects of psychiatric practice has not yet been accompanied by a comparably increased attention to the teaching of ethics to psychiatric trainees.

The growth of interest in psychiatric ethics since the 1980s, and the number of different subjects packed into psychiatric training, make it important not to overinterpret the failure to develop these programs. However, there are some special problems that emerge when including the teaching of ethics in psychiatric training. First, a great deal of this training occurs in monstrously immoral social institutions—outdated, uncomfortable, inhumane, and reflecting the fear and stigma of mental illness, as well as the political refusal to recognize and accept the inevitable costs if the mentally ill are regarded as full citizens and members of the community. The psychiatric trainee participating in these institutions—whether hospitals, community programs, prisons, homes for the elderly, schools for the retarded, or the network of social services that usually fails to integrate them—feels the discomfort that has marked the entire profession's relation to the mental health system. There are several possible responses to this discomfort: guilt, anger at the profession, political activism, cynical nihilism, or withdrawal from involvement in mental health. However, whatever the specific form of the response, it is not usually a comfortable time to think about the basic ethical issues involved. Fortunately, the problem seems to be diminishing, with the growing interest and awareness in the profession of the social, political, and ethical significance of its work, and, perhaps, the beginning of a recognition that consideration of these is an essential component of a training program.

A second problem in teaching ethics in psychiatric training programs relates to the subject matter itself. Trainees are struggling to acquire a new paradigm, to think of behavior as determined by biological, psychological, and social forces. This requires a suspension of their more customary framework for regarding the same behavior, the everyday common-sense approach that includes a considerable amount of moral judgment. An important theme of psychiatric training is learning to suspend moral judgments in areas where they would naturally be employed. At times, this can lead to an unfortunate generalization outside the clinical setting, a kind of amorality that seeks to understand all behavior while judging nothing. Optimally, good psychiatric training eventually leads students to recognize that in certain carefully specified clinical situations there are advantages to suspending moral judgments in order to create a field of inquiry that will make it possible to dissect the determinants of behavior—and indeed of morality itself. If not, the emotional atmosphere necessary for the inquiry process can not be established. Similarly, good training in ethical reasoning should lead students to recognize the advantage of temporarily suspending familiar moral judgments, so that the principles underlying these judgments can be elucidated and compared with alternative moral principles. The conflict of two such principles, or 'goods', defines an ethical dilemma, and the analysis of such a dilemma requires students to make explicit those everyday moral judgments that they have previously held implicitly or unconsciously.

Thus, both ethical and clinical reasoning require the suspension of familiar moral judgments, and ideally they can reinforce each other. However, the problem in training is that a student who is struggling with the unsettling new paradigm of psychiatry may use the more familiar paradigm of morality as a resistance, and impose moral judgments which interfere with the optimal neutrality of the clinician. In the jargon of the field, ethical reasoning is confused with moral passion, and morality is used as a resistance against clinical understanding. While ethics is by no means incompatible with clinical reasoning, they are different, and there may be interactions between them that have educational significance. In a sense, learning psychiatry can be like learning a new language, and it may be useful to stop using one's native tongue for a while. This interaction can work in both directions, and just as learning a new language can enhance one's understanding of a familiar one, so these two different frameworks for considering human behavior can clarify and explicate the characteristics of the other.

Ethics in continuing education

Psychiatric education extends beyond the formal training program, and psychiatric ethics has an important role to play in continuing education. Seminars and symposia have received wide attention, especially the conferences of the Hastings Center on ethical aspects of psychiatric treatment and research. There has also been a growing awareness of ethical issues by those psychiatrists who completed their formal training before these topics were included in educational programs.[26] Some novel techniques have been tried, such as role-playing,[27] hypotheticals, and mock disciplinary procedures,[28] in addition to the traditional 'ethics rounds', which use a case-conference format and usually address staff at various levels, including graduate psychiatrists.[29]

The American Psychiatric Association has become increasingly active in promoting ethics education for graduate psychiatrists, as well as trainees, especially with respect to the issue of sexual misconduct. In addition to its code of ethics,[30] the association has published an anthology on the topic of professional sexual misconduct,[31] a compendium of the legal consequences of sexual misconduct,[32] and a series of videotapes on the issue.[33,34] These resources are designed to be particularly useful in the ethics education of practicing psychiatrists.

What to teach?

Metaethics

The content of the curriculum in psychiatric ethics can be considered on three levels. First is the basic introduction to ethics, the philosophical basis of moral discourse, or meta-ethics. For a psychiatrist to have more than opinions on right and wrong, to understand the place of these views in the larger sphere of moral reasoning, the types of justification that are being used or discarded, and the history of these views in general ethics—in short, to have an ethical understanding of moral positions—requires some education in meta-ethics. This necessity is analogous to the need for training in basic biochemistry and pharmacology for the psychiatrist to understand psychoactive medications, both those currently in use and those not yet developed.

Few psychiatrists are prepared to teach meta-ethics; if it is to be taken seriously, it requires the collaboration of philosophers, ethicists, or others with similar backgrounds. It can be taught as a distinct body of knowledge with the advantage of emphasizing the inherent structure and relationships of the discipline itself, but with the disadvantage of being given low priority by trainees who are preoccupied with more immediate and practical concerns. Alternatively, the meta-ethical dimensions of specific ethical issues can be explored in the context of discussing those specific issues. For example, a discussion of the relationship between individual autonomy, involuntary treatment, and the right to treatment in psychiatric settings can be used to explore the relationship between utilitarian and absolutist modes of ethical reasoning. This second approach reverses the advantages and disadvantages of the first; the material is organized in categories that 'feel' more relevant to the students, but at the risk of diluting and fragmenting the critical issues in the underlying philosophical dialogue. There are practical problems that also must be considered: if qualified teachers are scarce, the first mode of presentation—a systematic review of ethical theory—requires less of their time, while the second format is more likely to encourage interaction between psychiatrists and professional philosophers.

Codes of ethics and the profession

The second level of the curriculum in psychiatric ethics would involve discussions of the normative rules, standards, and codes of the profession: what psychiatrists and psychiatry ought to do and why.[35,36] Students should be educated about what it means to be a member of a profession;[37] how the profession decides on a code of conduct or ethics for its members and enforces it; and the history, evolution, and current status of psychiatry's ethical codes. This material also can be taught in a separate discussion or integrated with the teaching of specific issues. This level of ethics is closely related to issues of law, politics, and social policy, and their teaching can be integrated into the curriculum. The teaching of rules of conduct can easily degenerate into moralistic sermons; such a fate is best prevented by serious efforts to explore professional codes or prescriptions in a meta-ethical framework, while at the same time considering their application to concrete situations and their practical consequences for society and for the profession.

The discussion of the codes and standards of the profession will also offer an opportunity to explore the nature of professionals and their relationship to the general society. Many of the recent controversies about psychiatric ethics focus on this theme: the dilemmas of providing treatment in a managed-care setting, the assumptions and mechanisms of peer review, and the issue of reporting a colleague who breaches the profession's code would all be examples. Trainees should be made aware of the varying systems for regulation of the profession, including criminal sanctions, civil suits, and government licensing bodies, as well as the profession's own code of self-governance, and of the interaction of these systems.

Specific topics

The third level of the curriculum in psychiatric ethics would be the consideration of specific issues in the field. The list of potential subjects is long enough that any course would have to make selections, but certain topics might be considered essential, either because they embody theoretical issues which are widely applicable to other situations, or because they present important dilemmas which clinicians face frequently. The following topics should be addressed, in some form, in any thorough curriculum in psychiatric ethics:

- *Involuntary treatment* is perhaps the quintessential issue of psychiatric ethics. In general medicine we make the assumption that the patient is free to make autonomous decisions about diseases of the body and their treatment, but this assumption is routinely called into question when the disease process affects the mind, as is the rule in psychiatry. The discussion of involuntary treatment will lead naturally into questions of the patient's autonomy, the physician's beneficence, the meaning of informed consent, the assessment of competence, and the problem of who should make decisions for the incompetent patient.

- The term '*double-agent problem*'[38] has been applied to situations in which the psychiatrist faces a dilemma because of obligations to a third party (an individual, an institution, or society at large) which conflict with the obligation to the patient. The assessment of dangerousness is the most obvious example of this problem, but the category also includes such issues as the distribution of limited resources (Chapter 18), the social and political abuse of psychiatry (Chapter 4), the distinction between illness and deviance (Chapter 9), and political activism by psychiatrists.

- *Confidentiality* has historically been a central ethical category in all of medicine, but especially in psychiatry because of the stigma attached to psychiatric diagnosis and treatment, and the importance of truth in the conduct of psychotherapy. The discussion of confidentiality will overlap with that of the double-agent problem, since the claim to override confidentiality is frequently made in the name of the interests of a third party. Perhaps the most common and gripping example of this problem currently is the dilemma of informing third parties who might be at risk because of contact with an HIV-infected patient. In the course of considering confidentiality, related issues which can be addressed include: the reasons for the principle of confidentiality (deontological vs. utilitarian arguments), the values which might override confidentiality, the effects of labeling and stigma, and dealings with third-party payers.

- *Economic issues* in psychiatry have generated some of the most pressing of current ethical problems, and recent changes in the financing of health care have brought these issues from the level of abstract social policy to the everyday experience of trainees caring for individual patients. The discussion of these issues might begin with a general consideration of the problem of distributive justice, and proceed to an exploration of the dilemmas involved in caring for a patient whose economic resources do not cover the recommended treatment. Related issues include the role of various social institutions in designing health-care payment systems, the tradition of caring for indigent patients, and the question of the physician's personal economic interests.

- *Sexual misconduct* is clearly the ethical issue which currently attracts the most attention from the public and the profession alike. The issue itself deserves thorough discussion, but it should also provide an opportunity to consider the reasons for maintaining professional boundaries (especially the possibility of harm to the patient versus harm to the treatment), the data on the incidence and effects of sexual misconduct (cf. ref. 31), other forms of boundary violation, the relationship of psychiatry to other areas of medicine and other professions, and the issue of reporting a colleague's misconduct.

- *The insanity defense* is an extremely rare occurrence, and one with which very few psychiatrists will ever deal directly. However, it is a crucially important topic because it presents so clearly the issue of guilt and responsibility, the conflict between the profession's paradigm of determinism and the society's paradigm of free will, and the need to decide which of these irreconcilable paradigms to employ in a given situation. Students should be familiar with the history of the defense, the actual incidence and outcome of insanity pleas, the role of the psychiatrist as expert witness, and the social and political effects of these arguments on the profession.

Besides these central topics, some related or subsidiary issues which might be regarded as elective include: the right to treatment; irreversible or invasive treatments; institutions, total institutions and deinstitutionalization; values, neutrality, and coercion in psychotherapy; guardianship and proxy for children and the retarded; psychopharmacology for recreation or performance enhancement; and consent and risk in psychiatric research. Each of these topics could be explored in terms of the values and choices they entail, the history of the profession's response, the arguments that have been presented on behalf of various positions, the basic ethical issues implicit in these arguments, and the pattern of views on the entire array of topics that reflect more general ethical positions.

Goals and objectives

The common confusion of ethics with morality leads to a fundamental tension between different objectives, often unstated, for teaching programs in ethics. Most students and many educators (particularly those who have had little formal exposure to ethical reasoning, but who appreciate the difficulty and importance of ethical dilemmas) tend to see training in ethics as a means of instilling or protecting idealism and 'human values' in students, or of offering them humane and reasonable guidelines for resolving ethical dilemmas in practice. Others, more inclined to value ethical discourse as an intellectually rigorous discipline, tend to see the objectives as educating students in the history and current status of the discipline and cultivating habits of critical reasoning about these issues. These different views are not incompatible, but neither are they identical; the failure to recognize, if not to resolve, the tension between them can seriously undermine the effectiveness of a teaching program in ethics. Thus, while any particular program is likely to pursue several different goals at the same time, the goals should be articulated as clearly as possible. Goals related to knowledge include understanding major systems of ethical reasoning and their similarities and differences, learning the terms and concepts used in ethical discourse, and learning the history of the contemporary ethical dilemmas in psychiatry, with the positions and arguments that have developed around them. Among the attitude-related goals are sensitizing the student to the ethical aspects of issues that might otherwise be seen as scientific or technical in nature, and acquainting him or her with the subtlety and complexity of ethical reasoning, often seen by those who are not familiar with it as little more than 'common sense'. The goals defined in terms of skill would include the student's ability to recognize ethical problems in psychiatry; to reason about them in a coherent, systematic, and useful way; and to understand the reasoning of others and participate with them in ethical discourse. Finally, the goals might involve modifying the professional behavior of students so that it is informed and guided by their understanding of psychiatric ethics.

The selection of goals for a specific curriculum will be determined by the stage in the student's professional education, the time available, the setting, and the faculty. Generally, programs that aim exclusively at modifying the student's behavior in a specific direction without attending to knowledge and attitude have little lasting impact, while those that focus on knowledge without attention to skill have difficulty involving more pragmatically oriented students.

Constructing curricula

Pedagogic principles

Educational programs are most successful if the students acquire knowledge that helps them to accomplish tasks in which they are currently engaged, and if they are given opportunities to apply the knowledge they are acquiring while they are acquiring it. When these principles are applied to the subject matter of psychiatric ethics, some general guidelines for constructing curricula emerge. First, although lectures about ethical issues may impart information about terms, concepts, and the history of arguments and positions, the student will gain familiarity with moral reasoning only by participating more actively through dialogue and discussion. Second, although the 'classic' issues of psychiatric ethics should be explored, and the student has much to learn about them and from participating in discussions of them, a valuable dimension is added if the underlying themes and problems are traced in the student's current professional experience. For example, the 'double agent' problem is clearly articulated in discussions of the psychiatrist's obligation to warn potential victims of violent patients in general, but the question will have additional meaning to the trainee who discusses it in terms of a psychotic patient who wants to return to an occupation involving public safety, or of an adolescent patient whose sexual or drug-related behavior is not acceptable to family or society.

Psychiatric ethics involves intellectual areas in which psychiatrists have no special claim to expertise, and there are advantages to constructing programs that will bring psychiatrists together with other mental health professionals, lawyers, sociologists, and philosophers, both in the student body and on the faculty. The broader meaning of one's routine and daily decisions is experienced dramatically when seen through the eyes of an intelligent observer who has been socialized into a different perspective. For example, courses including psychiatric trainees and law students provide each of these groups with an opportunity to explore ethical questions in involuntary treatment or criminal responsibility which greatly enlarges the perspective that either group meeting alone would have.[39]

Finally, like any other curriculum, attention to evaluation enriches the program. Not only does it force the faculty to specify goals and objectives (all too often ignored when the subject matter is obviously relevant, but necessarily vague and amorphous), but it also forces a dialogue between students and faculty members about these goals. Students often approach programs in psychiatric ethics with the assumption that the intent is to teach them what to do in difficult or special situations. A well-constructed curriculum and evaluation procedure can convey that the goal is to help students identify alternatives and analyze the ethical aspects of the choices they face in their daily professional activities, to discuss these intelligently with their colleagues, and to clarify and, when appropriate, resolve differences and conflicts.

A curricular model

The following is presented as a model program for teaching one specific topic in psychiatric ethics, the issue of sexual misconduct. The illustration assumes that the faculty has adequate appropriate expertise, relevant clinical opportunities for students, and time in the curriculum; it would have to be modified to an extent if these resources are limited.

Before beginning clinical work, medical students should be told clearly that sexual relationships with patients are prohibited by the profession. For practical reasons, this principle must be stated before the students start seeing patients, but the presentation of the rule also provides an opportunity for an introductory discussion of how and why the profession makes such rules, and why the student must be willing to substitute the profession's judgment in some matters for his or her own. The topic can also be used as a vehicle to introduce a general framework for the consideration of ethical dilemmas, since the question of sex between a physician and a consenting adult patient leads naturally into a consideration of the conflicts involving respect for the patient's autonomy, the duty to protect the patient from unforeseen harm, the physician's personal interest, and the physician's responsibility to the profession and its future patients. In this fashion, ethics can be presented as a rigorous intellectual discipline, and as a basic science of medicine. Later in medical school, clinical supervisors should be attentive to boundary issues in their discussion of the student's work with patients, and should take the initiative in addressing these issues explicitly, as students are likely to avoid raising them out of ignorance or discomfort.

In the early years of residency in psychiatry, the issue of sexual misconduct should be addressed again in a seminar format, but this time with attention to the profession's explicit statements on the subject (including, for example, the Hippocratic Oath and the code of the American Medical Association, as well as that of the American Psychiatric Association), the history of these statements and the arguments about them, and the profession's mechanisms for enforcing its code (including the requirement to report allegations of misconduct and the procedures for professional sanction, as well as licensing procedures and civil and criminal penalties). Later in residency, a more advanced seminar might consider the data on the incidence and effects of sexual misconduct (cf. ref. 31), the evolution of the profession's position on the issue, the relationship to other forms of boundary violations, and the central role of transference and countertransference in these considerations. Perhaps the most compelling learning experience for the student in this area, as in others, will come in the individual supervision of work with patients, and supervisors must be trained and encouraged to open the issue for discussion. The supervisor should create an atmosphere in which the presentation of boundary dilemmas, and especially of countertransference difficulties, is a natural and expected part of the work, rather than a source of shame for the trainee, and in which the ethical principles discussed in the classroom can be applied directly and explicitly to the student's work with specific patients.

The same issues should be revisited regularly in continuing education beyond residency training, because clinicians will face them regularly, because the issues and arguments will likely evolve over time, and because the individual practitioner may avoid thinking about them without reinforcement from the profession to keep them in continual focus. Ethics rounds, peer supervision, and didactic presentations in continuing education settings all provide opportunities for this necessary ongoing education.

Conclusion

Interest in the teaching of psychiatric ethics has lagged behind the growing interest in the ethical issues themselves, but will surely continue to increase. Such teaching is more likely to occur in psychiatric and continuing education programs than in pre-medical or medical school curricula. It should include discussion of meta-ethics, or the basic principles of ethical reasoning; normative codes of professional conduct, or the rules for psychiatrists facing choices; and the specific situations and problems that interest and trouble psychiatrists today.

References and notes

1. McCartney, J. R.: Consultation–liaison psychiatry and the teaching of ethics. *General Hospital Psychiatry* **8**:411–14, 1986.
2. Hayes, J. R.: Consultation–liaison psychiatry and clinical ethics: a model for consultation and teaching. *General Hospital Psychiatry* **8**:415–18, 1986.
3. Perl, M.: Response to the articles 'Consultation–liaison psychiatry and the teaching of ethics' by J. R. McCartney and 'Consultation–liaison psychiatry and clinical ethics' by J. R. Hayes. *General Hospital Psychiatry* **8**:419–21, 1986.
4. Bursztajn, H.: 'Ethicogenesis': response to the articles 'Consultation–liaison psychiatry and the teaching of ethics' by J. R. McCartney, and 'Consultation–liaison psychiatry and clinical ethics' by J. R. Hayes. *General Hospital Psychiatry* **8**:422–4, 1986.

5. Case vignette: teaching ethics and psychotherapy. *Ethics and Behavior* **8**:69, 1996.
6. Lazarus, A. A.: Fixed rules vs. idiosyncratic needs. *Ethics and Behavior* **6**:80-1, 1996.
7. Gabbard, G. O.: Teacher of the year? *Ethics and Behavior* **6**:82–5, 1996.
8. Culver, C. M., Clouser, K. D., Gert, B., *et al.*: Special report: basic curricular goals in medical ethics. *New England Journal of Medicine* **312**:253–6, 1985.
9. Cf.: Teaching medical ethics, a special edition of *Academic Medicine* **64**:699–788, 1989.
10. Bloch, S.: Teaching psychiatric ethics. *Medical Education* **22**:550–3, 1988.
11. Sondheimer, A. and Martucci, C.: An approach to teaching ethics in child and adolescent psychiatry. *Journal of the American Academy of Child and Adolescent Psychiatry* **31**:415–22, 1992.
12. Schnapp, W. B., Stone, S., Van Norman, J., and Ruiz, P.: Teaching ethics in psychiatry: a problem-based learning approach. *Academic Psychiatry* **20**:144–9, 1996.
13. Hassenfeld, I. N. and Grumet, B.: Fifteen years of teaching psychiatric law and ethics to residents. *Academic Psychiatry* **20**:165–75, 1996.
14. Self, D. J. and Olivarez, M.: Retention of moral reasoning skills over the four years of medical education. *Teaching and Learning in Medicine* **8**:195–9, 1996.
15. Bickel, J.: Human values teaching programs in the clinical education of medical students. *Journal of Medical Education* **62**:369–78, 1987.
16. Wolstenholme, G.: Teaching medical ethics in other countries. *Journal of Medical Ethics* **11**:22–4, 1985.
17. Pellegrino, E. D., Hart, R. J., Henderson, S. R., Loeb, S. E., and Edwards, E. G.: Relevance and utility of courses in medical ethics. *Journal of the American Medical Association* **253**:49–53, 1985.
18. Cf. a special issue of *Academic Medicine* on 'The humanities and medical education'. Vol. **70**, 1995.
19. Radwany, S. M. and Adelson, B. H.: The use of literary classics in teaching medical ethics to physicians. *Journal of the American Medical Association* **257**:1629–31, 1987.
20. Sider, R. and Clements, C.: Psychiatry's contribution to medical ethics education. *American Journal of Psychiatry* **139**:498–501, 1982.
21. Perl, M. and Shelp, E. E.: Psychiatric consultation masking moral dilemmas in medicine. *New England Journal of Medicine* **307**:618–21, 1982.
22. Coverdale, J. H., Bayer, T., Isbell, P., and Moffic, C.: Are we teaching psychiatrists to be ethical? *Academic Psychiatry* **16**:199–205, 1992.
23. Coverdale, J. H.: The status of ethics education in Australasian psychiatry. *Australian and New Zealand Journal of Psychiatry* **30**:813–18, 1996.
24. Roberts, L. W., McCarty, T., Lyketsos, C., *et al.*: What and how psychiatry residents at ten training programs wish to learn about ethics. *Academic Psychiatry* **20**:131–43, 1996.
25. *The principles of medical ethics, with annotations especially applicable to psychiatry.* Washington, DC, American Psychiatric Association, 1995.
26. Handelsman, M.: Ethics training at mental health centers. *Community Mental Health Journal* **25**:42–50, 1989.
27. Roman, B. and Kay, J.: Residency education on the prevention of physician patient sexual misconduct. *Academic Psychiatry* **21**:26–34, 1997.
28. Levine, S. and Pinsker, H.: The mock trial in psychiatric staff education. *Bulletin of the American Academy of Psychiatry and the Law* **22**:127–32, 1994.

29. Appelbaum, P.: Solving clinical puzzles: strategies for organizing mental health ethics rounds, in S. J. Reiser, H. J. Bursztajn, P. S. Appelbaum, and T. G. Gutheil (ed.), *Divided staffs, divided selves: a case approach to mental health ethics.* Cambridge, Cambridge University Press, 1987, pp. 41–59.

30. *The principles of medical ethics, with annotations especially applicable to psychiatry.* Washington, DC, American Psychiatry Association, 1995.

31. Gabbard, G. (ed.): *Sexual exploitation in professional relationships.* Washington, DC, American Psychiatric Press, 1989.

32. Legal sanctions for mental health professional–patient sex. Washington, DC, American Psychiatric Association, 1993.

33. Subcommittee on Education of Psychiatrists on Ethical Issues, American Psychiatric Association: *Ethical concerns about sexual involvement between psychiatrists and patients—videotaped vignettes for discussion.* Washington, DC, American Psychiatric Association, 1986.

34. Subcommittee on Education of Psychiatrists on Ethical Concerns, American Psychiatric Association: *Reporting ethical concerns about sexual involvement with patients* (videotape). Washington, DC, American Psychiatric Association, 1990.

35. Moore, R. A.: Ethics in the practice of psychiatry—origins, functions, models,and enforcement. *American Journal of Psychiatry* **135**, 157–63, 1978.

36. Michels, R.: The physician and medical education. *P&S Quarterly* **19**:13–15, 1974.

37. Michels, R.: Professional ethics and social values. *International Review of Psychoanalysis* **3**:377–84, 1976.

38. *American Psychiatric Association and the Institute of Society, Ethics, and the Life Sciences: a conference on conflicting loyalties.* Special supplement, 1978. Hastings-on-Hudson, New York, the Institute, 1978.

39. Himmelstein, J. and Michels, R.: The right to refuse psychoactive drugs. *Hastings Center Report* **3**:8–11, June, 1973.

Appendix

Codes of ethics

Codes for the ethical guidance of physicians have been promulgated over many centuries and in many different countries. In this appendix we offer a selection which we believe are relevant to the psychiatrist. Included are the *Hippocratic Oath*, and the *Declaration of Geneva* of the World Medical Association.

Two codes for the ethical conduct of biomedical research are provided—the *Declaration of Helsinki* and the *Nuremberg Code*.

There are few specific codes of ethics for psychiatrists. We cite three—*The Principles of medical ethics with annotations especially applicable to psychiatry* of the American Psychiatric Association, the World Psychiatric Association's *Declaration of Madrid*, and the *Code of Professional Ethics of the Psychiatrist* of the Russian Society of Psychiatrists.

The Hippocratic Oath

I swear by Apollo Physician and Asclepius and Hygieia and Panaceia and all the gods and goddesses, making them my witnesses, that I will fulfil according to my ability and judgment this oath and this covenant:

To hold him who has taught me this art as equal to my parents and to live my life in partnership with him, and if he is in need of money to give him a share of mine, and to regard his offspring as equal to my brothers in male lineage and to teach them this art—if they desire to learn it—without fee and covenant; to give a share of precepts and oral instruction and all the other learning to my sons and to the sons of him who has instructed me and to pupils who have signed the covenant and have taken an oath according to the medical law, but to no one else.

I will apply dietetic measures for the benefit of the sick according to my ability and judgment; I will keep them from harm and injustice.

I will neither give a deadly drug to anybody if asked for it, nor will I make a suggestion to this effect. Similarly I will not give to a woman an abortive remedy. In purity and holiness I will guard my life and my art.

I will not use the knife, not even on sufferers from stone, but will withdraw in favor of such men as are engaged in this work.

Whatever houses I may visit, I will come for the benefit of the sick, remaining free of all intentional injustice, of all mischief and in particular of sexual relations with both female and male persons, be they free or slaves.

What I may see or hear in the course of the treatment or even outside of the treatment in regard to the life of men, which on no account one must spread abroad, I will keep to myself holding such things shameful to be spoken about.

If I fulfil this oath and do not violate it, may it be granted to me to enjoy life and art, being honored with fame among all men for all time to come; if I transgress it and swear falsely, may the opposite of all this be my lot.

[Reprinted by permission from *Ancient Medicine: Selected Papers of Ludwig Edelstein*, edited by Oswei Temkin and C. Temkin, Baltimore, Johns Hopkins University Press, 1967]

The Declaration of Geneva

Physician's Oath

At the time of being admitted as a member of the medical profession:

I solemnly pledge myself to consecrate my life to the service of humanity;

I will give to my teachers the respect and gratitude which is their due;

I will practise my profession with conscience and dignity; the health of my patient will be my first consideration;

I will maintain by all the means in my power, the honor and the noble traditions of the medical profession; my colleagues will be my brothers;

I will not permit considerations of religion, nationality, race, party politics or social standing to intervene between my duty and my patient;

I will maintain the utmost respect for human life from the time of conception; even under threat, I will not use my medical knowledge contrary to the laws of humanity;

I make these promises solemnly, freely and upon my honor.

[Adopted by the General Assembly of the World Medical Association, Geneva, 1948, amended 1968. Reprinted by permission]

The Nuremberg Code

The judgment by the war crimes tribunal at Nuremberg laid down 10 standards to which physicians must conform when carrying out experiments on human subjects.

PERMISSIBLE MEDICAL EXPERIMENTS

The great weight of the evidence before us to effect that certain types of medical experiments on human beings, when kept within reasonably well-defined bounds, conform to the ethics of the medical profession generally. The protagonists of the practice of human experimentation justify their views on the basis that such experiments yield results for the good of society that are unprocurable by other methods or means of study. All agree, however, that certain basic principles must be observed in order to satisfy moral ethical and legal concepts:

1. The voluntary consent of the human subject is absolutely essential. This means that the person involved should have legal capacity to give consent; should be so situated as to be able to exercise free power of choice, without the intervention of any element of force, fraud, deceit, duress, overreaching, or other ulterior form of constraint or coercion; and should have sufficient knowledge and comprehension of the elements of the subject matter involved as to enable him to make an understanding and enlightened decision. This latter element requires that before the acceptance of an affirmative decision by the experimental subject there should be made known to him the nature, duration, and purpose of the experiment; the method and means by which it is to be conducted; all inconveniences and hazards reasonably to be expected; and the effects upon his health or person which may possibly come from his participation in the experiment. The duty and responsibility for ascertaining the quality of the consent rests upon each individual who initiates, directs, or engages in the experiment. It is a personal duty and responsibility which may not be delegated to another with impunity.

2. The experiment should be such as to yield fruitful results for the good of society, unprocurable by other methods or means of study, and not random and unnecessary in nature.

3. The experiment should be so designed and based on the results of animal experimentation and a knowledge of the natural history of the disease or other problem under study that the anticipated results justify the performance of the experiment.

4. The experiment should be so conducted as to avoid all unnecessary physical and mental suffering and injury.

5. No experiment should be conducted where there is an a priori reason to believe that death or disabling injury will occur; except, perhaps, in those experiments where the experimental physicians also serve as subjects.

6. The degree of risk to be taken should never exceed that determined by the humanitarian importance of the problem to be solved by the experiment.

7. Proper preparations should be made and adequate facilities provided to protect the experimental subject against even remote possibilities of injury, disability or death.

8. The experiment should be conducted only by scientifically qualified persons. The highest degree of skill and care should be required through all stages of the experiment of those who conduct or engage in the experiment.

9. During the course of the experiment the human subject should be at liberty to bring the experiment to an end if he has reached the physical or mental state where continuation of the experiment seems to him to be impossible.

10. During the course of the experiment the scientist in charge must be prepared to terminate the experiment at any stage, if he has probable cause to believe, in the exercise of the good faith, superior skill and careful judgment required of him, that a continuation of the experiment is likely to result in injury, disability, or death to the experimental subject.

[Reprinted by permission from Mitscherlich A, Mielke F. *Doctors of infamy: the story of the Nazi medical crimes.* New York, Schuman, 1949]

Declaration of Helsinki

Recommendations guiding medical doctors in biomedical research involving human subjects

INTRODUCTION

It is the mission of the physician to safeguard the health of the people. His or her knowledge and conscience are dedicated to the fulfilment of this mission.

The Declaration of Geneva of the World Medical Association binds the physician with the words, "The health of my patient will be my first consideration," and the International Code of Medical Ethics declares that, "A physician shall act only in the patient's interest when providing medical care which might have the effect of weakening the physical and mental condition of the patient."

The purpose of biomedical research involving human subjects must be to improve diagnostic, therapeutic and prophylactic procedures and the understanding of the aetiology and pathogenesis of disease.

In current medical practice most diagnostic, therapeutic or prophylactic procedures involve hazards. This applies especially to biomedical research.

Medical progress is based on research which ultimately must rest in part on experimentation involving human subjects.

In the field of biomedical research a fundamental distinction must be recognised between medical research in which the aim is essentially diagnostic or therapeutic for a patient, and medical research the essential object of which is purely scientific and without implying direct diagnostic or therapeutic value to the person subjected to the research.

Special caution must be exercised in the conduct of research which may affect the environment, and the welfare of animals used for research must be respected.

Because it is essential that the result of laboratory experiments be applied to human beings to further scientific knowledge and to help suffering humanity, the World Medical Association has prepared the following recommendations as a guide to every physician in biomedical research involving human subjects. They should be kept under review in the future. It must be stressed that the standards as drafted are only a guide to physicians all over the world. Physicians are not relieved from criminal, civil and ethical responsibilities under the law of their own countries.

I. BASIC PRINCIPLES

1. Biomedical research involving human subjects must conform to generally accepted scientific principles and should be based on adequately performed laboratory and animal experimentation and on a thorough knowledge of the scientific literature.

2. The design and performance of each experimental procedure involving human subjects should be clearly formulated in an experimental protocol which should be transmitted to a specially appointed independent committee for consideration, comment and guidance.

3. Biomedical research involving human subjects should be conducted only by scientifically qualified persons and under the supervision of a clinically competent medical person. The responsibility for the human subject must always rest with a medically qualified person and never rest on the subject of the research, even though the subject has given his or her consent.

4. Biomedical research involving human subjects cannot legitimately be carried out unless the importance of the objective is in proportion to the inherent risk to the subject.

5. Every biomedical research project involving human subjects should be preceded by careful assessment of predictable risks in comparison with foreseeable benefits to the subject or to others. Concern for the interests of the subject must always prevail over the interests of science and society.

6. The right of the research subject to safeguard his or her integrity must always be respected. Every precaution should be taken to respect the privacy of the subject and to minimize the impact of the study on the subject's physical and mental integrity and on the personality of the subject.

7. Physicians should abstain from engaging in research projects involving human subjects unless they are satisfied that the hazards involved are believed to be predictable. Physicians should cease any investigation if the hazards are found to outweigh the potential benefits.

8. In publication of the results of his or her research, the physician is obliged to preserve the accuracy of the results. Reports of experimentation not in accordance with the principles laid down in this Declaration should not be accepted for publication.

9. In any research on human beings, each potential subject must be adequately informed of the aims, methods, anticipated benefits and potential hazards of

the study and the discomfort it may entail. He or she should be informed that he or she is at liberty to abstain from participation in the study and that he or she is free to withdraw his or her consent to participation at any time. The physician should then obtain the subject's freely given informed consent, preferably in writing.

10. When obtaining informed consent for the research project the physician should be particularly cautious if the subject is in a dependent relationship to him or her or may consent under duress. In that case the informed consent should be obtained by a physician who is not engaged in the investigation and who is completely independent of this official relationship.

11. In case of legal incompetence, informed consent should be obtained from the legal guardian in accordance with national legislation. Where physical or mental incapacity makes it impossible to obtain informed consent, or when the subject is a minor, permission from the responsible relative replaces that of the subject in accordance with national legislation. Whenever the minor child is in fact able to give consent, the minor's consent must be obtained in addition to the consent of the minor's legal guardian.

12. The research protocol should always contain a statement of the ethical considerations involved and should indicate that the principles enunciated in the present declaration are complied with.

II. MEDICAL RESEARCH COMBINED WITH CLINICAL CARE (CLINICAL RESEARCH)

1. In the treatment of the sick person, the physician must be free to use a new diagnostic and therapeutic measure, if in his or her judgement it offers hope of saving life, re-establishing health or alleviating suffering.

2. The potential benefits, hazards and discomfort of a new method should be weighed against the advantages of the best current diagnostic and therapeutic methods.

3. In any medical study, every patient including those of a control group, if any, should be assured of the best proven diagnostic and therapeutic method. This does not exclude the use of inert placebos in studies where no proven diagnostic or therapeutic method exists.

4. The refusal of the patient to participate in a study must never interfere with the physician-patient relationship.

5. If the physician considers it essential not to obtain informed consent, the specific reasons for this proposal should be stated in the experimental protocol for transmission to the independent committee (1, 2).

6. The physician can combine medical research with professional care, the objective being the acquisition of new medical knowledge, only to the extent

that medical research is justified by its potential diagnostic or therapeutic value for the patient.

II. NON-THERAPEUTIC BIOMEDICAL RESEARCH INVOLVING HUMAN SUBJECTS (NON-CLINICAL BIOMEDICAL RESEARCH)

1. In the purely scientific application of medical research carried out on a human being, it is the duty of the physician to remain the protector of the life and health of that person on whom biomedical research is being carried out.

2. The subjects should be volunteers—either healthy persons or patients for whom the experimental design is not related to the patient's illness.

3. The investigator or the investigating team should discontinue the research if in his/her or their judgment it may, if continued, be harmful to the individual.

4. In research on man, the interest of science and society should never take precedence over considerations related to the well-being of the subject.

[Adopted by the 18th World Medical Assembly, Helsinki, June 1964, amended by the 29th World Medical Assembly, Tokyo, October 1975, and the 35th World Medical Assembly, Venice, October 1983]

The Declaration of Madrid

In 1977, the World Psychiatric Association approved the Declaration of Hawaii, setting out ethical guidelines for the practice of psychiatry. The Declaration was updated in Vienna in 1983. To reflect the impact of changing social attitudes and new medical developments in the psychiatric profession, the World Psychiatric Association has once again examined and revised these ethical standards.

Medicine is both a healing art and a science. The dynamics of this combination are best reflected in psychiatry, the branch of medicine that specialises in the care and protection of those who are infirm because of a mental disorder or impairment. Although there may be cultural, social and national differences within and between countries, the need for ethical conduct and continual review of ethical standards is universal.

As practitioners of medicine, psychiatrists must be aware of the ethical implications of being a physician, and of the specific ethical demands of the specialty of psychiatry. As members of society, psychiatrists must advocate fair and equal treatment of the mentally ill, and social justice and equity for all.

Ethical behaviour is based on the psychiatrists' individual sense of responsibility towards the patient and their judgement in determining what is correct and appropriate conduct. External standards and influences such as professional codes of conduct, the study of ethics, or the rule of law by themselves will not guarantee the ethical practice of medicine.

Psychiatrists should, at all times, keep in mind the boundaries of the psychiatrist–patient relationship, and be primarily guided by respect for patients and concern for their welfare and integrity.

It is in this spirit that the General Assembly of the World Psychiatric Association approved the following guidelines concerning ethical standards that should govern the conduct of psychiatrists worldwide.

1. Psychiatry is a medical discipline concerned with the provision of the best treatment for mental disorders, with the rehabilitation of individuals suffering from mental illness and with the promotion of mental health. Psychiatrists serve patients by providing the best therapy available in consistence with accepted scientific knowledge and ethical principles. Psychiatrists should devise therapeutic interventions that are the least restrictive to the freedom of the patient, and seek advice in areas of their work in which they do not have primary expertise. While doing so, psychiatrists should be aware of and concerned with the equitable allocation of health resources.

2. It is the duty of psychiatrists to keep abreast of scientific developments of the specialty and to convey updated knowledge to others. Psychiatrists trained in research should seek to advance the scientific frontiers of psychiatry.

3. The patient should be accepted as partner by right in the therapeutic process. The therapist–patient relationship must be based on mutual trust and respect, to allow the patient to make free and informed decisions. It is the duty of psychiatrists to provide the patient with relevant information so as to empower the patient to come to a rational decision according to his or her personal values and preferences.

4. When the patient is incapacitated and/or unable to exercise proper judgement because of a mental disorder, the psychiatrist should consult with the family and, if appropriate, seek legal counsel to safeguard the human dignity and the legal rights of the patient. No treatment should be provided against the patient's will, unless withholding treatment would endanger the life of the patient and/or those who surround him or her. Treatment must always be in the best interest of the patient.

5. When psychiatrists are requested to assess a person, it is their duty to first inform and advise the person being assessed about the use of the findings and about the possible repercussions of the assessment. This is particularly important when psychiatrists are involved in third party situations.

6. Information obtained in the therapeutic relationship should be kept in confidence and used only for the purpose of improving the mental health of the patient. Psychiatrists are prohibited from making use of such information for personal reasons, or for financial or academic benefits. Breach of confidentiality may only be appropriate when serious physical or mental harm to the patient or to a third person could ensue if confidentiality were maintained; in these circumstances psychiatrists should, whenever possible, first advise the patient about the action to be taken.

7. Research that is not conducted in accordance with the canons of science is unethical. Research activities should be approved by an appropriately constituted ethical committee. Psychiatrists should follow national and international rules for the conduct of research. Only individuals properly trained for research should undertake or direct it. Because psychiatric patients are particularly vulnerable research subjects, extra caution should be taken to safeguard their autonomy as well as their mental and physical integrity. Ethical standards should also be applied in the selection of population groups, in all types of research, including epidemiological and sociological studies, and in collaborative research involving other disciplines or several investigating centres.

[Adopted by the World Psychiatric Association, Madrid, August 1996. Reprinted by permission]

Principles of Medical Ethics with Annotations Especially Applicable to Psychiatry.

Preamble

The medical profession has long subscribed to a body of ethical statements developed primarily for the benefit of the patient. As a member of this profession, a physician must recognize responsibility not only to patients but also to society, to other health professionals, and to self. The following Principles, adopted by the American Medical Association, are not laws but standards of conduct, which define the essentials of honorable behavior for the physician.[1]

Section 1

A physician shall be dedicated to providing competent medical service with compassion and respect for human dignity.

   1. The patient may place his/her trust in his/her psychiatrist knowing that the psychiatrist's ethics and professional responsibilities preclude him/her gratifying his/her own needs by exploiting the patient. The psychiatrist shall be

---

[1] Statements in italics are taken directly from the American Medical Association's Principles of Medical Ethics

ever vigilant about the impact that his/her conduct has upon the boundaries of the doctor/patient relationship, and thus upon the well being of the patient. These requirements become particularly important because of the essentially private, highly personal, and sometimes intensely emotional nature of the relationship established with the psychiatrist.

2. A psychiatrist should not be a party to any type of policy that excludes, segregates, or demeans the dignity of any patient because of ethnic origin, race, sex, creed, age, socioeconomic status, or sexual orientation.

3. In accord with the requirements of law and accepted medical practice, it is ethical for a physician to submit his/her work to peer review and to the ultimate authority of the medical staff executive body and the hospital administration and its governing body. In case of dispute, the ethical psychiatrist has the following steps available:

   a. Seek appeal from the medical staff decision to a joint conference committee, including members of the medical staff executive committee and the executive committee of the governing board. At this appeal, the ethical psychiatrist could request that outside opinions be considered.
   b. Appeal to the governing body itself.
   c. Appeal to state agencies regulating licensure of hospitals if, in the particular state, they concern themselves with matters of professional competency and quality of care.
   d. Attempt to educate colleagues through development of research projects and data and presentations at professional meetings and in professional journals.
   e. Seek redress in local courts, perhaps through an enjoining injunction against the governing body.
   f. Public education as carried out by an ethical psychiatrist would not utilize appeals based solely upon emotion, but would be presented in a professional way and without any potential exploitation of patients through testimonials.

4. A psychiatrist should not be a participant in a legally authorized execution.

Section 2

A physician shall deal honestly with patients and colleagues, and strive to expose those physicians deficient in character or competence, or who engage in fraud or deception.

1. The requirement that the physician conduct himself/herself with propriety in his/her profession and in all the actions of his/her life is especially important in the case of the psychiatrist because the patient tends to model his/her behavior after that of his/her psychiatrist by identification. Further, the necessary intensity of the treatment relationship may tend to activate sexual

and other needs and fantasies on the part of both patient and psychiatrist, while weakening the objectivity necessary for control. Additionally, the inherent inequality in the doctor-patient relationship may lead to exploitation of the patient. Sexual activity with a current or former patient is unethical.

2. The psychiatrist should diligently guard against exploiting information furnished by the patient and should not use the unique position of power afforded him/her by the psychotherapeutic situation to influence the patient in any way not directly relevant to the treatment goals.

3. A psychiatrist who regularly practices outside his/her area of professional competence should be considered unethical. Determination of professional competence should be made by peer review boards or other appropriate bodies.

4. Special consideration should be given to those psychiatrists who, due to illness, jeopardize the welfare of their patients and their own reputations and practices. It is ethical, even encouraged, for another psychiatrist to intercede in such situations.

5. Psychiatric services, like all medical services, are dispensed in the context of a contractual arrangement between the patient and the treating physician. The provisions of the contractual arrangement, which are binding on the physician as well as on the patient, should be explicitly established.

6. It is ethical for the psychiatrist to make a charge for a missed appointment when this falls within the terms of the specific contractual agreement with the patient. Charging for a missed appointment or for one not cancelled 24 hours in advance need not, in itself, be considered unethical if a patient is fully advised that the physician will make such a charge. The practice, however, should be resorted to infrequently and always with the utmost consideration for the patient and his/her circumstances.

7. An arrangement in which a psychiatrist provides supervision or administration to other physicians or nonmedical persons for a percentage of their fees or gross income is not acceptable; this would constitute fee-splitting. In a team of practitioners, or a multidisciplinary team, it is ethical for the psychiatrist to receive income for administration, research, education, or consultation. This should be based upon a mutually agreed upon and set fee or salary, open to renegotiation when a change in the time demand occurs. (See also Section 5, Annotations 2, 3, and 4.)

Section 3

A physician shall respect the law and also recognize a responsibility to seek changes in those requirements which are contrary to the best interests of the patient.

1. It would seem self-evident that a psychiatrist who is a law-breaker might be ethically unsuited to practice his/her profession. When such illegal activities bear directly upon his/her practice, this would obviously be the case. However, in other instances, illegal activities such as those concerning the right to protest

social injustices might not bear on either the image of the psychiatrist or the ability of the specific psychiatrist to treat his/her patient ethically and well. While no committee or board could offer prior assurance that any illegal activity would not be considered unethical, it is conceivable that an individual could violate a law without being guilty of professionally unethical behavior. Physicians lose no right of citizenship on entry into the profession of medicine.

2. Where not specifically prohibited by local laws governing medical practice, the practice of acupuncture by a psychiatrist is not unethical per se. The psychiatrist should have professional competence in the use of acupuncture. Or, if he/she is supervising the use of acupuncture by nonmedical individuals, he/she should provide proper medical supervision. (See also Section 5, Annotations 3 and 4.)

Section 4

A physician shall respect the right of patients, of colleagues, and of other health professionals, and shall safeguard patient confidences within the constraints of the law.

1. Psychiatric records, including even the identification of a person as a patient, must be protected with extreme care. Confidentiality is essential to psychiatrist treatment. This is based in part on the special nature of psychiatric therapy as well as on the traditional ethical relationship between physician and patient. Growing concern regarding the civil rights of patients and the possible adverse effects of computerization, duplication equipment, and data banks makes the dissemination of confidential information an increasing hazard. Because of the sensitive and private nature of the information with which the psychiatrist deals, he/she must be circumspect in the information that he/she chooses to disclose to others about a patient. The welfare of the patient must be a continuing consideration.

2. A psychiatrist may release confidential information only with the authorization of the patient or under proper legal compulsion. The continuing duty of the psychiatrist to protect the patient includes fully apprising him/her of the connotations of waiving the privilege of privacy. This may become an issue when the patient is being investigated by a government agency, is applying for a position, or is involved in legal action. The same principles apply to the release of information concerning treatment to medical departments of government agencies, business organizations, labor unions, and insurance companies. Information gained in confidence about patients seen in student health services should not be released without the students' explicit permission.

3. Clinical and other materials used in teaching and writing must be adequately disguised in order to preserve the anonymity of the individuals involved.

4. The ethical responsibility of maintaining confidentiality holds equally for the consultations in which the patient may not have been present and in which

the consultee was not a physician. In such instances, the physician consultant should alert the consultee to his/her duty of confidentiality.

5. Ethically the psychiatrist may disclose only that information which is relevant to a given situation. He/she should avoid offering speculation as fact. Sensitive information such as an individual's sexual orientation or fantasy material is usually unnecessary.

6. Psychiatrists are often asked to examine individuals for security purposes, to determine suitability for various jobs, and to determine legal competence. The psychiatrist must fully describe the nature and purpose and lack of confidentiality of the examination to the examinee at the beginning of the examination.

7. Careful judgment must be exercised by the psychiatrist in order to include, when appropriate, the parents or guardian in the treatment of a minor. At the same time, the psychiatrist must assure the minor proper confidentiality.

8. Psychiatrists at times may find it necessary, in order to protect the patient or the community from imminent danger, to reveal confidential information disclosed by the patient.

9. When the psychiatrist is ordered by the court to reveal the confidences entrusted to him/her by patients, he/she may comply or he/she may ethically hold the right to dissent within the framework of the law. When the psychiatrist is in doubt, the right of the patient to confidentiality and, by extension, to unimpaired treatment, should be given priority. The psychiatrist should reserve the right to raise the question of adequate need for disclosure. In the event that the necessity for legal disclosure is demonstrated by the court, the psychiatrist may request the right to disclosure of only that information which is relevant to the legal question at hand.

10. With regard for the person's dignity and privacy and with truly informed consent, it is ethical to present a patient to a scientific gathering, if the confidentiality of the presentation is understood and accepted by the audience.

11. It is ethical to present a patient or former patient to a public gathering or to the news media only if the patient is fully informed of enduring loss of confidentiality, is competent, and consents in writing without coercion.

12. When involved in funded research, the ethical psychiatrist will advise human subjects of the funding source, retain his/her freedom to reveal data and results, and follow all appropriate and current guidelines relative to human subject protection.

13. Ethical considerations in medical practice preclude the psychiatric evaluation of any person charged with criminal acts prior to access to, or availability of, legal counsel. The only exception is the rendering of care to the person for the sole purpose of medical treatment.

14. Sexual involvement between a faculty member or supervisor and a trainee or student, in those situations in which an abuse of power can occur, often takes advantage of inequalities in the working relationship and may be unethical because: (a) any treatment of a patient being supervised may be

deleteriously affected; (b) it may damage the trust relationship between teacher and student; and (c) teachers are important professional role models for their trainees and affect their trainees' future professional behavior.

Section 5

A physician shall continue to study, apply, and advance scientific knowledge, make relevant information available to patients, colleagues, and the public, obtain consultation, and use the talents of other health professionals when indicated.

1. Psychiatrists are responsible for their own continuing education and should be mindful of the fact that theirs must be a lifetime of learning.

2. In the practice of his/her specialty, the psychiatrist consults, associates, collaborates, or integrates his/her work with that of many professionals, including psychologists, psychometricians, social workers, alcoholism counselors, marriage counselors, public health nurses, etc. Furthermore, the nature of modern psychiatric practice extends his/her contacts to such people as teachers, juvenile and adult probation offices, attorneys, welfare workers, agency volunteers, and neighborhood aides. In referring patients for treatment, counseling, or rehabilitation to any of these practitioners, the psychiatrist should ensure that the allied professional or paraprofessional with whom he/she is dealing is a recognized member of his/her own discipline and is competent to carry out the therapeutic task required. The psychiatrist should have the same attitude toward members of the medical profession to whom he/she refers patients. Whenever he/she has reason to doubt the training, skill, or ethical qualifications of the allied professional, the psychiatrist should not refer cases to him/her.

3. When the psychiatrist assumes a collaborative or supervisory role with another mental health worker, he/she must expend sufficient time to assure that proper care is given. It is contrary to the interests of the patient and to patient care if he/she allows himself/herself to be used as a figurehead.

4. In relationships between psychiatrists and practising licensed psychologists, the physician should not delegate to the psychologist or, in fact, to any nonmedical person any matter requiring the exercise of professional medical judgment.

5. The psychiatrist should agree to the request of a patient for consultation or to such a request from the family of an incompetent or minor patient. The psychiatrist may suggest possible consultants, but the patient or family should be given free choice of the consultant. If the psychiatrist disapproves of the professional qualifications of the consultant or if there is a difference of opinion that the primary therapist cannot resolve, he/she may, after suitable notice, withdraw from the case. If this disagreement occurs within an institution or agency framework, the differences should be resolved by the mediation or arbitration of higher professional authority within the institution or agency.

Section 6

A physician shall, in the provision of appropriate patient care, except in emergencies, be free to choose whom to serve, with whom to associate, and the environment in which to provide medical services.

1. Physicians generally agree that the doctor-patient relationship is such a vital factor in effective treatment of the patient that preservation of optimal conditions for development of a sound working relationship between a doctor and his/her patient should take precedence over all other considerations. Professional courtesy may lead to poor psychiatric care for physicians and their families because of embarrassment over the lack of a complete give-and-take contract.

2. An ethical psychiatrist may refuse to provide psychiatrist treatment to a person who, in the psychiatrist's opinion, cannot be diagnosed as having a mental illness amenable to psychiatric treatment.

Section 7

A physician shall recognize a responsibility to participate in activities contributing to an improved community.

1. Psychiatrists should foster the cooperation of those legitimately concerned with the medical, psychological, social, and legal aspects of mental health and illness. Psychiatrists are encouraged to serve society by advising and consulting with the executive, legislative, and judiciary branches of the government. A psychiatrist should clarify whether he/she speaks as an individual or as a representative of an organization. Furthermore, psychiatrists should avoid cloaking their public statements with the authority of the profession (e.g., "Psychiatrists know that . . .").

2. Psychiatrists may interpret and share with the public their expertise in the various psychosocial issues that may affect mental health and illness. Psychiatrists should always be mindful of their separate roles as dedicated citizens and as experts in psychological medicine.

3. On occasion psychiatrists are asked for an opinion about an individual who is in the light of public attention, or who has disclosed information about himself/herself through public media. In such circumstances, a psychiatrist may share with the public his/her expertise about psychiatric issues in general. However, it is unethical for a psychiatrist to offer a professional opinion about that specific individual unless he/she has conducted an examination and has been granted proper authorization for such a statement.

4. The psychiatrist may permit his/her certification to be used for the involuntary treatment of any person only following his/her personal examination of that person. To do so, he/she must find that the person, because of mental illness, cannot form a judgment as to what is in his/her own

best interests and that, without such treatment, substantial impairment is likely to occur to the person or others.

The Code of Professional Ethics of the Psychiatrist

Preamble

Since ancient times and until now professional ethics has been an essential part of medicine. Professionalism in medicine has always meant a combination of special knowledge and the art of healing with high ethical standards.

The role of ethics is especially important in the professional activities of a psychiatrist, owing to the delicate nature of the therapist-patient relationship and the unique nature of the moral problems encountered.

As psychiatry has at its disposal means of affecting the human mind, it is an object of intense scrutiny by society. Though a psychiatrist, like any other physician, should be guided in his activity by compassion, kindness, and charity, it is necessary to draw up a documentary version of generally accepted rules of professional psychiatric ethics.

This code is based on humanistic traditions of Russian psychiatry as well as on fundamental principles of human rights and freedoms. It was developed in accordance with ethical standards acknowledged by the international professional community.

The purpose of the Code is to highlight moral perspectives, to provide psychiatrists with a "key" to making decisions in situations that present difficult problems from ethical, legal, and medical points of view; to minimize the risk of making mistakes; and to protect psychiatrists from possible unlawful demands. The Code is also to contribute to consolidation of the professional psychiatric community of Russia.

Article 1

The main aim of the professional activity of the psychiatrist is to provide psychiatric care to anyone who needs it and to contribute to the promotion and protection of the mental health of the population.

The health and the welfare of the patient are the paramount value for the psychiatrist in his professional activity.

The psychiatrist must always be ready to help every patient irrespective of his age, sex, race, nationality, social or financial status, religious affiliations, political beliefs, or other differences.

The psychiatrist ought not to show superiority to patients or to give preference to some of them for non-medical reasons.

The psychiatrist must take care to protect the mental health of the people; to participate in the development and improvement of psychiatric care; to draw the attention of the public and mass media to its problems, achievements, and drawbacks; and to contribute to public education on problems of mental health.

Each psychiatrist is morally accountable for the activities of the professional psychiatric community the psychiatrist belongs to.

Article 2

Professional competence of the psychiatrist—encompassing his special knowledge and the art of healing—is the essential prerequisite for psychiatric activity.

The psychiatrist must always develop his professional knowledge and skills using all accessible sources of medical knowledge, results of scientific research, personal experience and the experience of his colleagues. Professional competence gives the psychiatrist the moral right to make important decisions independently and to guide other specialists and the staff.

The psychiatrist should seek assistance from his colleagues in case of difficulties encountered in providing psychiatric care and should help his colleagues if they have similar problems.

Article 3

The psychiatrist must not violate the ancient ethical rule of the doctor: "First of all do no harm!"

The psychiatrist must not harm his patient, causing moral, physical or financial injury, either intentionally or through neglect. The psychiatrist must not be indifferent to the actions of other persons who may be instrumental in causing such injury to the patient.

If an examination or treatment is associated with side effects, pain sensations, possible complications, application of coercive measures, and other negative phenomena, the psychiatrist must carefully balance the risk of damage and the expected positive effect.

Psychiatric intervention can be morally justified only if realistically attainable benefits for the patient outweigh the possible negative effects: "The medicine must not be worse than the disease."

Article 4

Any abuse of psychiatric knowledge or the position of the doctor is incompatible with professional ethics.

The psychiatrist must not use his professional knowledge and abilities against the medical interests of patients or in order to distort the truth; nor should the psychiatrist either take medical measures or refuse them to those in need, without sufficient grounds.

The psychiatrist must not thrust his philosophical, religious, or political views on the patient. Personal prejudices or other nonprofessional motives must not influence diagnosis and treatment. The diagnosis of mental illness cannot be based only on the differences between the patient's beliefs and opinions and the generally accepted ones.

When providing psychiatric care, the psychiatrist must not take advantage of the patient's mental disability or his position as a doctor to make commercial transactions with the patient, to use the patient's labor for his own purposes, or to have sexual relations with the patient.

The psychiatrist must not assist in the patient's suicide.

The psychiatrist must not use medical methods for punishing the patient or for the convenience of the staff or other persons; and the psychiatrist must not take part in tortures, executions, or other forms of cruel and inhumane treatment towards human beings.

Article 5

The psychiatrist is morally obligated to respect the patient's autonomy, honor, and dignity and to look after the patient's rights and legal interests.

Humiliation of the patient and inhumane and unmerciful attitudes towards him are serious violations of professional ethics.

The psychiatrist must be extremely careful with the private life of his patient: he must not interfere in it without the patient's consent, and if there are medical indications for controlling the patient's behaviors, the interference should be confined to clinical necessity; in such cases the psychiatrist should inform the patient about the nature of the measures taken and the reasons for them.

In caring for his patients, the psychiatrist should follow the principle of minimal constraint of freedom and should help develop the patient's responsibility for his actions.

In case of conflicting interests, the psychiatrist must give preference to the interests of the patient, unless their realization could cause serious damage to the patient and threaten the rights of other persons.

Article 6

The psychiatrist aspires to a "therapeutic relationship" with the patient, based on mutual agreement, trust, honesty, and mutual responsibility.

In case the patient fails to establish such a relationship because of his mental status, it is established with his legal representative, a relative, or other close person acting in the patient's interests. If and when the relationship is established for nontherapeutic purpose, such as for a forensic examination, its nature must be thoroughly explained to the person concerned.

The psychiatrist must discuss with the patient his mental health problems, the proposed plan of examination and treatment, and the advantages and disadvantages of relevant medical methods, without concealing from the patient any side effects and complications that have a significant probability of occurring. The psychiatrist should spare the patient psychological trauma and aspire to instil optimism for the future.

The psychiatrist must not promise his patient the impossible and must keep his word to the patient. His task is to turn the patient into an ally for achieving his health and well-being.

Article 7

The psychiatrist must respect the patient's right to consent to or to refuse the offered psychiatric care after having been provided with the necessary information.

Psychiatric intervention cannot be used against or irrespective of the patient's own will, except where, because of severe mental disorder, the patient is incapable of forming a judgment as to what is beneficial for him and when lack of such an interference might cause serious damage to the patient or to other people. Application of involuntary measures is necessary in such cases and is morally justified, though it is acceptable only within the limits defined by such a necessity.

Absence of a legal foundation for the application of involuntary measures to a patient whose mental condition seems problematic for the psychiatrist does not relieve the psychiatrist of the moral duty to search for other actions that are devoid of coercive elements. A patient's refusal of psychiatric care is a matter of concern for the doctor's conscience.

In special cases, when the psychiatrist is responsible for a compulsory examination of the patient or for other compulsory psychiatric measures ordered by the court or by another authorized body, the psychiatrist must implement such measures in strict accordance with law. If the psychiatrist does not find medical indications for compulsory measures, his moral duty is to inform the body that has made such a decision.

Article 8

Whatever the psychiatrist has been told by the patient in the course of examination and treatment, including the very fact of the provision of psychiatric care, must not be disclosed without permission of the patient or his legal representative.

The psychiatrist must not divulge confidential information obtained from another doctor, from medical documents, or from other sources, without proper permission.

The patient's death does not relieve the psychiatrist of the obligation to preserve confidentiality.

The psychiatrist is permitted to disclose confidential information to other persons irrespective of the patient's or his representative's consent only in cases specified by law or when the psychiatrist has no other means to prevent serious harm to the patient or other persons. In these cases, the patient should be informed of the disclosure whenever possible.

Article 9

In research or clinical trials of new medical methods or agents involving the patients, the parameters and conditions of the study should be determined beforehand by means of meticulous balancing of the risks for the patient and the positive effect expected.

The patient's welfare must always be more important to the researcher than public benefits or scientific interests.

Research and experiments may be carried out only with the informed consent of the patient or his legal representative, after all relevant information has been given, and it must comply with other regulations established by law.

The psychiatrist should respect the patient's right to refuse to take part in a research project for any reason. The refusal must never adversely affect the patient's psychiatric care.

Article 10

It is the moral right and duty of the psychiatrist to uphold professional independence.

When taking care of patients and participating in commissions and consultations, acting as an expert, the psychiatrist must openly declare his opinion, defend his point of view, and, if subjected to outside pressures, should demand legal and public protection.

The psychiatrist should refuse to collaborate with the representatives of patients or other persons who are seeking actions that contradict ethical principles or law.

The right of the psychiatrist to defend his point of view should be combined with high personal standards and the ability to acknowledge and to correct his own mistakes, whether he discovers them himself or they are pointed out by colleagues.

Article 11

Honesty, justice, decency, respect for the knowledge and experience of others, as well as readiness to share one's own experience and knowledge, constitute the ethical foundation for relationships with colleagues.

The psychiatrist must do his best to consolidate the professional community inspired by moral principles, and to defend the honor and dignity of colleagues as one's own.

The psychiatrist is obliged to analyze impartially his own mistakes as well as the mistakes of colleagues. The psychiatrist's disagreement or criticism concerning the judgments and the actions of his colleagues should be objective, well grounded, and polite. The psychiatrist should avoid negative statements about the work of one's colleagues in the presence of patients or their relatives, except in cases of legal proceedings concerning the doctor's actions. Any attempt to enhance one's reputation by casting discredit on one's colleagues is not ethical.

The psychiatrist has a moral duty to restrain dishonest and incompetent colleagues, as well as any nonprofessionals, from doing harm to the health of the patient.

Article 12

The responsibility for violation of the professional ethical code of the psychiatrist is regulated by the charter of the Russian Psychiatric Society (the charter of a professional community that adopts the present code).

[Adopted by the Russian Society of Psychiatrists, April 1994. Reprinted by permission]

Name index

Subject index

Subject index